S0-BGM-022

STRABISMUS II

A Grune & Stratton Rapid Manuscript Reproduction

STRABISMUS II

Proceedings of the Fourth Meeting
of the International Strabismological Association
October 25–29, 1982
Asilomar, California

Edited by

Robert D. Reinecke, M.D.
Ophthalmologist-in-Chief
Wills Eye Hospital
Philadelphia, Pennsylvania
Professor and Chairman
Department of Ophthalmology
Jefferson Medical College of
Thomas Jefferson University
Philadelphia, Pennsylvania

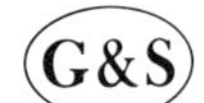

Grune & Stratton, Inc.
(Harcourt Brace Jovanovich, Publishers)
Orlando San Diego San Francisco New York London
Toronto Montreal Sydney Tokyo São Paulo

Library of Congress Cataloging in Publication Data

International Strabismological Association. Meeting
(4th : 1982 : Asilomar, Calif.)
Strabismus II.

"A Grune & Stratton rapid manuscript reproduction."
Bibliography: p.
Includes index.
1. Strabismus—Congresses. I. Reinecke, Robert D.,
1929– II. Title. [DNLM: 1. Strabismus—Congresses.
W3 IN904M 4th 1982s / WW 415 I615 1982s]
RE771.I484 1982 617.7'62 84-47739
ISBN 0-8089-1424-3

Grune & Stratton, Inc.
Orlando, FL 32887

Distributed in the United Kingdom by
Grune & Stratton, Ltd.
24/28 Oval Road, London NW 1

Library of Congress Catalog Number 84-47739
International Standard Book Number 0-8089-1424-3
Printed in the United States of America

84 85 86 87 10 9 8 7 6 5 4 3 2 1

CONTENTS

Preface

The papers in this book represent the majority of the papers presented at the fourth meeting of the International Strabismological Association, which was hosted by the American Association for Pediatric Ophthalmology and Strabismus and was held at Asilomar, California, on October 25–29, 1982. This was the largest meeting to date of the ISA and these proceedings are in proportion to that large meeting. The authors are to be thanked for their reasonably prompt submission of the papers. The increased number of papers delayed final publication to a small extent, which we hope will be acceptable to the organization and the many authors. I have been privileged to serve as editor.

ROBERT D. REINECKE, M.D.

Acknowledgments

Special thanks go to the many authors who have supplied their manuscripts, and to Alan Scott, M.D., who arranged the meeting and coordinated the abstracts and submission of the papers to me. Due to computer and other problems, an extraordinary amount of work was done by my assistants, Margie Harron and Sheryl Wizov. A special note of thanks goes to the Wills Eye Hospital Librarian, Fleur Weinberg, and her assistant, Gloria Lewis, who checked the many references in the papers. Also, thanks to Kurt Simons, Ph.D., and Clark Robbins, who solved many of the word processing computer problems that we encountered.

INTRODUCTION

Opening Remarks

Honored Colleagues, Ladies and Gentlemen, it is a great pleasure to greet you in this delightful place. Fortunately, the majority of those attending are young enough to be interested in the origin of this Association and the rationale of its meetings.

Only a few decades ago strabismus was thought of as just a cosmetic problem by many ophthalmologists. International organizations for the prevention of blindness were concerned with the prevention and treatment of infective, traumatic, or inherited lesions only. It was Charles Thomas, then President of the European Strabismus Council, who persuaded WHO to include prevention and treatment of amblyopia among its objectives. Strabismus was one of the main themes at the 1958 World Congress. Despite reports of valuable work carried out in various areas in the preceding years, reconciliation of diagnostic methods, criteria of cure, and fundamental principles was difficult. It was realized that productive cooperation could only be based on a common scientific language. A meeting was organized by Cuppers of specialists from all continents, prior to the 1966 World Congress. Its goals were to dispel this confusion due to diversity in terminology, to agree on methods of examination, and to evaluate therapeutic methods. In addition, papers were selected to familiarize participants with recent advances in research and therapy. No one could expect these goals to be reached within the frame of a six-day meeting. Yet, a promising start was made. It was clear that continuance of communication at an international level would be beneficial. We owe to Jampolsky the creation of the ISA with this objective. Keith Lyle took charge of organizing its structure. Its aims were to improve early diagnostic and treatment procedures, to agree on common terminology and standardization of diagnostic methods, to disseminate knowledge, and to foster research on strabismus. Every four years the Association would hold a meeting. Here we are now to commence our fourth Congress. Far from entirely fulfilling our objects, our meetings have been useful, having contributed to the dissemination of knowledge, rapidly providing information that would otherwise have taken longer to reach us. Most important is the uniformity attained in strabismological language. This is noteworthy when one compares today's strabismus literature with that of a few years ago.

This is the first ISA meeting in this country and also the first time its Congress is held in the form of a joint meeting with the AAPOS. It is a great pleasure to share this Congress with AAPOS and I would like to thank the members of its Council for the important contribution of their group, which will add to the success of the meeting.

We owe special thanks to the ISA Organizing Committee for arranging the Congress so efficiently, and to the Program Committee for the responsibility of selecting topics and papers.

Congratulations to Drs. von Noorden (Chairman of the Bielschowsky Committee) and Parks (Chairman of the Linksz Award Committee) and their collaborators on their excellent choice in selecting our Bielschowsky Lecturer and Linksz Awardee. As if his amazing activity, plus the tasks I have mentioned were not enough, Marshall Parks was asked to review our By-Laws. This he has done with his well known efficiency, and for this we must thank him again.

The members of our Bureau have been most cooperative and understanding in the preparatory meetings and through postal contacts, helping in every possible way. To them, deepest thanks.

What shall I say of our Secretary-Treasurer, Alfred Huber? As Secretary, only those who have occupied this post in world-wide associations can realize what amount of labor it involves, contacting members spread all over the world. During his period of office, these problems have been increased because areas where usually things function normally have "enjoyed" postal strikes, which made his work still more overtiring. To him and his efficient secretary, Margrit Sheerer, our deep gratitude. As Treasurer, he fulfills his task perfectly; he collects the treasure, keeps it in safe Banhofstrasse vaults and, as an honest Bernese citizen, he returns it to the last penny.

Our thanks to all participants, lecturers, and moderators for their effort in making the meeting a fruitful one. Our special thanks to our younger colleagues. In England they say that "a man should retire when he can no longer learn from his registrars," and a Spanish proverb says that "only he whose greatest wish is to be surpassed by his pupils deserves to be called a teacher." Those from whose experience you might have benefited expect to profit from your measured enthusiasm.

I wish too to thank our secretaries, hostesses, and those people who you may never see but on whose work the success of a meeting depends so greatly.

There is always a sad moment in these meetings when we have to recall those members and friends who have passed on. I beg of you to stand and keep in silence for a minute as a tribute to their memory.

Now on behalf of those of us who come from oversees, I wish to express to our American colleagues our warmest thanks for their reception. Many of us have enjoyed the hospitality of this country before and are happy to be on these blessed shores again.

I declare the fourth ISA Congress open and wish you all a pleasant and fruitful meeting.

ALFREDO ARRUGA, M.D.
President ISA

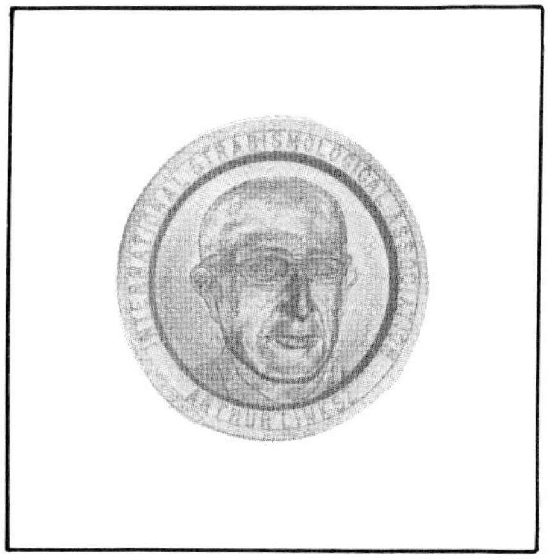

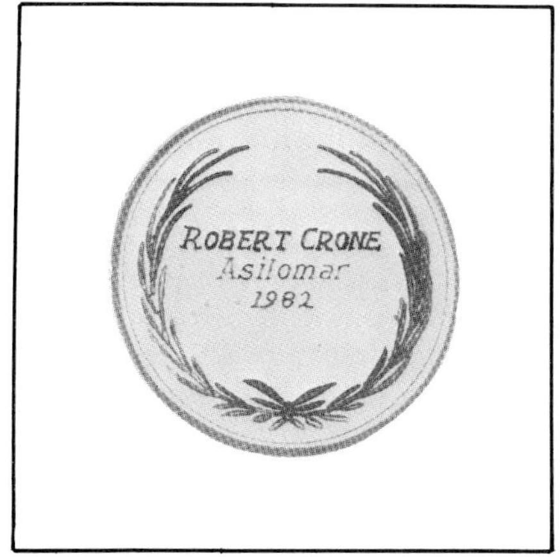

THE LINKSZ MEDAL AND PRIZE

Dr. Arthur Linksz was born in Czechoslovakia and earned his medical degree in Hungary. He immigrated to the United States in 1939 and was a member of the famous Dartmouth Eye Institute faculty in Hanover, New Hampshire.

Dr. Linksz is a foremost authority in the field of visual physiology and color vision, renowned for his many contributions in optics, sensory physiology and reading disabilities. The Linksz Medal and Prize, first presented to Dr. Alfredo Arruga at the 1982 meeting of the International Strabismological Association, honors outstanding contribution to our knowledge of oculomotor physiology and strabismus.

The Linksz Medal and Prize is made possible by Smith-Kettlewell Eye Research Foundation, San Francisco, California.

A special recognition of the contributions of Professor Crone will be made by the Linksz Committee.

THE 1982 BIELSCHOWSKY LECTURE

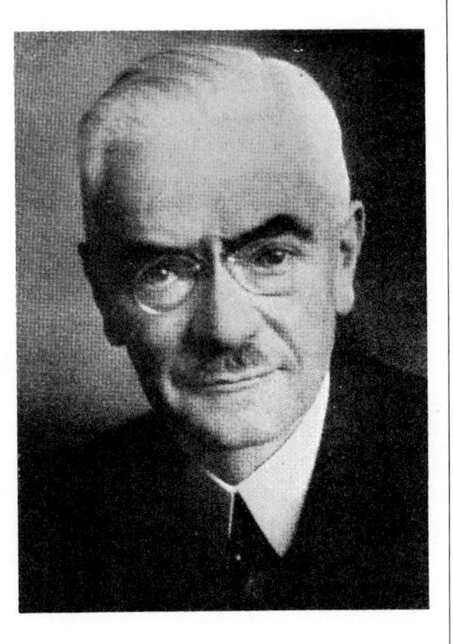

The 1982 Bielschowsky Lecturer is Mr. Kenneth Wybar, surgeon and Director of the Orthoptic Department at Moorfields Eye Hospital in London. He is also affiliated with the Hospital for Sick Children and Royal Marsden Hospital in London.

Mr. Wybar has made strabismus intelligible to us through his marvelous summary in Duke Elders' *System*. We honor him also for his original research on the pupil and other subjects.

This lecture, traditionally one of the highlights of the ISA Congress, is dedicated to the memory of Professor Alfred Bielschowsky (1871-1940), one of the great masters of the science of ocular motility disorders. His extraordinary impact on European, and after his immigration, on American ophthalmology was based on an immense clinical acumen built on the broad and deep foundation of sensory and motor physiology.

Past Bielschowsky Lecturers:

1970 G.K. von Noorden
1974 H. Harms
1978 A. Jampolsky

Introduction to Bielschowsky Lecture

It is appropriate that the name of Alfred Bielschowsky is honored by dedicating the principal lecture presented at this Congress to the memory of this great scientist and teacher. Few of us assembled here will remember him in person, as Bielschowsky died in 1940; but all of us are aware that his heritage forms a substantial segment of our science as we know it today.

The fourth Bielschowsky lecture will be presented by a man who is worthy, indeed, of this honor; for as Bielschowsky before him, he has based his approach to ocular motility on sound scientific principles, aided by a strong background in neuro-ophthalmology. He has been a beacon of common sense in our science throughout the years, years during which strabismology was often obfuscated by fashionable trends, conjecture and adulation of unproven hypotheses.

A Scotsman by heritage, by wit and by personal charm, Kenneth Wybar received his early training in Glasgow where he received his medical doctorate in 1956. For many years now he has been associated with Moorfields Eye Hospital as the Director of the Orthoptic Department, and with the Hospital for Sick Children and the Royal Marsden Hospital, as ophthalmic surgeon. His numerous scientific contributions are well known to us. Perhaps his masterpiece was Volume 6 of Duke-Elder´s System, co-authored with Sir Stewart, which has become an indispensable source of reference.

I understand from any of his former orthoptists that he has also been the idol of generations of orthoptic students at Moorfields. In addition to his talents as a teacher, his good looks and keen wittedness must have contributed to this adulation. Many years ago I, myself, became the subject of his jesting. At one of the first International Strabismus Congresses I ever attended, we had just finished an elegant dinner at the ancient Royal Apothecary Hall of London. I was in the process of lighting my pipe when I was reprimanded by a splendidly liveried servant that this act was entirely reprehensible as the Queen had yet to be toasted. Whereupon Kenneth Wybar, seated at the head table, leaned over to Keith Lyle and commented audibly, with the usual twinkle in his eyes: "You see, old man, this is precisely why we had to fight those Huns." As a young and aspiring strabismologist of Teutonic heritage, I would have been devastated by this comment had it not been for the consoling observation that my own charming dinner companion, who happened to be Mr. Wybar´s daughter, had lit up her cigarette minutes earlier.

Members and guests of the Association, it is with distinct pleasure that I present to you the 4th Bielschowsky lecturer, Mr. Kenneth Wybar.

GUNTER K. VON NOORDEN, M.D.
October 25, 1982

The 4th Bielschowsky Lecture
Asilomar Conference Center—October 1982

KENNETH WYBAR

OCULAR MOTILITY DISORDERS IN PEDIATRIC DISEASE

Mr. President, Ladies and Gentlemen, I should like to express my great awareness of the honor which has been bestowed on me by being invited by the International Strabismological Association to deliver the 4th Bielschowsky Lecture, an occasion which is being shared with the American Association for Pediatric Ophthalmology and Strabismus.

Alfredo Arruga, I am glad that you are presiding on this occasion. We have enjoyed a friendship over many years, and particularly since the inauguration of the CESSD (The European Concilium Dedicated to the Study of Strabismus) in 1954. There are many highlights which are worthy of mention, but the outstanding event is reflected in a delightful weekend which was spent at your charming villa (Fig 1) in Bagur in Northern Spain some years ago. I know that this is a place of special significance to your family, because looking across the bay from the villa is the house in the village (Fig 2) in which you were born, and I know also how much your father, Count Hermenegilde Arruga, an ophthalmologist of great distinction (Fig 3), loved the villa which provided him with relaxation from his ardous work in Barcelona, particularly as a pioneer in the surgical treatment of retinal detachment.

There are many happy memories of the weekend, but perhaps the peak was reached in the early hours one morning after an excellent dinner and in the midst of an interesting discussion when Arthur Jampolsky made a profound remark that "if abnormal retinal correspondence had never been invented the world would be a happier place." Needles to say that, having been brainwashed in my formative years by such a remark, it is my firm intention to avoid any mention in this lecture of the sensory anomalies which occur in strabismus!

Gunter von Noorden, I should like to thank you very sincerely for your introduction to this lecture. I have always regarded as a great bonus my friendship with you over the years, because of the warmth of your personality and also because of your great enthusiasm in your chosen spheres of interest which have contributed so much over so many years to an increase in the knowledge of the many problems in the sensory and motor anomalies of ocular motility. This was expressed most aptly by Sir Stewart Duke-Elder (Fig 4) in Volume VI of the System of Ophthalmology in the introduction to Chapter IX - "Throughout this volume his (that is, Gunter von Noorden's) name appears many times and he has made the subject of ocular motility particularly his own". As a co-author of the volume (Duke-Elder and Wybar, 1973) I fully endorsed this sentiment, and I am very conscious at this time that I have been introduced by Gunter, who was the first Bielschowsky Lecturer in 1970; it is obvious that I am faced with a formidable task in attempting to maintain the high standards which have been set in the past.

The name Bielschowsky has a very special place in ophthalmology. Alfred Bielschowsky (Fig 5), a native of a Silesian village, studied medicine in Breslau, Leipzig and Berlin where he graduated in 1894, and became a distinguished and much revered ophthalmologist with an essentially scientific approach to his main interest, the anomalies of ocular motility, which was almost certainly fostered by his early associations with F. B. Holfmann and Ewald Hering. With great distinction he filled the Chairs of Ophthalmology at Marburg and Breslau, and, for personal reasons, but undoubtedly with religious and political overtones, he came to the United States of America in 1936, and within a short time found his niche at the Dartmouth Medical School where he became Director of the Eye Institute and Professor of Ophthalmology of the Medical School, so that he was able to continue the momentum of his previous career with many further advances in knowledge until his death in 1940. Perhaps his emigration to American represented a great personal tragedy, but it proved to be a fortunate one for America because he entered into a congenial atmosphere which was essential for his work, and many American Ophthalmologists came under the magic of his spell, so that his influence has continued in a way which would have fulfilled his highest ambition.

When I started in ophthalmology the name Bielschowsky came to my attention at an early stage, but this was without any great depth, although subsequently his name signified two distinct landmarks in my career; first, when I mastered the correct spelling of his name so that I could lambast people working in my clinic who failed to spell it correctly, and secondly, when I came to understand the true interpretation of his head tilting test. This illustrates the fundamental truth that a full understanding of the disorders of ocular motility must be based on a sound knowledge of the function of the extrinsic ocular muscles, and not simply on a mindless learning by rote of a series of complicated actions without any knowledge of how to apply them in a practical way, but it must seem odd to such a distinguished audience that I should take any pride in understanding the Bielschowsky head tilting test. However, in many years as a teacher of postgraduate students and as an examiner in the diploma and fellowship examinations I recall only too well the look of horror when I asked a candidate about the basis of the Bielschowsky head tilting test to realize that such knowledge is in no way universal among ophthalmologists as a whole.

I have enjoyed a full life in ophthalmology, and from a very early stage I have nurtured a particular interest in the problems of ocular motility. This started towards the end of the Second World War when I joined the Royal Navy as a Surgeon Lieutenant with general responsibilities, but I was in contact with batches of trainees whose strabismus had been neglected in the early years of the war, and this provided me with considerable surgical experience. However, my main interest stems from my contact with Keith Lyle as a Resident at Moorfields Eye Hospital, High Holborn, when I marvelled at his skill in the management of so many different forms of strabismus, often of a complicated nature. I am delighted that he is present at this lecture, and he is to me a very special colleague and friend.

Despite my early interest in strabismus I have never devoted myself exclusively to this topic. Perhaps the opportunity was not there at the right time, but even if it had, I think I should have embraced the topic of strabismus within the wider sphere of pediatric ophthalmology, and this has gradually evolved over the years whilst retaining some interest in certain aspects of adult ophthalmology. It is of interest to recall that during the Giessen and Grunberg Meetings in 1966, which initiated the foundation of the International Strabismological Association, I had several discussions with Marshall Parks and Frank Costenbader, who were urging me to become a pediatric ophthalmologist.

I have been fortunate in being in close contact over a period of many years with the problems of ocular motility in a children's hospital - The Hospital for Sick Children, Great Ormond Street as it was (Fig 6) and as it is now (Fig 7), in a cancer hospital - The Royal Marsden Hospital at Fulham Road (Fig 8) and in the country branch at Belmont (Fig 9), and in an eye hospital - Moorfields Eye Hospital, High Holborn (Fig 10) which is part of Moorfields Eye Hospital as a whole (Fig 11).

It is my intention in this Bielschowsky lecture to deal with certain disorders of ocular motility in children which I have experienced at my various hospitals, particularly these which are associated with some general pediatric disorder. These topics are of a diverse nature - congenital ocular motor apraxia, cranio-facial dysostosis, Moebius's syndrome, benign intracranial hypertension, and the retinopathy of prematurity (retrolental fibroplasia).

I think there should be a sense of modesty in giving an eponymous lecture, and this is illustrated very clearly by the introduction which the late Sir Robert Jones, who is regarded in England as the Father of Orthopaedics, gave in his address to the London Medical Society in 1914: "When your Council graciously invited me to deliver the oration before this distinguished Society, I fear I had not the courage to refuse. The honor was such that for a time I did not realize my grave responsibility and now I deplore the consciousness that I do not possess those gifts of erudition and imagination which have charmed while they have enlightened you in the past". How must I feel at this moment when such a man felt that way, and I can only hope that this lecture will prove to be worthy of the occasion.

CONGENITAL OCULAR MOTOR APRAXIA

Congenital ocular motor apraxia is a term which is used to describe a particular anomaly of ocular movement in childhood, and it was put forward by David Cogan in 1952 (Fig 12) as a new condition; this is correct as regards the use of term "congenital ocular motor apraxia". However, it is of interest to note that such an anomaly was described to some extent by Gowers (1879) in a general discussion on the mechanism of reflex fixation of the eye. Sir William Richards Gowers (Fig 13) occupies a unique place in the establishment of neurology as a special aspect of medicine; a man of great intellect he applied his special skills in relating carefully documented clinical observations to the basic knowledge at that time of the structure and function of the brain, so that he provided an immense impetus in establishing clinical neurology on a scientific basis. This anomaly has also been described as "a spasm of fixation"

(Holmes, 1930) and "a locking of fixation" (Hacaen, Ajuriaguerra, de Roques, David and Dell, 1950).

Furthermore, it is of particular interest in the context of this lecture to take account of the fact that Bielschowsky (1903) provided one of the earliest accounts of this peculiar form of loss of voluntary control of ocular movement, but with a retention of the vestibulo-ocular reflex, which became known as the Roth-Bielschowsky syndrome, because of a description of a similar condition by Roth (1901) two years previously.

It is significant to take regard of the definition of "apraxia" by Nathan (1947), although not in the context of ocular motor apraxia, as "an inability to move a certain part of the body in accordance with a proposed purpose, the mobility of this part being otherwise preserved".

The condition is characterized by an abnormality of conjugate lateral gaze when attempts are made to induce this by a command (through the mediation of the frontal motor cortex) or by a visual stimulus (through the mediation of the occipital visual cortex). This abnormality may take the form of an absence of these movements at all times, or of a defect of these movements at certain times, particularly during emotion, excitement, or fatigue. This is illustrated by a "freezing" of the eyes which may occur in a child on encountering a stranger. This defect of conjugate lateral gaze may be mitigated by a compensatory head thrust, which is of a quick and jerky nature in the direction of the intended gaze.

It is evident that the condition of congenital ocular motor apraxia demonstrates the close and fundamental relationship which exists between the function of the movements of the head and the directional orientation of the eyes which is mediated by the special senses, in particularly those of a visual nature, so that there is an intimate and complementary relationship between head movements and eye movements (Ben-Zur, Feldman and Bender, 1970); this has been discussed in detail by Taylor (1980) and by Gresty, Halmagyi and Taylor (1983). There are two main mechanisms which are concerned in the maintenance of a constant relationship between the eyes and the visual field, and which are dictated by the position of the head.

First, it is dependent on a movement of the environment which creates a slow pursuit movement of the eyes, and it is considered that the stimulus for such a movement is the so-called "retinal slip" which has different connotations, but in this context implies a disparity between the position of the image of the target and its predicted position on the retina. This reflex movement is dependent on a feedback system in which the input signals are related to the retinal slip, and this has been demonstrated in optokinetic nystagmus (Collewijin, 1969).

Secondly, it is dependent on the highly developed vestibulo-ocular reflex which maintains the eyes in all three orthogonal planes (horizontal, frontal and sagittal) of freedom (Jones, 1966). The angular acceleration of the head provides the control signal for the vestibulo-ocular reflex, and this is transduced by the semicircular canals into a neural signal which is in proportion to the velocity of the head (Robinson, 1972). In this way a normal head movement in any direction is accompanied by a movement of the eyes to an equal extent in the opposite direction.

It follows from an understanding of this relationship between the head movements and the ocular movements, that the quick and jerky compensatory head thrust which is a characteristic feature of congenital ocular motor apraxia has certain unusual features. The head thrust of necessity must go far beyond the object of fixation because the head thrust towards the object of fixation is followed inevitably by a conjugate lateral movement of the eyes in the opposite direction as the result of the influence of the vestibulo-ocular reflex. Ultimately, however, the head thrust achieves a position which is sufficient to enable a fixation of the eyes on the object, and the head is then moved back gradually until it faces the object of fixation so that the eyes and head once more become aligned. This seems to be a prolonged process because of its complex descriptive nature, but in fact it is completed within a second or even less (Cogan, 1952).

In congenital ocular motor apraxia there is a retention of optokinetic nystagmus, but it tends to be of an abnormal type so that the two phases of the nystagmus are more or less equal in speed with an absence of the usual distinction of fast and slow phases in the optokinetic response.

This form of compensatory head thrust is illustrated by a boy of 4 years who developed a persistent conjugate lateral deviation of the eyes to the left at the age of 2 months, but from the age of 4 months he showed an ability to move the eyes into the midline by a vigorous shaking of the head. This ultimately changed into a series of peculiar jerky movements of the head with an ability to obtain an unsteady movement of the eyes to the midline with fixation on a straight-ahead target. There was some degree of ataxia with an unsteady gait. Another typical form of oculomotor apraxia was seen in a child of 5 years who had moved her head from an early age in a jerky way in order to carry out fixation of a particular object with some degree of overshooting of the target which was then adjusted by a small movement of the eyes in the reverse direction. It is interesting that this had been observed by the parents, particularly when the child was attempting to identify them from a distance, but they had attached no significance to these peculiar head movements.

Ocular motor apraxia may occur in isolation, but quite frequently it is associated with reading difficulties (Altrocch and Menkes, 1960) which are overcome to a limited extent by learning to move the head rather than the eyes when scanning lines of print. It is also sometimes associated with other apractic dysfunctions such as a difficulty in walking or an occurrence of brief and abrupt involuntary contractions of individual muscles or of groups of muscles of the face or upper extremities. There is also sometimes a kinetic disturbance of the mechanism of speech.

As a general rule the disorder of ocular movements which occurs in ocular motor apraxia is in a lateral direction, and this is invariable as far as the congenital form of the condition is concerned. However, in the acquired type of the condition the anomaly may rarely be of a vertical nature. This is illustrated in a girl of 7 years with Niemann-Pick disease (Sanders and Wybar, 1970) which was confirmed by liver biopsy; this case was first described at the meeting of the European Consilium Dedicated to the Study of Strabismus (CESSD) in London in September 1969.

The child showed an established ataxia with a positive Romberg sign, a reduction in the power and tone of the upper extremities, and an extensor response to the plantar reflexes. There was evidence of an alternating exotropia on near and on distant fixation with a preference for fixing with the left eye. There was no abnormality of lateral movements of the eyes of a voluntary nature, to a command (command movements) or to a moving target (following movements), but there was an absence of any random vertical movements.

There was also an abnormality of optokinetic movements in a vertical direction with a loss of typical saccadic movements, but there were variable movements in the direction of rotation of the drum (that is, a partial retention of the slow phase of the optokinetic nystagmus). There was, however, a retention of normal vertical movements which were mediated by proprioceptive mechanisms (the so-called doll's head phenomenon). It is interesting that the use of this phenomenon was made in everyday life so that thrusting head movements occurred to induce upward and downward movements of gaze, and these were preceded by a lid closure to abolish fixation. Sometimes the eyes would remain "stuck" in a position of elevation (so that there was an appearance similar to the position of the eyes which occurs during an oculogyric crisis), but this was overcome by vigorous head movements in upward and downward directions.

It is interesting that her elder sister developed similar features with a disturbance of balance and a hepatosplenomegaly at the age of 7 years. There was an impairment of conjugate elevation of the eyes, and the diagnosis of juvenile Niemann-Pick disease was confirmed at the age of 8 years by bone marrow biopsy, and also subsequently at post mortem when she succumbed to the disease at the age of 10 years.

Craniofacial Dysostosis

The condition of craniofacial dysostosis refers to a developmental anomaly of the skull and face, and there are various forms of the condition (the craniosynostosis syndromes). The development of the craniofacial complex becomes determined at an early stage of intrauterine life with a spread of cells in the third week of embryonic life laterally from an area between the ectoderm and endoderm in the region of the primitive streak; this appears as a midline thickening of the embryonic ectoderm to form the mesoderm. The cranial extension of the mesoderm is concerned in the formation of the primordium of the notochord, and the ectoderm which is associated with the notochord proliferates to form the neural plate; neural crest cells develop at the junction between the neural plate and the surface ectoderm, and some of the neural crest cells migrate in lateral directions into the maxillary, mandibular and frontonasal processes (Collin, 1983). It is evident that craniofacial development is influenced during the first 9 weeks of embryonic life by intrinsic factors which control the migration from the neural crest. The intrinsic genetic factors also control induction which is the process by which certain groups of cells are able to exert an effect on the differentiation of adjacent groups of cells. Subsequently other factors become more important, and this is illustrated by the control which the primordial eye exerts on the development of the orbit.

A proliferation of the neural plate results in the formation of the neural tube, and the bulge which is created cranially overhangs the buccopharyngeal membrane which is concerned with the development of the primitive mouth (stomodeum). In the fourth week of embryonic life the mesoderm in the region of the stomodeum forms a series of elevations which become the facial processes and pharyngeal arches; a facial cleft is avoided as a general rule because the grooves between the facial processes become obliterated by differential rates of growth under normal conditions of the cells in the region. The cranial base develops in the seventh week of embryonic life.

The craniosynostosis syndromes follow essentially a premature fusion of the cranial sutures which is a deformity of a non-specific nature; it may occur as an isolated anomaly (simple craniosynostosis) or in association with other abnormalities, such as in Apert´s syndrome (Collin, 1983). This was described originally by Virchow (1851) who considered that the premature stenosis limits expansion of the skull in a direction at right angles to the line of the suture and this has come to be regarded as Virchow´s law.

In early childhood the expanding brain has an indirect influence on the cranial bones so that the cerebral expansion which causes a separation of the cranial sutures is followed by the deposition of new bone at the sutural edges to fill the inevitable bony defects. However, when there is a premature fusion of some of the cranial sutures, there is an undue separation of the cranial sutures which have been spared from the premature stenosis, in order to accommodate the expanding brain, so that there is an increased compensatory growth across the wide sutures. This is an important factor in preventing an increase in the intracranial pressure, because if it fails to occur the previously unaffected sutures will become closed with an inevitable increase in the intracranial pressure. This is a serious event because in the earlier stages it leads to ocular complications - papilledema and optic atrophy - and in the later stages it leads to neurological complications - headaches, epilepsy and a 6th. nerve palsy which tends to be bilateral.

The increased intracranial pressure causes a downward displacement of the posterior parts of the orbits and also the anterior cranial fossa so that the roofs of the orbits assume a more vertical direction than usual. This contributes to a shallowness of the orbits which is accentuated by a displacement forwards of the greater wings of the sphenoid, and also by a hypoplasia of the maxillae. The increased intracranial pressure also exerts an effect on the cribriform plate which is displaced downwards, with an expansion in a lateral direction of the ethmoids so that there is an undue separation of the orbits with the production of a state of hypertelorism.

There are many different forms of the cranio-facial dysostoses, but in this communication discussion is limited to two main forms of the condition - oxycephaly and Crouzon´s disease - with a discussion also of hypertelorism which has certain special considerations. These conditions have been recognized for many years, but more recently there has been a fresh impetus in the search for knowledge following the development of elaborate and to some extent heroic reconstructive surgical procedures (Tessier, 1967), in view of the morbidity and even the mortality which may follow such extensive surgical interference. This surgical approach demands a multidisciplinary team: a plastic surgeon; a neuro-surgeon; a maxillo-facial surgeon; an ear, nose and throat surgeon; and an ophthalmic surgeon. It is, I am afraid, a reflection of the frailty of man - and I am using man in a strictly masculine sense, rather than in a generic sense--that some years ago when Paul Tessier came to the Hospital for Sick Children, Great Ormond Street, to demonstrate the techniques of the operation, because at that time my colleagues, David Matthews and Ivor Broomhead (plastic surgeons) and Kenneth Till (neuro-surgeon) were keen to embark on such surgical treatment, particularly in view of the many cases of this kind attending the hospital, on the day following the first case dealt with by Paul Tessier the main comment centered on the theater sister, who accompanied Paul Tessier from Paris who was undoubtedly a very chic Parisian young lady. However, this diversion did not detract from the recognition of the brilliance of Paul Tessier´s surgical abilities.

The timing of the surgical treatment of craniofacial dysostoses imposes a difficult problem; but sometimes the ophthalmologist plays an important role, particularly when there are obvious ocular signs of an increased intracranial pressure. This may be determined by an involvement of the optic nerve as the result of a direct pressure or as the result of an indirect pressure due to the development of papilloedema. This may also be determined by corneal exposure because of the shallowness of the orbits.

Oxycephaly

This form of craniofacial dysostosis has been given various terminologies--acrocephaly, tower skull, steeple skull, and turricephaly.

In this condition a premature synostosis of the craniofacial sutures results in a vertical elongation of the head with a shortening of its antero-posterior diameter and to a lesser degree of its transverse diameter (Fig. 14). The synostosis of the base of the skull determines the upward expansion of the brain towards the patent anterior fontanelle with a formation of a dome-shaped head with tapers to its summit (sometimes with the production of a meningocele or even a cerebral hernia) and the associated upward displacement of the optic nerves is liable to cause optic atrophy as the result of a disruption of the nutrient vessels in the optic canals. Optic atrophy may also follow papilledema as the result of an increased intracranial pressure, and rarely it may be induced simply by a narrowing of the optic canals. The vertical direction of the forehead is accentuated by the absence of obvious supracilliary arches and the face shows characteristic features; prominence of the nose, hypoplasia of the maxillae (flatness of the cheeks) and prognathism (prominence of the lower jaw). The orbits are shallow with a marked loss of the roofs so that the eyes appear to be unduly prominent and, although this is not a true form of exophthalmos, because it is the result simply of the restricted space within each orbit, it is liabile to cause varying degrees of exposure keratitis.

Sometimes oxcephaly may be associated with syndactylism and this constitutes the so-called acrocephalo-syndactyly syndrome of Alpers (Fig. 15).

Crouzon´s Disease

Crouzon´s disease (the craniofacial dysostosis of Crouzon) represents a disorder of the development of the skull which is to a large extent a variant between oxycephaly (as described above) and scaphocephaly in which there is a long and narrow head so that there is an elongation of the antero-posterior diameter of the skull with a narrowing of the transverse diameter. There are certain other characteristic features; a marked frontal bossing, a prominent hooked nose, a pronathism of the lower jaw with irregularly spaced dentition and a tendency for a persistent salivation, some degree of proptosis, and a sloping of the palpebral apertures in outward and downward directions (Fig. 16).

Hypertelorism

The term hypertelorism was put forward by Greig in 1924 to denote the form of dysostosis of the skull which is characterized by an unduly wide separation of the two eyes (Fig. 17). The condition was recognized long before the observations of Greig: Giovanni Battista della Porta in 1586 depicted such a case in a drawing in his book, de humana physiognomonia, and he aptly accompanied this with a drawing of a cow (Fig. 18) to emphasize the bovine appearance of hypertelorism. It is legitimate to include hypertelorism in a discussion of the craniofacial dysostoses, but it may be admitted that to some extent it is a descriptive term; and, although Greig (1924) considered that it is the result simply of an enlargement of the lesser wings of the sphenoid bone, the wide spearation of the orbits is seldom an isolated event so that it may be an accompanying feature of oxycephaly or Crouzon´s disease. It may be associated with some form of congenital cleft of the face (such as a cleft palate or cleft lip) or of the cranium (such as a meningo-encephalocele). In the main hypertelorism is produced by an expansion of te ethmoids in temporal directions (Bertelson, 1958).

It is pertinent to pause at this stage and consider David Middleton Greig (Fig. 19) who devoted so much of his working life to an understanding of the deformities of the skull with a particular emphasis on hypertelorism. As an ophthalmic surgeon he was based at the University of St. Andrew´s, which is one of the oldest Universities in Great Britain (Fig. 20). I sense some rumblings of disquiet from the golfing fraternity of the International Strabismological Association, and before there is a walk-out of these members in protest, perhaps headed by Phil Knapp, who is well-known in Pro-Am golfing circles in the United States, quite apart from his distinction in many aspects of ocular motility disorders, I hasten to show a photograph of what may be regarded as the real St. Andrew´s (Fig. 21) and may be considered to be of much greater importance than the University!

Greig took a particular interest in a home for mentally defective children, many of whom had cranial deformities, and

Duke-Elder (1964) with his supreme ability to manipulate words in such an apt way described how Greig "possessed of a remarkable flair for discerning the rare and curious manifestations of disease and sleuth-like pertinacity in tracing them backwards to their origins and onwards to their ultimate results, gathered a unique collection of pathological material which he studied and annotated with punctilious care and rare insight". Greig also was able to make use of words and in his lecture on hypertelorism, which was published in the Edinburgh Medical Journal in 1924, he opened with a cogent quotation form Walter de la Mare; "any event in this world--any human being for that matter--that seems to wear even the faintest cast or warp of strangeness, is apt to leave a disporportionately sharp impression on one´s senses".

Strabismus in the Craniofacial Dysostoses

Some form of strabismus is a common feature in the craniofacial dysostoses, as illustrated in the occurrence of a strabismus in 29 of the 35 cases in a series described by Greaves, Walker and Wybar (1979); in this series the craniofacial dysostoses represented oxycephaly (10 cases), Crouzon´s disease (5 cases) and hypertelorism (20 cases) (Fig. 22), and the Tessier procedure was carried out in 19 of the 35 cases. It is usually assumed that an exotropia is the invevitable type of strabismus in the craniofacial dysostoses, but this is not correct. In this series an esotropia occurred in 7 of the 10 cases of oxycephaly with an exotropia in only one case; an esotropia occurred in 2 of the 5 cases of Crouzon´s disease with an exotropia in 2 cases; an esotropia occurred in 4 of the 20 cases of hypertelorism with an exotropia in 10 cases; and in 3 other cases there was a hypertropia (Fig. 23). In 6 cases there was an absence of any significant deviation (Fig. 23).

Particular attention must be paid to the frequent occurrence of the V phenomenon in association with a strabismus; in 27 of the 29 cases of strabismus in the series (Fig. 24). This was emphasized by Limon de Brown (1974) who found consistent evidence of the V phenomenon in a series of 10 cases of oxycephaly and Crouzon´s disease. She considered that the V phenomenon is the result of a mechanical defect rather than the result of a neurogenic lesion. This was based on the assumption that the shallowness of the orbits in an anteroposterior direction results in a diminished support of the eyeball so that a greater reliance is placed on the supporting role of the inferior transverse ligament of Lockwood (suspensory ligament of the eyeball) with an overaction of the inferior oblique and inferior rectus muscles, which are associated anatomically with the ligament, in an attempt to try and enhance the effectivity of the ligament. In this way it is postulated that any underaction of the superior oblique and superior rectus in such cases is secondary to the overaction of the inferior oblique and inferior rectus. This conclusion, however, may have only a limited application.

It is well established that in the V phenomonen in general the overaction of the inferior oblique is of a primary nature due to a sagittalisation of the superior and inferior obliques so that the line of pull of the superior oblique, instead of being in a similar plane to that of the inferior oblique (Fig. 25) makes a significantly greater angle with the vertical meridian when the eye is in the primary position as compared with the angle which is made by the inferior oblique (Fig. 26) and this enhances the vertical influence of the inferior oblique as compared with the superior oblique hence the progressively greater updrift or upshoot of the eye as it moves into a position of adduction.

In contrast, it seems more likely that in the V phenomenon which occurs in the craniofacial dysostoses the weakness of the superior obliques is of a primary nature so that the overaction of the inferior obliques is a secondary event. It is likely that the restricted anteroposterior diameter of the orbit in oxycephaly and Crouzon's disease, and also to some extent an anomalous development of the bony structures in the region of the trochlea, result in an underaction of the tendinous part of the superior oblique which may be purely of a mechanical nature, or there may even be some developmental anomaly of the muscle.

In hypertelorism a weakness of the superior oblique plays a significant role in the V phenomenon which is a common feature of the condition (Figs. 27a-e) but the mechanism of this weakness may be variable. In hypertelorism there is a displacement laterally of each orbit, but this displacement does not affect the orbital apex. It follows that a displacement of the eye laterally without any real change in the position of the trochlea increases the angle of the line of pull of the superior oblique with the vertical meridian (Fig. 28) with a decrease in its effectiveness as a depressor of the eye. Furthermore, the even greater incidence of the V phenomenon in hypertelorism after the Tessier operation (Fig. 29) (14 of the 19 cases before the Tessier operation and 10 of the 19 cases after the Tessier operation) may be regarded as the result of an increased weakness of the action of the superior oblique which is prone to occur because of some degree of interference with its normal function in the region of the trochlea. These figures are of greater significance when regard is taken of the fact that in hypertelorism the increased incidence of the V phenomenon is much greater when in the presence of an esotropia as compared with the presence of an exotropia.

The weakness of the superior obliques in the craniofacial dysostoses may not necessarily be obvious on an assessment of the degree of resticted movement of the eye in a position of depression in adduction, and in such cases it is more readily detected by the Bielschowsky head-tilting test (a most appropriate test to mention in the context of this lecture) which provides a positive response in the presence of a superior oblique paresis; a forcible tilting of the head to the side of the affected eye results in an updrift of the affected eye because of the elevating influence of the superior rectus is not neutralized by the depressing influence of the superior oblique when an attempt is made by the superior rectus and superior oblique to compensate for the excyclotropic position of the eye which follows the forcible head tilting. A positive response is readily apparent in each eye when the strabismus is essentially of the alternating type, but it is less easy to demonstrate in the dominant eye in a strabismus when there is an obvious preference to fix with the dominant eye. It is evident, however, that in such a case the bilateral nature of the superior oblique paresis is detected on careful examination and certainly it becomes apparent when surgical treatment is incorrectly limited to the assumedly affected eye, so that a recession (with sometimes an anteroposition) of the inferior oblique of one eye is followed within a short time by an obvious overaction of the inferior oblique of the other eye.

Moebius Syndrome

This syndrome was described originally by Graefe (1880) but the name of Moebius has become associated with the syndrome because of his extensive study of the condition with publications in 1888 and 1892. There is seldom any element of inheritance but occasionally it may occur in more than one member of the family (Harrison and Parker 1960). In general terms the condition represents a congenital bilateral facial diplegia with a defective bilateral form of lateral gaze.

The presenting feature of the condition is usually the parent's awareness of a lack of any significant alteration in the facial expression, even on an emotional occasion, so that there is a persistence of a bland facial appearance, despite obvious other bodily changes in keeping with the emotion of the moment; occasionally the repesenting feature may be awareness by the mother of a difficulty in feeding. The failure of a closure of the eyelids during sleep is usually noticed at a later stage and this may be somewhat asymmetrical.

The typical feature of the syndrome is a complete loss or a fairly marked deficiency of abduction which is of a bilateral nature, but this is seldom noticed by the parent at an early age unless it is associated with an obvious strabismus. This failure of the abducted eye on lateral gaze to generate horizontal saccades is a feature of the syndrome irrespective of the nature of the stimulus for such a movement--ocular or vestibular (Wollensak, Fleischer-Peters and Hovels, 1962). The loss (or more or less complete loss) of bilateral abduction induces a compensatory head posture so that the head is moved in an exaggerated way in order to achieve fixation of an object in the right or left lateral field, or in order to maintain fixation of an object which is moving to the right or to the left. There is only occasionally a disturbance of vertical movement. When this occurs, it takes the form of a limitation of elevation or depression of one eye. The movements of convergence are normal in the few cases which show an absence of a strabismus. A defect of adduction is an unusual feature of the syndrome; in four of the 16 cases reported by Bannister, Walker and Wybar (1976). This defect of adduction is rarely so extreme that there is a virtual loss of all lateral movements of both eyes, but it has been reported as a characteristic feature (Duke-Elder 1964); and when it occurs, it necessitates a persistent movement of the head in any form of change of fixation.

A strabismus is a common feature of Moebius syndrome and in view of the characteristic bilateral loss of abduction, this has been assumed to be almost invariably an esotropia. But this is not a valid assumption and in the 16 cases reported by Bannister, Walker and Wybar (1976) various forms of strabismus occurred: an esotropia occurred in seven cases--two with an associated A phenomonen, one with a hypotropia of one eye, and two with a dissociated vertical divergence; an exotropia occurred in four cases, but in one of the four cases, the exotropia was of a consecutive nature following surgical treatment for an esotropia, in one of the three other cases there was an associated A phenomenon, and in another case there was a hypertropia of one eye; in one case there was an isolated hypertropia of one eye; and in one case there was an isolated dissociated vertical divergence; in the three remaining cases there was no evidence of strabismus, but one of the three cases had had corrected surgical treatment for an esotropia at an early age so that binocular function was retained in only two cases spontaneously.

A lack of potential binocular function is a feature of cases of the Moebius snydrome when there is a manifest strabismus despite appropriate therapeutic measures. The cases which are described above showed a restoration of binocular function after surgical treatment at an early age in only one case, and binocular function was present in two cases in which there had never been any form of strabismus. This frequent loss of binocular function is related to the congenital nature of the disorder, but it is fostered also to some extent by the high incidence of anisometropia and astigmatism which fosters the development of amblyopia of the more affected eye. This is confirmed by the higher incidence of amblyopia and defective stereopsis in the Moebius syndrome as compared with a group of isolated strabismics in a similar age range.

The facial weakness is variable in severity and it is also variable in its symmetry so that the extent of the facial weakness is inconsistent in individual cases. It is interesting that an asymmetry of the facial paresis is frequently associated with a similar asymmetry of the ocular motility disorder. The facial weakness is somewhat difficult to define because as a general rule it tends to show a blend of upper and lower motor neurone involvement. Characteristically the facial weakness is detected at an early age because it is accompanied by a difficulty in feeding (sucking) and subsequently the facial weakness becomes noticeable by the lack of any emotional facial expression, such as in laughing or crying. This is illustrated very clearly when the facial palsy is bilateral and symmetrical (Fig. 30), but even more when it is bilateral and asymmetrical because it tends to produce an unfortunate grimace (Fig. 31). Sometimes, however, the facial weakness is of a partial nature so that there is a relatively normal response of the facial muscles to emotional stimuli, but otherwise there is rather an inert or bland appearance of the face. The facial palsy (or paresis) causes a failure of a complete closure of the eyelids during sleep, but it is rare for the cornea of either eye to be involved in a serious way because of a turning up of the eyes on an attempted lid closure due to an intact Bell's phenomenon (Fig. 32).

However, there is a reduction in corneal sensitivity in some cases and a superficial punctate corneal erosion may occur, but this is seldom of a progressive nature and relatively free from any symptoms, except occasionally for some photophobia.

Furthermore, the facial weakness may be associated with epiphora. This is seldom, if ever, the result of any significant degree of ectropiion of the lower eyelid with a failure of the lower punctum to be in reasonable apposition to the globe and there is little doubt that it is the result essentially of a defect of the pumping mechanism of the lacrimal sac which is dependent on the integrity of the components of the orbicularis muscle which embrace the lacrimal sac.

A different anomaly of lacrimation has been reported (Henderson 1939). This takes the form of so-called crocodile tears, which is a form of paradoxical lacrimation which occurs on eating--the term is derived from the legend that crocodiles weep before devouring their victims! It is likely that the abnormal lacrimation is the result of a paradoxical innervation of the lacrimal gland by the parasympathetic nerve fibres which are normally concerned in the function of salivation. It would seem that this results from a dysplasia of the lacrimal nucleus in the brain-stem as a developmental anomaly.

A deformity of the tongue is a frequent feature of the Moebius syndrome. This takes the form of an inability to protrude the tongue a normal distance beyond the teet (Fig. 33) and this lack of protrusion may be asymmetrical so that one side of the tongue protrudes more than the other side. In this context it is of interest to note an undue incidence of dental caries in the series of cases described by Bannister, Walker and Wybar (1976). This is almost certainly the result of a stagnation of saliva. It is likely that this congenital anomaly of the tongue musculature contributes to the difficulty of the suckling of the infant, although the facial paresis probably plays an important role in this, as discussed earlier.

There is sometimes a variable degree of hypotonia in early childhood so that they are essentially "floppy babies".

There is also sometimes a delay in certain of the motor milestones in early life, such as a holding up of the head, sitting or walking; an absence of the pectoral muscles occurs rarely.

Deformities of the hands may occur, such as an absence of one or more fingers, a webbing of the fingers, a claw hand, and an asymmetry of the fingers so that the fingers of one hand are much shorter than those of the other hand (Fig. 34). Deformities of the feet may occur, such as a club foot, a duplication of the big toe, and a webbing of the toes (Fig. 35). There may be a defect of hearing which may take the form of deafness or a partical loss of hearing. Sometimes there is an anomaly of the pinna of the ear.

It is of interest to take regard of the intellectual difficulties which may be found in the Moebius syndrome. In the series of 16 cases reported by Bannister, Walker and Wybar (1976), five patients had a low intelligence quotient (IQ) and a further three were difficult to assess. The remainder had a normal level of intelligence, although two of these were regarded initially as having a low IQ, but were later considered to have an average or even above average level of intelligence. It is of interest to note that the milestones of those found to have a normal level of intelligence appeared to be delayed if the method of assessment involved an activity requiring normal muscle tone, so that care must be exercised in choosing appropriate methods when assessments are made of young children with the Moebius syndrome.

In this context it is also of interest to take note of the difficulties in communication which may occur in cases of Moebius syndrome. It is evident that the peculiar apearance of the face with a general lack of facial expression even on attempting to smile when the facial palsy is symmetrical, and by the development of an unsightly grimace when the facial palsy is asymmetrical, creates difficulties of communication because of the intuitive reliance which is placed on facial expression during normal conversation. This disturbance of the facial expression imposes practical and emotional difficulties on the patients and also in the case of children on their parents. Obviously any difficulty in communication is increased when there is also a form of deafness.

A benign intracranial hypertension occurred in a boy of 15 years with Moebius syndrome (Nelson and Huppert 1980). This case is discussed in detail but no evidence is put forward which shows an association between the two conditions.

The etiology of the Moebius snydrome is not known precisely despite recognition of the condition for 100 years. This is largely because it is relatively rare and few cases have undergone detailed investigation at autopsy. The main finding is an atrophy of the brain-stem nuclei and their related nerves (Heubner 1900; Rainey and Fowler 1903; Spatz and Ullrich 1931) and the clinical features of the condition and the electromyographic investigations indicate that the brain-stem dysfunction is of a widespread nature.

It is difficult to understand the nature of the defective adduction which is sometimes a feature of the syndrome. It seems most unlikely that it is the result of any lesion of the third cranial nucleus or nerve because of the isolation of the involvement to the medial rectus. There is, however, a disturbance of vestibular nystagmus in the Moebius syndrome which suggests an interruption of the pathways in the medial (posterior) longitudinal bundle (fasciculus) so that the loss of adduction may be akin to that which occurs in an internuclear ophthalmoplegia, and such a suggestion is supported by the finding of a defective development of the medial longitudinal bundle in a brain-stem in a two year old boy with Moebius syndrome (Heubner 1900).

A teratogenic etiology is a reasonable assumption in cases of the Moebius syndrome in which there are also multiple congenital deformities (Papst 1963).

An interesting and unusual suggestion has been put forward recently by Ramsay and Walker (1983) that the evidence of certain overlapping clinical features of Moebius syndrome and Duane´s snydrome may be an indication that they are essentially similar conditions. In this way Duane´s snydrome represents a mild form of Moebius syndrome, although it differs by being characterized by an element of paradoxical innervation.

The management of strabismus in the Moebius syndrome imposes great difficulties when trying to achieve a satisfactory result. The provision of a spectacle correction has no significant influence on the degree of the strabismus and is of value only in trying to obtain good vision in each eye, particularly when there is a significant degree of ametropia or anisometropia so that the spectacle correction facilitates the carrying out of occlusion.

Surgical treatment should be carried out when there is an esotropia with a full recession of both medial rectus muscles.

This may only give a limited result and a further recession of each medial rectus should be carried out using looped sutures so that each muscle retains an effective action in the region of the functional equator (Fig. 36). Rarely a resection of one or both lateral rectus muscles is of value in the treatment of an esotropia. Surgical treatment is seldom required when there is an exotropia unless it is unduly noticeable.

Benign Intracranial Hypertension

This is a complex condition of doubtful etiology, despite its recognition for about a quarter of a century, and it is unusual in early childhood. I am introducing the subject simply to give details of an unusual case.

A boy who had suffered severe eczema from an early age (Fig. 37) had been treated extensively by topical steroids with some amelioration of the eczema (Fig. 38). He presented with an apparent convergent strabismus of the right eye at 4 1/2 years of fairly sudden onset, but on examination the right eye was found to be blind (no perception of light) and he was also found to have partial loss of abduction of the left eye due to a paresis of the left VIth cranial nerve. The vision of the left eye was reduced to a level of 6/18. He had a benign intracranial hypertension with marked bilateral papilledema and it was considered that the condition had resulted from an absorption of steroids through the skin over a prolonged period of time. He was treated by dexamethasone by mouth followed by prednisolone by mouth with dramatic improvement so that within three weeks his vision had improved to 6/12 in the right eye and 6/9 in the left one.

I saw him again recently at the age of 10 years. He has a normal level of vision in each eye for distance and near (6/5 and N5) with full visual fields on a simple confrontation test, and yet there is a marked degree of pallor of both optic discs (Figs. 39 and 40). This pallor is so great that it is almost incompatible with the levels of his visual acuity and it must be assumed that there is a general depression of the function of the optic nerves without causing any absolute loss of visual function.

The Retinopathy of Prematurity-- Retrolental Fibroplasia

It might seem rather anachronistic to include the subject of retrolental fibroplasia in a lecture given in 1982 because nearly three decades ago the problem if its etiology appeared to be resolved in a scientific manner and it seemed at that time that the condition would cease to be a clinical entity, except only as an isolated event.

Retrolental fibroplasia was described originally by Theodore Terry in 1945 in a paper in the Archives of Ophthalmology headed "Retrolental Fibroplasia in Premature Infants". However, he had described various aspects of the condition during the previous three years (Terry 1942a&b; 1943a&b). Terry was then Assistant Professor of Ophthalmology at Harvard University but this was his final position because he died tragically in 1946 at the relatively young age of 47 years before he had time to do more than lay the groundwork of his dicovery of this unusual retinal disorder of the premature infant. Terry was in a unique position to be involved in the unravelling of such a discovery because he had received formal trainings in both pathology and ophthalmology.

In general terms retrolental fibroplasia is the result of an obliteration of the developing retinal vessels, which are in an immature state because of the prematurity and this obliteration is essentially the result of an unduly high concentration of oxygen in the arterial blod. This is followed by a profuse proliferation of new vessel formations when the infant is removed from the rich oxygen atmosphere with the development usually of some form of retrolental membrance of fibrous tissue. This was confirmed by experimental investigation and I shall be sufficiently chauvinistic to mention Ashton, Ward and Serpell (1953) who wrote such a brilliant preliminary report on the role of oxygen in the genesis of retrolental fibroplasia which was based on detailed experimental work on kittens in the Department of Pathology at the Institute of Ophthalmology in London. I say "chauvinistic" because I know that other workers in other countries were working along similar lines with the formulation of similar conclusions. It was natural to assume that a careful monitoring of oxygen administration to the premature infant and a detailed assessment of the changes occurring in the retina would result in a virtual elimination of the condition and indeed there was a dramatic decrease in the incidence of the condition in the late 1950′s.

However, the incidence of retrolental fibroplasia seems once again to be on the increase, at least to some extent, and Silverman (1977) warned that the waning of interest which followed the investigations in the 1950′s was misplaced because "many of the challenges of experience had not yet been confronted". This is endorsed by Flynn (1983) who agrees with the original conclusion that the occurrence of retrolental fibroplasia is inversely related to the birth weight, but he emphasized that this is only one aspect and that there is a type of premature infant who can be recognized almost intuitively by experience as a likely candidate for the condition; a tiny infant who is critically ill for weeks or even months after birth and who demands all the skill and care from a team of experts to remain alive because of the presence of life-threatening conditions of the pulmonary system (the respiratory distress syndrome), of the central nervous system (convulsions, hydrocephaly), of the cardiac system (bradycardia-apnoea, congestive cardiac failure), of the hematological system (anemia as the result of the presence of premature enzymes), and sometimes other features.

There is evidence that the abrupt termination of vascularisation in the peripheral part of the retina in the premature infant is seen particularly in the temporal region (Flynn, O-Grady, Herrera, Kushner, Cantolino and Milam, 1977; Kushner, Essner, Cohen and Flynn, 1977) and there is little doubt that this accounts for the predilection for the involvement of the temporal part of the retinal in cases of retrolental fibroplasia when the condition is not widespread. This may take the form of a raised mass of disorganized retinal tissue which extends from the region of the optic nervehead to the temporal periphery with a complete disruption of macular function, but sometimes these changes are less severe with a traction of the macular part of the retina in a temporal direction. These changes which occur in the temporal part of the retina because of a failure of the premature retinal vessels to extend as far as the temporal periphery of the retina support the hypothesis put forward by Flynn (1983) that the stimulus, which leads to the essential structural anomaly of retrolental fibroplasia, is created within the avascular part of the retina rather than within an already vascularised retina or within neovascular membranes.

The traction of the retina in a temporal direction creates an unusual form of exotropia which may be designated as a pseudo-exotropia. This is illustrated by a boy whom I saw recently at the age of 5 1/2 years. He was referred to me from abroad for surgical treatment of a right exotropia. He was born 10 weeks prematurely with a birth weight of slightly less than 1 1/2 kilograms and he was maintained in an oxygen incubator for six weeks. The precise concentrations of oxygen in the incubator and particularly the concentration of oxygen in the arterial circulation were not recorded.

On a straight-forward observation, the boy who was sitting with his mother during the taking of the history showed an obvious well-marked right exotropia (Figs. 41 and 42) and it was slightly odd, therefore, to find on subsequent examination that he had levels of vision in the right eye of 6/18 and N5 whereas the left eye, which appeared to be in a "straight" position, was virtually blind (no perception of light or perhaps at times a vague recognition of a bright light). This apparent anomaly was explained readily on an examination of the fundus of the right eye which showed a marked traction of the macular area in a temporal direction (Fig. 43) so that he was forced to fix with his only sighted eye in a position of exotropia, with the typical changes of a partial form of retinopathy of prematurity (retrolental fibroplasia) in the temporal periphery. There were marked changes in the blind left eye involving the whole of the temporal part of the retina with an extensive fibro-vascular membrane which had caused a disruption of the optic nervehead.

Needless to say, I did not embark on surgical treatment for this pseudo-exotropia!

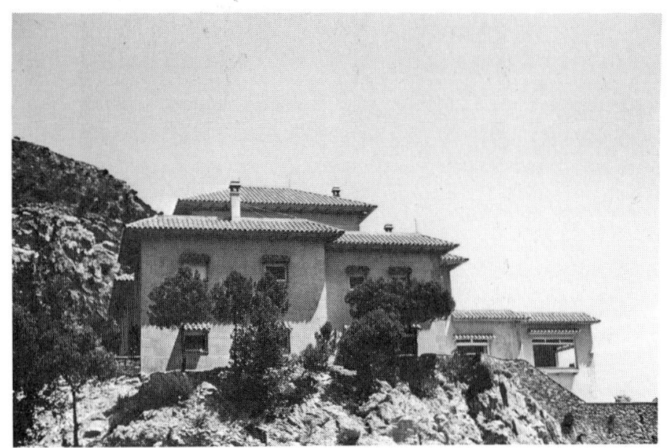

Fig. 1 The "Arruga" villa in Bagur, Spain

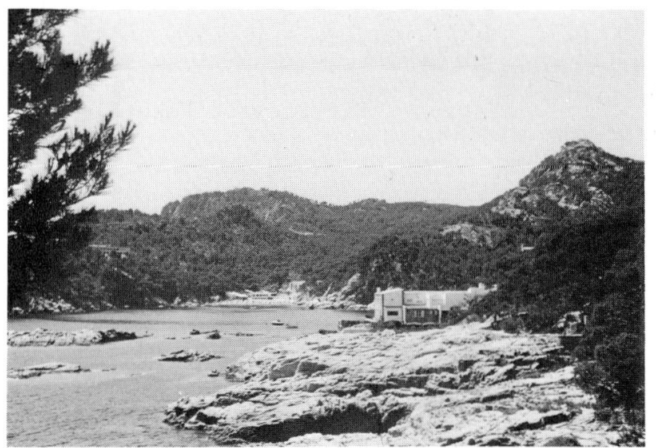

Fig. 2 The birthplace of Alfredo Arruga

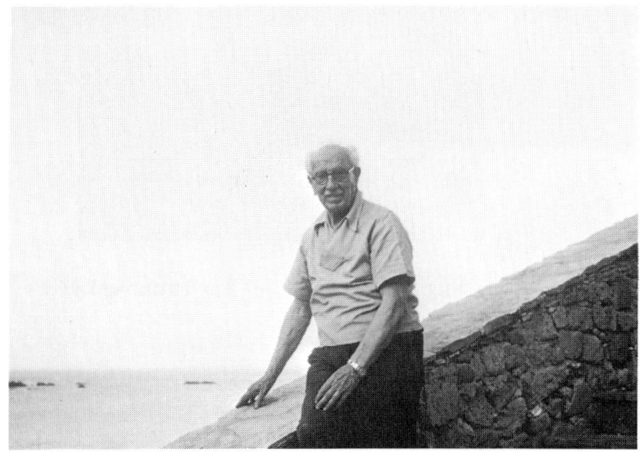

Fig. 3 Count Hermenegilde Arruga

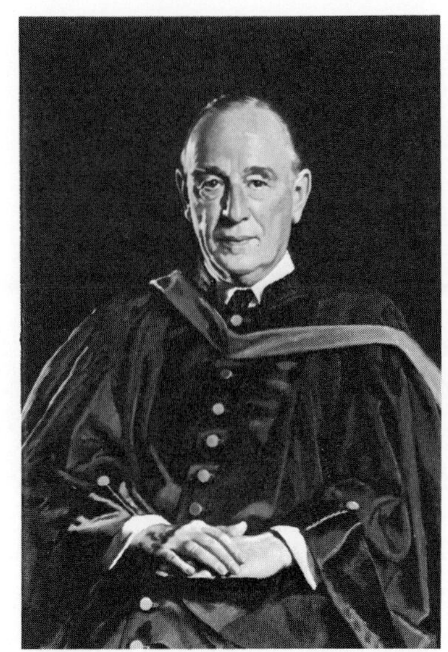

Fig. 4 Sir Stewart Duke-Elder

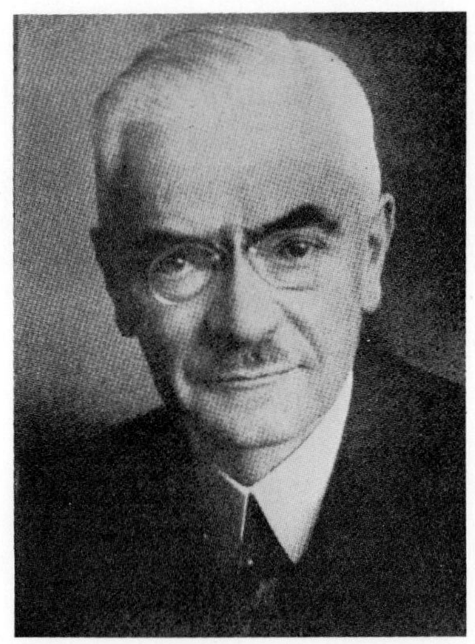

Fig. 5 Alfred Bielschowsky

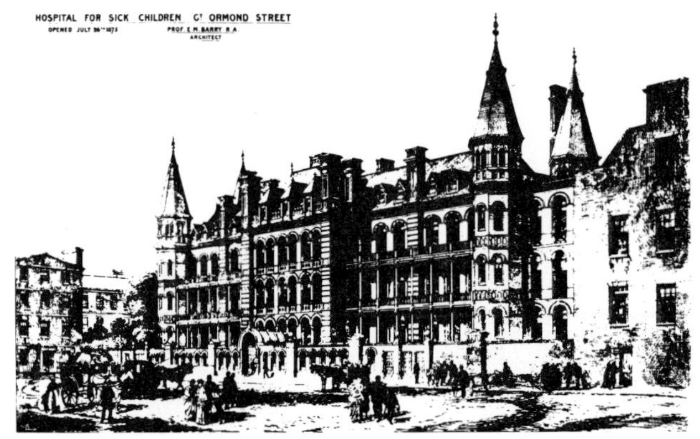

Fig. 6 The Hospital for Sick Children, Great Ormond Street, London--as it was

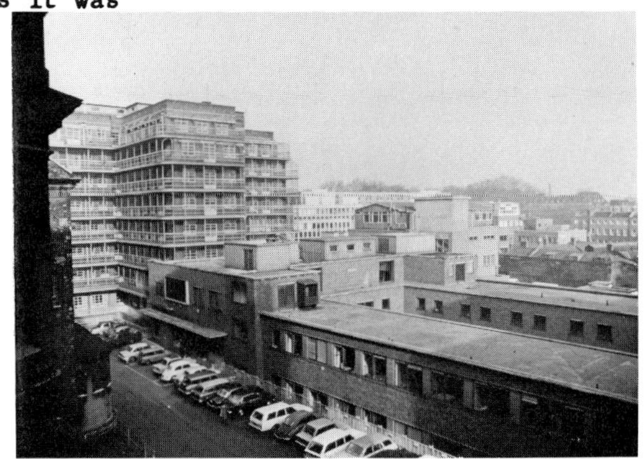

Fig 7. The Hospital for Sick Children, Great Ormond Street, London--as it is now

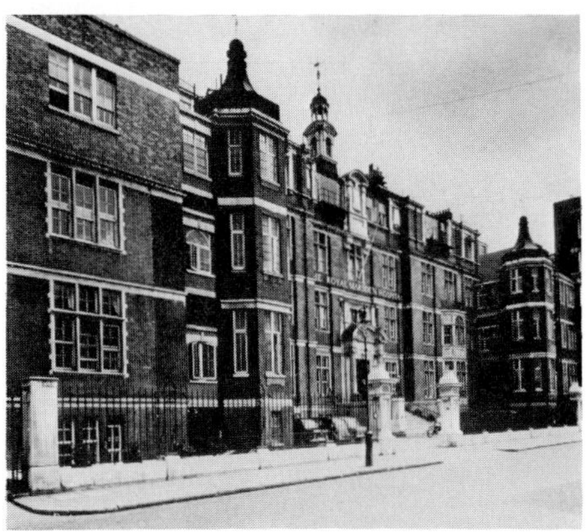

Fig. 8 The Royal Marsden Hospital, Fulham Road, London

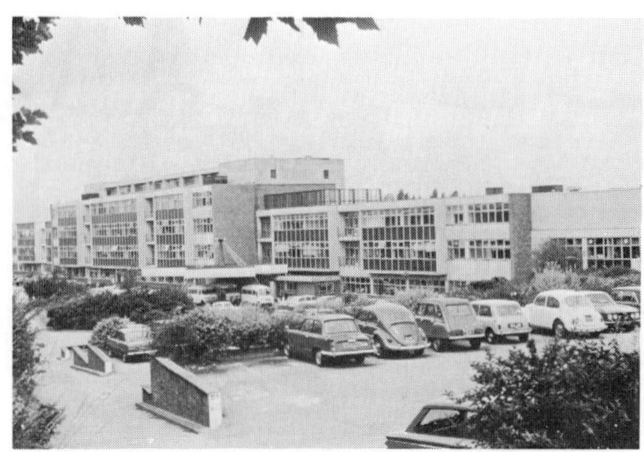

Fig. 9 The Royal Marsden Hospital, Belmont, Surrey

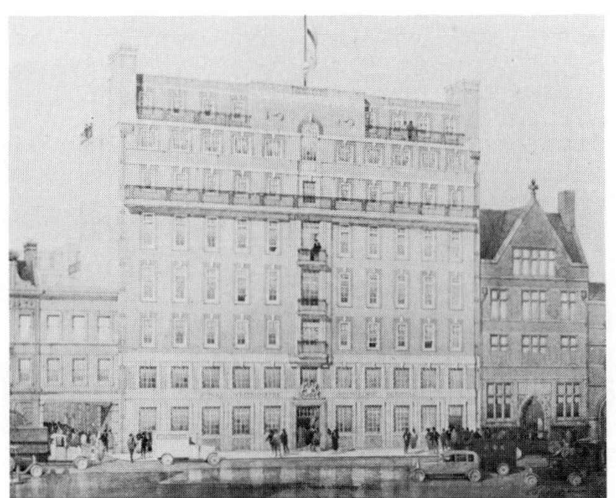

Fig. 10 Moorfields Eye Hospital, High Holborn, London

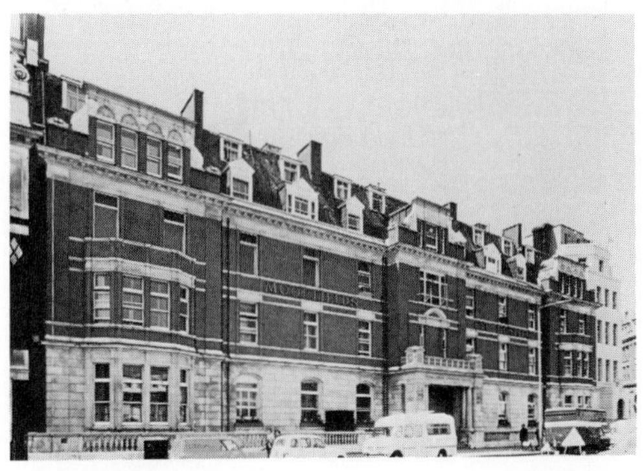

Fig. 11 Moorfields Eye Hospital, City Road, London

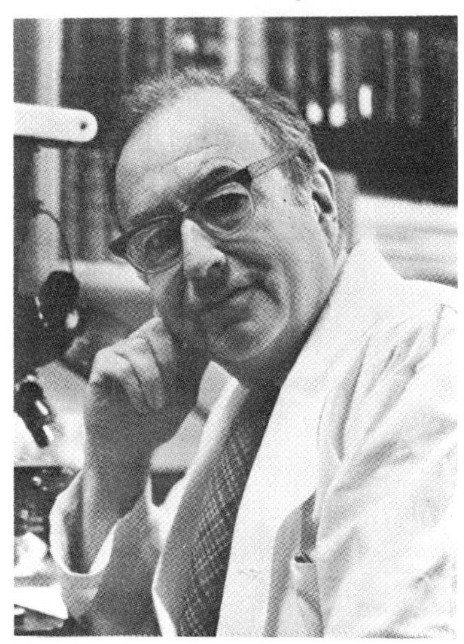

Fig. 12 David Cogan

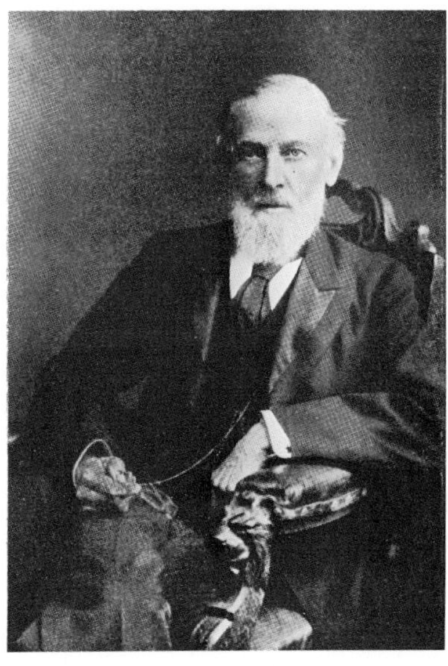

Fig. 13 Sir William Richard Gowers

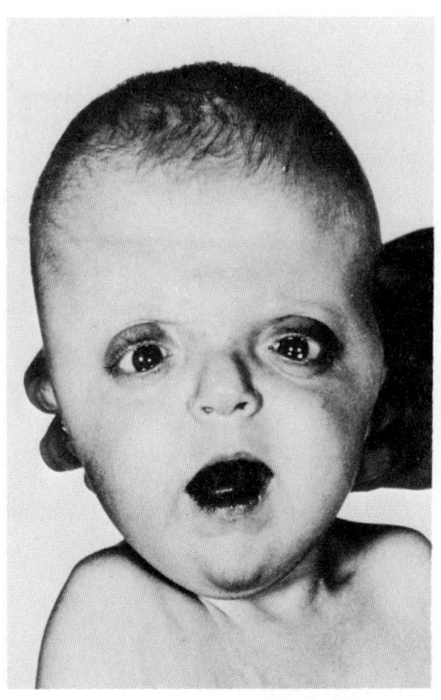

Fig. 14 Oxycephaly

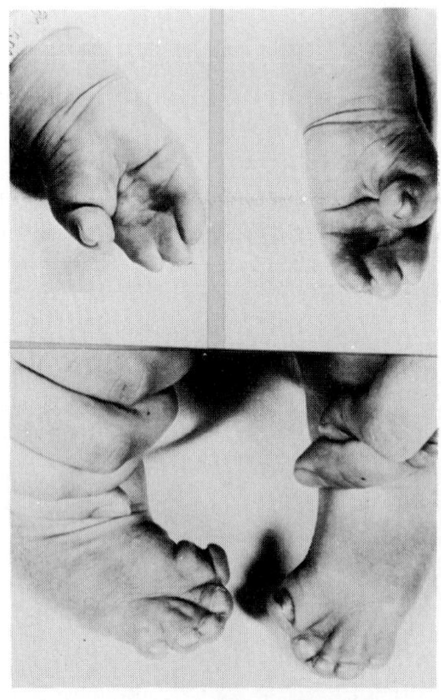

Fig. 15 The acrocephalo-syndactyly syndrome of Alpert

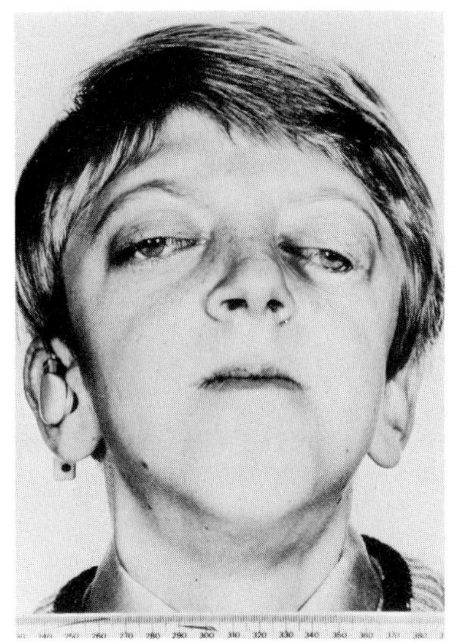

Fig. 16 Crouzon's disease

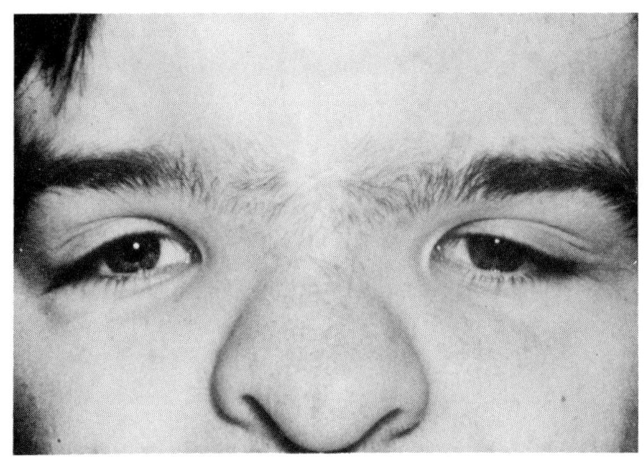

Fig. 17 Hypertelorism

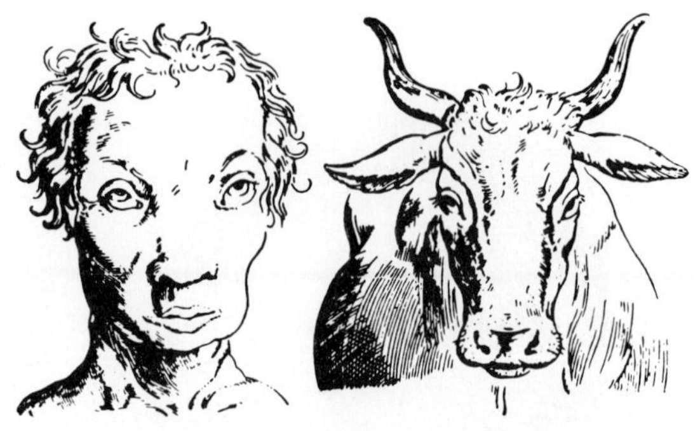

Valdè magni oculi.

Fig. 18 Hypertelorism--cow-like appearance

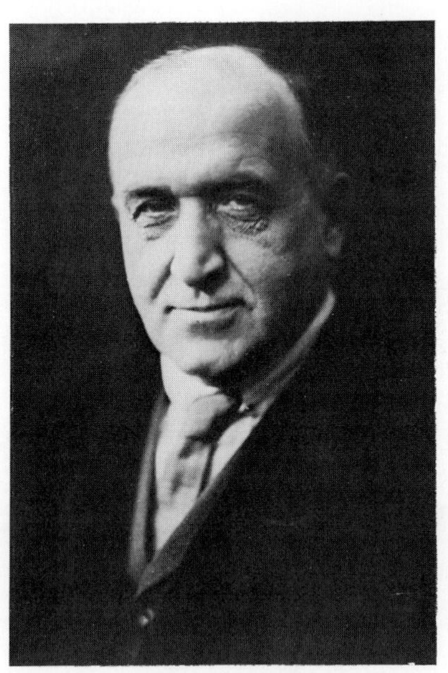

Fig. 19 David Middleton Greig

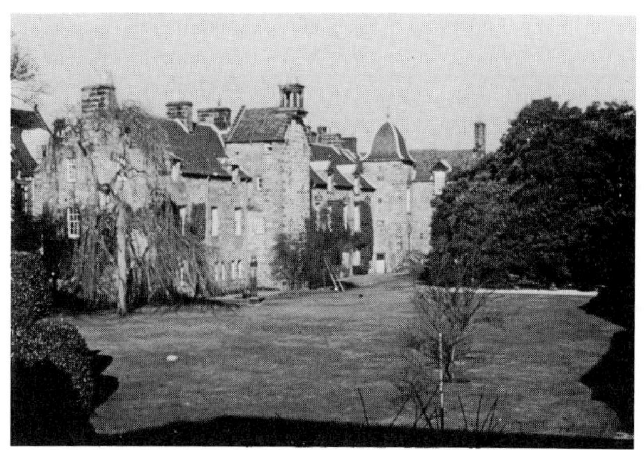

Fig. 20 The University of St. Andrews, Scotland

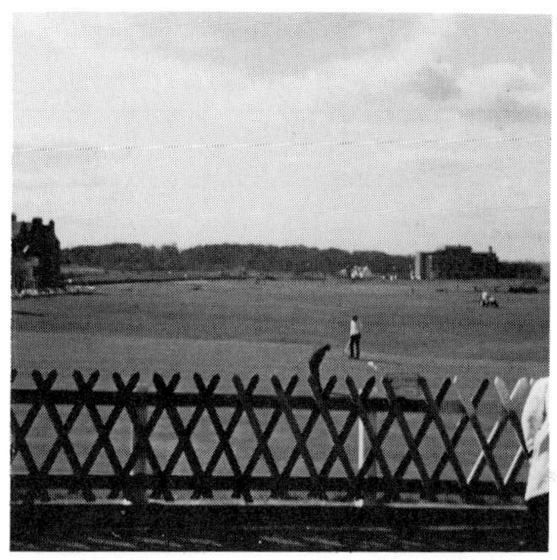

Fig. 21 The Old Course, St. Andrews, Scotland

	OXYCEPHALY	CROUZON'S DISEASE	HYPERTELORISM	TOTAL
NUMBER OF CASES IN SERIES	10	5	20	35
NUMBER OF CASES INVOLVED IN TESSIER PROCEDURE	4	3	12	19

Fig. 22 Craniofacial dysostosis; oxycephaly; Crouzon's disease; and hypertelorism

	OXYCEPHALY	CROUZON'S DISEASE	HYPERTELORISM	TOTAL
ESOTROPIA	7	2	4	13
EXOTROPIA	1	2	10	13
HYPERTROPIA	1	-	2	3
ORTHOTROPIA	1	1	4	6

Fig. 23 Craniofacial dysostosis--nature of strabismus

	OXYCEPHALY	CROUZON'S DISEASE	HYPERTELORISM	TOTAL
ESOTROPIA	7	2	4	13
EXOTROPIA	1	1	10	12
HYPERTROPIA c̄ ESOTROPIA	1	-	1	2
				27

Fig. 24 Craniofacial dysostosis--incidence of V phenomena

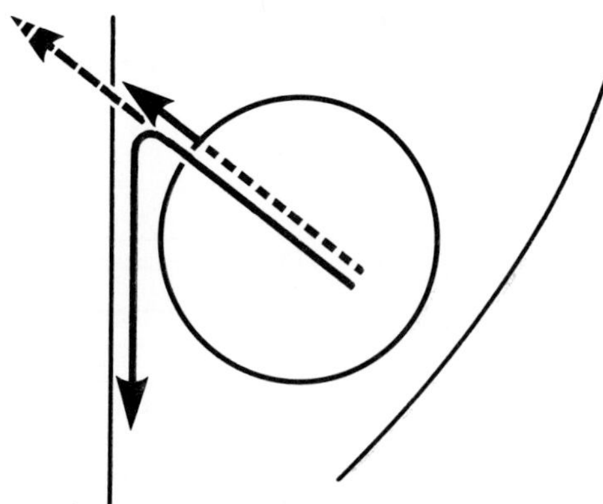

Fig. 25 Similar directions of lines of pull of superior and inferior obliques in normal eye

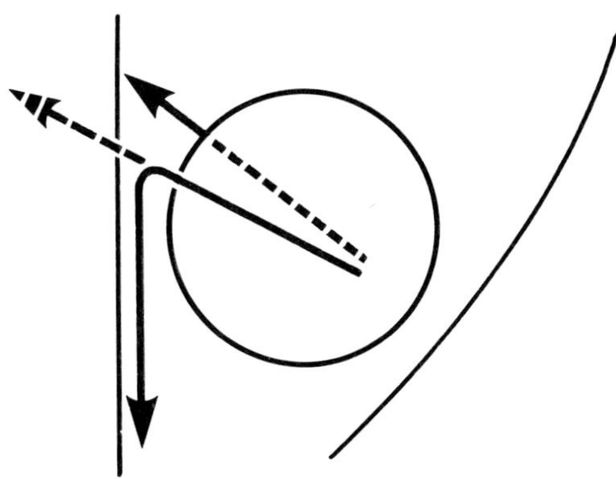

Fig. 26 Different directions of lines of pull of superior and inferior obliques in V phenomenon

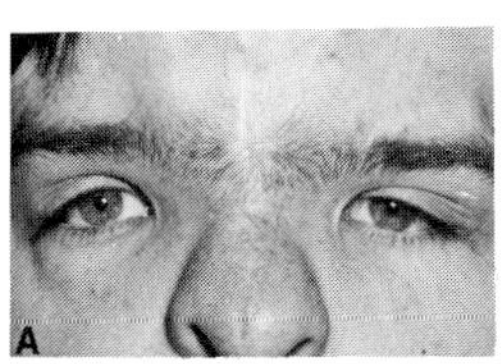

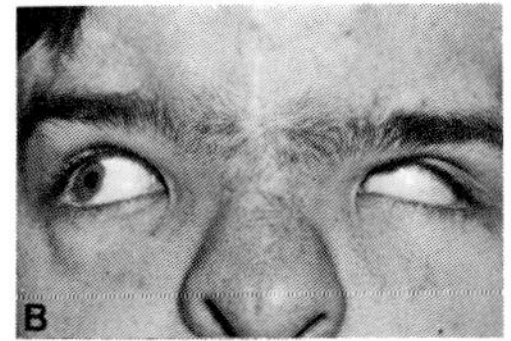

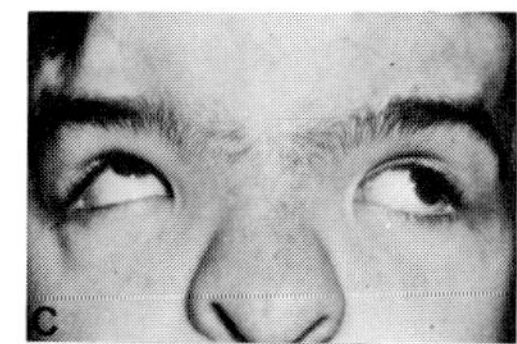

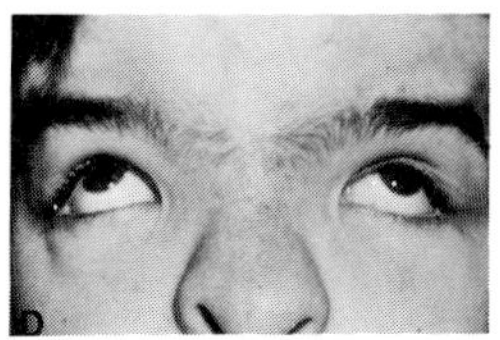

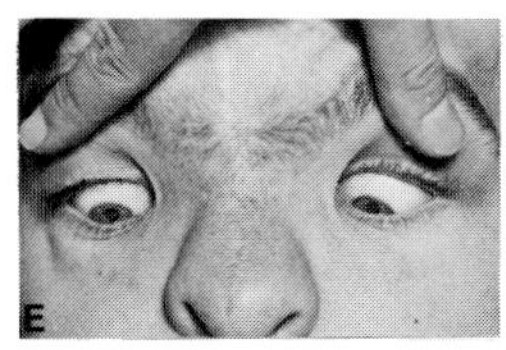

Fig. 27 Hypertelorism--exotropia with V phenomenon: (a) eyes in primary position; (b) eyes in dextroversion; (c) eyes in laevoversion; (d) eyes in elevation; (e) eyes in depression

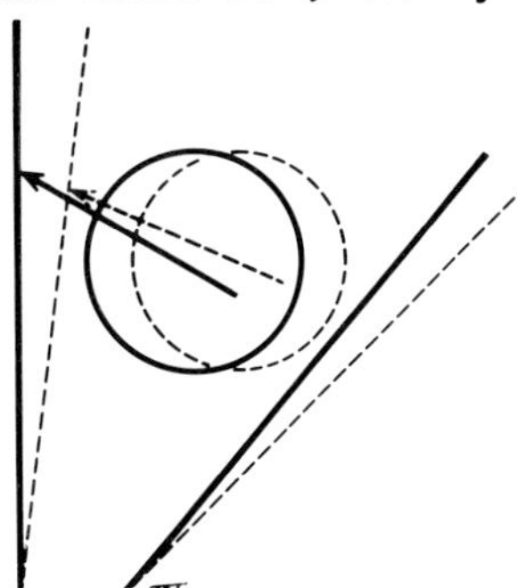

Fig. 28 Hypertelorism--alteration in direction of line of pull of superior oblique (dotted lines), in contrast to the line of pull in normal eye

	OXYCEPHALY		CROUZON'S DISEASE		HYPERTELORISM	
	BEFORE	AFTER	BEFORE	AFTER	BEFORE	AFTER
ESOTROPIA	3	3	1	1	1	9
EXOTROPIA	1	1	1	-	7	2

Fig. 29 Craniofacial dysostosis--V phenomenon before and after Tessier operation

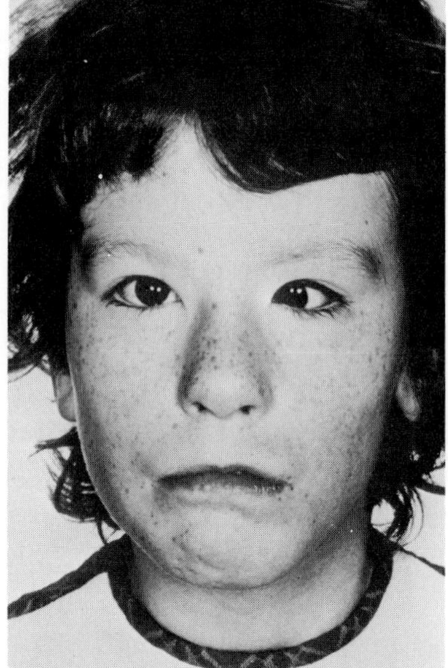

Fig. 30 Moebius syndrome--expressionless face even on attempting to smile when facial palsy bilateral and symmetrical

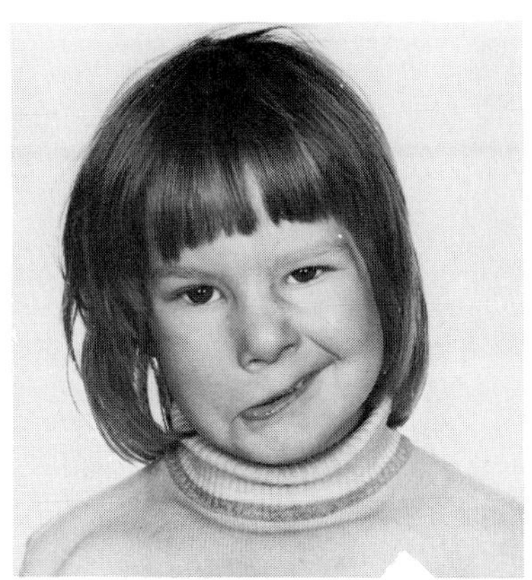

Fig. 31 Moebius syndrome--facial grimace on attempting to smile when facial palsy bilateral but asymmetrical

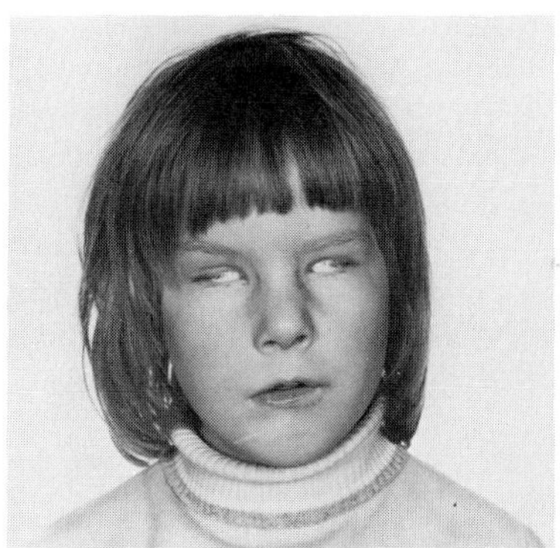

Fig. 32 Moebius syndrome--defective lid closure but retention of Bell´s phenomenon

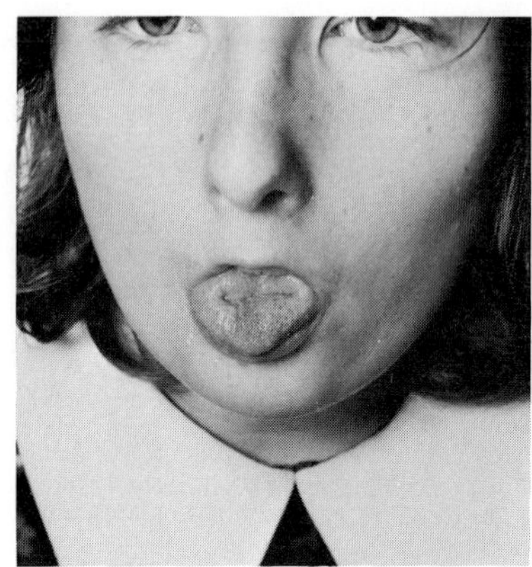

Fig. 33 Moebius snydrome--partial atrophy of tongue with limited protrusion beyond teeth

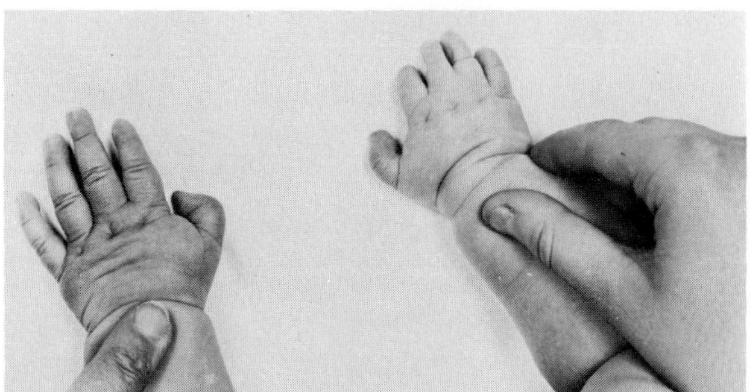

Fig. 34 Moebius snydrome--shortening of fingers and thumb of right hand

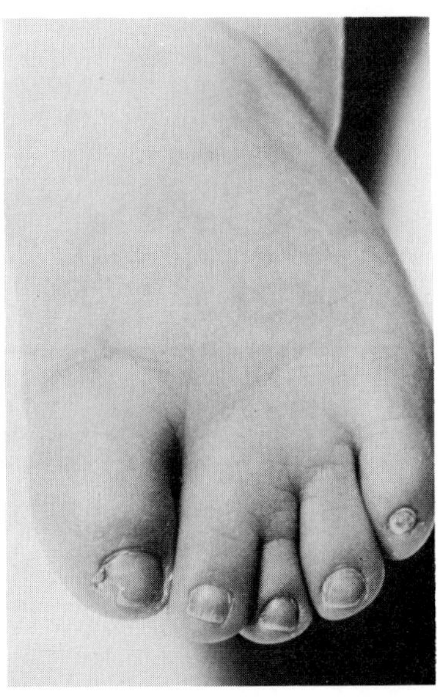

Fig. 35 Moebius syndrome--partial webbing of toes of left foot

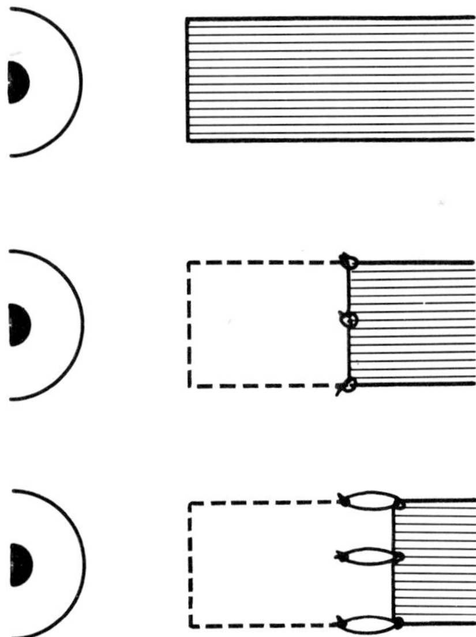

Fig. 36 Recession of medial rectus muscle and recession combined with looped sutures

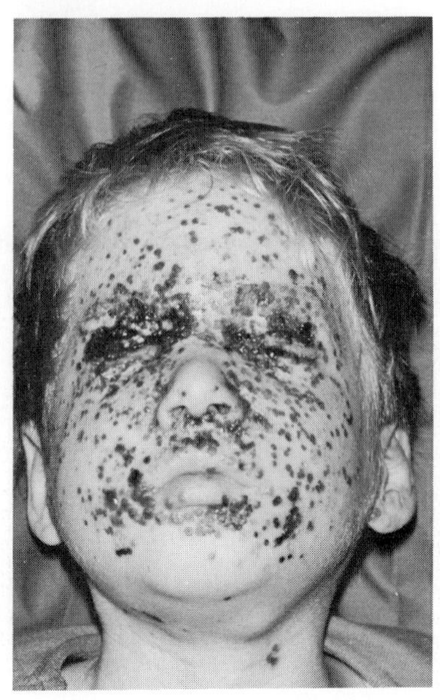

Fig. 37 Severe eczema of face

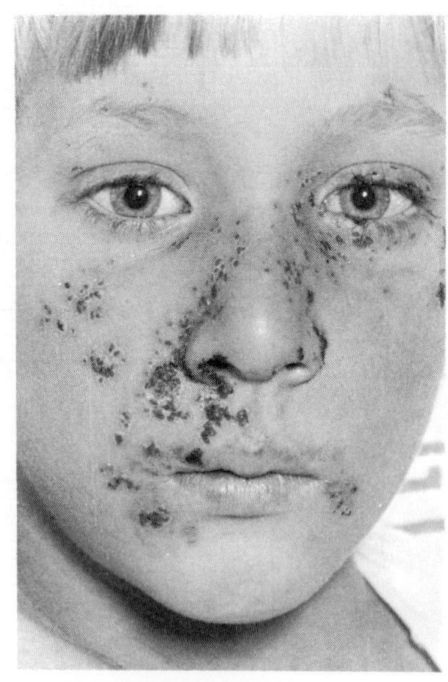

Fig. 38 Improvement of eczema of face after use of topical steroids

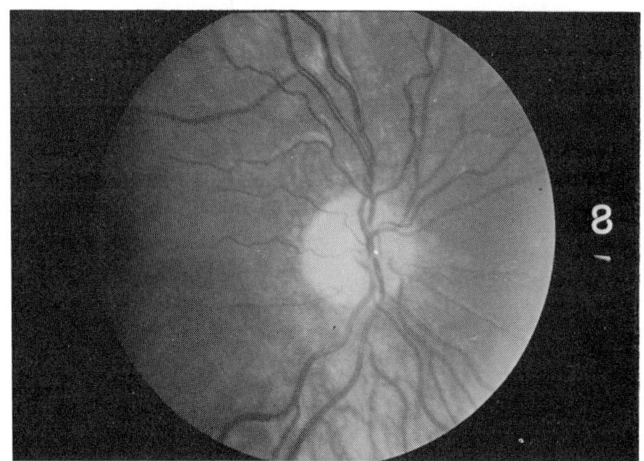

Fig. 39 Right eye--consecutive optic atrophy in benign intracranial hypertension

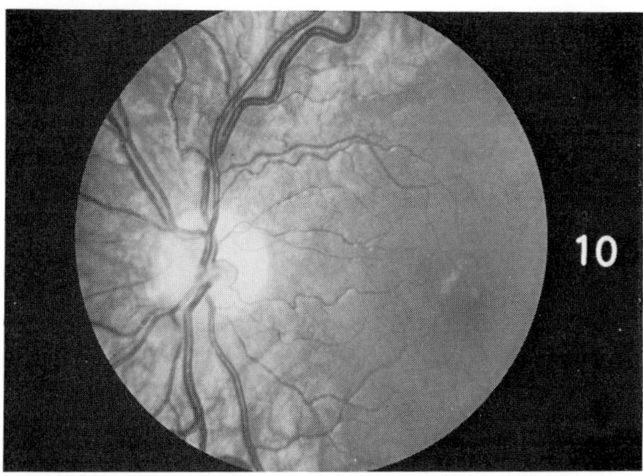

Fig. 40 Left eye--consecutive optic atrophy in benign intracranial hypertension

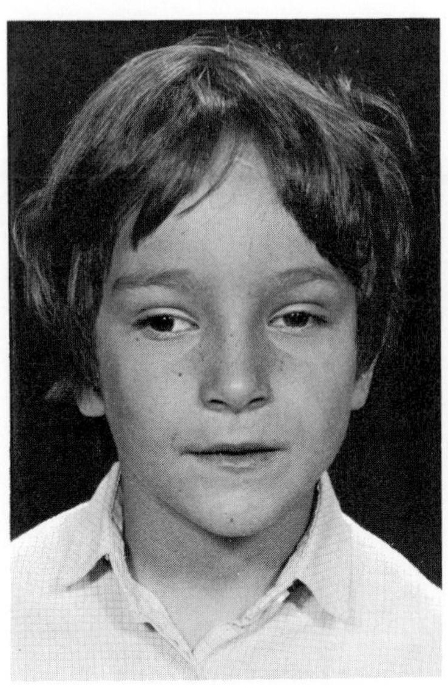

Fig. 41 Retrolental fibroplasia--apparent (but false) right exotropia

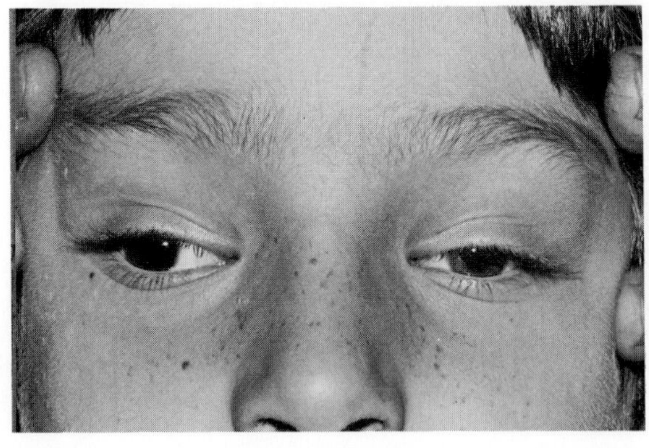

Fig. 42 Retrolental fibroplasia--apparent (but false) right exotropia

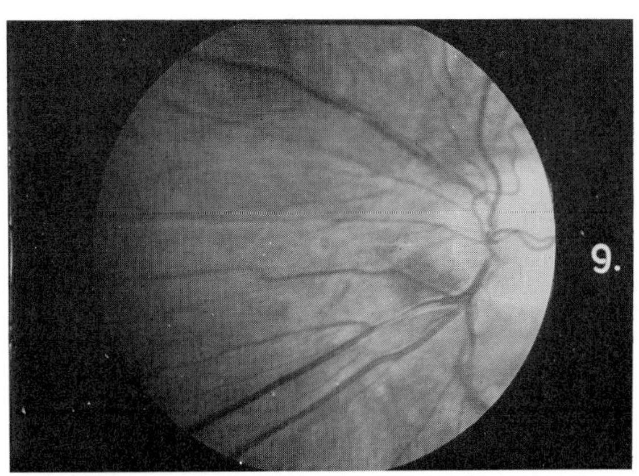

Fig. 43 Retrolental fibroplasia--traction of macular area of right eye

References

1. Altrocchi PH, Menkes JH: Congenital ocular motor apraxia. Brain 83:579-588, 1960

2. Ashton N, Ward B, Serpell G: Role of oxygen in the genesis of retrolental fibroplasia. Brit J Ophthalmol 37:513-520, 1953

3. Bannister PH, Walker J, Wybar KC: Moebius syndrome. Brit Orthopt J 33:67-77, 1976

4. Ben-Zur PH, Feldman PM, Bender MB: Eye and head coordination of normal subjects and patients with defective oculomotor output. Physiologist 13:148, 1970

5. Bertelsen TI: The premature synostosis of the cranial sutures. Acta Ophthalmol 36 (suppl 51):9-176, 1978

6. Bielschowsky A: Das klinische bild der assziierten blicklahmung und seine bedeutung fur die topische diagnostik. Munchen Med Wehnschr 50:1666, 1903

7. Brown, Limon de E: Trans 2nd Cong Internat Strabismological Assoc. Fells P (ed), Diffusion Generale de Librairie, Paris-Marseille (France), 1976, pp 371

8. Cogan DG: A type of congenital ocular motor apraxia presenting jerky head movements. Trans Am Acad Ophthalmol Otolaryngol 56:853-862, 1952

9. Collewijn H: Optokinetic eye movements in the rabbit: input-output relations. Vision Res 9:117-132, 1969

10. Collin R: In: Pediatric Ophthalmology; Current Aspects. Wybar K, Taylor D (eds) Marcel Dekker Inc., New York, 1983 (in press)

11. Duke Elder S: System of Ophthalmology, Vol III--Normal and Abnormal Development, Part 2: Congenital Deformities, Henry Kimpton, London, 1964, p. 1032

12. Duke Elder S: System of Ophthlamology, Vol III--Normal and Abnormal Development, Part 2: Congenital Deformities, Henry Kimpton, London, 1964, p. 1035

13. Duke Elder S, Wybar K: System of Ophthalmology, Duke Elder S (ed) Vol VI--Ocular Motility and Strabismus, Henry

Kimpton, London, 1973, p. 642

14. Flynn JT: In: Pediatric Ophthalmology; Current Aspects. Wybar K, Taylor D (eds) Marcel Dekker Inc., New York, 1983 (in press)

15. Flynn JT, O'Grady GE, Herrera J, Kushner BJ, Cantolino S, Milam W: Retrolental fibroplasia. I. Clinical Observations. Arch Ophthalmol 95:217-223, 1977

16. Gowers WR: Note on a reflex mechanism in the fixation of the eyeballs. Brain 2:39-41, 1879

17. Graefe A: In: Handbuch der gesammten Augenheikunde, No. 6, Wilhelm eugelman, Leipzig, 1880, p. 60

18. Greaves B, Walker J, Wybar K: Disorders of ocular motility in craniofacial dysostosis. J Roy Soc Med 72:21-24, 1979

19. Gresty M, Halmagy GM, Taylor D: In :Pediatric Ophthalmology; Current Aspects. Wybar K, Taylor D (eds), Marcel Dekker Inc., New York, 1983 (in press)

20. Gresty M, Halmagy GM, Taylor D: In: Pediatric Ophthalmology; Current Aspects. Wybar K, Taylor D (eds), Marcel Dekker Inc., New York, 1983 (in press)

21. Harrison M, Parker N: Congenital facial diplegia. Med J Aust 1:650-653, 1960

22. Hecaen H, Ajuriaguerra J De, Rougues L, David M, Dell MB: Psychical paralysis of vision (balint) during the development of a Leuco-encephalitis of Balo type. Rev Neurol 83:81-104, 1950

23. Henderson JL: The congenital facial diplegia syndrome: clinical features, pathology and etiology. Brain 62:381-403, 1939

24. Heubner O: Ueber Angeborenen kernmangel. Char Ann 25:211-243, 1900

25. Holmes G: Spasm of fixation. Trans Ophthalmol Soc U K 50:253-262, 1930

26. Jones GM: Interactions between optokinetic and vestibulo-ocular responses during head rotation in various

planes. Aerospace Med 37:172-177, 1966

27. Kushner BJ, Essner D, Cohen IJ, Flynn JT: Retrolental fibroplasia: II pathologic correlation. Arch Ophthalmol 95:29-38, 1977

28. Moebius PJ: Ueber angeborene doppelseitige abducens-facialis lahmung. Munch Med Wochenschr 35:91-94, 1888

29. Moebius PJ: Ueber infantilen kernschwund. Munch Med Wochenschr 39:17-21, 1892

30. Nathan PW: Facial apraxia an apraxic dysarthria. Brain 70:449-478, 1947

31. Nelson L, Huppert L: Moebius syndrome associated with benign intracranial hypertension. Ann Ophthalmol 12:296-300, 1980

32. Porta della GB: De humana physiognomonia, Hanover, 1586, p. 189

33. Rainy H, Fowler JS: Congenital facial diplegia due to nuclear lesion. Rev Neurol 1:149-155, 1903

34. Ramsay JH, Walker JW: In: Pediatric Ophthalmology, Current Aspects. Wybar K, Taylor D (eds), Marcel Dekker, Inc., New York, 1983 (in press)

35. Robinson DA: On the nature of visual oculomotor connections. Invest Ophthalmol 11:497-502, 1972

36. Rodin EA: Impaired ocular pursuit movements. Diagnostic value. Arch Neurol 10:327-330, 1964

37. Roth WC: Demonstration von kranken mit ophthalmoplegie. Neurologisches Centralblatt 20:921-924, 1901

38. Sanders MD, Wybar KC: Vertical supranuclear ophthalmoplegia with compensatory head movements. Report of a case with lipidosis in: Strabismus ´69, St. Louis, Mosby, 1970, pp. 63-69

39. Silverman WA: The lesion of retrolental fibroplasia. Sci Am 236:00-107, 1977

40. Spatz H, Ullrich O: Klinischer und anatomischer beitrag

zu den angeborenen beweglichkeitsdefekten im hirn-nervenbereich. Ztschr F Kinderheilkd 51:579-597, 1931

41. Taylor D; Disorders of head and eye movements in children. Trans Ophthalmol Soc U K 100:489-494

42. Taylor D: In: Pediatric Ophthalmology; current aspects. Wybar K, Taylor D (eds), Marcel Dekker Inc., New York, 1983 (in press)

43. Terry TL: Extreme prematurity and fibroblastic overgrowth of persistent vascular sheath behind each crystalline lens. Am J Ophthalmol 25:203-204, 1942

44. Terry TL: Fibroblastic overgrowth of persistent tunica vaculosa lentis in infants born prematurely. III. Studies in development and regression of hyaloid artery and tunica vasculosa lentis. Am J Ophthalmol 25:1409-1423, 1942

45. Terry TL: Fibroblastic overgrowth of persistent tunica vasculosa lentis in premature infants. II. Report of cases--clinical aspects. Arch Ophthalmol 29:36-53, 1943

46. Terry TL: Fibroblastic overgrowth of persistent tunica vasculosa lentis in premature infants. IV. Etiologic factors. Arch Ophthalmol 29:54-68, 1943

47. Terry TL: Retrolental fibroplasia in premature infants. V. Further studies on fibroplastic overgrowth of persistent tunica vasculosa lentis. Arch Ophthalmol 33:203-208, 1945

48. Tessier P: Osteotomies totales de la face syndrome de crouzon syndrome d'apert oxcephalies. Scaphocephalies. Turricephalies. Annales Chirurgie Plastique 12:273-286, 1967

49. Virchow R: Ueber den cretinismus, namentlich in franken, und uber pathologische schadelformen. Vhdl Phys-Med Ges Wurzburg 2:241-256, 1851

50. Wollensak J, Fleischer-Peters A, Hovels O: Congenital oculo-facial palsies. Klin Monatsbl Augenheilkd 140:383-396, 1962

KENNETH WYBAR, M.D., ChM, FRCS

Surgeon, Moorfields Eye Hospital

Director of the Orthoptic Department, Moorfields Eye Hospital, High Holborn

Ophthalmic Surgeon, The Hospital for Sick Children, Great Ormond Street

Ophthalmic Surgeon, The Royal Marsden Hospital (formerly the Royal Cancer Hospital)

Civilian Consultant in Ophthalamology to the Royal Navy

Member of the Court of Examiners of the Royal College of Surgeons

Fellow of the Royal Society of Medicine (past President of the Section of Ophthalmology)

Member of the Ophthalmological Society of the United Kingdom (past Vice President)

Fellow of the Faculty of Ophthalmologists (past Vice President)

Books

1. System of Ophthalmology (edited by Sir Stewart Duke-Elder) Volume II: The Anatomy of the Visual System. Kimpton, London. 1961. (Jointly with Duke-Elder, Stewart)

2. Lyle and Jackson's Practical Orthoptics in the Treatment of Squint. Fifth Edition: H.K. Lewis, London. 1967. (Jointly with Lyle, T.K.)

3. Ophthalmology--Concise Medical Textbooks. Bailliere, Tindall and Cassell, London. 1966.

Ophthalmology--Concise Medical Textbooks. (2nd Edition). Bailliere, Tindall, London. 1974.

Ophthalmology--Concise Medical Textbooks. (3rd Edition). Bailliere, Tindall, London. (in press) (Jointly with Kerr-Muir, M.)

4. System of Ophthalmology (edited by Sir Stewart Duke-Elder) Volume VI: Ocular Motility and Strabismus. Kimpton, London. 1973. (Jointly with Duke-Elder, Stewart)

5. Pediatric Ophthalmology--Current Aspects. (Wybar, K. and Taylor, D., editors). Marcel Dekker, Inc., New York. (in press)

<u>Contributions to Books</u>

1. The Nature of Endocrine Exophthalmos. In Advances in Ophthalmology, Vol. VII, 119. S. Karger, Basel, New York, 1957.

The Eye Lesion in Hyperthyroidism.

2. Current Medicine and Drugs, I, 1. Butterworths, London. 1961. (Brit. Med. Encycl. Med. Pract., 12, 73, 1961)

3. Neoplasms of the Cornea. International Ophthalmology Clinics (edited by P.D. Trevor-Roper). Vol II, p. 657. Little Brown and Co., Boston, 1962.

4. The Eye in Relation to Endocrine Disturbance, In Clinical Surgery; The Eye. p. 89, Butterworth, London, 1964.

5. The Eyes in the Early Years of Life. In National Society of Children's Nurseries, London, 1963.

6. Cancer of the Eye. In Prevention of Cancer. Edited by R. W. Raven and F.J.C. Roe, Butterworth, London, 1967.

7. Squint in Relation to Malignant Disease. In International Ophthalmology Clinics. Edited by A. Schlossman, Little, Brown and Co., Boston, Vol. 6, No. 3, 1966.

8. Symposium on the Problems of Strabismus. The Aetioloy of Motor Disturbance of Squint. Strabismus Symp. Giessen. Edited by A. Arruga. Karger, Basel, New York, 130, 1968.

9. Nystagmus in Childhood. Trans. First Internat. Con. Orthopt., 249, 1968. Henry Kimpton, London.

10. Some Developmental Eye Disorders Present at Birth and in the Neonatal Period. In Aspects of Developmental and Pediatric Ophthalmology. Edited by P.A. Gardiner, R.C. MacKeith and V.H. Smith. Clinics in Developmental Medicine No. 32. Spastics International Medical Publications and

Heinemann Medical, p. 75, London, 1969. (Jointly with Harcourt, R.B.)

11. Ocular Myopathy in Childhood. In Strabismus ´69--Transactions of the Consilium Europaeum Strabismi Studio Deditum Congress, London, 1969. p. 78, Henry Kimpton, London, 1970.

12. Vertical Supranuclear Ophthalmoplegia with Compensatory Head Movements. Report of a case with a lipidosis. In Strabismus ´69--Transactins of the Consilium Europaeum Strabismi Studio Deditum Congress, London, 1969. p. 63. Henry Kimpton, London, 1970. (Jointly with Sanders, M.D.)

13. The Use of Prisms in Pre-Operative and Post-Operative Treatment. The First Congress of the International Strabismological Association, Acapulco, 1970. p. 243. Henry Kimpton, London, 1971.

14. Dissociated Ocular Deviation. In International Ophthalmology Clinics (edited by O.M. Ferrer) Vol. II, p. 182, Little, Brown and Co., Boston, 1971.

15. Nystagmus in Early Childhood. In International Ophthalmology Clinics (edited by O.M. Ferrer) Vol. II, p. 177, Little, Brown and Co., Boston, 1971.

16. Disorders of Ocular Motility in Craniopharyngiomata. Proc. Sec. Internat. Cong. Orthopt. Amsterdam, 1971. Excerpta Medica, p. 272, Amsterdam, 1971.

17. Acquired Optic Atrophy in Early Childhood. In the Optic Nerve, Proceedings of Second William MacKenzie Memorial Symposium, Glasgow, 1971 (edited by J.S. Cant), p. 12, henry Kimpton, London, 1972.

18. The Management of Nystagmus. In Aspects of Neuro-Ophthalmology (edited by S.I. Davidson), p.31, Butterworth, London, 1974.

19. Other Tumors of the Eye and Orbit. In Cancer in Children, Clinical Management (edited by H.J.G. Bloom, J. Lemerle, M.K. Neidhardt and P.A. Voute), p. 128, Springer-Verlag, Berlin, Heidelberg, New York, 1975. (Jointly with Dalley, V.)

20. Disorders of Ocular Motility in Hydrocephalus in Early Childhood. Trans. 2nd Cong. Internat. Strabismological Assoc.

p. 366. Diffusion Generale de Librairie, Marseille, 1974.

21. The Surgery of Ptosis. In Operative Surgery, Fundamental International Techniques, Third Edition. General Editors: C. Rob and R. Smith. Eyes (Edited by S.J.H. Miller), p. 92, Butterworths, London, Boston, 1976.

22. Ocular Motility Problems in Craniofacial Dysostosis. Trans. 3rd Internat. Cong. Orthopt., p. 299. Stratton Intercontinental Medical Book Corporation, New York, 1976. (Jointly with Walker, J.W.)

23. Disorders of Ocular Motility in Children. In: Medical Ophthalmology. Ed. F. Clifford Rose, p. 119, Chapman and Hall, London, 1976.

24 (a) Sensory Aspects of Normal Binocular Vision in Scientific Foundations of Ophthalmology. Edited by Edward S. Perkins and David W. Hill, p. 223. William Heinemann Medical Books. Ltd., 1977. (Jointly with Taylor, D)

(b) Sensory Aspects of Deranged Binocular Vision in Scientific Foundations of Ophthalmology. Edited by Edward S. Perkins and David W. Hill, p. 231. William Heinemann Medical Books, Ltd., 1977. (Jointly with Taylor, D.)

25. La Conduite Partique dans le Traitement du Nystagmus. In: Les Chiers de L'Orthoptie. A.F.I.M. Toulouse, p. 15.

26. Surgical Procedures in A and V Pattern Strabismus. Trans. 4th Internat. Cong. Orthopt., 34, 1981. Henry Kimpton, London. (Jointly with Calcutt, C., Mathalone, B., and Walker, J.W.)

27. Anomalies of Ocular Motility in Pediatric Disorders. Bielschowsky Lecture. Trans. 4th Congress Internat. Strabismological Assoc., San Francisco, 1982.

28. Amblyopia and Disorders of Ocular Motility in Craniosynostosis. Collin, R., Walker, J., and Wybar, K. (Paper read by Walker, J., in Sydney, October 1980)

29. (a) Delayed Visual Development. In: Pediatric Ophthalmology; Current Aspects. Edited by Kenneth Wybar and David Taylor. Marcel Dekker, Inc., New York. (in press) (Jointly with Karseras, A.)

(b) The A and V Phonomena. In: Pediatric Ophthalmology;

Current Aspects. Edited by Kenneth Wybar and David Taylor. Marcel Dekker, Inc., New York. (in press)

(c) Malignant Disease. In: Pediatric Ophthalmology; Current Aspects. Edited by Kenneth Wybar and David Taylor. Marcel Dekker, Inc., New York. (in press)

30. Strabismus in Cerebral Palsy. Strabismus Symposium, Amsterdan. September 1981, p. 87. Dr. W. Junk Publishers: The Hague, Boston, London. 1982.

CONTRIBUTORS

Emiko Adachi-Usami, M.D.
Department of Ophthalmology
Chiba University School of Medicine
Chiba, Japan

Miguel Alvares, M.D.
Moorfields Eye Hospital
London, England

Leonard Apt, M.D.
Department of Ophthalmology
Jules Stein Eye Institute
University of California at Los Angeles School of Medicine
Los Angeles, California

Penny A. Asbell, M.D.
Lions Eye Research Laboratories
Louisiana State University Eye Center
Louisiana State University School of Medicine
New Orleans, Louisiana

Cynthia W. Avilla, C.O.
Ophthalmology Service
Cullen Eye Institute
Baylor College of Medicine
Houston, Texas

Shinobu Awaya, M.D.
Department of Ophthalmology
Nagoya University School of Medicine
Nagoya, Japan

Bruno Bagolini, M.D.
Clinica Oculistica
Policlinico
Modena, Italy

Evan Ballard, M.D.
Jules Stein Eye Institute
University of California at Los Angeles School of Medicine
Los Angeles, California

J. Bronwyn Bateman, M.D.
Department of Ophthalmology
Jules Stein Eye Institute
University of California at Los Angeles School of Medicine
Los Angeles, California

Robert H. Bedrossian, M.D.
Bedrossian Eye Clinic, P.S.
Vancouver, Washington

Pierre Vital Berard, M.D.
University Clinic of Ophthalmology
Motility Department
Hospital Nord
Marseilles, France

Maria de Huerto Bernasconi, M.D.
Montevideo, Uruguay

Wayne W. Bixenman, M.D.
Strabismus and Pediatric Ophthalmology
El Dorado Medical Plaza
Tucson, Arizona

William P. Boger, III, M.D.
Department of Ophthalmology
Harvard Medical School
Boston, Massachusetts

Julio Cesar Bottos, M.D.
Department of Ophthalmology
Faculdade de Ciencias Medicas da Santa Casa de Misericordia
São Paulo, Brazil

J. Raymond Buncic, M.D.
Hospital for Sick Children
Toronto, Ontario, Canada

Fernando Cabrera, M.D.
Department of Ophthalmology
San Juan de Dios Hospital
University of Chile Medical School
Santiago, Chile

Carolyn Calcutt, M.D.
Royal Eye Unit
Kingston Hospital
Surrey, England

Jorge Alberto F. Caldeira, M.D.
Ophthalmological Clinic
Faculty of Medicine
São Paulo University School of Medicine
São Paulo, Brazil

Joseph Calhoun, M.D.
Pediatric Ophthalmology Department
Wills Eye Hospital
Philadelphia, Pennsylvania

A. Cammorota, M.D.
Instituto de Oftalmologia Pediatrica
Buenos-Aires, Argentina

Emilio C. Campos, M.D.
Department of Ophthalmology
University of Modena
Modena, Italy

Ulysses M. Carbajal, M.D.
Andrews University Medical Clinic
Berrien Springs, Michigan

C. Chiesi, M.D.
Department of Ophthalmology
University of Modena
Modena, Italy

Andrew Choy, M.D.
Jules Stein Eye Institute
University of California at Los Angeles Center for the Health Sciences
Los Angeles, California

Fred C. Chu, M.D.
Neuroophthalmology Department
National Eye Institute
Bethesda, Maryland

Alberto O. Ciancia, M.D.
Instituto de Oftalmologia Pediatrica
Buenos-Aires, Argentina

Gerhard W. Cibis, M.D.
Children's Mercy Hospital
Kansas City, Missouri

Kenneth J. Ciuffreda, M.D.
Neurological Unit
University of California
Berkeley, California

M. Claramunt
Department of Ophthalmology
San Juan de Dios Hospital
Unviersity of Chile Medical School
Santiago, Chile

David G. Cogan, M.D.
Neuroophthalmology Department
National Eye Institute
Bethesda, Maryland

Gerald Cohen, Ph.D.
Department of Ophthalmology
University of Rochester
Rochester, New York

J. R. O. Collin, F.R.C.S.
Moorfields Eye Hospital
London, England

Raymond J. Connolly, M.D.
Tufts-New England Medical Center
Boston, Massachusetts

H. G. Conrad, M.D.
Orthoptic Department
University Eye Hospital
Kiel, West Germany

Robert A. Crone,
Oogheelkundige Kliniek
Amsterdam, The Netherlands

Earl R. Crouch, Jr., M.D.
Department of Ophthalmology
Eastern Virginia Medical School
Norfolk, Virginia

Luiz A. Peduti Cunha, M.D.
São Paulo University School of Medicine
São Paulo, Brazil

Henderson de Almeida, M.D.
Department of Ophthalmology
School of Medicine UFMG
Belo Horizonte, MG, Brazil

Emma Limon deBrown, M.D.
Department of Ophthalmology
Hospital Manuel Gea Gonzalez
Mexico City, Mexico

W. de Decker, M.D.
Orthoptic Department
University Eye Hospital
Kiel, West Germany

Monte Del Monte, M.D.
Department of Ophthalmology
Children's Hospital National Medical Center
Washington, D.C.

Teresa Diaz, M.D.
Department of Ophthalmology
San Juan de Dios Hospital
University of Chile Medical School
Santiago, Chile

James B. Dickson, M.D.
Department of Ophthalmology
United States Regional Hospital
Sheppard Air Force Base
Wichita Falls, Texas

S. Dobsky, M.D.
Montevideo, Uruguay

Donald B. Dunlop, M.D.
Newcastle, Australia

Kuniaki Egi, M.D.
Department of Ophthalmology
Okayama University Medical School
Okayama-shi, Japan

Allan M. Eisenbaum, M.D.
Department of Pediatric Ophthalmology
Aurora Presbyterian Hospital
Aurora, Colorado

David K. Emmel, M.D.
Department of Pathology
Jules Stein Eye Institute
University of California at Los Angeles School of Medicine
Los Angeles, California

Peter Fells, M.D.
Moorfields Eye Hospital
London, England

Edison J. Geraisate Filho, M.D.
Centro Oftalmologico Pacaembu
São Paulo, Brazil

John T. Flynn, M.D.
Department of Ophthalmology
Bascom Palmer Eye Institute
University of Miami School of Medicine
Miami, Florida

Robert Y. Foos, M.D.
Department of Pathology
Jules Stein Eye Institute
University of California at Los Angeles School of Medicine
Los Angeles, California

John Forestner, M.D.
Department of Ophthalmology
Emory University School of Medicine
Atlanta, Georgia

Monica Fornander, M.D.
Department of Ophthalmology
Danderyds Sjukhus
Danderyd Sweden

R. Scott Foster, M.D.
Jules Stein Eye Institute
University of California at Los Angeles Center for the Health Sciences
Los Angeles, California

Douglas Freely, M.D.
Department of Ophthalmology
Fitzsimmons Army Medical Center
Aurora, Colorado

Thomas Frey, M.D.
Department of Ophthalmology
George Washington University
Washington, D.C.

Sakuko Fukai, M.D.
Department of Ophthalmology
Division of Neuroophthalmology
Kawasaki Medical School
Okayama, Japan

Masafumi Fukushima, M.D.
Department of Ophthalmology
Kawasaki Medical School
Kurashiki, Japan

J. Allen Gammon, M.D.
Department of Ophthalmology
Emory University School of Medicine
Atlanta, Georgia

H. Garcia, M.D.
Instituto de Oftalmologia Pediatrica
Buenos-Aires, Argentina

William E. Gillies, M.D.
Orthoptic Department
Royal Victorian Eye and Ear Hospital
Melbourne, Australia

Gary Gitschlag, M.D.
Pediatric Ophthalmology and Strabismus
Knoxville, Tennessee

M. H. Gobin, M.D.
Orthoptic Department
University Eye Clinic of Leiden, and
Clinic of Ophthalmology
University Academy
Leiden, Netherlands

D. Godde-Jolly, M.D.
CNO Des Quinze-Vingts
Paris, France

H. Goossens, M.D.
Orthoptic Department
University Eye Clinic, Hamburg
Hamburg, Germany

John L. Grady, M.D.
United States Naval Regional Medical Center
Charleston, South Carolina

Peter P. Gruenberg, M.D.
Jules Stein Eye Institute
University of California at Los Angeles
Center for the Health Sciences
Los Angeles, California

S. Gur, M.D.
Occupational Health and
Rehabilitation Institute at
Loewenstein Hospital
Raanana, Israel

David L. Guyton, M.D.
The Wilmer Ophthalmological Institute
Johns Hopkins Hospital
Johns Hopkins University School of
Medicine
Baltimore, Maryland

W. Haase, M.D.
Orthoptic Department
University Eye Clinic, Hamburg
Hamburg, West Germany

Oscar Ham, M.D.
Department of Ophthalmology
San Juan de Dios Hospital
University of Chile Medical School
Santiago, Chile

David Hamedo, M.D.
Department of Ophthalmology
San Juan de Dios Hospital
University of Chile Medical School
Santiago, Chile

Mary K. Hammock, M.D.
Department of Neurosurgery
Children's Hospital National Medical
Center
Washington, D.C.

Brian Harcourt, M.D.
Ophthalmic Department
General Infirmary
Leeds, England

Hiram H. Hardesty, M.D.
University Suburbian Health Center
Cleveland, Ohio

Roger L. Hiatt, M.D.
Department of Ophthalmology
University of Tennessee Center for
Health Sciences
Memphis, Tennessee

David A. Hiles, M.D.
University of Pittsburgh
Pittsburgh, Pennsylvania

Midoriko Hitomi, M.D.
Department of Ophthalmology
Okayama University Medical School
Okayama-shi, Japan

Barry Holland, M.D.
Royal Eye Unit
Kingston Hospital
Surrey, England

Fukue Horibe, M.D.
Department of Ophthalmology
Nagoya University School of Medicine
Nagoya, Japan

Creig S. Hoyt, M.D.
Department of Ophthalmology
University of California Medical
School
San Francisco, California

Alfred Huber, M.D.
University Eye Clinic
Zurich, Switzerland

Rie Ichikawa, M.D.
Department of Ophthalmology
Okayama University Medical School
Okayama-shi, Japan

Akahiro Inatomi, M.D.
Depoartment of Ophthalmology
Shiga University of Medical Science
School of Medicine
Shiga-ken, Japan

Malcolm R. Ing, M.D.
Department of Ophthalmology
John A. Burns School of Medicine
University of Hawaii at Manoa
Honolulu, Hawaii

Satoshi Ishikawa, M.D.
Department of Ophthalmology
Kitasato University, Sagamihara
Kanagawa, Japan

Shyun Jeng, M.D.
Department of Ophthalmology
National Taiwan University Hospital
Taipei, Taiwan, Republic of China

D. Jordan, M.D.
Clinique Ophthalmologique
Hopital Nord
Marseilles, France

Louise C. Kaldis, M.D.
Department of Ophthalmology
Houston Eye Associates
Houston, Texas

Kazutaka Kani, M.D.
Department of Ophthalmology
Hyogo College of Medicine
Hyogo-ken, Japan

Osamu Katsumi, M.D.
Department of Ophthalmology
Keio University
Tokyo, Japan

Norman Katz, M.D.
Ophthalmology Service
Walter Reed Army Medical Center
Washington, D.C.

Herbert E. Kaufman, M.D.
Louisiana State University Eye Center
Louisiana State University School of
Medicine
New Orleans, Louisiana

C. G. Keith, F.R.A.C.O., F.R.A.C.S.
Royal Children's Hospital
Melbourne, Australia

Robert V. Kenyon, M.D.
Neurological Unit
University of California
Berkeley, California

Ellen M. Keough, M.D.
Tufts-New England Medical Center
Boston, Massachusetts

R. Kies, M.D.
Children's Mercy Hospital
Kansas City, Missouri

Hisashi Kimura, M.D.
Department of Ophthalmology
Kawasaki Medical School
Kurashiki, Japan

W. H. Kitchen, M.D., F.R.A.C.P.
The Royal Women's Hospital
Melbourne, Australia

G. Kluge, M.D.
Department of Orthoptics and
Pleoptics
University Eye Clinic
Keil, West Germany

Guntram Kommerell, M.D.
Abteilung Schielbehandlung
Universitats-Augenklinik
Freiburg, FRG, Denmark

Krystyna M. Krzystkowa, M.D.
Ophthalmological Clinic
Department of Pathophysiology of
Vision and Neuroophthalmology
Copernicus Academy of Medicine
Cracow, Poland

Anna Kubato-Zielinska, M.D.
Department of Pathophysiology of Vision and Neuroophthalmology
Copernicus Academy of Medicine
Cracow, Poland

Masanori Kubo, M.D.
Department of Ophthalmology
Tokushima University
Tokushima, Japan

Nobue Kubota, M.D.
Department of Ophthalmology
Teikyo University School of Medicine
Tokyo, Japan

Burton J. Kushner, M.D.
University Hospitals Center for Health Sciences
Madison, Wisconsin

Joseph Lang, M.D.
Department of Orthoptics
University Eye Clinic
Zurich, Switzerland

David Lasley, M.D.
Department of Ophthalmology
Bascom Palmer Eye Institute
University of Miami School of Medicine
Miami, Florida

Ted Lawwill, M.D.
University of Kansas Medical Center at Kansas City
Kansas City, Kansas

John P. Lee, F.R.C.S.
Moorfields Eye Hospital
London, England

Gunnar Lennerstrand, M.D.
Department of Ophthalmology
University Hospital
Linkoping, Sweden

Luke Long-Kuang Lin, M.D.
Department of Ophthalmology
National Taiwan University Hospital
Taipei, Taiwan, Republic of China

Donna N. Loupe, C.O.T., C.O.
Lions Eye Research Laboratories
Louisiana State University Eye Center
Louisiana State University School of Medicine
New Orleans, Louisiana

T. Keith Lyle, M.D.
London, England

V. Macellari, M.D.
Laboratories of Biomedical Technologies
Instituto Superiore di Sanita
Roma, Italy

Sergio Martinez-Oropeza, M.D.
Department of Ophthalmology
Hospital Manuel Gea Gonzalez
Mexico City, Mexico

Bruce Mathalone, M.D.
Royal Eye Unit
Kingston Hospital
Surrey, England

S. Mattheus, M.D.
Abteilung Schielbehandlung
Universitats-Augenklinik
Freiburg, FRG, Denmark

Toshio Mauro, M.D.
Teikyo University School of Medicine
Tokyo, Japan

Edward Mawas, M.D.
Fondation Ophthalmologique A. de Rothschild
Paris, France

Lucie J. Mawas, M.D.
Fondation Ophthalmologique A. de Rothschild
Paris, France

James G. May, Ph.D.
Lions Eye Research Laboratories
Louisiana State University Eye Center
Louisiana State University School of Medicine
New Orleans, Louisiana

Malcolm L. Mazow, M.D.
Department of Ophthalmology
Hermann Eye Center
Houston, Texas

Anne McIndoe, M.D.
Lincoln Institute
Melbourne, Australia

Keith W. McNeer, M.D.
Department of Ophthalmology
Medical College of Virginia
Richmond, Virginia

Henry S. Metz, M.D.
Department of Ophthalmology
University of Rochester School of Medicine
Rochester, New York

Ewy Meyer, M.D.
Department of Ophthalmology
Rambam Medical Center
Haifa, Israel

Yukihiko Mitsui, M.D.
Tokushima University School of Medicine
Tokushima, Japan

David Mittelman, M.D.
Department of Ophthalmology
Strich School of Medicine
Loyola University
Maywood, Illinois

Motoya Miura, M.D.
Department of Ophthalmology
Nagoya University School of Medicine
Nagoya, Japan

Fernando Ortiz Monasterio, M.D.
Department of Plastic Surgery
Hospital Manuel Gea Gonzalez
Mexico City, Mexico

Thomas F. Moore, M.D.
Department of Pediatric Ophthalmology and Ocular Motility
St. Joseph's Hospital
Phoenix, Arizona

Keith S. Morgan, M.D.
Lions Eye Research Laboratories
Louisiana State University Eye Center
Louisiana State University School of Medicine
New Orleans, Louisiana

Reiko Mori, M.D.
Department of Ophthalmology
Okayama University Medical School
Okayama-shi, Japan

Richard S. Muchnick, M.D.
Manhattan Eye, Ear, and Throat Hospital
New York, New York

Kazuo Mukuno, M.D.
Department of Ophthalmology
Kitasato University, Sagamihara
Kanagawa, Japan

Maria A. Musarella, M.D.
Hospital for Sick Children
Toronto, Ontario, Canada

Takashi Nakagawa, M.D.
Department of Ophthalmology
Sapporo Medical College
Sapporo, Japan

Leonard B. Nelson, M.D.
Department of Pediatric Ophthalmology
Wills Eye Hospital
Philadelphia, Pennsylvania

Pinhas Nemet, M.D.
Department of Ophthalmology
Ichilov Hospital
Tel-Aviv, Israel

Karl G. Nyman, M.D.
Department of Ophthalmology
Danderyds Sjukhus
Danderyd, Sweden

Per Odenrick, M.D.
Department of Clinical Neurophysiology and Biomedical Engineering
University Hospital
University of Linkoping
Linkoping, Sweden

Emiko Ohmi, M.D.
Ohmi Eye Clinic
Osaka, Japan

Hiroshi Ohtsuki, M.D.
Department of Ophthalmology
Okayama University Medical School
Okayama-shi, Japan

Takashi Ohzeki, M.D.
Department of Ophthalmology
Yokohama City University School of Medicine
Yokohama, Japan

John F. O'Neill, M.D.
Department of Ophthalmology
Children's Hospital National Medical Center
Washington, D.C.

A. Pacheco, M.D.
Montevideo, Uruguay

Y. Palma, M.D.
Montevideo, Uruguay

Earl A. Palmer, M.D.
The Oregon Health Sciences University
Portland, Oregon

Marshall M. Parks, M.D.
Department of Ophthalmology
Children's Hospital National Medical Center
Washington, D.C.

I. Perlman, M.D.
Department of Physiology and Biophysics
Faculty of Medicine
Haifa, Israel

Thomas C. Prager, Ph.D.
Department of Ophthalmology
Neumann Eye Institute
DeLand, Florida

John A. Pratt-Johnson, M.D., F.R.C.S.(C.)
Department of Ophthalmology
University of British Columbia, and
Vancouver General Hospital
Vancouver, British Columbia, Canada

Cindy Pritchard, M.D.
Department of Ophthalmology
Bascom Palmer Eye Institute
University of Miami School of Medicine
Miami, Florida

Miguel Puentes, M.D.
Department of Ophthalmology
San Juan de Dios Hospital
University of Chile Medical School
Santiago, Chile

Edward L. Raab, M.D.
Department of Ophthalmology
Mount Sinai Hospital
New York, New York

B. Rapp, M.D.
Clinique D'Ophthalmologie
Hopital Cantonal Universitaire de Geneve
Geneve, Switzerland

Stefan Rethy, M.D.
Augenarzt
Dinslaken, Germany

S. Rethy-Gal, M.D.
Augenarzt
Dinslaken, Germany

Roger Reydy, M.D.
Clinique Ophthalmologique
Faculté de Medcine
Marseilles, France

James D. Reynolds, M.D.
University of Pittsburgh
Pittsburgh, Pennsylvania

E. Rivas, M.D.
Montevideo, Uruguay

Richard M. Robb, M.D.
Department of Ophthalmology
The Children's Hospital Medical Center
Boston, Massachusetts

Peter Roggenkamper, M.D.
Augenklinik Tech. Universitat
Munchen, Germany

Philip Roholt, M.D.
Department of Ophthalmology
University of Florida College of Medicine
Gainesville, Florida

Paul E. Romano, M.D.
Department of Ophthalmology
University of Florida College of Medicine
Gainesville, Florida

David Romero-Apis, M.D.
Department of Ophthalmology
Hospital Manuel Gea Gonzalez
Mexico City, Mexico

S. Ron, M.D.
Occupational Health and Rehabilitation Institute at Loewenstein Hospital
Raanana, Israel

Teresa Rosales, M.D.
Jules Stein Eye Institute
University of California at Los Angeles Center for the Health Sciences
Los Angeles, California

Arthur L. Rosenbaum, M.D.
Jules Stein Eye Institute
University of California at Los Angeles Center for the Health Sciences
Los Angeles, California

Andre Roth, M.D.
Clinique D'Ophthalmologie
Hopital Cantonal Universitaire de Geneve
Geneve, Switzerland

Mark Ruttum, M.D.
Cullen Eye Institute
Baylor College of Medicine
Houston, Texas

Agneta Rydberg, M.D.
Department of Ophthalmology
Danderyds Sjukhus
Danderyd, Sweden

A. B. Safran, M.D.
Clinique D'Ophthalmologie
Hopital Cantonal Universitaire de Geneve
Geneve, Switzerland

Per Sandstedt, M.D.
Department of Pediatrics
University Hospital
Linkoping, Sweden

Robert A. Sargent, M.D.
Department of Ophthalmology
The Children's Hospital
Denver, Colorado

A. Daniele Sargentini, M.D.
Laboratories of Biomedical
Technologies
Instituto Superiore di Sanita
Roma, Italy

Jeanne-Marie Sarniguet-Badoche, M.D.
Attachee de Strabologie
a l'Hopital Lariboisiere
Paris, France

Richard A. Saunders, M.D.
Storm Eye Institute
Medical University of South Carolina
Charleston, South Carolina

Peter J. Savino, M.D.
Department of Neuroophthalmology
Wills Eye Hospital
Philadelphia, Pennsylvania

Abraham Schlossman, M.D.
Manhattan Eye, Ear, and Throat
Hospital
New York, New York

Elisabeth Schulz, M.D.
University Eye Clinic
Hamburg, Germany

Alan B. Scott, M.D.
Smith-Kettlewell Institute of Visual
Sciences
San Francisco, California

William E. Scott, M.D.
Department of Ophthalmology
University Hospitals
Iowa City, Iowa

David Sevel, M.D.
Veterans Administration Medical
Center
San Diego, California

Maria Luz Silva, M.D.
Department of Ophthalmology
San Juan de Dios Hospital
University of Chile Medical School
Santiago, Chile

Gur Singh, M.D., Ph.D.
Department of Ophthalmology
Danderyds Sjukhus
Danderyd, Sweden

Teresita Sison-Diego, M.D.
Andrews University Medical Clinic
Berrien Springs, Michigan

Carlos Souza-Dias, M.D.
Department of Ophthalmology
Faculdade de Ciencias Medicas
Santa Casa de Misericordia
São Paulo, Brazil

Filao Spencer, M.D.
Ophthalmic Department
General Infirmary
Leeds, England

Annette Spielmann, M.D.
Department of Ophthalmology
Nancy, France

Lawrence Stark, M.D.
University of California
Berkeley, California

Kathleen S. Stern, M.D.
Department of Ocular Motility
Manhattan Eye, Ear, and Throat
Hospital
New York, New York

Ian M. Strachan, F.R.C.S.Ed.
Royal Hallamshire Hospital
Sheffield, England

Miyuki Sugawara, M.D.
Department of Ophthalmology
Nagoya University School of Medicine
Nagoya, Japan

Fusako Takahashi, M.D.
Department of Ophthalmology
Shiga University of Medical Science
School of Medicine
Shigen-Ken, Japan

Osamu Tamura, M.D.
Ophthalmology Department
Tokushima University
Tokushima, Japan

Geraldine Tillson, D.B.O.
Department of Ophthalmology
University of British Columbia
Vancouver General Hospital
Vancouver, British Columbia, Canada

Christine Timms, D.B.O.
Moorfields Eye Hospital
London, England

H. Treumer, M.D.
Department of Orthoptics and
Pleoptics
University Eye Clinic
Kiel, West Germany

Jun Tsutsui, M.D.
Department of Ophthalmology
Division of Neuroophthalmology
Kawasaki Medical School
Kurashiki, Japan

Yasuo Uemura, M.D.
Department of Ophthalmology
Keio University School of Medicine
Tokyo, Japan

Justin L. Van Selm, M.D.
Department of Ophthalmology
University of Cape Town
Groote Shcuur Hospital
Cape Town, South Africa

G. Varghese, M.D.
University of Kansas Medical Center
at Kansas City
Kansas City, Kansas

Guillermo Velez, M.D.
Department of Ophthalmology
Antioquia University Hospital
San Vincente de Paul
Medellin, Colombia

Suzanne Veronneau-Troutman, M.D.
Cornell University Medical College
New York, New York

Gunter K. von Noorden, M.D.
Department of Ophthalmology
Texas Children's Hospital
Houston, Texas

Elizabeth Waddell, M.D.
Moorfields Eye Hospital
London, England

Yoshimasa Watanabe, M.D.
Department of Ophthalmology
Sato Eye Clinic
Okayama University Medical School
Okayama-ken, Japan

Jean-Berard Weiss, M.D.
Laboratoirie de l'Ecole Pratique des
Hautes Etudes
Fondation Ophthalmologique de
Rothschild
Paris, France

David B. Werner, M.D.
State College, Pennsylvania

Noel Wheeler, Ph.D.
University of California at Los Angeles
School of Medicine
Los Angeles, California

Lloyd M. Wilcox, Jr., M.D.
New York Hospital
Cornell Medical Center
New York, New York

Stewart M. Wolff, M.D.
The Wilmer Institute
Baltimore, Maryland

Kenneth W. Wright, M.D.
Division of Ophthalmology
Children's Hospital of Los Angeles
Los Angeles, California

Kenneth Wybar, M.D.
Department of Orthoptics
Moorfields Eye Hospital
London, England

Thaddeus A. Zak, M.D.
Children's Hospital
Buffalo, New York

ETIOLOGY OF EARLY STRABISMUS

O. Ham, M. Puentes, F. Cabrera, D. Hamedo,
T. Diaz, M. L. Silva, and M. Claramunt

ABSTRACT

In 100 children, it was proved that perinatal conditions, be they normal or pathological, do not determine either the quality of binocular vision nor neurological motor alterations.

Perinatal pathology data was not more frequent in children with strabismus than in those having normal binocular vision.

Thus, the authors, conclude that perinatal pathology is not responsible for the etiology of early strabismus.

INTRODUCTION

The cause of strabismus, in the first months of life, remains unknown.(1) Nevertheless, we frequently have found perinatal problems, related to deficient oxygen administration, in the history of patients with infantile strabismus. Occasionally, we also see strabismus associated with early neurological damage. The neurological damage is usually attributed to maternal hypoxia, infection or bleeding during pregnancy or labor, or similar pathology occurring in the infant during labor or the neonatal period.(2)

Literature has confirmed the relationship between cerebral problems and perinatal difficulties. Thus Birch(3) reported subnormal mental conditions and Myers(4) have demonstrated cerebral damage and cerebral palsy related to hypoxia and other perinatal complications.

In 1947, Heinonen(5) opined that after inheritance, birth trauma was the second leading cause of strabismus. By promoting a deficient development of fusion, it was suspected that even small trauma could cause infantile strabismus. In relation to such data, other authors reported strabismus in 25% of the cases. Later, Unger and other authors(6) found early cerebral damage in 60% of strabismic patients, this

STRABISMUS II
ISBN 0-8089-1424-3

damage expressed itself as mental deficiency, psycopathic traits, somatic and general motor retardation, which were attributed to complicated deliveries. These findings were more frequent in patients with strabismus than in those of the control group.

In 1958, Doden(7) stated that strabismus was caused by a primary anomaly of optomotor coordination which could be determined genetically, or by acquired anomalies occurring during birth. An accessory factor was necessary such as hypermetropia, diminished fusion capacity of anatomical anomalies. Recent authors studied the relationship betwen perinatal conditions, early strabismus and neurologic damage.(8-12)

Quere(13), based on electro-oculographic findings, has also pointed out, that the majority of cases with infantile strabismus are due to a supranuclear innervational disorder.

Kalbe, Berndt and de Decker(14) point out that neurological damage is not the only responsible factor for the etiology of strabismus, unless the infants are prematures with a birth weight under 1000 gr or have damaged structures that control motor coordination. This may also occur if there is inherited weakness. They suggest this should be confirmed looking for minimal cerebral dysfunction or a "minimal cerebral palsy" in patients with strabismus.

Meanwhile, Klier has denied that mental physical retardation has a greater incidence in strabismic children.(15)

Spivey(16) and other authors(17) have reemphasized in the last years the role and importance of inheritance, even in congenital strabismus.

From our own clinical observations, we believe that etiology of early strabismus is predominantly perinatal complications, that selectively damage structures controling fusion capacity of the oculomotor coordination system (the same as we see in adults after a brain trauma).(18) If true, the infant would not be able to develop binocular vision, and thus, a fusion lock to assure a long lasting ocular alignment. Thus, strabismus could develop anytime after birth. Such damage could be expressed as a deficit of fusion capacity only, or soft signs of neurological damage.

In this paper, we aimed to answer the following two questions:

1. Do perinatal conditions influence and determine the quality of binocular vision?

2. Is perinatal pathology more frequent in infants with strabismus than those with normal binocular vision?

MATERIAL AND TECHNIQUES

To answer these questions, we have divided our investigation in two parts:

1. Comparative study of binocular vision (B.V.) in two groups of patients: one group formed by those born under normal perinatal conditions and another group formed by those born under pathological conditions.

2. Comparative study of perinatal conditions in children with infantile strabismus and children with normal binocular vision.

To study the first aspect we reviewed obstetrical data and ophthalmology conditions in 100 children 5 to 7 years old, chosen by chance and having been born at the maternity ward of San Juan de Dios Hospital. The ophthalmological assessment included nystagmus detection, cover test, fusional vergences with prisms, Titmus stereo test, Worth test for distance and Bagolini striated glasses for distance and near. The family history of strabismus was evaluated. Neurological assessment as any motor retardation or neurological anomaly was simultaneously done without the examiner knowing the perinatal data.

The second aspect was studied by a review of the obstetrical data of 36 cases of early onset strabismus, chosen consecutively and compared with the data of children with normal binocular vision.

We considered binocular vision normal if monocular vision was 5/8, Titmus stereo acuity up to circle number 8 and fusional convergence was at least of 15 prism diopters for distance and 20 prism diopters for near.(19)

We considered binocular vision abnormal if stereopsis was no better than circle number 6 on the Titmus test, even if the fusional vergences were normal or if amblyopia or strabismus was present. Ill defined cases (subnormal cases) that could neither be included in the previous groups, were excluded from the comparative study.

RESULTS

A. Relationships between binocular vision and perinatal conditions: 100 children were examined. Two groups were distinguished according to their perinatal conditions.

1. Children born under normal conditions with a normal Apgar score (8-10): 36 cases. We considered normal conditions the following situations: elective cesarean section, reductible umbilical cord circular, premature labor with child of adequate weight for his gestational age, spinal or general anesthesia (without respiratory depression).

2. Children with perinatal pathology data: 64 cases. We did not include late pathology during the perinatal period.

TABLE 1

Normal Perinatal Conditions and Quality of Binocular Vision

Binocular Vision	Cases
Normal	10
Subnormal	7
Abnormal	19
Total	36

TABLE 2

Neurological Examination Results In Children with Normal Perinatal Conditions

Neurological Conditions		Cases
Normal	(NE 1)	12
Fine motricity retardation	(NE 2)	1
Fine and gross motricity retardation	(NE 3)	2
Gross motricity and mental retardation	(NE 4)	1
Not examined		20
Total		36

TABLE 3

Neurological Condition and Quality of Binocular Vision in Children with Normal Perinatal Conditions

Neurological Condition	Binocular Vision Quality: Normal	Binocular Vision Quality: Abnormal
NE1	3	6
NE2	0	1
NE3	0	1
NE4	1	0
Not examined	6	11
Total	10	19

In the second group was born under pathological conditions and the B.V. condition can be seen on Table 4.

In the cases showing abnormal B.V., three cases with strabismus were included.

TABLE 4

Pathologic Perinatal Conditions and Quality of Binocular Vision

Binocular Vision	Cases
Normal	26
Subnormal	12
Abnormal	26
Total	64

If we consider the incidence of each pathological perinatal factor separately in the two classes of B.V., we did not find a clear difference between both groups.

TABLE 5

Neurological Examination Results in Children with Pathological Perinatal Conditions

Neurological Condition		Cases
Normal	(NE 1)	32
Fine motricity retardation	(NE 2)	2
Fine and gross motoricity retardation	(NE 3)	6
Gross motricity and mental retardation	(NE 4)	2
Not examined		22
Total		64

Table 6 shows the relationship between the neurological conditon and the different visual classes.

TABLE 6

Neurological Condition and Quality of Binocular Vision in Children with Pathological Perinatal Conditions

Neurological	Binocular Vision Quality	
Condition	Normal	Abnormal
NE1	13	13
NE2	0	2
NE3	3	2
NE4	0	2
Not examined	11	6
Total	27	25

B. Comparative study of perinatal conditions in children with strabismus and children with normal B.V.

TABLE 7

Perinatal Conditions and Strabismus or Normal Binocular Vision (BV)

Perinatal Conditions	Strabismus	Normal BV
Normal	11 (31%)	10 (27%)
Pathologic	25 (69%)	27 (73%)
Total	36 (100%)	37 (100%)

1. Children with strabismus. The obstetrical data in 36 cases with early strabismus revealed no obstetrical pathology in 11 cases and obstetrical pathology in 25 cases (Table 7).

Ten cases with perinatal pathology had intrapartum hypoxia: in 5 cases, cesarean section was performed with resultant normal Apgar score in 3 cases. Other associated pathology present included eclampsia, premature membrane rupture, twin pregnancy, delayed pregnancy, disruptia placenta, forceps, premature labor, delayed labor, induced labor, umbilical cord circular, infection and large fetus for gestational age. Apgar score was not available in 8 cases. In the rest of the cases, the Apgar score at one minute was 4 or less in two cases and normal in 26 cases. Apgar score at five minutes was 6 in one patient and normal in 27 patients.

2. Children with normal B.V., we registered 37 cases. Their perinatal data was normal in 10 cases and pathological in 27 cases (Table 7). Intrapartum hypoxia was diagnosed in 13 cases. Other pathological cases as previously mentioned had lower incidence than in the first group.

DISCUSSION

In analysing binocular vision in children born under normal conditions, we found the majority of them had abnormal B.V., contrary-wise to what could be expected if perinatal conditions really influence B.V. quality. Furthermore, those children born under pathological conditions, instead of increasing the rate of abnormal B.V. were found to have the same as those born under normal perinatal conditions. In each group, significant difference in the incidence of each perinatal complication was found. Not even fetal distress determined the quality of B.V.

The neurological examination was normal in 75% of the cases born under normal conditions and 76% of the cases born under pathological conditions, thus making us doubt about the real influence perinatal conditions have on motor development. Perhaps too much time had elapsed between the neurological examination and the perinatal damage. It is well known, that neurological examination changes with the age and depends on the emotional conditions of the child.

In the second part of this paper, we studied and compared the obstetrical data of 36 children with strabismus and 37 children with normal B.V.

The data revealed that most of the children were born under pathological conditions both in the group of patients with strabismus (69%) and in the group with normal B.V. (73%). This can be seen on Table 7. The factor having greatest incidence was fetal distress which amazingly, was present in 28% of children with strabismus and 35% of visually normal children. Apgar score was the same in both groups.

These findings oppose and contradict reports from authors such as Unger(6) and confirm von Noorden's(18) point of view and other authors,(14,17) that state, that in the genesis of strabismus multiple factors are responsible. We believe it noteworthy that we did not have cases with birth weight under 1000 gr and we did not have cases with cerebral palsy. Thus, we do not dispute the relationship between early strabismus and both low birth weight and cerebral palsy.(10,11,14)

CONCLUSIONS

Even though our data is limited, we conclude that they negate the hypothesis that stimulated this investigation. The following seems to be true:

1. Children born under normal perinatal conditions demonstrated abnormal fusion capacity. This is not worse if perinatal problems including intrapartum hypoxia were present,

but we did not consider children with birth weight less than 1000 gr.

2. The neurological examination especially concerned with ocular motility, is not worse in children born under pathological perinatal conditions than those born under similar normal conditions. A normal neurological examinations was not more frequent in children having normal binocular vision.

3. The incidence and type of pathologic perinatal data, including fetal distress, are similar in children with strabismus and children with normal binocular vision. Therefore, the reported perinatal conditions are not responsible of the etiology of early strabismus nor binocular vision deficiency.

REFERENCES

1. Lang J: Strabismus. Diagnostick Schielformen, Therapie. Bern Hans Huber 1976, pp 143-144.

2. Denhoff E, Robinault IP: Cerebral Palsy and Related Disorders. New York, McGraw-Hill Book Co., 1960.

3. Birch HG: Perinatal Factors and Mental Subnormality, in Pan American Health Organizations: Perinatal Factors Affecting Human Development. Washington, D.C., 1969, p. 45-50.

4. Myers RE: Fetal Asphyxia and Perinatal Brain Damage, in Pan American Health Organization: Perinatal Factors Affecting Human Development. Washington, D.C., 1969, p. 205-214.

5. Heinonen O: Das Geburstrauma als ursache des Schielens. Acta Ophthalmol 25:19-28, 1947.

6. Unger L: Begleitschielen und fruhkindlicher Hirnschaden. Klin Monatsbl Augenheilkd 130:642-659, 1957.

7. Doden W: Zur Enstehung des Begleitschielens. Ber Dtsch Ophthalmol Ges 61:294, 1958. Cited in von Noorden GK. Burian-von Noorden's Binocular Vision and Ocular Motility, 2nd edition. St. Louis, CV Mosby Co, 1980, p 158.

8. Hiles DA: Results of strabismus therapy in cerebral palsied children. Am Orthp J 25:46-53, 1975.

9. Fisher NF: The relationships between esotropia and neurological dysfunction. J Pediatr Ophthalmol 11:184-187, 1974.

10. Fledelius H: Prematurity and the Eye. Acta Ophthalmol, Supplementum 128, 1976. Chapter 9, Binocularity, pp 127-158.

11. Fabiszewka-Gorna D: Squint in children born before term. Klin oczna 48:25-27, 1978. Abstract, Ophthalmic Lit 1978, 32(6), March 1980, p. 616.

12. Buckley E, Seaber JH: Dyskinetic strabismus as a sign of cerebral palsy. Am J Ophthalmol 91:652-657, 1981.

13. Quere MA: Le traitement precoce des strabismus infantiles. Paris, Doin, 1973, p. 18-21.

14. Kalbe U, Berndt K, de Decker W: Strabismus bei zerebralparetischen und ungeschadigten kindern. Vergleich der motorischen Symptome. Klin Monatsbl Augenheilkd 175:367-374, 1979.

15. Klier P: Entwicklung und Intelligenz schielender Kinder. Klin Monatsbl Augenheilkd 154:699-706, 1969.

16. Spivey BE: Strabismus: Factors in anticipating its occurrence. Aust J Ophthalmol 8:5-9, 1980.

17. Griffin JR, Asano GW, Somers RJ, Anderson CE: Heredity in congenital esotropia. J Am Optom Assoc 50:1237-1242, 1979.

18. von Noorden GK: Burian von Noorden's Binocular Vision and Ocular Motility. 2nd ed, St Louis, CV Mosby Co., 1980, p. 150-165.

19. Parks MM: Ocular Motility and Strabismus. Hagerstown, Harper & Row, 1975, p. 44 and 63.

GAIT AND POSTURAL SWAY EXAMINATIONS IN STRABISMIC CHILDREN WITH CONVERGENCE EXCESS

G. Lennerstrand, P. Odenrick, and P. Sandstedt

ABSTRACT

Twenty children (10 girls and 10 boys) aged 4-10 years with esotropia, convergence excess type, were examined. Fifteen had useful binocular vision and were supplied with bifocal glasses, which they had been wearing for at least six months prior to the testing. The others were wearing adequate distance correction. Gait was examined on a 10 m walkway. Velocity, stride frequency, stride length, and duration of stride phases were calculated from recordings obtained with footswitches. Postural sway was examined on a forceplate, both with eyes closed and with eyes open (fixation maintained at 5 m). Gait and sway parameters were calculated on a computer. Reference values were obtained from a large group of age-matched healthy children without strabismus.

Nine (45%) of the strabismic children showed abnormally short single support time in their gait. Six (30%) showed increased postural sway, all with eyes open and two also with eyes closed. A total of 12 (60%) of the children showed abnormal results in gait and/or postural sway.

We conclude that sensitive examination of gait and posture can reveal abnormal motor control in a high proportion of children with esotropia of the convergence excess type. The results indicate a visuo-motor disturbance in these children of ocular motility and motor systems for locomotion and posture.

INTRODUCTION

Strabismus is seen in a high proportion of patients with motor dysfunctions due to lesions of the central nervous system.(1-3) However, most strabismic children do not show any clinical signs of abnormal skeletal muscle control.(3) It is possible that more sensitive laboratory methods could reveal low grade motor dysfunctions.

STRABISMUS II
ISBN 0-8089-1424-3

We performed gait and postural sway examination on children with strabismus of the convergence excess type. This type of strabismus reflects a disproportion between the accomodative effort and the convergence signal. An additional aim of the study was to test for visuo-motor abnormalities that could be revealed also in the skeletal muscle control of these patients.

MATERIALS

Patients. Twenty children with esotropia of the convergence excess type participated in the study, 10 girls and 10 boys (Table 1). The mean age was 7.8 years (range 4-10). Only one of them (patient 13), showed any signs of delayed mental and motor development. All had passed public health care and school examinations without remarks, and apart from strabismus none showed any abnormalities in physical examinations prior to the present tests.

The convergence excess type of strabismus is defined as a strabismus, which, at near fixation (0.33 m), exceeds the distance deviation by at least 15 prism diopters.(4) One child (patient 11) did not reach this level but was included since she benefitted from bifocal glasses.

All patients had a basic deviation of convergent latent or manifest strabismus (esophoria or esotropia) at distance fixation, ranging between one and 18 prism diopters. The angle of strabismus increased at near fixation except in one girl (subject 19, Table 1), who had been operated on for esotropia and convergence excess two years prior to the test. In seven other operated children the deviation at near fixation had been reduced (see Table 1). The operations had been performed more than six months before the testing. The convergence excess at the examinations and the maximal convergence excess at any time previously have been listed in Table 1.

In all children the visual acuity (VA) was 0.6 or better with adequate correction for refractive errors. 14 children had moderate or good binocular vision with bifocal glasses, which had been worn successfully for 6 months or more before the tests. The near additions were between +1 and +3 diopters. Five of the children had no binocular functions (no fusion) and bifocals were not prescribed.

In eight of the children, the AC/A (accommodative convergence/accommodation) was determined and it ranged between 6 and 15 prism diopters per diopter of accommodation (normal value is 3-5), confirming the diagnosis of convergence excess.

Reference values for gait analysis were obtained from 75 healthy children, 29 girls and 46 boys, mean age 7.2 years (range 4-10). For postural sway examination, 25 healthy children served as a reference series, 12 girls and 13 boys, mean age 6.8 years (range 4-10). For gait analysis, the results were adjusted for age (Norlin et al, 1981) and for postural sway adjusted for sex.(5)

METHODS

The children were wearing their glasses during all examinations.

Gait examination. Foot-switches were placed under the heal and the ball of both feet. The patients were walked on a 10 m walkway at five different velocities, ranging from very slow to very fast. Velocity, stride frequency, stride length, and duration of stride phases were calculated.(6) The detailed description of the method has been published. Results from the patients were compared to age-matched reference values at corresponding speed or stride duration. The reference values were expressed as prediction intervals at the 95% level. Normalization to velocity or stride duration was done by linear interpolation.(7)

Postural sway examination. The patients were standing barefoot with the feet in 45 degrees fanshaped position on a Kistler forceplate in a dark room. A vertical light rod 5 m in front of the patient served as a fixation point. The examinations were done with eyes open and eyes closed; each recording lasted 15 seconds. The signals from the plate were filtered by a low-pass filter at 11 Hz and A/D-converted with a sampling rate of 40 Hz. The signals were processed on line in a computer (PDP 11/34). The sway of the body was described by the coordinates in the horizontal plane of the total force on the forceplate. The total sway amplitude was quantified as the area of a confidence ellipse at the 61% level for the mean position of the sway in the transverse and the sagittal place.(8) The relation between total sway with eyes open and eyes closed is presented as Romberg's quotient(9)

Statistical methods. A pathological sway was defined as an area exceeding the mean value +2 S.D. for the reference

TABLE 1. Clinical data and results of examinations.

					Orthoptic Data						
						Convergence excesses (prism diopters)			Postural sway examination		
									Area		
Pat. No.	Age (Years)	Sex Girls=G Boys=B	Bifocals Yes/No	Operation Yes/No	Binocular functions (1)	Max measured	At examination	Gait examination, (2) Single support 10^{-3} (s)	Eyes open 10^{-6} (m^2) (3)	Eyes closed 10^{-6} (m^2) (4)	Romberg's quotient (%)
1	4.5	B	No	No	0	21	18	340 (320-400)	224p	103	46
2	4.5	B	Yes	No	+	29	29	350 (330-440)	116	no value	no value
3	5.0	G	Yes	Yes	+	37	6	360 (320-430)	233p	64	27
4	5.0	G	Yes	No	+++	22	22	350 (330-460)	205p	204	100
5	5.5	G	Yes	No	+++	19	14	280p (300-390)	77	26	34
6	6.5	G	Yes	No	+++	19	7	420 (340-590)	44	57	130
7	7.0	B	Yes	No	+++	16	15	420 (340-500)	27	47	174
8	7.0	G	Yes	No	+++	23	18	440 (380-670)	65	131	202
9	8.0	B	Yes	No	+	23	20	310p (410-580)	142	127	89
10	8.5	B	Yes	Yes	++	20	14	470 (410-560)	42	57	136

11	8.5	G	Yes	No	+	12	12	330p (360-430)	120p	65	54
12	8.5	G	Yes	Yes	++	23	12	370p (380-470)	175p	231p	132
13	9.0	B	No	Yes	0	22	18	380p (520-600)	460p	429p	93
14	9.0	B	No	Yes	0	20	6	640 (630-750)	46	53	115
15	9.0	B	No	Yes	0	20	15	550 (530-610)	44	46	105
16	9.5	G	Yes	No	+++	18	16	440p (460-520)	76	27	36
17	10.0	B	No	No	0	23	19	460p (470-620)	52	42	81
18	10.0	G	Yes	Yes	+++	25	12	390p (490-660)	47	50	106
19	10.5	G	No	Yes	++	20	-4	510 (450-570)	59	22	37
20	10.5	B	Yes	No	++	15	15	380p (460-590)	92	115	125

Notes: (1) +++ = stereoacuity > 240 sec of arc (normal)
++ = stereoacuity < 240 sec of arc
+ = positive Bagolini test but no stereopsis
0 = no fusion (no binocularity)
(2) Values at very slow velocity, normal range within brackets
(3) Normal range for boys: 25-149 and girls: 3-102
(4) Normal range for boys and girls: 0-229

series. Differences between mean values were tested according to Student's t-test.

RESULTS

Gait examination. Nine (45%) of the children showed pathologically short single support (quadrant I and III in Fig 1), especially at slow velocities. No other significant abnormalities in gait parameters measured were found.

Results of gait and postural sway examinations

The relative deviations from normal limits for single support (SS) and the area of sway with eyes open are shown for all patients (numbers refer to Table 1). The scales are expressed as a quotient:

$$\frac{V - L}{M - L}$$

where V = measured value
L = for SS: lower limit of prediction interval at 95% level
for area: mean value + 2 standard deviations
M = mean value for reference group

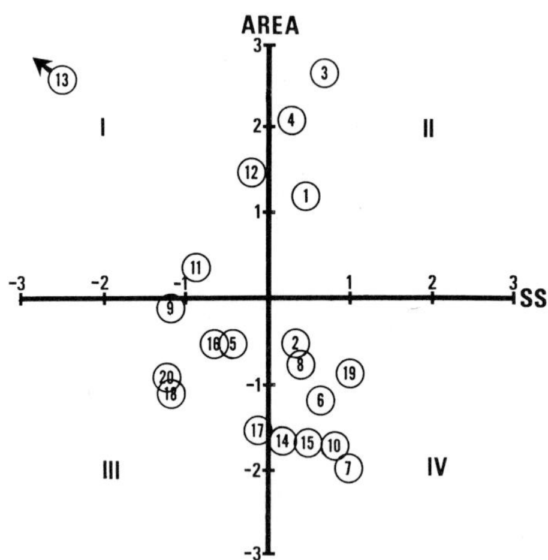

fig.1

Quadrant I: Pathological results of both SS and sway area.
Quadrant II: Pathological results of sway area and normal results of SS.
Quadrant III: Pathological results of SS and normal results of sway area.
Quadrant IV: Results within normal limits.

Postural sway examination. Six (30%) of the children showed a pathologically increased sway, all six with eyes open, and two also with eyes closed (quadrant I and II in Fig 1). The mean value of Romberg's quotient (Table 1) for the patient series was 96% (S.D. 49), and for the reference group 147% (S.D. 85; $p<0.05$). No significant differences between sway amplitude in lateral and sagittal plane, and no lateral displacement of the mean position of the sway were found.

A total of 12 (60%) of the children showed abnormal results at gait and/or postural sway examinations (quadrant I, II, and III, Fig 1). No correlations were found between variables describing anomalies in the eyes and variables from the gait and postural examinations.

DISCUSSION

The present study has shown that a high proportion of mentally and physically healthy children with esotropia of the convergence excess type have abnormal gait and abnormal postural sway. Routine clinical examination did not reveal any neurological deficits, like increased skeletal muscle tonus or ataxia. However, performance in sensitive laboratory tests of gait and postural sway was abnormal in 60% of the children.

The patients walked, especially at slow velocities, with an abnormally short single support, as if they had difficulties in keeping the dynamic equilibrium. During the single support phase of gait only one foot is in contact with ground. Thus, the demand for postural control is most pronounced in this phase, especially at slow velocities.

Abnormal postural sway was more often seen in the test situation with eyes open when vision played a role for maintenance of dynamic equilibrium than when motor control was performed with eyes closed. This is clearly demonstrated by the significant differences between normal children and children with convergence excess in the Romberg's quotient, i.e., the ratio between sway areas with eyes open and closed.

It seems unlikely that the gait and postural abnormalities were due to peripheral visual disturbances. The children had been wearing glasses for a long time. All strabismus operations had been performed more than six months prior to the testing and sensory adaptation to the new eye position probably was developed fully. During the testing of gait and postural sway the children fixated a distant target which eliminated confusion induced by the bifocal glasses. Furthermore, pathological motor control was equally common in children with and without bifocal glasses.

The abnormal control of gait and posture is more likely dependent on central dysfunction. This is further supported by the notion that convergence excess is a central abnormality of the accommodation convergence coupling and not a peripheral dysfunction of the eye muscles. However, a direct relation between the degree of convergence excess and the gait and postural abnormalities was not found in this study or in an extended investigation including children with non-accommodative esotropia.(10) An attempt to delineate the structural basis of the central abnormality must be speculative. Since the gait and postural disturbances in the strabismic children resembled ataxia, the brainstem-cerebellar complex would seem implicated. Visual influences on motor control of skeletal muscle could be mediated by the connections between visual cortical and subcortical areas and structures in the brainstem and cerebellum.(11) However, such interaction also is known to occur at many other levels of the central nervous system. For example, in postural imbalance from deficiences of visual localization, direct influence on spinal structure has been suggested,(12) and further investigation is needed to elucidate the mechanisms for the abnormal motor control in strabismus.

ACKNOWLEDGEMENTS

The skillful assistance of Gun Kvarnstrom and Karin Wranne, orthoptists, is gratefully acknowledged.

This study was supported by grants from the Swedish Medical Research (nos. 4751 and 4497), the Research Committee of Ostergotlands lans landsting and Vivian L. Smith Foundation for Restorative Neurology, Houston, Texas.

REFERENCES

1. Unger L: Begleitschielen and fruhkindlicher Hirnshaden. Klin Monatsbl Augenheilkd. 130:642-659, 1957.

2. Levine MS: Cerebral palsy diagnosis in children over age 1 year: standard criteria. Arch Phys Med Rehabil 61:385-389, 1980.

3. von Noorden GK, Burian HM: Binocular vision and ocular motility. St. Louis, CV Mosby, 1981.

4. Parks MM: Ocular Motility and Strabismus. Hagerstown, Harper & Row, 1975.

5. Odenrick and Sandstedt

6. Larsson LE, Odenrick P, Sandlund B, Weitz P, Oberg PA: The phases of the stride and their interaction in human gait. Scand J Rehabil Med 12:107-112, 1980.

7. Norlin R, Odenrick P, Sandlund B: Development of gait in the normal child. J Pediatr Orthop 1:261-266, 1981.

8. Sahlstrand T, Ortengren R, Nachemson A: Postural equilibrium in adolescent idiopathic scoliosis. Acta Orthop Scand 49:354-365, 1978.

9. Njiokiktjien CJ, van Parys JA: Romberg's sign expressed in a quotient. Agressologie 17 specno:95-99, 1976.

10. Odenrick P, Sandstedt, Lennerstrand G

11. Hoyt WF, Frisen L: Supranuclear ocular motor control. Some clinical considerations - 1974, in Lennerstrand G, Bach-y-Rita P (eds): Basic Mechanisms of Ocular Motility and Their Clinical Implications. Oxford, Pergamon Press, 1975, pp 379-392.

12. Brandt TH: The relationship between retinal image slip, oscillopsia, and postural imbalance, in Lennerstrand G, Zee D, Keller EL (eds): Functional Basis of Ocular Motiliy Disorders. Oxford, Pergamon Press, 1982, pp 379-389.

MICROTROPIA: COMPARISON OF TWO GEOGRAPHICALLY DIFFERENT GROUPS

L. A. P. Cunha, M.D. and J. A. F. Caldeira, M.D.

ABSTRACT

Microtropia (MT) has received attention recently, and particularly microexotropia (MXT). Secondary MT is frequently observed following a surgery for strabismus, hence, it is common. Two geographically diffent groups are analysed in this paper.

PATIENTS AND METHODS

Seventy patients with microtropia (MT) as defined by Lang(1,2) have been analysed from a population seen at Leeds General Infirmary (LGI) in Leeds, England (Group 1). Results are compared to a series of a 135 MT patients seen at the Division of Ophthalmology (D.O), Sao Paulo University School of Medicine, Brazil (Group 2). In the LGI series, a total of 35 with microexotropia (MXT), and were seen at LGI, the remaining 35 were the microesotropia (MET) who returned from September, 1979, till February 1980. Group 2 were the 135 with MT seen at D.O. from October 1975 till October 1980.

Analysis of MTs have been published elsewhere.(3,4) The following factors were examined:

1. Types of MT
2. Sex distribution
3. Age at presentation
4. Fixating eye
5. Vertical component
6. Amblyopia
7. Refraction
8. Fusion
9. Stereopsis
10. Amblyopia treatment

The atypical responses to the four-diopter prism test(5) were sought when examining all patients with presumed MT in keeping with current concepts.(6)

STRABISMUS II
ISBN 0-8089-1424-3

RESULTS

The data may be seen in Tables 1 to 9.

1. Types of microtropia: MXT occurred in 37 of the 135 patients seen at D.O. in Sao Paulo. Secondary MT was observed frequently after a surgery for esotropia (ET) - even secondary MXT. But in Leeds all secondary MT came from the same name tropia (Table 1). Seondary MET (consecutive to surgery) was twice as frequent as secondary MXT in Leeds, but at D.O. each type was about 25%.

2. Sex distribution: No difference in sex distribution between primary MXT in Leeds and in both primary and secondary MET in Sao Paulo. Males predominated in primary MET and females in secondary MET in Group 1. In Group 2, primary MXT was more frequently seen in females. In both populations secondary MXT occurred slightly more frequently in males (Table 2).

3. Age at presentation: In both series secondary MT was seen and primary MXT was seen at a later age. In Leeds almost all secondary MT were seen before the age of six with the mean age lower than age six. The mean age at presentation was older in Sao Paulo (Table 3). The first consultation of secondary MT was considered the original deviation.

4. Fixating eye: No difference between OD and OS was found in MET at D.O., while both males and females with MXT preferred to fixate with OS. At LGT males preferred to fixate with OS and females preferred OD in all MT. In both series, males with MXT preferred to fixate with OS (Table 4).

5. Vertical component (up to 5 degrees): No vertical component was seen at LGI but was in secondary MT at D.O. where a primary MTs had small vertical components (Table 1).

6. Amblyopia density: Mild amblyopia (i.e., less than one full line in visual acuity between eyes hasn't occurred at LGI but it was twice as frequent in MET than in MXT at D.O. The incidence of moderate amblyopia (i.e., one to up three tenths difference in visual acuity was three times higher in group 1 than in group 2. Severe amblyopia (i.e., more than three-tenths of difference in visual acuity between eyes) was seen in about 20% of all patients in both series. No amblyopia was found in 25% of MET and in 35.14% of MXT in group 2 and in 5.71% of MET and 14.26% of MXT in group 1. Absence of amblyopia was consistently higher in MXT (Table 5).

7. Refraction: Emmetropia OU was found only in MXT in group 2. No patient in the series had emmetropia OU in MET. Spherical and cylindrical anisometropia were more frequent in MXT than in MET at LGI. The difference was more striking when spherical anisometropia higher than 2 diopters was considered in MXT patients in group 2. In most cases the more ametropic eye was the nonfixating one. Hypermetropic astigmatism was the more frequent in both series in both eyes, but myopic astigmatism was more frequent in MXT in both groups. Mixed astigmatism in the fixating eye was present only in MXT patients in group 2. Astigmatism in the nonfixating eye had a higher incidence in the Sao Paulo series but was also frequent in the fixating eye in this group, which did not occurred in Leeds. The incidence of more than 2 diopters of astigmatism was similar in fixating and nonfixating eyes in group 2. Such high astigmatism was seen only in nonfixating eyes of MXT patients at LGI (Table 6).

8. Fusion and its range: Absence or nonsustained fusion was common in primary MT and secondary MT in group 2. In group 1 this was seen only in 4% of primary MET. Convergence amplitude was normal in more than 50% of primary MT subjects in both groups. In the Leeds series almost all MET patients had normal convergence amplitude and more than 50% of MXT subjects had a normal divergence amplitude. In group 2 convergence and divergence amplitudes were better in primary MT (Table 7).

9. Stereopsis: Streopsis was absent frequently in group 2, mainly in secondary MT, whereas in primary MXT it was frequently better than 120" for distance. In group 1, the higher incidence of good stereopsis for near was seen also in primary MXT. In the Leeds series, all secondary MT had at least some stereopsis, while almost all in the Sao Paulo series had none. In both groups, the better stereopsis was seen in MXT. The number of secondary MXT patietns was small in both series. A small number of patients in both groups was not reliable for sensory tests and their responses have not been included (Table 8).

10. Treatment for amblyopia: In both series treatment has been instituted in MXT less frequently than in MET. Reasons for nontreatment included absence of amblyopia, late age at presentation and noncompliance. Results after treatment have shown improvement in both groups, but only at D.O. did visual acuity become equal OU and this was observed in 20% of the treated subjects (Table 9).

TABLE 1 - Types of Microtropia

Total Number of Subjects	Group 1 70	Group 2 135
MET	35 (50%)	98 (72, 59%)
MXT	35 (50%)	37 (27, 41%)
1° MT	55 (78, 57%)	102 (75, 55%)
2° MT	15 (21, 43%)	33 (24, 45%)
1° MET	25 (71, 43% of MET)	76 (77, 55%)
1° MXT	30 (85, 72% of MXT)	26 (70, 27%)
2° MET	10 (28, 57% of MET)	22 (22, 45%)
2° MXT	5 (14, 28% of MXT)	11 (29, 73%)
2° MET consecutive to ET	10 (100% of 2° MET)	20 (90, 91%)
2° MET consecutive to XT	0 (0% of 2° MET)	2 (9, 09%)
2° MXT consecutive to ET	0 (0% of 2° MXT)	8 (72, 73%)
2° MXT consecutive to XT	5 (100% of 2° MXT)	3 (27, 27%)
MT associated with HT	0 (0%)	21 (15, 56%)
1° MT associated with HT	0 (0% of 1° MT)	8 (7, 84%)
2° MT associated with HT	0 (0% of 2° MT)	13 (39, 39%)

MET = microesotropia
MXT = microexotropia
1° = primary
2° = secondary
MT = microtropia
ET = esotropia
XT = exotropia
HT = hypertropia

TABLE 2 - Sex Distribution

	Group 1	Group 2
M MET	18 (51, 43% of MET)	49 (50%)
F MET	17 (48, 57% of MET)	49 (50%)
M 1° MET	15 (60% of 1° MET)	38 (50%)
F 1° MET	10 (40% of 1° MET)	38 (50%)
M 2° MET	3 (30% of 2° MET)	11 (50%)
F 2° MET	7 (70% of 2° MET)	11 (50%)
M MXT	19 (54, 28% of MXT)	13 (35, 14%)
F MXT	16 (45, 72% of MXT)	24 (64, 86%)
M 1° MXT	16 (53, 33% of 1° MXT)	6 (23, 07%)
F 1° MXT	14 (46, 67% of 1° MXT)	20 (76, 92%)
M 2° MXT	3 (60% of 2° MXT)	7 (63, 64%)
F 2° MXT	2 (40% of 2° MXT)	4 (36, 36%)
M 1° MT	31 (56, 36% of 1° MT)	44 (43, 14%)
F 1° MT	24 (25, 45% of 1° MT)	58 (56, 86%)
M 2° MT	6 (40% of 2° MT)	18 (54, 55%)
F 2° MT	9 (60% of 2° MT)	15 (45, 45%)

M = Male
F = Female

TABLE 3 - AGE AT PRESENTATION

		Group 1	Group 2
Under 6 years	1° MET	19 (76% of 1° MET)	26 (34, 21%)
	1° MXT	17 (56, 67% of 1° MXT)	4 (15, 58%)
	2° MET	10 (100% of 2° MET)	11 (50%)
	2° MXT	4 (80% of 2° MXT)	5 (45, 45%)
6 till 10 years	1° MET	6 (24% of 1° MET)	24 (31, 58%)
	1° MXT	12 (40% of 1° MXT)	10 (38, 46%)
	2° MET	0 (0% of 2° MET)	4 (18, 18%)
	2° MXT	1 (20% of 2° MXT)	3 (27, 27%)
Older than 10 years	1° MET	0 (0% of 1° MET)	26 (34, 21%)
	1° MXT	1 (3, 33% of 1° MXT)	12 (46, 15%)
	2° MET	0 (0% of 2° MET)	7 (31, 82%)
	2° MXT	0 (0% of 2° MXT)	3 (27, 27%)
Mean age at presentation	MET	4 yrs, 7 mos	7 yrs, 5 mos
	MXT	6 yrs	8 yrs, 1 mo
	1° MET	5 yrs, 1 mo	7 yrs, 8 mos
	1° MXT	6 yrs, 6 mos	8 yrs, 9 mos
	2° MET	3 yrs, 4 mos	7 yrs
	2° MXT	3 yrs, 4 mos	6 yrs, 9 mos

TABLE 4 - The Nonfixating Eye

		Group 1	Group 2
MET			
males	-OD	11 (61, 11% of males with MET)	23 (46, 94%)
	-OS	7 (38, 89% of males with MET)	26 (53, 06%)
females	-OD	5 (29, 41% of females with MET)	24 (48, 98%)
	-OS	12 (70, 59% of females with MET)	25 (51, 02%)
Total	-OD	16 (45, 72% of MET subjects)	47 (47, 96%)
	-OS	19 (54, 28% of MET subjects)	51 (52, 04%)
MXT			
males	-OD	12 (63, 16% of males with MXT)	7 (53, 85%)
	-OS	7 (36, 84% of males with MXT)	6 (46, 15%)
females	-OD	6 (37, 50% of females with MXT)	14 (58, 33%)
	-OS	10 (62, 50% of females with MXT)	10 (41, 67%)
Total	-OD	18 (51, 43% of MXT subjects)	21 (56, 76%)
	-OS	17 (48, 57% of MXT subjects)	16 (43, 24%)

TABLE 5 - Amblyopia Density

	Group 1	Group 2
MILD		
in MET	0 (0% of MET)	26 (27, 08%)
in MXT	0 (0% of MXT)	5 (13, 51%)
MODERATE		
in MET	28 (80% of MET)	26 (27, 07%)
in MXT	22 (62, 86% of MXT)	8 (21, 62%)
SEVERE		
in MET	5 (14, 28% of MET)	20 (20, 83%)
in MXT	8 (22, 86% of MXT)	11 (29, 73%)
ABSENCE OF AMBLYOPIA (at last consultation)		
in MET	2 (5, 71% of MET)	24 (25%)
in MXT	5 (14, 28% of MXT)	13 (35, 14%)

TABLE 6 - Refraction (1)

	Group 1	Group 2
Emmetropia OU		
in MET	0 (0% of MET)	0 (0%)
in MXT	0 (0% of MXT)	3 (8, 11%)
Spherical anisometropia (SA)		
in MET	18 (51, 43% of MET)	39 (40, 21%)
in MXT	25 (71, 43% of MXT)	14 (37, 84%)
SA above 2sph		
in MET	3 (16, 67% of MET with SA)	10 (25, 64%)
in MXT	19 (76% of MXT with SA)	6 (42, 86%)
Cylindrical anisometropia (CA)		
in MET	10 (28, 57% of MET)	21 (21, 65%)
in MXT	22 (62, 86% of MXT)	10 (27, 03%)
CA above 2 cyl		
in MET	0 (0% of MET with CA)	4 (19, 05%)
in MXT	8 (36, 36% of MXT with CA)	2 (20%)
Type of astigmatism (Ast) in the nonfixating eye (NFE)		
Hyperopic		
in MET	16 (94, 12% of NFE with Ast and MET)	69 (94, 52%)
in MXT	20 (86, 96% of NFE with Ast and MXT)	20 (80%)
Myopic		
in MET	0 (0% of NFE with Ast and MET)	2 (2, 74%)
in MXT	2 (8, 70% of NFE with Ast and MXT)	4 (16%)
Mixed		
in MET	1 (5, 88% of NFE with Ast and MET)	2 (2, 74%)
in MXT	1 (4, 35% of NFE with Ast and MXT)	1 (4%)

TABLE 6 - Refraction (II)

	Group 1	Group 2
Type of astigmatism (Ast) in the fixating eye (FE)		
Hyperopic		
in MET	8 (100% of FE with Ast and MET)	65 (98, 48%)
in MXT	9 (90% of FE with Ast and MXT)	15 (75%)
Myopic		
in MET	0 (0% of FE with Ast and MET)	1 (1, 52%)
in MXT	1 (10% of FE with Ast and MXT)	2 (10%)
Mixed		
in MET	0 (0% of FE with Ast and MET)	0 (0%)
in MXT	0 (0% of FE with Ast and MXT)	3 (15%)
Incidence of anisometropia		
in MET	19 (54, 29% of MET)	46 (46, 94%)
in MXT	30 (85, 71% of MXT)	20 (54, 05%)
in MT	49 (70% of MT)	66 (48, 89%)
Ast in the NFE		
in MET	18 (51, 43% of MET)	73 (75, 26%)
in MXT	23 (65, 71% of MXT)	25 (67, 57%)
Ast in the FE		
in MET	7 (20% of MET)	66 (68, 04%)
in MXT	10 (28, 57% of MXT)	20 (54, 05%)
Ast above 2 cyl in the NFE		
in MET	0 (0% of the NFE with Ast and MET)	15 (20, 55%)
in MXT	16 (69, 57% of the NFE with Ast & MXT)	5 (20%)
Ast above 2 cyl in the FE		
in MET	0 (0% of the FE with Ast and MET)	9 (13, 64%)
in MXT	0 (0% of the FE with Ast and MXT)	3 (15%)

TABLE 7 - Fusion and Its Range*

	Group 1	Group 2
Fusion		
1° MET	25 (100% of 1° MET)	59 (90,77%)
2° MET	10 (100% of 2° MET)	14 (73, 68%)
1° MXT	30 (100% of 1° MXT)	23 (95, 83%)
2° MXT	5 (100% of 2° MXT)	2 (50%)
No fusion or nonsustained fusion		
1° MET	1 (4% of 1° MET)	6 (12%)
2° MET	0 (0% of 2° MET)	8 (61, 54%)
1° MXT	0 (0% of 1° MXT)	1 (4, 76%)
2° MXT	0 (0% of 2° MXT)	2 (50%)
Normal range of convergence		
1° MET	23 (92% of 1° MET)	32 (64%)
2° MET	10 (100% of 2° MET)	3 (23, 08%)
1° MXT	20 (66, 67% of 1° MXT)	12 (57, 14%)
2° MXT	4 (80% of 2° MXT)	1 (25%)
Normal range of divergence		
1° MET	6 (24% of 1° MET)	18 (36%)
2° MET	4 (40% of 2° MET)	1 (7, 69%)
1° MXT	17 (56, 67% of 1° MXT)	8 (38, 10%)
2° MXT	4 (80% of 2° MXT)	0 (0%)

*Only of patients who gave reliable responses

TABLE 8 - Stereopsis*

	Group 1	Group 2
No stereopsis		
MET	(8, 57% of MET)	44 (61, 12%)
MXT	3 (9, 09% of MXT)	13 (46, 43%)
1° MET	3 (12% of 1° MET)	32 (56, 14%)
2° MET	0 (0% of 2° MET)	12 (80%)
1° MXT	3 (11, 11% of 1° MXT)	7 (31, 82%)
2° MXT	0 (0% of 2° MXT)	6 (100%)
Stereopsis better than 120"		
MET	7 (20% of MET)	5 (6, 94%)
MXT	17 (51, 52% of MXT)	10 (35, 71%)
MT	24 (35, 29% of MT)	15 (15%)
1° MET	4 (16% of 1° MET)	4 (7, 02%)
2° MET	3 (30% of 2° MET)	1 (6, 67%)
1° MXT	16 (57, 14% of 1° MXT)	10 (45, 45%)
2° MXT	1 (20% of 2° MXT)	0 (0%)

*In Group I, stereopsis was measured for near (Titmus, Frisby and TNO tests) and in Group 2, for distance (polaroid vectographic). Only reliable responses have been included.

TABLE 9 - Treatment for Amblyopia

	Group 1	Group 2
Total MET treated subjects	29 (82, 86% of MET)	77 (78, 57%)
Total MXT treated subjects	22 (62, 86% of MXT)	20 (54, 05%)
Reason for nontreatment in MET:		
a) absence of amblyopia	3 (8, 57% of MET)	8 (8, 16%)
b) late age at presentation	0 (0% of MET)	13 (13, 27%)
c) others	3 (8, 57% of MET)	0 (0%)
Reason for nontreatment in MXT:		
a) absence of amblyopia	4 (11, 43% of MXT)	8 (21, 62%)
b) late age at presentation	1 (2, 86% of MXT)	9 (24, 32%)
c) others	8 (22, 86% of MXT)	0 (0%)
Positive results (after treatment VA improved at least 0.1 or more)		
in MET	25 (86, 21% of treated MET)	61 (81, 33%)
in MXT	18 (81, 82% of treated MXT)	14 (70%)
Equal VA in OU after treatment		
in MET	0 (0% of treated MET)	16 (21, 33%)
in MXT	0 (0% of treated MXT)	4 (20%)

DISCUSSION

Both groups showed similarities between: (1) MET and MXT; (2) primary MT and secondary MT; (3) primary MET and primary MXT; (4) secondary MET and secondary MXT.

(1) MET and MXT:

a. MET occurred with a similar frequency in either sex.
b. Absence of a significant amblyopia was seen more commonly in MXT.
c. Spherical anisometropia greater than 2 diopters is more commonly seen in MXT. Emmetropia in OU has not occurred in MET.
d. Both spherical and cylindrical ametropias are normally higher in the nonfixating eye in MET and MXT.
e. Both in the nonfixating and fixating eye with astigmatism the hypermetropic type is the commonest.
f. Myopic astigmatism has a higher incidence in patients with MXT.
g. Anisometropia occurred in more than 50% of the MXT patients.
h. High incidence of astigmatism in the nonfixating eye in both MET and MXT was found.
i. Good stereopsis was more frequently associated with MXT.
j. MET patients were given amblyopia treatment more frequently than MXT patients.
k. The response to amblyopia treatment was good in most cases of MET and MXT.

(2) Primary MT and secondary MT:

a. Secondary MT represented about one fourth of all MT patients.
b. Secondary MT patients normally are seen earlier than primary MT.

(3) Primary MET and primary MXT:

a. In both series primary MET patients were seen earlier than primary MXT subjects.
b. Good stereopsis was present in most primary MXT patients.

(4) Secondary MET and secondary MXT:

a. Secondary MXT was more commonly seen in male than in female subjects.

The most striking differences between both groups have been pointed out. Could racial and/or geographical components explain them? The easiest explanation would be a social difference causing subjects to be referred earlier in Leeds. A higher miscegenation rate in Brazil than in England could be an important factor to explain why in five years 37 MXT have been seen in Sao Paulo and 35 was the total number of MXT at LGI. That could also mean a higher rate of MT in Sao Paulo, but we do not know MT prevalence in Leeds. In Sao Paulo, MT respresents at least 1% of all patients referred to the Eye Division.

Overcorrections may occur less frequently at LGI and that could partially explain why secondary MT in group 1 always came from the respective tropia. The number of secondary MXT is too small in group 1 to be of statistical significance.

Possibly a lower compliance rate in the Sao Paulo series caused severe amblyopia to be present more commonly in this group. Anisometropia, although frequent in both populations, was more severe in group 1 where a higher incidence of astigmatism in the nonfixating eye was also present.(7)

Sensorial findings are better in group 1 probably due to an earlier treatment with less severe amblyopia in the nonfixating eye. Compliance with the treatment being probably higher in this series a better result is to be expected. Even so, good stereopsis in both populations in primary MXT patients, which to present themselves later for consultation, is consistently high. Scotoma density is normally lighter in exo than in esotropia(8) even if it has a larger area. That could probably explain the difference in stereopsis level in both groups.

SUMMARY

Findings in two geographically different series of patients with microtropia, one from Leeds (England) and the other from Sao Paulo (Brazil), are compared and differences and similarities stressed and commented upon.

ACKNOWLEDGEMENTS

The authors wish to thank Mr. R.B. Harcourt, Consultant to the Eye Department, Leeds General Infirmary, for allowing them to quote his cases and the orthoptists at Leeds General Infirmary for their help and cooperation.

REFERENCES

1. Lang J: Microstrabismus. Br Orthopt J 26:30-37, 1969.

2. Lang J: Management of microtropia. Br J Ophthalmol 58:281-292, 1974.

3. Cunha LAP: Microeso e microexotropias: Comparacoes em uma amostragem de Yorkshire. Arq Brasil Oftalmol 45:93-97, 1982.

4. Cunha LAP, Caldeira JAF, Moises CMA, Mattiussi GMC: Analise retrospectiva de microtropias. Arq Brasil Oftalmol 44:202-209, 1981.

5. Romano PE, von Noorden GK: Atypical responses to the four- diopter prism test. Am J Ophthalmol 67:935-941, 1969.

6. von Noorden GK: Burian-von Noorden's Binocular Vision and Ocular Motility. Saint Louis, Mosby Co., 1980, pp 303-307.

7. Johnson F, Cunha LAP, Harcourt RB: The clinical characteristics of microexotropia. Br Orthop J 38:54-59, 1981.

8. Parks MM: Ocular Motility and Strabismus. Hagerstown, Harper & Row, 1975, p 73.

BINOCULAR VISION AND OKN ASYMMETRY IN STRABISMIC PATIENTS

J. T. Flynn, C. Pritchard, and D. Lasley

ABSTRACT

Optokinetic asymmetry has been noted in strabismic and amblyopic subjects. We studied a group of 28 early-onset esotropic subjects with OKN asymmetry and latent nystagmus. EOG recordings documented their OKN asymmetry. Binocular vision was determined by standard free space and synoptophore tests. In addition, the tilt transfer test was performed on a group of these subjects. Results indicate that some form of peripheral fusion is present in 50% of these patients.

INTRODUCTION

Monocular optokinetic nystagmus (OKN) asymmetry probably was first described in humans with strabismus and amblyopia by Nicolia(1) in 1959. In such a patient, an asymmetry is seen in the monocular response to an optokinetic target traveling in a nasal compared to temporal direction. In the OKN nasal moving target, the eye either makes no movement or a slow, irregular pursuit in the direction of the target without a refixation saccade (Fig 1). The asymmetric response disappears under binocular conditions.

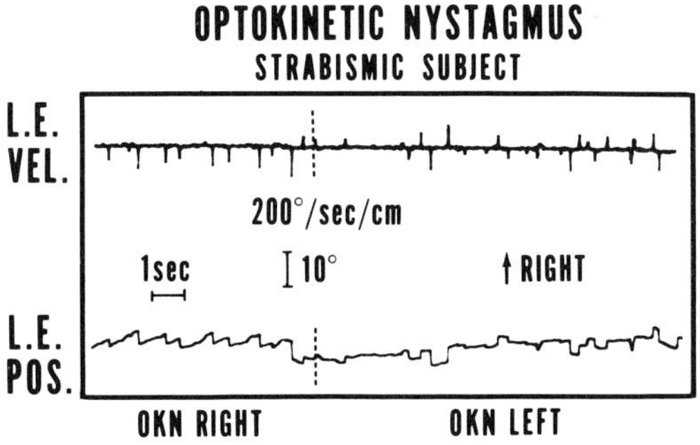

1. Monocular OKN asymmetry in a strabismic patient. The response when targets are taken in a temporal to nasal direction is normal. The response when targets are taken in a nasal to temporal direction is abnormal or absent.

STRABISMUS II
ISBN 0-8089-1424-3

In animals(2-4) and humans(5,6) the development of symmetry of the monocular OKN response is a maturational phenomenon. The later development of the nasal to temporal response thought to be due to binocular connections made via the visual cortex down to the optokinetic centers in the pre-tectum.

At the 1981 ARVO Meeting, Rosenberg, Pritchard and Flynn(7) described what seemed a related asymmetry. Briefly, if a normal subject is rotated while fixating a target which rotates with him, the vestibular ocular reflex (VOR) is suppressed. Strabismic subjects with OKN asymmetry develop a nystagmus with the fast component in the direction in which they are being rotated (Fig 2). In our series of patients we have studied, 25 have both asymmetries, 6 have at least one and 2 patients originally thought to have the OKN asymmetry proved, on further recording, not to have it (Table 1).

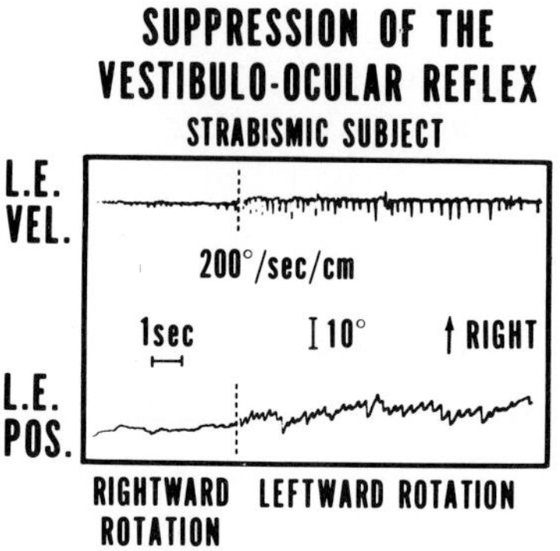

2. VOR reflex suppression abnormality demonstrated monocularly in a strabismic patient. When the subject is rotated to the left with the fixation target, VOR suppression occurs. When the subject is rotated to the right with the rotating target, VOR cannot be suppressed and the subject develops a right-beating nystagmus.

In a preliminary study(8) we reasoned that if OKN asymmetry were due to an absence or failure of cortical binocular neurones to develop, then as a first step in documenting this failure, we might look for absence of binocular vision. The full anatomical details of the hypothesis are spelled out in the above citation.(8) To test the hypothesis we used the ordinary clinical tests for binocular single vision in strabismic patients (Table 2). The results of that study can be summarized. We found, contrary to the predictions of the hypothesis and our expectations, a significant portion of thess patients had binocular single vision as evidence of some form of cortical binocularity (Table 3).

TABLE 1

OKN ASYMMETRY
(n= 33)

		YES	NO
ABNORMAL VOR SUPPRESSION	YES	25	5
	NO	1	2

TABLE 2

BINOCULAR VISION TESTS
Free Space
Worth 4 dot
Bagolini Lenses
Titmus stereo test
Synoptophore
Simultaneous perception
Fusion targets

TABLE 3

SUMMARY OF BINOCULAR FUNCTIONS IN VOR-OKN ASYMMETRIC STRABISMIC PATIENTS (N=17)

Patient #	W4 Dot	Bagolini	Stereo	SMP	Fusion
1	-	-	-	*	*
2	-	-	-	*	*
3	-	-	-	-	-
4	-	-	-	+	+
5	-	-	-	*	*
6	+	+	-	+	+
7	+	+	+	-	-
8	-	-	*	*	*
9	-	+	*	*	*
10	+	+	-	+	-
11	+	-	-	+	+
12	-	-	*	+	-
13	-	*	*	+	-
14	-	-	-	+	+
15	+	-	-	+	-
16	-	+	-	+	+
17	+	+	+	+	+

* = no information or unreliable information

Because these tests are clinical tests applicable to large clinical populations of all ages, we might be missing evidence of cortical dysbinocularity that might be revealed by a more subtle psychophysical test of binocular vision in a group of these patients. We chose the tilt transfer after-effect as representative of an adaptation effect relying on a pool of binocular neurones in the cortex to transfer the effect from one eye to the other. The method has been well described in the psychophysical literature(9-11) as a method of quantifying cortical binocularity by transfer of the adaptation effect from one eye to the other via a pool of binocular cortical neurones (Fig 3).

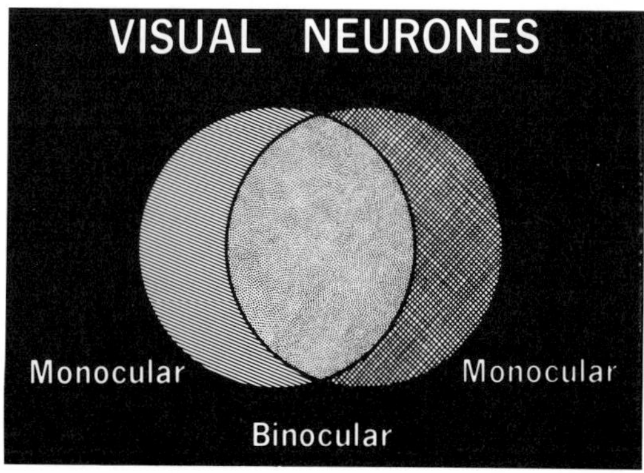

3. Venn diagram of binocular neurone pool responsible for tilt transfer effect.

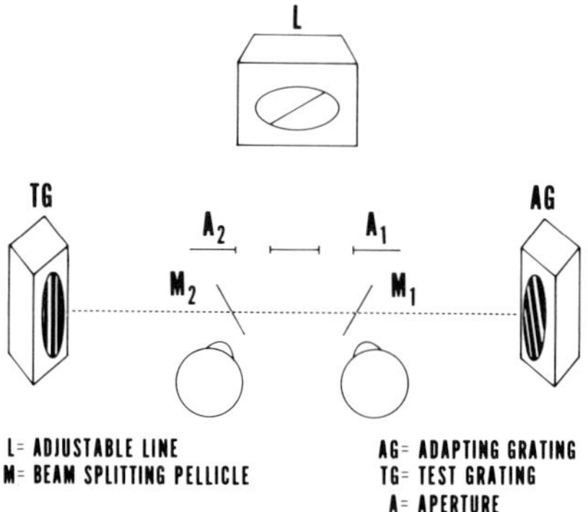

4. Schematic diagram of the tilt transfer after-effect testing apparatus.

METHOD

The test was performed as described by Mitchell and Ware.(9) Briefly, the subject was seated before a beam-splitting haploscope (Fig 4) 66 cm from his eye. In the first part of the test, the subject made ten settings of the vertical line monocularly for each eye. This monocular eye was then adapted for two minutes to a grating tilted 100 degrees from the vertical. Following this adaptation, the subject viewed a vertical grating while being required to set a line projected to the side of the vertical grating parallel to this grating. The subject was allowed as many trials as necessary. The test grating was viewed for 2 seconds followed by the adapting (tilted) grating for 10 seconds. When the line was set parallel to the grating to the satisfaction of the subject, this was taken as his monocular tilt. Ten such settings were made monocularly and the degree of the tilt of the vertical line was a measure of the monocular tilt after-effect.

The procedure was then repeated under binocular conditions with the tilted (adapting) grating in the one eye and the vertical (test) grating in the other eye. The task was the same and measure of the tilt of the vertical line was a measure of the adaptation effect transferred from right to left or left to right. This was expressed as a percentage or fraction of the tilt effect observed under monocular testing conditions.

RESULTS

Data was gathered on 14 patients. Many others were tested but naive strabismic subjects often were unable to perform the test. Ten of the tested subjects had congential or early-acquired strabismus. All 10 had monocular OKN asymetry both clinically and demonstrable on their eye movement recordings. All 10 had failed to suppress their VOR. Six of the 10 had definite latent nystagmus and in 3 subjects, the evidence was equivocal. Four subjects, 3 with acquired strabismus and one normal subject, were included as controls.

The data showed marked internal variability and some surprising responses (Table 4). First of all, 7 subjects showed evidence of an abnormal monocular adaptation effect. That is, they tilted the line in the same direction as the adaptation grating. Of these subjects, 2 were amblyopes. We believe the reason for this response was the inability of the amblyopes, at least, to fix the grating rather than the line. This is the responses a normal control subject will give when instructed to fix the line rather than the grating in performing this monocular tilt test.

Second, the number of subjects who were able to successfully transfer the effect in this group of subjects was small. Of the 20 potential transfers, right to left and left to right among our 10 subjects, the tilt effect was transfered seven times. Two subjects transfered in both directions and 3 subjects were able to transfer in one direction only. Interestingly, 2 of the 3 subjects who were able to transfer the effect from the right eye to the left eye were amblyopes in the right eye, yet were still able to effect the behavior of the non-amblyopic left eye with an adapting stimulus in the amblyopic eye. The numerical values of the tilt transfer effect for all our subjects are shown in the Figure 5.

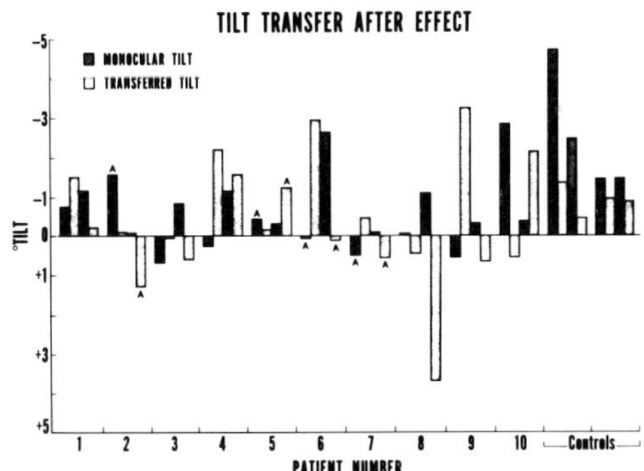

5. Histogram of the tilt transfer for the monocular and binocular tilt transfer effect (expressed as a percentage of the monocular tilt effect) for all subjects. Data below the horizontal line represents strabismic subjects whose data showed no monocular adaptation effect. The data from the normal subjects is to the right of the figure.

TABLE 4

TILT TRANSFER EFFECT: BINOCULAR RESULTS (N=10)

DIRECTION	#
R→L	1/10
L→R	2/10
R↔L	2/10

DISCUSSION

We had hoped to find a psychophysical test which would clearly show an absence of binocularity to parallel the results of our OKN and VOR asymmetries. Clearly, the tilt transfer after-effect test is such an appropriate test. The tilt transfer is dependent on a pool of binocular neurones which can be influenced by an adapting grating in one eye to affect the sensation of the vertical in the other unadapted eye. The fact that 5 of our 10 subjects showed some ability to transfer the effect from the adapting eye to the testing eye demonstrates that this effect is probably dependent on a different pool of cortical binocular neurones than is the OKN-VOR effect. In a sense, though disappointing, these negative findings demonstrate the complexity of the information processing task performed by various pools of cortical neurones which guide the behavior of the visual sensory and motor system. We will continue to search for a psychophysical test whose results will parallel the results we are observing on the motor side with our OKN and VOR reflex abnormalities.

ACKNOWLEDGEMENTS

Supported in part by the Fight for Sight Children's Diagnostic Eye Clinic, Bascom Palmer Eye Institute, University of Miami School of Medicine, Miami, Florida and a research grant from the National Institutes of Health EYO 3580-02.

REFERENCES

1. Nicolai H: Differenzen zwischen optokinetischem Rechts und Links nystagmus bei einseitiger-(Schiel) Amblyopie. Klin Monatsbl Augenheild 134: 245-250, 1959.

2. Van Hof-Van Duin J: Early and permanent effects of monocular deprivation on pattern discrimination and visuomotor behavior in cats. Brain Res 111:261-276, 1976.

3. Atkinson J: Development of OKN nystagmus in human infant and monkey infant, in Freeman RD (ed): Developmental Neurobiology of Vision. NY, Plenum Pub, 1979, p 277-287.

4. Hoffman KP: OKN nystagmus and single cell responses in the nucleus tractus opticus, in Freeman RD (ed): Developmental Neurobiology of Vision. NY, Plenum Pub, 1979, p 63-72.

5. Naegele JR, Held R: Monocular optokinetic nystagmus shows directional asymmetry in human infants. Invest Ophthalmol & Vis Sci (ARVO Abstracts) Supplement, 1980, p 210.

6. Naegele JR, Held R: The postnatal development of monocular optokinetic nystagmus in infants. Vision Res 22:341-346, 1982.

7. Rosenberg ML, Pritchard C, Flynn J: Asymmetry of the optokinetic response and visual suppression of vestibulo-ocular reflex in strabismic patients. ARVO Abstracts, Supplement to Investigative Ophthalmology, Visual Science 20: March 1981, p 26.

8. Flynn J: Vestibulo-optokinetic interactions in strabismus. Publication pending.

9. Mitchell DE, Ware C: Intraocular transfer of a visual after-effect in normal and stereoblind humans. J Physiol (Lond) 236:707-721, 1974.

10. Blake R, Overton R, Stern SL: Interocular transfer of visual after-effects. J Ex Psychol (Human Percep) 7:367-381, 1981.

11. Movshon JA, Chambers BE, Blakemore C: Interocular transfer in normal humans and those who lack stereopsis. Percept 1:483, 1971.

OCULAR MORBIDITY IN VERY LOW BIRTHWEIGHT INFANTS

C. G. Keith and W. H. Kitchen

ABSTRACT

In the years 1977-78, 258 infants weighing less than 1500g were born at, or transfered to, the Royal Women's Hospital Melbourne; 177 (68.5%) survived, and 111 of these received an ophthalmic examination. Significant ocular pathology was found in 37 (33%): 21 (19%) children had strabismus, 19 (17%) had a significant refractive error, eleven (10%) had cicatricial retrolental fibroplasia (RFL), and three (2.7%) had poor vision due to optic atrophy associated with cerebral palsy. No children were blind due to RLF, indicating that the recent increase in survival rate of very-low-birth weight (VLBW) infants has not been accompanied by an increase in the prevalence of severe RLF. In those children with neither cerebral palsy nor RLF, the prevalence of strabismus was 11%, and of refractive errors 13%. Myopia was found mainly in children who had shown RLF changes in the neonatal period. VLBW infants should continue to be screened in the premature nursery for RLF, and at the age of two for the detection of refractive errors and strabismus.

INTRODUCTION

The introduction of intensive care units into neonatal nurseries has caused a significant increase in the survival rate of VLBW infants (500g - 1500g), and considerable concern has been expressed that a parallel increase in the prevalence of children with severe neurosensory disorders may be occurring. In order to assess this, a collaborative study has been carried out on the neurosensory status status, age two years, of surviving VLBW infants born in the years 1977-78. The general data has been published elsewhere,(1) and we report here the ocular findings from one of the two participating hospitals.

MATERIALS AND METHODS

In the years 1977-78, 258 VLBW infants were born in, or transfered in the neonatal period, to the Royal Women's Hospital, Melbourne. Seventy-four children succumbed in the

STRABISMUS II
ISBN 0-8089-1424-3

hospital, and seven children later died at home, giving a total mortality of 81 (31.5%). Of the 177 long term survivors, two (1.1%) were untraced and reliable reports on three children (1.7%) suggested no ocular abnormality, and 172 (97.2%) were reviewed by the developmental pediatrician at two years of age. Although appointments were offered to all families, only 111 (63%) appeared for ophthalmic examination by one of the authors (CGK). Eighty of these 111 had been screened in the premature nursery for retrolental fibroplasia methods previously described.(2) Twenty-one children weighed <1000g at birth, and 90 weighed between 1000g and 1500g.

The ocular examination consisted of visual acuity assessment with the Catford drum, inspection and cover test for the detection of strabismus, refraction after instillation of cyclopentolate 1% drops, and scrutiny of the fundus for cicatricial RLF and arteriolar tortuosity. All data were prepared for computer analysis.

TABLE 1

Strabismus	21 (19%)
RLF	11 (10%)
Optic Atrophy	3 (2.7%)
Refractive Error	19 (17%)

Significant ocular defects found in 37 children out of 111 reviewed.

RESULTS

Among the 111 children reviewed, one or more significant ocular defects were found in 37 (33%) (Table 1). Twenty-one (19%) had strabismus, 19 (17%) had a significant refractive error, and eleven (10%) had cicatricial RLF. Fifteen children had cerebral palsy, seven had strabismus, and three had poor vision due to optic atrophy. In a prior report,(1) only two of these children had been detected.

TABLE 2

I	9
II	7
III	2
IV	1
11 Cases	19 Eyes

The grades of RLF found 11 children (19 eyes). Three eyes were clinically normal.

Cicatricial RLF was found in 19 eyes of 11 children (Table 2). Grade I was found in nine, Grade II in seven, Grade III in two, and Grade IV in one. These changes were sometimes assymetric, as in a case, who had a retinal fold in the right eye (Grade IV), while the left was normal. Eight (7%) of the children had Grade II-IV RLF in one or both eyes. No obvious difference in the severity of RLF occurred in those weighing <1000g at birth, and those weighing between 1000g and 1500g. However, RLF was significantly more common in the former group, being found in six out of 21 (19%), but in five out of 90 (5.5%) in the latter group (p>.01). In eight of the eleven children, developing RLF had been detected in the nursery, two had not been screened, and in the remaining child, the retinal periphery was not seen clearly when examined in the special care nursery. Six of the eleven children had myopia, and the refractive errors were mainly high (Table 3); one child had hypermetropic astigmatism, and four were emmetropic. Two children had strabismus, one convergent, one vertical. No children were blind because of RLF, and only one eye had severely reduced vision, due to a retinal fold (Grade IV).

TABLE 3

R.	-2	-9	-7	-7	-0	-4
L.	-4	-9	-0	-9	-7	-9

The refractive errors in diopters found in the six cases of RLF with myopia.

TABLE 4

STRABISMUS
20 CONVERGENT - 1 VERTICAL

			Cerebral Palsy
No Refractive Error		13	(5)
Hypermetropia	>3D	2	
Myopia/Astigmatism	>2D	3	(1)
Hypermetropic Astigmatism	>2D	3	(1)
TOTAL		21	

The refractive status of the 21 children with strabismus. The number with cerebral palsy are indicated separately.

Of the 21 children with strabismus, in 20 it was convergent, and one was vertical. The refractive data of these children are shown in Table 4, in which it can be seen that no significant refractive error was found in thirteen, hypermetropia in two, myopia with or without astigmatism in three, and simple hypermetropic astigmatism in three. Seven of the children with strabismus had cerebral palsy and RLF was present in two.

TABLE 5

Hypermetropia	>3D	3
Myopia	>2D	6
Myopic/ Astigmatism	>2D	2
Hypermetropic/ Astigmatism	>2D	8

The refractive errors found in 19 children.

The refractive errors found in 19 children showed a predominance of myopia and hypermetropic astigmatism (Table 5), but myopia was particularly associated with cicatricial RLF, being found in six out of the eight cases. The prevalence of refractive errors in children without RLF was 13%.

DISCUSSION

The ocular morbidity was high in this group of VLBW infants, and this may be due to the considerable bias for those children with known, or easily recognizable defects, to have responded to the offer of an examination. Thus the figures may be artificially high, but on scrutinizing the available data on the 66 children who did not have an eye examination, six had developing RLF when examined in the premature nursery, six had cerebral palsy, and a further four children had strabismus diagnosed by other ophthalmologists. Thus the group of children not examined would not have been free from ocular problems. In view of this, the group examined is thought to be a representative sample of VLBW infants, and that the given figures are a valid estimate of the prevalence of ocular defects.

The incidence and severity of RLF has fluctuated greatly over the past forty years. It is relevant to compare the present state with that pertaining before intensive care procedures were in common use, but when oxygen levels were monitored by arterial sampling, and some transcutaneous monitoring was performed. Gunn et al(3) reported on babies born 1975-76, none of whom had assisted respiration, and found a 60.5% survival rate of infants weighing 501g - 1500g, 80 of the 95 survivors had an ophthalmological examination after discharge from hospital, and 27 (33.8%) were found to have RLF. Eight (10%) of these were in Grades II-V, and two (2.5%) were completely blind.

In the present paper, cicatricial RLF was found in eleven (10%) of VLBW infants, eight (7%) of whom were in Grade II-IV, and significant ocular problems occurred in seven, but none was blind. This latter finding does not seem to be fortuitous, as, todate (September 1982), no case of blindness, caused by RLF, in any of the VLBW infants born and treated at this hospital since the beginning of the study in 1977, has been found. A prevalence of RLF similar to ours was reported recently(4) in a control trial of vitamin E for prevention of RLF in which a total of eight cases (8%) of cicatricial RLF occurred in 99 control and treated children.

When we consider only babies weighing <1000g at birth; in our series 19% had cicatricial RLF, which is slightly higher than the figure of 16% reported by Pape et al,(5) for babies born in 1974, but two of their babies (5%) were blind. So the prevalence of cicatricial RLF following the introduction of intensive care units does not seem to have increased significantly, and a decrease in the severity of the disease seems to have occurred.

Myopia has been recognized as a common ocular feature in premature infants,(6) but it has long been suspected that it is mainly associated with RLF. Zacharias et al(7) reported that RLF of all degrees would produce myopia, and Kalina(8) found that myopia was not prevalent when RLF was excluded. Gunn et al(3) found myopia in 37% of cases with RLF and 2% of cases without RLF. Scharf et al(9) did not find any difference in the prevalence of myopia in a group of children weighing between 1000g and 2000g, and those weighing between 2000g and 2500g at birth, but he found an incidence of approximately 43% of myopia in both, which does not accord with other reports. Shapiro et al(10) compared the refractive status in babies weighing between 1750g and 2000g with those weighing less than 2000g at birth, and found no increase in myopia, but the mean weight of his premature babies was over 1600g, so any tendency for myopia in the smaller ones may not have been apparent. Kushner(11) found no significant difference in the refractive errors found in VLBW infants who were free from RLF changes at 36 weeks gestational and chronological age, and those found in full term infants when examined at two years of age. The results in our series tend to support the association between RLF and myopia, as seven of the eight myopic children had been screened in the premature nursery, and in six of them developing RLF had been noted, one was thought to be normal, but later became myopic (R -3.0 D.S., L -5 D.S.) and it is not impossible that minor changes were missed in this infant. The difficulties in detection and interpretation of fundus appearances is highlighted by the considerable discrepancy in reports of the prevalence of developing RLF among premature babies. Hittner et al(12) found that 65% of babies weighing <1500g showed the changes of developing RLF, while Finer et al (4) found a prevalence of 28% in those weighing under 1000g and 20% of those weighing between 1000g and 1500g. Keith et al(2) found that 23.3% of those weighing <1000g and 6% of those between 1000g - 1500g showed RLF changes. The staging classifications for developing RLF differed slightly in the three papers, but the difference was mainly in the grading rather than changes observed, so the results should be comparable. However, it seems that the majority of cases of myopia can be predicted from examination in the premature nursery, and only the odd case will be unexpected.

Strabismus is common among VLBW infants, being found in 21 (19%) out of the 111 children reviewed, and it was reported (by other ophthalmologists) to be present in four of the 66 children not seen by us. Assuming no other cases of strabismus were present, the gross prevalence in the whole cohort is 25 out of 177 (14%). If the 21 cases of cerebral palsy are excluded (fifteen reviewed, and six not reviewed), because of the high prevalence of strabismus and if the 11 cases of RLF are also excluded (two with strabismus) because of the known existence of ocular abnormalities; only sixteen (11%) cases of strabismus remain among the 145 VLBW infants. The 11% is comparable with Kushner's(11) figure of 13% for strabismus among premature babies without RLF or cerebral palsy, while in the group of comparable full-term infants, strabismus was present only in 2.7%.

Children who developed cerebral palsy were found to have a high ocular morbidity, particularly optic atrophy and strabismus. Three children in this group had severe optic atrophy causing blindness, and these were the only blind children in the series.

At the Royal Women's Hospital, Melbourne, a significant increase in survival has been achieved, together with a downward trend in the prevalence of strabismus and blindness. This has been reported(13) in a recent study of three cohorts of inborn VLBW infants. For those managed at the time when intensive care was in its early stage of development (1966-70), the long term survival rate was 37%; 21.6% had strabismus, and 3.9% were blind. For the cohort treated in 1973-74, when intensive care was more sophisticated, the long term survival rate changed little (37.3%), but the incidence of strabismus was reduced to 13.4% and 3% of children were blind. In the most recent era (1977-78), 68.5% of the cohort survived to the age of two years, 12.4% had strabismus, and 1.2% were blind. Blindness was due to RLF in 1.3% of children in the first cohort, 1.5% in the second cohort, and in none of the children in the third cohort. We wish to stressed that these results related to inborn infants only, since the figures are not strictly comparable with those of our present study.

The purpose of this survey was to assess the degree of ocular morbidity in VLBW infants, assess the value of the screening in the premature nursery for RLF, and at two years for the detection of ocular morbidity. From the results we may conclude that if a premature baby does not have cerebral palsy, and is free from RLF changes, then one can expect normal vision, but strabismus or astigmatism will occur in approximately 18%. For this reason, it seems reasonable to continue examinations at two years of age, but if RLF, particularly Stage III, has been seen, then the child should be more closely monitored after discharge from hospital.

ACKNOWLEDGEMENTS

We are grateful to the pediatricians at the Royal Women's Hospital, Dr. F.R. Betheras, Dr. L. Markman, Dr. K. Mountain, Dr. L. Murton, and Dr. P. Wearne, for allowing us access to their patients. To Miss Kate Hobson for technical assistance and Mrs. Gayle Poor for secretarial assistance.

REFERENCES

1. Kitchen WH, Yu VFH et al: Collaborative study of very-low-birthweight infants: Outome of two-year-old survivors. Lancet(I):1457-1460, 1982.

2. Keith CG, Smith ST, Lansdell BJ: Retrolental fibroplasia: A study of the incidence and aetiological factors, 1977-1979 Med J Aust 2:589-592, 1981.

3. Gunn TR, Easdown J, Outerbridge EW, Aranda JV: Risk factors in retrolental fibroplasia. Paediatrics 65:1096-1100, 1980.

4. Finer NN, Schindler RF, Grant G, Hill GB, Peters KL: Effect of intramuscular vitamin E on frequency and severity of retrolental fibroplasia. A controlled trial. Lancet (I):1087-1091, 1982.

5. Pape KE, Buncic RJ, Ashby S, Fitzhardinge PM: The status at two years of low-birth-weight infants born in 1974 with birth weights less than 1001gm. J Paediatr 92:253-260, 1978.

6. Fletcher MC, Brandon S: Myopia of prematurity. Am J Ophthalmol 40:474-481, 1955.

7. Zacharias L, Chisholm JF, Chapman RB. Visual and ocular damage in retrolental fibroplasia. Am J Ophthalmol 53:337-345, 1962.

8 Kalina R: Ophthalmic examination of children of low birth weight. Am J Ophthalmol 67:134-136, 1969.

9. Scharf J, Zonis S, Zeltzer M: Refraction in premature babies. Metabolic Ophthalmol 2:395-396, 1978.

10. Shapiro A, Yanko L, Nawratzki I, Merin S: Refractive power of premature children at infancy and early childhood. Am J Ophthalmol 90:234-238, 1980.

11. Kushner BJ: Strabismus and amblyopia associated with regressed retinopathy of prematurity. Arch Ophthalmol 100:256-261, 1982.

12. Hittner HM, Godio LB, Rudolph AJ et al: Retrolental fibroplasia; efficacy of vitamin E in a double-blind clinical study of preterm infants. New Eng J Med 305:1365-1371, 1981.

13. Kitchen WH, Ryan MM, Richards A et al: Changing outcome over 13 years of very-low-birthweight infants. Semin Perinatol 6:373-389, 1982.

EARLY SURGICAL ALIGNMENT FOR CONGENITAL ESOTROPIA

M. R. Ing

ABSTRACT

To provide sufficient numbers of patients varying in age of initial adequate surgical alignment for congenital esotropia, over 150 patients managed by seven ophthalmologists in three countries were personally examined by the author and the results compiled for a clinical study. From this population group, 106 patients were chosen who had reliable answers, satisfactory alignment and an ophthalmologist's confirmation exam of the congenital nature of the problem by at least one year of age.

The results of sensory testing showed that those adequately aligned by the age of 6 months versus 12 months versus 24 months wee not statistically different, but those patients aligned after 24 months of age demonstrated a significantly lower percentage with evidence for binocularity ($p <.001$).

The results of the present clinical study demonstrate that the initial adequate surgical alignment in the congenital esotropic patient should be accomplished by 2 years of age to attain the highest yield of binocular function.

INTRODUCTION

Previous clinical studies have not agreed concerning the optimum time for surgical ocular alignment in congenital esotropia.

Recall that it wasn't until 1958 that the first cure for congenital esotropia was reported by Costenbader.(1) He described a patient whom he had surgically aligned by the age of 16 months who demonstrated, 5 years later, the ability to fuse Worth 4 lights at 13 inches and phoria responses on cover testing. Costenbader recommended surgical alignment after esotropia found in infancy (which included congenital esotropia) by 6 to 18 months age age.(2) The recommendation

STRABISMUS II
ISBN 0-8089-1424-3

of early surgery was supported by the published series by Taylor(3,4) and Ing et al(5) in the United States, Stumpf(6) in Germany, Gale(7) in Australia, and Uemura(8) in Japan. The advice to operate before 18 months of age, however, was challenged by von Noorden et al,(9) and Fisher et al(10) contested the concept that surgery between 6 to 12 months led to statistically significant better results than surgery performed on infants between the ages of 12 to 24 months. Nevertheless, Foster et al(11) and Reinecke(12) have concluded that the prognosis for a functional result was better when surgical treatment was performed by 2 years of age.

Somewhat belatedly, the laboratory studies in the development of the mammalian visual system, particularly those of the recent Nobel prizewinning laureates Hubel and Wiesel(13-17) have supported the concept that earlier rather than later surgical alignment should provide a better developed neurophysiologic matrix for a binocular result following strabismus surgery. In addition, psychophysical investigations in human subjects bridged the gap between animal experiments in the laboratory and clinical studies by ophthalmologists. Banks et al(18) in their investigations of the interocular transfer of the tilt after-effect, concluded that "...the sensitive period for the development of binocularity begins several months after birth and peaks between one and three years of age. In cases of congenital esotropia, early corrective surgery appears to be indicated for the development of cortical binocularity..."

Among the difficulties facing the investigator who attempts to evaluate the results of treatment has been the controversy as to what group of strabismic infants have "congenital" esotropia and what criteria denote a cure of the condition. Different tests used by different researchers have been given different relative importance in the previous evaluations, leading to further confusion about the results. Furthermore, the results of treatment have been reported on relatively small numbers of patients so that even the statistical evaluations have been subject to question.

SUBJECTS AND METHODS

To avoid the various pitfalls of previous clinical studies, the author conducted a multi-center study in which the following criteria were used for selection of patients: (1) a history of esotropia by 6 months of age, (2) confirmation by an ophthalmologist's diagnosis by 1 year of age, (3) first surgical alignment achieved to within 10 prism diopters of orthophoria (as opposed to first surgery) for a minimum of 6 months, (4) sufficient maturity to reliably respond to sensory testing. Patients with neurological abnormalities were excluded.

The author personally performed the examination on all patients except those previously treated by him. The tests were uniformly performed on all patients using the same testing instruments and these tests were done prior to obtaining any information concerning the clinical history in order to minimize prejudical bias. Corrected Snellen visual acuities were obtained. Cover testing was performed with strict accommodation control techniques that included wearing full refractive correction and fixating 20/30 letter targets at distance and near. Cover tests included the cover-uncover, simultaneous prism and cover, and the alternate cover test. The sensory tests were: (1) Bagolini striated glasses with fixation target at 1/3 meter, (2) Worth 4 lights at 1/3 meter, and (3) the Polaroid Titmus vectographic stereotest.

A total of 162* patients from eight centers in three countries were examined but all patients were eliminated who did not have a confirming ophthalmologist's examination by 12 months of age, whose history was unreliable or conflicting, who had high hyperopia and a history suggesting acquired esotropia and who had a history of never being adequately aligned. Of the 106 patients retained for the study, there were 54 males and 52 females.

RESULTS

The patients were divided into four subgroups according to the age of initial adequate surgical alignment:

1) Aligned by age 6 months. (Cases 1 through 20)
2) Aligned by age 7 to 12 months. (Cases 21 through 66)
3) Aligned by age 13 to 24 months. (Cases 67 through 90)
4) Aligned by age 25 to 79 months.(Cases 91 through 106)

*Eight of the author's patients were included in the study and report but were examined by one of the participating strabismologists under the same condition of no previous knowledge of patient history.

The subgroups were analyzed and compared., and were found similar in:

(1) Confirmation age by ophthalmologist's exam (average: 7 months overall).

(2) Length of follow-up from initial adequate surgical alignment (average: 8 years, 4 months, for the groups as a whole).

(3) Length of follow-up from the last surgical procedure (average: 7 years).

(4) Initial refraction (average: +1.6 diopters).

(5) Initial deviation (average: 55 prism diopters).

(6) Number of horizontal muscle procedures (53% received satisfactory alignment from one procedure, 35% required two horizontal procedures and 13% required three or more).

(7) Number of patients who received vertical muscle surgery (33% of the group as a whole).

(8) Number of patients who received glasses or miotics to nurture the results (68% of the group as a whole).

(9) Incidence of residual amblyopia, defined as difference in corrected visual acuity of one line or more (46% of the group as a whole).

(10) Motor alignment. There was no statistically significant difference in the motor alignment results of the four subgroups (Table 1).*

(11) Incidence of dissociated divergence (62% of the group as a whole).

TABLE 1

Present Alignment

Alignment Age (mo)	Phoria or Intermittent Tropia (%)	Small-Angle Tropia (%)	Large-Angle Tropia (%)	No. Cases
0 - 6	6 (30%)	14 (70%)	0 (0%)	20
7 - 12	17 (37%)	26 (56%)	3 (7%)	46
13 - 24	11 (46%)	13 (54%)	0 (0%)	24
25 - 79	3 (18%)	11 (69%)	2 (13%)	16
Total	37 (35%)	64 (60%)	5 (5%0	106

*Chi square = 7.4, 6 degrees of freedom, not significant

TABLE 2

Results of Bagolini Striated Glasses Testing

Alignment Age (mo)	Binocularity %	No Binocularity %	No. Cases
0 - 6	20 (100%)	0 (0%)	20
7 - 12	46 (100%)	0 (0%)	46
13 - 24	23 (95%)	1 (5%)	24
25 - 79	7 (44%)	9 (56%)	16
Total	96 (91%)	10 (9%)	106

The evaluation of evidence for binocularity with Bagolini lenses did however reveal significant differences between the three earlier-aligned subgroups in contrast to the later-aligned one. Almost all patients aligned by 6, 12, or 24 months of age showed a binocular response while less than one-half of those aligned after the age of 24 months did so (Table 2).

The stereoacuity measurements, made the Polaroid Titmus vectograph overlay, were recorded in seconds or arc and reproducibility was continually checked throughout the exam. As noted by Reinecke,(19) validity of the stereopsis test is checked by simple reversal of the target, in which case the circle with disparity should appear to be recessed rather than standing out.

Results of the crucial sensory examination with Worth 4 lights and stereopsis testing are shown in Table 3. Since patients with both fusion and stereopsis are felt to have a more secure form of binocularity than those with only one of these qualities, the table displays the number, with these functions noted separately. Table 3 also shows the number from each subgroup who responded negatively to either sensory test. Alignment achieved by age 0 through 24 months results in a high percentage of patients with evidence for binocularity, but a much smaller percentage of those aligned after the age of 24 months show these functions (Figure 1). The differences between the first three subgroups (aligned by 24 months) compared with the latest-aligned subgroup reach a high level of statistical significance,* while the difference in results between each of the three earlier-aligned subgroups did not.**

DISCUSSION

As noted by Taylor,(4) it is unusual for an ophthalmologist to have the opportunity to make the diagnosis of "congenital" esotropia at birth. Generally however, despite the risk of some cases being extremely early "acquired esotropia", the diagnosis can be reasonably made if the onset is apparent before 6 months of age.(5,20,21)

Previous studies have sought to determine the optimum age of alignment for the congenital esotrope. Although these studies have reached some preliminary conclusions, they are usually based on the age of initial surgery rather than the age of initial adequate alignment, and have often lacked adequate controls. A prospective, randomized, blind study is not possible since the age of initial adequate alignment does not always correspond to the age of initial surgery and there is no way to prospectively determine the former. A retrospective study therefore is mandatory with the methods of examination and diagnosis standardized.

The present study clearly showed that the one major parameter in which there was a statistically significant difference was the evidence for binocularity. The yield of binocularity in patients aligned after the age of 24 months was substantially less than those aligned before that age ($p < .001$).

---

*Difference between the first three subgroups vs latest-aligned subgroup, chi square = 46.9, probability of error less than .001, 6 degrees of dreedom.

**Difference between each of the first three subgroups (6 months vs 12 months vs 24 months), chi square = 7.03, 4 degrees of freedom, not significant.

All patients aligned by the age of 6 months showed evidence for binocularity, and those aligned by the age of 12 months or 24 months had a high percentage of binocularity. There was no statistically significant difference in binocularity among the earlier-aligned subgroups. These results concur therefore with a smaller, less controlled series previously reported.(11)

Fusion of the Worth 4 lights can be demonstrated in patients with up to 8 prism diopters of heterotropia, and some investigators(5,22) have concluded with Costenbader that "the visualizing of four lights in the presence of bifoveal fixation, or even in the presence of a small manifest esotropia, suggests a more stable binocular relationship than if no fusion could be demonstrated."(2(p408)) Parks felt that these patients obtained peripheral fusion despite a foveal esodeviation by virture of the ability of Panum's visual space for peripheral binocular vision to encompass a retinal image disparity up to 5 degrees of esodeviation. Parks also pointed out that fusional vergence amplitudes in monofixation are comparable to those in bifoveal fixation.

Two previous studies(5,22) have shown that those enjoyed fusion of Worth 4 lights also had fusional ability with the major amblyoscope so the latter test was not used in this study.

As reported earlier, there was no exact correlation between fusion of either standard or micro Worth 4 lights and the finding of stereopsis. Some patients with one function did not demonstrate the other and this fact supports the concept that they are different facets of binocular function.

Of the few aligned after 24 months of age who demonstrated evidence for binocularity, only two patients showed both fusion and stereopsis and both of these were aligned before the age of 3 years. One patient in this group did however show evidence of gross stereopsis with a small residual angle of deviation, even though adequate alignment was not achieved until after 4-1/2 years of age. Therefore it is apparently possible to establish some, albeit weaker, evidence of binocularity even at that late age.

As previously noted by Taylor,(3) refined stereopsis (40 seconds of arc) was possible for the aligned congenital esotrope, but is extremely rare. Only two patients in this study demonstrated this degree of excellence in stereoacuity. Most patients achieved what has been designated as "gross" stereoacuity (200 to 3000 seconds of arc). The vast majority of patients who showed a functional cure with stereopsis fell within the confines of the monofixation syndrome.

FIGURE I

BINOCULARITY RESULTS OF PATIENTS ADEQUATELY ALIGNED

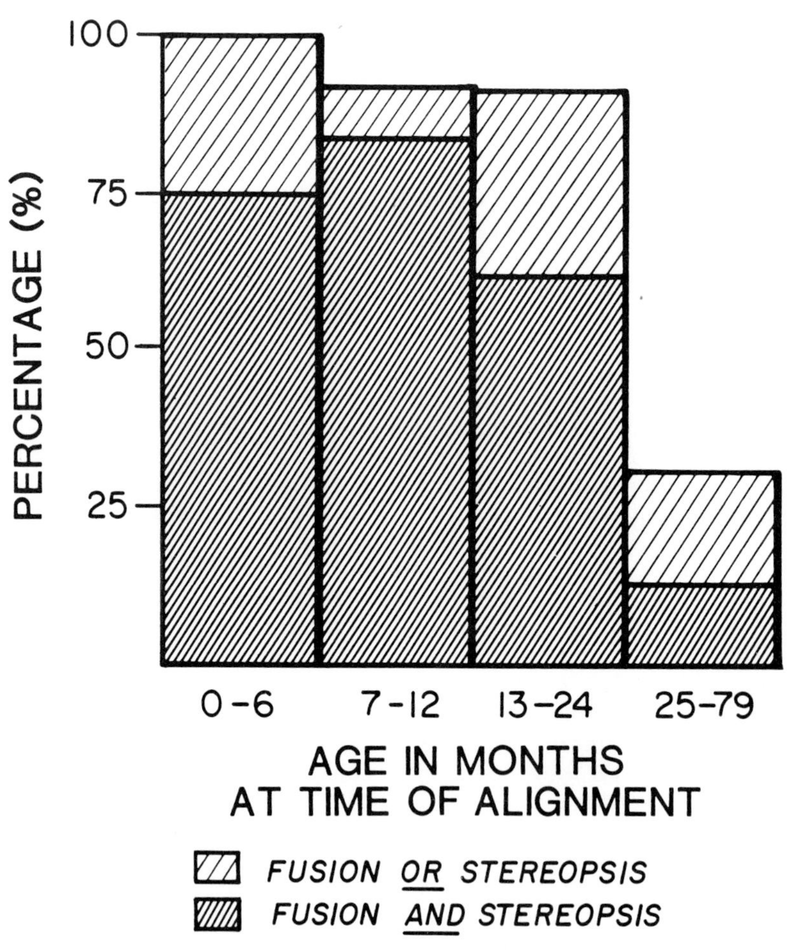

TABLE 3

Results of Worth 4 Light and Stereopsis Testing

Alignment Age (mo)	Fusion and Stereopsis	Fusion or Stereopsis	Neither	No. Cases
0 - 6	15	5	0	20
7 - 12	38	4	4	46
13 - 24	15	7	2	24
25 - 79	2	3	11	16
Total	70	19	17	106

Jampolsky(23) has called the cover test the "supreme court test" of binocularity, and this test was routinely performed in the present study. Jampolsky, however, had earlier concluded that there was a surprising mixture of tropia and phoria in his "fusional disparity" cases,(24) and up to 8 prism diopters of heterotropia can apparently co-exist with peripheral binocularity in the monofixation cases discussed by Parks.(22)

Absence of a manifest deviation may or may not indicate bifixation, and a more reliable indicator of bifixation appears to be refined stereoacuity. Many strabismologists have seen a presumably well-aligned congenital esotrope slip into an exotropic position and one might conclude that at some point these previously esotropic cases were close to or definitely "orthophoric" on their way to exotropia. Clearly, binocularity could only be demonstrated by relying on sensory tests to augment a clinical impression derived from motor tests alone.

ACKNOWLEDGEMENTS

A modification of a thesis submitted as partial fulfillment for membership in the American Ophthalmological Society, May 1981.

Acknowledgement is also given to Dr. Robert Worth, Professor of Public Health, University of Hawaii School of Medicine, who prepared the statistical analysis, and to the following strabismologists wihout whose patients this study could not have been accomplished:

Dr. David Hiles, Pittsburgh PA
Dr. Arthur Jampolsky, San Francisco CA
Dr. Joseph Lang, Zurich, Switzerland
Dr. Marshall Parks, Washington DC
Dr. John Pratt-Johnson, Vancouver BC, Canada
Dr. Alan Scott, San Francisco CA
Dr. Daniel Taylor, New Britain CT

REFERENCES

1. Costenbader FD: Clinical course and management of esotropia, in Allen JH (ed): Strabismus Ophthalmic Symposium II. St Louis, CV Mosby Co, 1958, pp 325-353.

2. Costenbader FD: Infantile esotropia. Trans Am Ophthalmol Soc 59:397-429, 1961.

3. Taylor DM: How early is early surgery in the management of strabismus? Arch Ophthalmol 70:752-756, 1963.

4. Taylor DM: Is congenital esotropia functionally curable? Trans Am Ophthalmol Soc 70:529-576, 1972.

5. Ing M, Costenbader FD, Parks MM, Albert DG: Early surgery for congential esotropia. Am J Ophthalmol 61:1419-1427, 1966.

6. Stumpf F: Is early surgery really necessary?, in Mein J, Bierlaagh JJM, Brummelkamp-Dons TEA (eds): Orthoptics: Proceedings of the Second International Orthoptic Congress. Amsterdam, Excerpta Medica, 1971, pp 220-223.

7. Gale D: The surgical management of esotropia in infancy. Trans Ophthalmol Soc UK 92:675-683, 1972.

8. Uemura Y: Surgical correction of infantile esotropia. Jpn J Ophthalmol 17:50-59, 1973.

9. von Noorden GK, Isaza A, Parks ME: Surgical treatment of congenital esotropia. Trans Am Acad Ophthalmol Otolaryngol 76:1465-1478, 1972.

10. Fisher NF, Flom MC, Jampolsky A: Early surgery for congenital esotropia. Am J Ophthalmol 65:439-443, 1968.

11. Foster RS, Paul TO, Jampolsky A: Management of infantile esotropia. Am J Ophthalmol 82:291-299, 1976.

12. Reinecke RD: Current concepts in ophthalmology: Strabismus. N Engl J Med 300:1139-1141, 1979.

13. Hubel DH, Wiesel TN: Receptive fields, binocular interaction and functional architecture in the cat's visual cortex. J Physiol (Lond) 160:106-154, 1962.

14. Hubel DH, Wiesel TN: Binocular interaction in striate cortex in kittens reared with artificial squint. J Neurophysiol 28:1041-1059, 1965.

15. Hubel DH, Wiesel TN: The period of susceptibility to the physiological effects of unilateral eye closure in kittens. J Physiol (Lond) 206:419-436, 1970.

16. Wiesel TN, Hubel DH: Effects of visual deprivation on morphology and physiology of cells in the cat's lateral geniculate body. J Neurophysiol 26:978-993, 1963.

17. Wiesel TN, Hubel DH: Comparison of the effects of unilateral and bilateral eye closure on cortical unit responses in kittens. J Neurophysiol 28:1029-1040, 1965.

18. Banks MS, Aslin RN, Letson RD: Sensitive period for the development of human binocular vision. Science 190:675-677, 1975.

19. Reinecke RD, Discussion of presentation by Drs Samuel C. Rawlings and J. Terry Yates. Ophthalmology 86:1471-1473, 1979.

20. Costenbader FD: Factors in the cure of squint, in Allen JH (ed): Strabismus Ophthalmology Symposium. St. Louis, CV Mosby Co, 1950, pp 367-376.

21. Parks MM: Operate early for congenital strabismus, in Brockhurst RJ, Boruchoff SA, Hutchinson BT, Lessell S (eds): Controversy in Ophthalmology. Philadelphia, WB Saunders Co, 1977, pp 423-433.

22. Parks MM: The monofixation syndrome. Trans Am Ophthalmol Soc 67:609-657, 1969.

23. Jampolsky A: A simplified approach to strabismus diagnosis, in Burian HM (ed): Strabismus: Proceedings of the New Orleans Academy of Ophthalmology. St Louis, CV Mosby Co, 1971, pp 34-92.

24. Jampolsky A: Management of small-degree esodeviations, in Haik GM (ed): Strabismus: Proceedings of the New Orleans Academy of Ophthalmology. St Louis, CV Mosby Co, 1962, pp 123-139.

RESULTS OF TREATMENT IN CONGENITAL "INFANTILE" ESOTROPIA

J.A. Pratt-Johnson and G. Tillson

ABSTRACT

Forty patients with infantile esotropia were treated throughout by the same ophthalmologist. The results, following treatment, are reported and discussed. Follow-up ranged from 5 to 14 years. All the patients had their initial surgery by the age of 2 years, 4 months. Thirty-four patients had their angle of deviation reduced to within 10 prism diopters of orthotropia. Twenty-six patients maintained this angle from the age of 2 years, 9 months or earlier. Only 6 patients showed evidence of binocular function on both the troposcope and the Wirt stereo test. The presence of DVD, nystagmus and amblyopia appeared to be the main reasons why patients did not develop fusion.

INTRODUCTION

Infants born with crossed eyes or who develop crossed eyes within the first few months of life are described as having congenital or infantile esotropia. In this paper we will use the term Infantile Esotropia. The majority of these patients have a syndrome which consists of convergent strabismus of large amount, usually in excess of 40 prism diopters and frequently cross fixate. A significant proportion of these patients later develop dissociated vertical divergent strabismus, overaction of both inferior oblique muscles and nystagmus.

There are occasional rare reports of central bifoveal sensory fusion being obtained after the treatment of patients with infantile esotropia but most authors agree that the best result that can be obtained is a monofixation syndrome with peripheral fusion. Excluding those patients with a marked accommodative factor and what appears to be an acquired accommodative strabismus within the first year of life, we have never seen a patient with the infantile esotropia syndrome who has developed central fusion. There are some reports in the literature which give details of sensory testing of patients who have had this syndrome.(1-3) Most of these reports record less than half the patients with some

STRABISMUS II
ISBN 0-8089-1424-3

peripheral fusion. This study was undertaken to examine those factors that would appear to influence whether or not a patient develops fusion.

PATIENTS AND METHODS

Forty patients were randomly selected provided they had fulfilled the following criteria:

1. Cross fixating esotropia confirmed by an ophthalmologist by the age of 9 months.
2. All patients were treated throughout by the same ophthalmologist and followed in his private office from the time of diagnosis until they were visually adult. (We have taken 6 years as being the age of visual maturity for the purposes of this paper.) The follow-up period ranged from 5 years to 14 years and 2 months.
3. All patients were capable of responding reliably to sensory tests of binocular function at the time of the final examination.
4. No other neurological abnormality was present.

All, except two (aged 5 and 9/12 years, and aged 5 and 11/12 years) of the patients were over the age of 6 years and the average age was 9 years, 2 months.

All patients, in our study, had their initial surgery before the age of 2 years, 4 months. Most patients were seen at least every 3 months from the time treatment was commenced until the age of 6 years. All patients were given a complete ophthalmological and orthoptic examination for the final assessment. The sensory tests for binocular function included the troposcope and the Wirt stereo test. The full optical correction was worn if there was a refractive error.

Peripheral fusion was considered to be present using the troposcope if a minimum of 4 prism diopters total fusional amplitude, using fusion slides with peripheral controls (Clement Clarke Ltd. F 113 and F 114 - Fig 1), were elicited. Most patients with peripheral fusion had 15 prism diopters or more of fusional amplitude. The amplitude of fusion did not necessarily relate to responses with the Wirt stereo test. Fusion slides with central controls (Clement Clarke Ltd. F 93 and F 94 - Fig 2) were also used to assess these patients but all of them suppressed one eye with these slides.

Stereopsis was considered to be present using the Wirt stereo test at near if the child could reliably and repeatedly identify stereo acuity of at least 3000 seconds of arc. No patient recorded better than 100 seconds of arc on this test.

The aim of treatment

Our aim in the mangagement of the infantile esotropia syndrome has been to reduce and maintain the deviation within 10 prism diopters of orthotropia because this is generally agreed to be the maximum angle of deviation which allows the development of peripheral fusion and the monofixation syndrome.(4-6) Treatment has included surgery, glasses, occlusion, miotics and prisms.

Surgical treatment

The amount of surgery was proportionate to the size of the esotropia (with full optical correction in place, if applicable). Bimedial recessions up to 6.0 mm were used for deviations up to 50 prism diopters. In addition one lateral rectus was resected up to 10 mm for deviations up 50 to 75 prism diopters and both lateral recti were resected additionally in deviations in excess of 75 prism diopters. The inferior cul de sac incision and approach in the conjunctiva were used in all cases.

In our previous study involving an analysis of 67 patients using the above technique 85% were reduced by the first surgery to within 10 prism diopters of orthotropia when examined within one week after surgery. In this study of 40 patients, 82% were within orthotropia immediately post surgery using the same technique. Hiles reported 85% of his patients achieved reduction of the angle to within 10 prism diopters of orthotropia.(7) Helveston noted that 91% of his patients were within 10 prism diopters of orthotropia immediately postoperatively, using the technique of bimedial recession combined with conjunctival recession.(8) It would, therefore, appear that a high percentage of patients are reduced to less than 10 prism diopters residual esotropia irrespective of the actual technique of initial surgery. If the initial surgery can align approximately 85% of patients satisfactorily and glasses, miotics, prisms and more surgery are available for the remainder, one can assume that satisfactory motor realignment in the treatment of infantile esotropia is not the main obstacle to obtaining fusion and stereopsis.

RESULTS

The sensory analysis of those patients with binocular function results, based on the troposcope and the Wirt stereo test, is shown in Table I.

TABLE 1

Sensory Results at Final Assessment (40 Patients)

Group	Sensory Results	Numbers
A	Fusion on troposcope Positive Wirt stereo test	6
B	Fusion on troposcope Negative Wirt stereo test	11
C	No fusion on troposcope Negative Wirt stereo test	23

The patients were divided into 3 groups on the basis of their sensory function. Group A represents those 6 patients who had fusion on the troposcope and stereopsis on the Wirt test as previously described whereas Group B represents those patients who had fusion only. In Group C although simultaneous macular perception was demonstrated on the troposcope in one patient and simultaneous foveal perception in another, none of the 23 patients in this group had demonstrable fusion or stereopsis. Seventeen, out of the 40 patients, thus showed some evidence of binocular function whereas the remainder showed no evidence.

TABLE 2

Deviation Always 10 Prism Diopters or Less (26 Patients)

Group	Sensory Results
A	6
B	11
C	9
Total	26

We have defined our aim of treatment as the reduction of the deviation to within 10 prism diopters of orthotropia and the maintenance of this position. Table II analyses the sensory results in those patients in which our aim was achieved. It can be seen that 26 patients fulfill the criteria of always being within 10 prism diopters of orthotropia following treatment. An additional 8 patients were reduced to within 10 prism diopters of orthotropia but failed to maintain this position. Only 6 patients in the series never achieved the goal of having their strabismus reduced to within 10 prism diopters of orthotropia despite intensive treatment involving glasses, miotics, prisms and further surgery.

A total of 34 patients had within 10 prism diopters of orthotropia although 8 did not maintain this position. a further analysis of these patients shows that 17 patients are in Groups A and B and have some evidence of binocular function. The other 17 patients are in Group C and do not show any binocular function on the tests described. This suggests that reducing the deviation to within 10 prism diopters of orthotropia may not be the significant factor which determines whether or not these patients develop binocular function. A recent study by Ing showed that surgical alignment should be accomplished by the age of 2 for the highest yield of binocular function.(9)

TABLE 3

Age Stable Reduction of Deviation to 10 Prism Diopters or Less Achieved (26 Patients)

Group	12m	18m	24m	30m	More than 30m	Total
A	3	2	0	1	0	6
B	5	1	0	2	1	9
C	4	2	1	0	4	11
Total	12	5	1	3	5	26

Table III analyses the age of the patient when the aim of treatment was achieved in our study. All 40 patients in our study had their initial surgery before the age of 2 years, 4 months and the large majority of these patients had their angle of deviation reduced to within 10 prism diopters of orthotropia by the age of 2. In our study the age at which motor alignment was achieved did not appear to be the significant factor in the sensory outcome.

TABLE 4

Sensory Results in Patients with D.V.D. Nystagmus, Amblyopia (Final Assessment)

Group	D.V.D.	Nystagmus	Nystagmus + D.V.D.	Amblyopia 2 Lines or More
A	1	0	0	0
B	6	8	6	3
C	15	17	12	9
Total	22	25	18	12

Table IV analyses the incidence of dissociated vertical divergence (DVD), nystagmus and amblyopia as it relates to the 3 groups. It can be seen that DVD, nystagmus, and amblyopia are much more common in Group C who never obtained fusion.

The incidence of amblyopia was particularly revealing to us. It is interesting that, out of the total number of 40 patients, 20 were amblyopic when visual acuity was first reliably recorded with the HVOT test. Eighteen responded to occlusion therapy, 8 achieving a visual acuity of 6/9 (20/30) in the amblyopic eye and 10 achieved 6/18 to 6/12 (20/60 to 20/40). Although the infantile esotropia syndrome is not thought to be commonly associated with significant amblyopia we had 2 cases of dense amblyopia of 6/120 (20/400) and 6/60 (20/200) that were resistant to repeated occlusion. It would seem to be important that an effort should be made to prevent or minimise the effects of amblyopia in patients with the infantile esotropia syndrome by determining which is their dominant eye so that this can be occluded on a part-time basis.

CONCLUSIONS

Our results indicate that the presence of dissociated vertical divergence, nystagmus or amblyopia of two lines or more are the main reasons why patients with infantile esotropia do not develop sensory fusion and stereopsis despite alignment within 10 prism diopters of orthotropia by age two.

REFERENCES

1. Ing M, Costenbader FD, Parks MM, Albert DG: Early surgery for congenital esotropia. Am J Ophthalmol 61:1419-1427, 1966.

2. Botet RV, Calhoun JH, Harley RD: Development of monofixation syndrome in congenital esotropia. J Pediatr Ophthalmol Strabismus. 18:49-51, 1981.

3. Fisher NF, Flom MC, Jampolsky A: Early surgery of congenital esotropia. Am J Ophthalmol 65:439-443, 1968.

4. Pratt-Johnson JA, Barlow JM: Stereoacuity and fusional amplitude in foveal suppression. Can J Ophthalmol 10:56-60, 1975.

5. Von Norden GK, Isaza A, Parks ME: Surgical treatment of congenital esotropia. Trans Am Acad Ophthalmol Otolaryngol 76:1465-1478, 1972.

6. Parks MM: Stereoacuity as an indicator of bifixation. In Arruga A (ed): International Strabismus Symposium. Glessen, 1966, Basel, S Karger, 1968.

7. Hiles DA, Watson BA, Biglan AW: Characteristics of infantile esotropia following early bimedial rectus recession. Arch Opthalmol 98:697-703, 1980.

8. Helveston EM: Personal communication (1981).

9. Ing M: Personal communication (1982).

NYSTAGMUS BLOCKAGE SYNDROME: REVISITED

G. K. von Noorden and C. W. Avilla

ABSTRACT

Controversy exists whether the nystagmus blockage syndrome (NBS) constitutes an entiry *sui generis* that must be distinguished from other forms of infantile esotropia with and without nystagmus. We review the clinical characteristics of NBS, as defined by Cuppers and his school, and show that some of these features are not pathognomonic for NBS as they occur also with other forms of strabismus. However, we also show EOG data that demonstrate that there exists a group of patients with congenital nystagmus and variable esotropia in whom the angle of strabismus is inversely related to the intensity of the nystagmus. It is likely that a pathophysiological relationship exists between esotropia and nystagmus in such patients. The diagnosis NBS was made in 92 (12%) of 781 consecutive patients with infantile esotropia. A review of the surgical results show a high incidence of over- and undercorrections. Recession of both medial rectus muscles combined with posterior fixation appears to be the optimal procedure.

It is well recognized that there exists a frequent association between latent or manifest nystagmus on the one hand and infantile esotropia on the other hand.(1) It has also been noted for a long time that the intensity of congenital nystagmus frequently increases in abduction and decreases in adduction.(2-4) In 1952, Franceschetti and Dieterle(5) provided the first electro-oculographic demonstration of this asymmetry of nystagmus intensity in different gaze positions. These authors suggested that patients who habitually hold their dominant eye in the postion of least nystagmus could develop suppression and esotropia in the fellow eye. They were first to imply that esotropia may then develop secondarily to nystagmus, namely on a sensory basis.

In 1962, Ciancia(6) described a syndrome that was present in one-third of his patients with infantile esotropia. This consisted of:

STRABISMUS II
ISBN 0-8089-1424-3

a. esotropia of early onset
b. rather large angle of deviation
c. bilateral limitation of abduction
d. jerky nystagmus increasing in abduction and practically disappearing in adduction
e. head turn toward the side of the fixating eye

In 1964, Adelstein and Cuppers(7) described a clinically similar entity and pointed out that the esotropia in patients with congenital nystagmus may develop on the basis of hypertonicity of the medial rectus muscles caused by the patient's sustained effort to block the nystagmus by adducting one or both eyes. In other words, the nystagmus was thought to be primary and the esotropia secondary. Thus the nystagmus blockage syndrome (NBS) was born and soon this new etiological concept of certain forms of infantile esotropia swept across Europe as attested by numerous publications on this subject. Whereas Adelstein and Cupper recognized the NBS in 10% of their patients with infantile esotropia, we found it in only 4.8% of ours in an initial report(8) but other authors have reported its incidence to be as high as 80%(9) After the initial wave of enthusiasm subsided, critical voices became audible. These ranged from the sobering question whether the blockage mechanism existed at all(10) to the suggestion that this mechanism may only be valid when an inverse relationship between the angle of esotropia and the nystagmus intensity can actually be demonstrated.(11) In view of the controversy, it is not surprising that confusion has arisen whether the nystagmus blockage mechanism exists at all and if so, when this diagnosis should be made. It is the purpose of this paper to clarify this issue.

METHODS

We reviewed the charts of 789 consecutive patiehts with infantile esotropia who were examined personally by the first author between 1973 and 1982. All had an onset of esotropia between birth and the first six months of life. Applying the diagnostic criteria set forth by Cianci(6) and Adelstein and Cuppers(7) and, using variability of the angle as an additional diagnostic feature, 92 patients (12%) in this group met the description of the NBS. Next, we asked the question in what respect these patients differed from others with infantile esotropia. It is well known that dissociated vertical deviation (DVD) and primary overaction of the inferior oblique (OAIO) are features commonly associated with congenial esotropia.(1,12-16) If the NBS is nosologically different from other forms of infantile esotropia, one would not expect these associated findings to occur in these patients with the same frequency as they do in other forms of infantile esotropia. We, therefore, compared the rate of occurrence of DVD and OAIO in our patients diagnosed as having the NBS (Group I) with asn age matched control group (Group II) of infantile esotropes without nystagmus of the abducting eye. The controls were selected at random (in alphabetical order) from our data pool of 789 patients. Table 1 shows that DVD and OAIO occurred about half as frequently in patients diagnosed as having NBS as in the control group.

TABLE 1

Associated Anomalies in Infantile Esotropes With (Group I) and Without (Group II) Nystagmus of the Abducting Eye

	OAIO	DVD	Albinism, Down's Syndrome, Hydrocephalus, Cerebral Palsy
Group I (84)	44%	23%	25%
Group II (80)	73%	46%	1%

Table 1 also shows a high rate of occurrence of associated ocular or neurological anomalies (25%) in Group I. These anomalies consisted of oculocutaneous albinism, 5 patients (6%); Down's syndrome, 4 patients (5%); congenital hydrocephalus, 7 patients (9%) and cerebral palsy, 5 patients (6%). These data contrast with those obtained from Group II which contained only one patient with Down's syndrome.

We surmise from these data that patients with infantile esotropia and nystagmus with increased amplitudes in abduction differ from patients with infantile esotropia without nystagmus in two aspects: (1) lower prevalence of DVD and OAIO and (2) frequent association of neurological anomalies. While this difference suggests a nosological distinction between infantile esotropes with and without nystagmus it does not answer the question whether there also exists a casual relationship between nystagmus and esotropia, as suggested by Adelstein and Cuppers.(7) The available evidence is insufficient to justify the assumption that the mere association between nystagmus and infantile esotropia suggests a nystagmus blocking mechanism. On the other hand, there are certain clinical situations where the concept of nystagmus blockage may well apply. For example, we have observed patients with large and variable angles of esotropia, usually in excess of 40 prism diopters, with an onset in early infancy. Frequently both eyes are adducted and the head is turned toward the side of the fixating, adducted eye. Spontaneous nystagmus is usually absent but bursts of manifest nystagmus may develop simultaneously with a decrease of the esodeviation. It appears likely that the nystagmus is dampened (blocked) by adduction or convergency innervation. Patching of either eye causes the head to be turned toward the non-patched eye which differentiates this group from cross-fixators. Abduction may be mildly limited but can always be elicited with the doll's head maneuver. Most importantly, a manifest nystagmus develops as soon as the fixating, adducted eye moves toward primary position and the amplitude of the nystagmus further increases as the eyes moves into abduction (Fig 1). This behavior is strikingly different and must be clearly distinguished from a jerky nystagmus that appears only in abduction (end point nystagmus).

The following case reports illustrate two other examples of acute nystagmus blockage:

Case 1: A 5-year-old boy presented with a history of having had a head turn to the right, nystagmus and a variable angle of esotropia since early infancy. His visual acuity was 20/60 when measured in primary position, 20/100 in dextroversion and 20/30 in levoversion. The patient had a marked head turn to the right, fused intermittently but developed a variable esotropia of up to 30 prism diopters when his head was straightened. There was no nystagmus with the eyes in levoversion but a jerky nystagmus with a fast phase toward the left developed as the eyes moved from levoversion toward the primary position. The remainder of

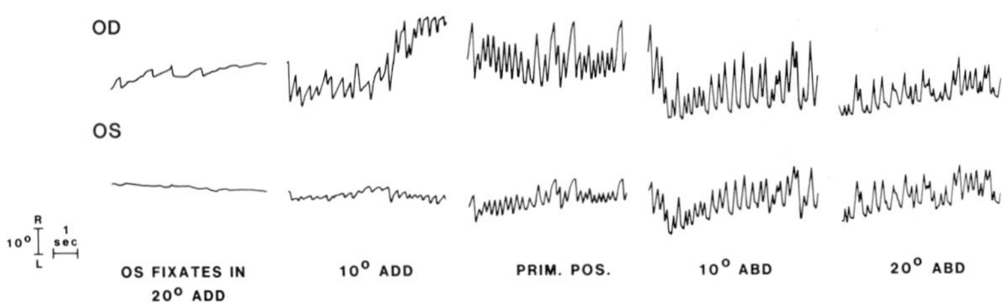

Figure 1. Electro-oculographic recordings show increasing nystagmus amplitudes as fixating OS moves in 10(o) increments from adduction toward abduction.

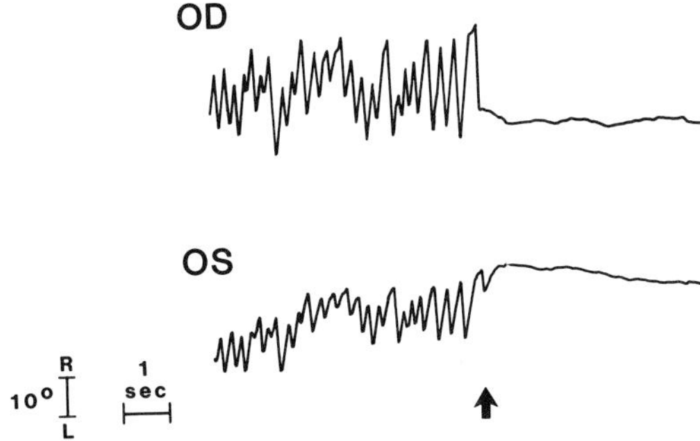

Figure 2. Electro-oculographic demonstration of acute nystagmus blockage (arrow) by adduction OS (see Figure 3).

the ocular examination, including cycloplegic refractions, was normal. The diagnosis of "asymmetric nystagmus" was made and a Kestenbaum-Anderson operation was performed to shift the neutral point from the left toward the primary position in order to eliminate the anomalous head posture.

Six months later the head turn had significantly decreased. However, there now was esotropia varying from orthophoria to 40 prism diopters with the eyes in primary position, as well as a jerky manifest nystagmus. The nystagmus disappeared as the esotropia increased (Fig 2) and

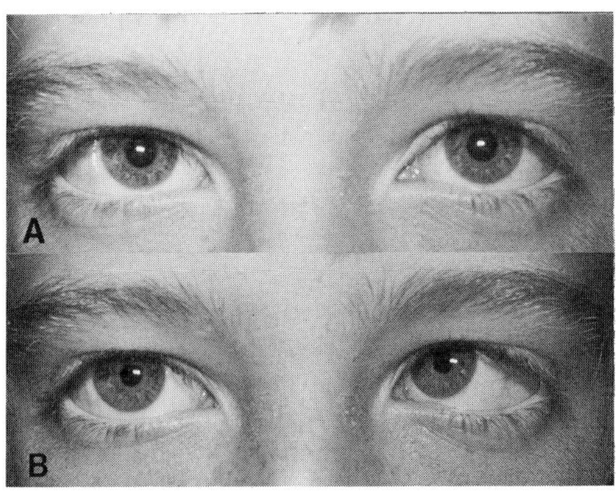

Figure 3. Acute esotropia with miosis in a patient with acute nystagmus blockage. Upper position: orthophoria with nystagmus (see Figure 2). Lower position: left esotropia develops as nystagmus disappears. Note miosis OU.

the pupils constricted simultaneously with the development of the esodeviation (Fig 3).

A second operation consisted of posteriorly fixating both medial rectus muscles 13 mm behind their original insertion. Six years later there was still variable esotropia in primary position. The patient had developed an alternate head turn. A manifest nystagmus was absent in primary position except when the patient performed pursuit movements with each adducted eye toward abduction.

Case 2: A 6-week-old girl presented with a history of congenital nystagmus. The ocular examination was negative except for findings consistent with oculocutaneous albinism and a pendular nystagmus which became jerky in lateroversion. Strabismus was absent. As an older sister had been treated by us for esotropia preceded, according to the history, by a congenital nystagmus, this patient was re-examined at frequent intervals and video recordings were obtained to demonstrate the absence of strabismus. The eyes remained orthophoric until the child was nearly 6 months old. At that time an esotropia of approximately 40 prism diopters at near and distance fixations developed suddenly and the amplitude of the nystagmus decreased. At the age of one year both medial rectus muscles were recessed 4 mm and posteriorly fixated 13 mm from their original insertion. At the age of 2-1/4 years the eyes were orthophoric but nystagmus in primary position persisted. The child had now developed head bobbing, synchronous with the frequency of nystagmus.

DISCUSSION

The two cases cited above are exceptions, however, inasmuch as an inverse quantitative relationship between the angle of esotropia and the amplitude of nystagmus could actually be demonstrated. For the majority of patients with infantile esotropia and nystagmus such a causal relationship remains presumptive and must be rejected unless supported by more convincing evidence than what has been presented in the literature.

We have shown that infantile esotropia with nystagmus which increases in abduction differs from other forms of infantile esotropia in several aspects. It appears reasonable to propose that such patients form a subgroup within the infantile esotropia syndrome. The characteristics of this subgroup were first described in 1962 by Ciancia.(6) Even though esotropia and nystagmus may be related to a common and still unknown factor, evidence is lacking that the esotropia is the result of nystagmus blockage in all such patients. We have also presented data to show that the nystagmus blocking mechanism, described four years later by Adelstein and Cuppers(5) should not be entirely rejected. However, we are in agreement with Kommerell(11) that this diagnosis should be reserved for patients in whom an inverse relationship between the angle of esotropia and the amplitude of nystagmus can actually be demonstrated.

The mechanism of nystagmus blockage in terms of adduction versus convergency innervation, the role of the near reflex in the dampening of the nystagmus amplitudes and the effect of nystagmus blockage on visual acuity and oscillopsia still remain unclear and deserve further investigation.

REFERENCES

1. von Noorden GK: Burian-von Noorden's Binocular Vision and Ocular Motility: Theory and Management of Strabismus, 2nd ed, St. Louis, CV Mosby, 1980, p. 296, 436

2. Lafon C: La vision des nystagmiques. Ann Ocul (Paris) 151:4, 1914

3. Ohm J: Das Ohrlabyrinth als Erzeuger des Schielens. Z Augenheilk 36: 253, 1916.

4. Kestenbaum A: Clinical Methods of Neuro-ophthalmological Examination, 2nd ed., New-York-London, Grune & Stratton, 1961, p. 334

5. Franceschetti A, Monnier M, Dieterle P: Analyse du nystagmus congenital par la methode electro-nystagmographique (ENG). Bull Schweiz Akad Med Wissensch 8:403-412, 1952

6. Ciancia A: Esotropia en el lactante, diagnostico y tratamiento. Arch Chil Oftalmol 19:117-124, 1962

7. Adelstein F, Cuppers C: Zum Problem der echten und der scheinbaren Abducens Lahmung (Das sogenannte "Blockierung ssyndrom"). Buech Augenarzt, 46:271-278, 1966

8. von Noorden GK: The nystagmus compensation (blockage) syndrome. Am J Ophthalmol 82:283-290, 1976

9. Muehlendyck H, Linnen HJ: Die operative behandlung nystagmusbedingter schwankender Schielwinkel mit der Fadenoperation nach Cuppers. Klin Mbl Augenheilk 167:273-290, 1975

10. Weiss J-B: Le 'blocage' existe-t-il? J Fr Ophtalmol 2:715-722, 1979

11. Kommerell G: Bezichungen zwischen Strabismus und Nystagmus, in Symposium Disorders of Ocular Motility Neurophysiological and Clinical Aspects, Munchen, J.F. Bergmann, 1978, pp. 367-373

12. Lang J: Der kongenitale oder fruhkindliche Strabismus. Ophthalmologica 154:201-208, 1967

13. Parks MM: Ocular Motility and Strabismus, Hagerstown, Harper and Row, 1974, p. 144

14. Helveston EM: Dissociated vertical deviation a clinical and laboratory study. Trans Am Ophthalmol Soc 78:734-779, 1980

15. Hiles DA, Watson BA, Biglan AW: Characteristics of infantile esotropia following early bimedial rectus recession. Arch Ophthalmol 98:697-703, 1980

16. Ing MR: Early surgical alignment for congenital esotropia. Trans Am Ophthalmol Soc 79:625-663, 1981

EARLY MEDICAL TREATMENT OF STRABISMUS BEFORE THE AGE OF 18 MONTHS

J.M. Sarniguet-Badoche

ABSTRACT

Strabismic children under eighteen months have been treated since 1974. Amblyopia could be avoided or cured in 90% of cases. A relative residual amblyopia was observed in only 9% of cases. Deviations < 30 prism diopters disappeared thanks to the mere medical treatment, more often with binocular vision normalization. Deviations > 30 prism diopters are often reduced with sectors treatment. Surgery is needed in 75% of the patients. The medical treatment consisted of wearing corrective glasses fitted with partial occlusive sectors. Daily motility exercises under parents supervision were also necessary for successful treatment.

INTRODUCTION

The medical treatment of strabismus before the age of 18 months gives a functional cure in a great number of cases. By early detection, effective prevention of amblyopia can be largely insured. When children are treated after the age of 18 months, the functional results are not as good in the control group of 100 cases.

METHODS

Detection

A. Detection of strabismus: We use the alternate screen test when possible, however, in most cases we used glasses with detection sectors, a personal method which we have used since 1976, to demonstrate even minimal deviation in infants.(1) A fixation object is presented to the child, if there is a symmetry of the iris on both sides of the detection sectors, there is no strabismus. Asymmetry suggests a monocular or alternating deviation. The iris of the deviated eye is hidden by the sector.

B. Detection of Amblyopia: We have completed the screening manuever and the test of tolerance to occlusion of

STRABISMUS II
ISBN 0-8089-1424-3

one eye by developing what we call the "right - left test". A toy is moved from right to left at the child's eyes level. The child is still wearing detection sector glasses. His reaction is observed. There are 3 possibilities:

1. Alternation: If the child fixes with the right eye to follow the object to the right, and fixates with the left eye to follow the object to the left, and does not significantly move the head, then there is no amblyopia.

2. Rotation of the head: If the child turns his head to maintain fixation with his normal eye in the visual field of his strabismic eye and the deviated eye only fixes in the extreme lateral field, then there is a strong preference for one eye and amblyopia risks developing in the other eye.

3. The top sign: If the child turns his head and then his body, like a top, to fix the toy with his healthy eye in the whole visual field then the strabismic eye cannot fix and amblyopia is present.

The clinical picture and the subsequent treatment should confirm the findings of this right-left test. Our experience confirms its reliability in more than 1000 children aged less than age 2 who have been tested. It is not necessary to quantify visual acuity in order to diagnose, presumptively or definitively, amblyopia in a young child.

Treatment

The method of partial occlusion sectors as developed by Berrondo(2) is used. A sector is a piece of translucent adhesive paper stuck to part of the lens to obstruct vision of that eye in a certain direction. The shape and size of the sectors are determined in terms of the preference of the normal eye. They are placed on the posterior surface of the glasses. The optical correction is the normal correction of the ametropia of each eye as measured after 8 days of atropinization.

Unlike prisms and optical penalization, this method alters neither the size, shape, nor the localization of objects. Unlike total occlusion, it produces a "division of visual attention", the first step towards binocular vision. The sectors must be modified at each follow-up visit in response to changes in the sensory and motor conditions caused by the treatment.

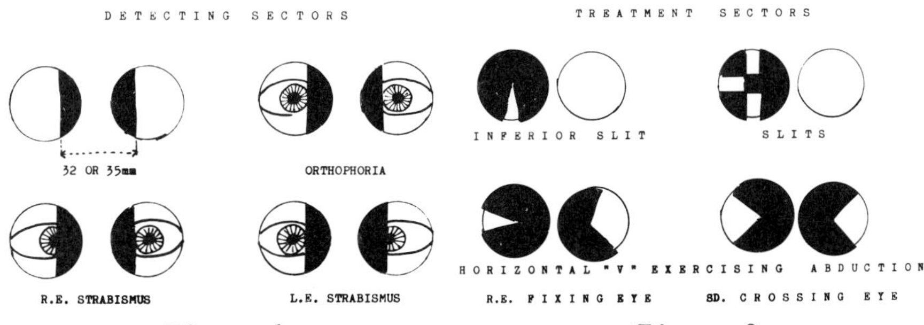

Figure 1 Figure 2

TREATMENT SECTORS

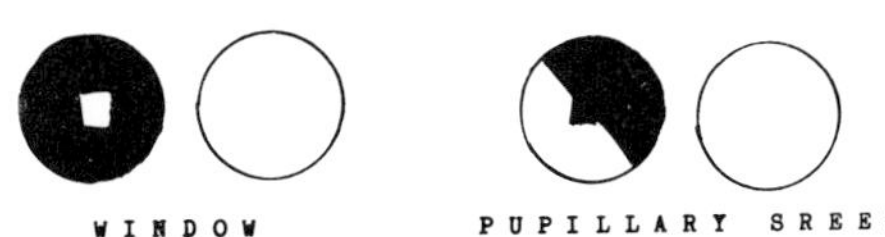

Figure 3

Sensory action: The sectors prevent neutralization and suppress the areas responsible for confusion or diplopia. Sectors tend not to actively inhibit monocular and binocular cortical cells. They prevent alternating amblyopia.

Motor action: Because of the continual change of the fixating eye, excessive contracture of the medial recti muscles is reduced and the lateral recti are stimulated.(3)

In pseudo-paresis of the external recti, the permanent motor action should be reinforced by the addition of motility exercising sectors 4 to 5 times a day under the supervision of the parents.(4) This mechanical therapy can normalize or considerably improve the abduction of eyes in fixed convergence. The cooperation of the parents is essential to supervise the wearing of the glasses and the exercises of the strabismic eye, several times a day.

The choice of the frame is important, as the sector occludes, it must remain in the correct position in front of the child's eyes for the treatment to be effective. If the glasses slide down the baby's nose, the sectors are no longer in the desired position. If the glasses are not large enough, the small child can cheat by looking over the lenses rendering the treatment ineffective.(5)

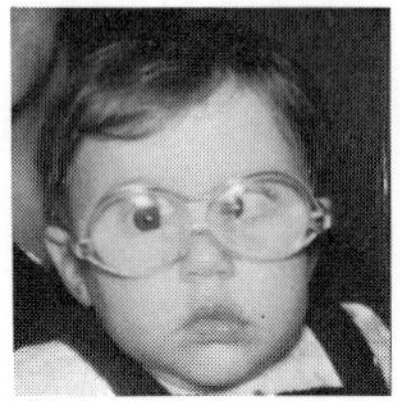
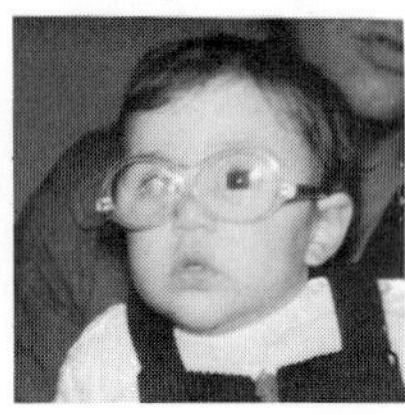

Figure 4

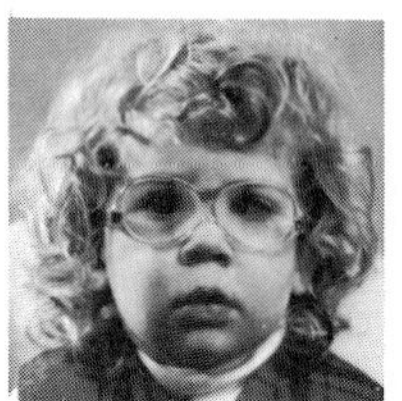
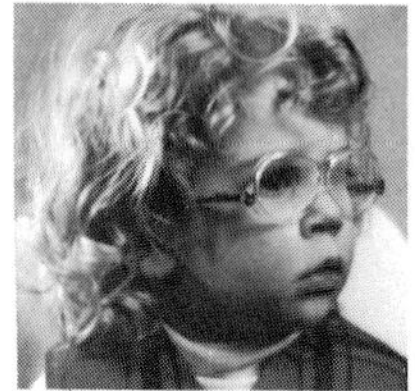

Figure 5

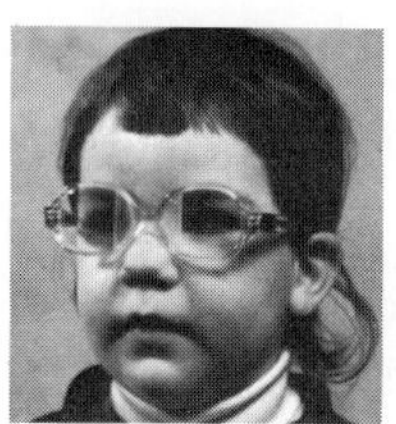
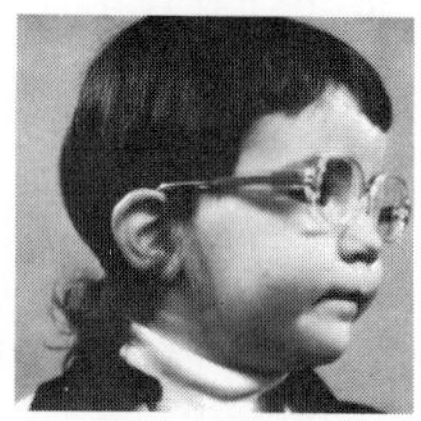

Figure 6

Treatment of Amblyopia. The treatment or prevention of amblyopia have absolute priority.

1. Severe amblyopia is treated by slits, associated with total occlusion for only 2 to 4 hours per day. The slits may be single or multiple. The triple slit is often used. It is essential to obtain "straight ahead" fixation of the strabismic eye.

2. Moderate amblyopia is treated by patching of the pupil and windows, central or off-centered.

The triangular window is effective as it allows abduction of the good eye and frequent changes in the fixating eye because of its tapered nasal point. The correct sector is the sector necessary and sufficient to make the child use his amblyopic eye as much as possible. The good eye is only used for reference vision. Without glasses, the good eye should remain dominant to avoid occlusion amblyopia.

Treatment of the deviation. When the amblyopia is corrected (or in cases of strabismus without amblyopia), bi-nasal sectors maintain good alternation until surgery or orthophorization. Equal or unequal, notched or oblique sectors are used according to the conditions of preference. Nasal sectors can be combined with carefully placed sectors which prevent gaze in the direction which causes upshoot or muscular over-activity.

Peripheral fusion can develop which, at this young age, favors significant reduction of the angle of deviation, or its disappearance, especially when the angle is less than 40 prism diopters before treatment. In cases with a small residual angle (< 20 diopters), prismatic treatment can lead to normalization of binocular vision and reduction of the angle.

RESULTS

The results have been analyzed of the 384 strabismic children aged less than 18 months, treated since 1974. The follow-up is greater than 4 years for 81 children, between 2 and 4 years for 152 children and between 1 and 2 years for 151 children. A group of 100 children treated between the age of 18 months and 3 years was taken as a control.

Amblyopia Treatment Results

Children treated before 18 months numbered 384 (35% with amblyopia before treatment). The prevention of amblyopia was effective, as only 1% had irreducible amblyopia, 9% had mild residual amblyopia (6/10 - 8/10), and 90% had equal acuity.

Children treated between the age of 18 months and 3 years - 100 cases (44% with amblyopia before treatment). The amblyopia was not treated as effectively for 9% had irreducible amblyopia, 21% had medium residual amblyopia (4/10 - 7/10), and 70% had equal acuity.

Angle of Deviation Treatment Results

(Not included in this study were those children with intermittent strabismus, in whom we obtained 90% functional cure. Only the cases of constant strabismus were retained.)

Children treated before 18 months numbered the same 384 cases. The cosmetic result without surgery was excellent in 59% of the children. Orthophoria was obtained in 169 children (44%), in 85% of cases where the angle of deviation before treatment was less than 30 prism diopters, in 25% of cases where the angle of deviation before treatment was between 30 and 50 prism diopters, and in only 3% of cases where the angle was more than 50 prism diopters (generally due to pseudoparesis of the lateral recti). A residual deviation less than 15 prism diopters (15%) was obtained (cosmetic cures) in 57 "aesthetic" children. 157 children (angle generally greater than 40 prism diopters before treatment) (41%) required surgery.

Of the children treated between the age of 18 months and 3 years (100 cases). Thirteen percent were orthophoric, 25% had a cosmetic result and 62% required surgery.

Binocular vision was obtained in each case where the child became orthophoric before the age of 2-1/2. Children treated before 18 months included 243 cases tested, but 141 children are still too young for testing. Of those tested, 107 children, now aged between 3 and 8, have normal stereoscopic binocular vision (44%). A further 34 children have peripheral fusion with poor stereoscopic vision but a good cosmetic results (14%) and 102 children have a persistent alternation or a orthotropic position (42%).

Children treated between the age of 18 months and 3 years included 100 cases. Binocular vision was only obtained in 18% and a peripheral fusion in another 18%.

CONCLUSIONS

The simplicity of the detection and the treatment, which are well accepted by children younger than 18 months, and the very favorable results, demonstrate the real value of early medical treatment of strabismus and amblyopia with the use of occlusion sectors.(6) Amblyopia can be prevented and there is a good probability of binocular vision. The success of this method depends on the cooperation of the parents, frequent follow-up and perfect adjustment of the sectors. It is desirable, therefore, that all strabismic children should be treated at this young age.

REFERENCES

1. Ardouin M, Urvoy M, Connault E: Experimentation of nasal sector glasses for screening of children 10 to 36 months old presenting strabismus and amblyopia. Fr Orth 12:35, 1980

2. Berrondo P: How to choose between the flip-flops and sectorial occlusions. Fr Orth 7:83, 1975

3. Sarniguet-Badoche JM: Management of blockage syndrome by sectors. Fr Orth 11:117, 1979

4. Sarniguet-Badoche JM: The medical treatment of pseudo paresis of lateral recti. Bull Soc Ophthalmol Fr 82:23-27, 1982

5. Julou J, Parent de Curzon H: Les principaux types de bascules par secteurs. Clin Ophthalmol 1:127, 1982

6. Badoche JM, Perroni C: From squint to orthophoria by heterophoria. J Fr Orth 11:44, 1979

DECREASING BEHAVIORAL FLEXIBILITY (OF ADJUSTMENT TO STRABISMUS) AS THE CAUSE OF RESISTANCE AGAINST TREATMENT DURING FIRST YEAR OF LIFE

S. Rethy and S. Rethy-Gal

ABSTRACT

Possibly immediate and full conservative treatment (glasses in special baby frame, binasal occlusion, and/or atropine ointment) was given from the 2nd to 10th month of life to babies with convergent strabismic angles from 25 to 60 prism diopters, in order to differentiate between the congenital inherited dispositions of strabismus or the acquired adjustments which become stabilized without treatment. The flexibility of adjustments to strabismus (sensory and motor inhibition, nystagmus, anomaly and overconvergence-Blockierung) was decreasing month after month during first year of life, as was shown by detailed case histories of 22 "congenital" cases becoming parallel without operation. The microstrabismus as an intermediate phase in all cases took longest to completely disappear. Refractive errors corrected were mostly astigmatic, sometimes low grade hyperopic and occasionally myopic. Most durable (therefore deep) adjustment was due to greatest flexibility of behavior patterns at an early start of strabismus. This and the seemingly inevitable period without treatment are analyzed as the factors of quickly developing resistance against treatment.

INTRODUCTION

One aspect that has not been covered in the present papers is the adaptation of the central nervous system to strabismus. Such adaptation stablizes the angle, making changes difficult with belated treatment. We may discover the unknown etiology of congenital strabismus, if we could document of the mechanism creating the resistance to a changed angle. The literature details most organic etiologies.(1,2)

Our hypothesis assumes that the resistance to change of the angle arises in early months of life quickly by developing anomalous retinal correspondence (ARC). The

STRABISMUS II
ISBN 0-8089-1424-3

anomalous movements of Bagolini are well known. They can keep the angle of strabismus stabilized.(3) We wish to pose two questions:

1. Can every functional strabismus acquire the therapeutic resistance during early weeks of life?
2. Can the stabilizing adaptation of early age, (by the initial plasticity of the brain) be responsible for quick development of resistance, a characteristic of every congenital strabismic case?

METHODS

We tried to break up the adaptation and to reverse the process of ARC development by the therapy of binasal occluding segments worn upon the glasses. Slight spherical overcorrection of the refractive errors found in cycloplegia was ordered.(4)

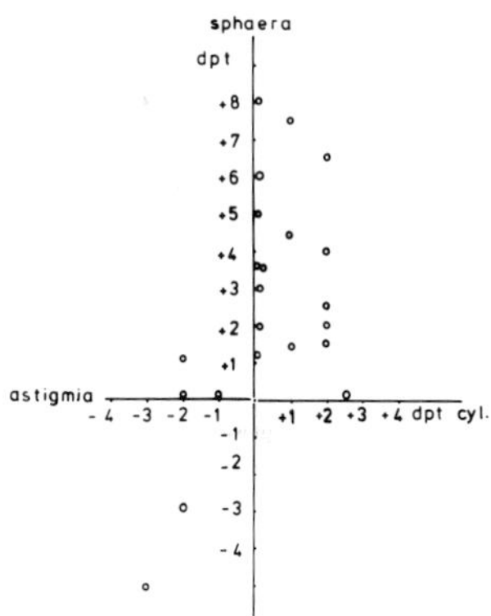

Figure 1. Cycloplegic refractive errors of babies with "congenital" strabismus, which started from 2nd month of life onward. Eight cases had spherical and 14 cases had an astigmatic refraction.

The gradual disappearance of the angle allowed later normal retinal correspondence (NRC) should occur if the plasticity of brain to readapt itselt was still present. We believe that the type of refractive error is not a determining factor as to whether the strabismus is an irreversible. The therapy resistance depends more on the long duration of adjustment than on the supposed origin of the strabismus. The therapy resistance can be best prevented by possibly immediate full conservative treatment. The prevention of adjustment must include the accepted modalities: motor, sensory and sensorimotor treatment. The patching of the eyes or the binasal segments in babies can eliminate the stimuli for suppression and for ARC.

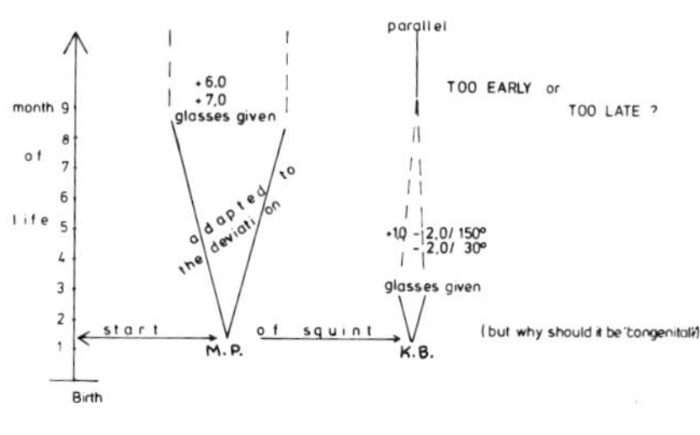

Figure 2. Different delay of treatment cause the difference in therapy-resistance in these 2 cases. Equal early onset was followed in the early case by long interval, until even +6.0 and +7.0 diopters could not remove the angle of strabismus stabilized by long adjustment. In contrast, the astigmatic correction straightened the eyes when only a short interval was allowed for unhindered adjustment in the 2nd case.

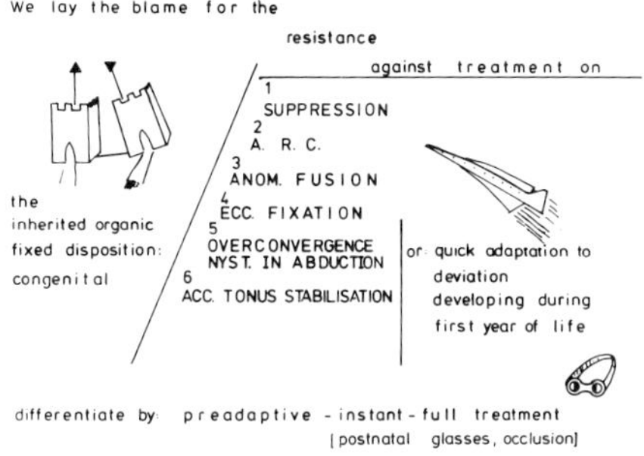

Figure 3. Comparison of the two possible groups of therapy-resistance and failures in strabismic therapy. Immediate treatment can distinguish between acquired adjustment or congenital organic resistance against therapy.

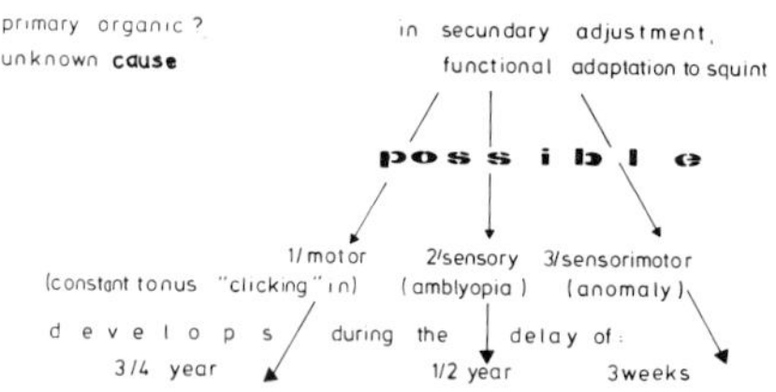

Figure 4. Effective prevention observes the different time factors of strabismic adjustment on motor, sensory and sensorimotor level.

SENSORIMOTOR BEHAVIOUR ADJUSTMENT OF THE BRAIN IN SQUINT

Disturbance: (stimulus)	response	retinal seat	quickness	duration	treatment
1. double vision	suppression (monofixation)	central	prompt	long	elimination of stimulus 1.
2. deplacement of objects (in one eye)	anomalous correspondence		age dependent	variable	binasal occlusion disconnection of anomaly 2.

Figure 5. Binasal segments eliminate the disturbing stimuli and stop the adaptation. Dominance can be influenced by the changing size of the segments.

The glasses can achieve two purposes at once:

1. to create sharp images at the fovea
2. to remove the stimulus for overaccommodation and overconvergence

MATERIALS

We report 22 cases treated since 1978, who attained bifoveal fixation and straight eyes after sometimes long, antiadaptive, full conservative therapy. All the cases initially had characteristic signs of congenital strabismus: nystagmus pseudoparesis in abduction, large unilateral or alternating esotropia with "V" or "A" patterns.

The angle was resistant at first. It was not corrected with the first glasses and binasal segments. The size of the binasal segment had to be greater on the dominant eye, smaller on the other eye. The patching segments were changed frequently to achieve alternate fixation.

RESIDUAL ANGLE RECEDING : Phases of unfolding binocular development

weeks of treatment	right- left	angle of squint	REMNANTS OF SENSO-RIMOTOR ADJUSTMENT
		pdpt	
1 - 4		r.+50	pseudoparesis of abduction with
5 - 8		l.+20	nystagmus
9 - 10		r. +10	
11 - 30		l. +6	microstrabismus
		dist. 0	
31 -		near: +20	(blockage) due to suppression for near
34 -			release point 0,5m
36 -			" " 0,3m
38-			" " 0,1m
40-		near: 0	no suppression

Figure 6. During the 40 weeks duration of segment occlusion the distinct phases of dominance and diminishing angle are shown with the changing pattern of segment-occlusion.

Prolonged atropinization assisted the constant wearing glasses that were frequently removed by the babies. We had better compliance with the glasses given to babies under 5 months of age and the best compliance were with those under 3 months.

All babies with gradually diminishing strabismus went through long phases of micro-strabismus. Later, with straight eyes for distance, they often had "blockage" or overconvergence for near vision. The overconvergence was treated by prescribing the usually one-sided sector on the dominant, not overconvergent eye. The nasal sector covered the pupil of the slowly convergent dominant eye to the moment as the other eye was ready to start the overconvergence. At this moment we could occasionally demonstrate the presence of a sudden suppression in the slave eye. The hologram slides worn on the eyes showed the suppression in one eye occuring only in binocular vision.(5) The nasal segment of the dominant side eliminated the binocular vision at the moment of overconvergence and thus the active suppression was hindered. Gradually the suppression became less and the overconvergence point came nearer, until the bifoveal fixation could be achieved for near and distance. Frequent recurrences with sudden disease and fever occurred in some cases or if the glasses were not worn constantly. The binasal segments and the continuous wear of the glasses proved helpful in such cases.

RESULTS

The time factors of the case history: age of onset, interval (or delay until the therapy was started) was plotted against the duration of necessary treatment until orthotropia was achieved.

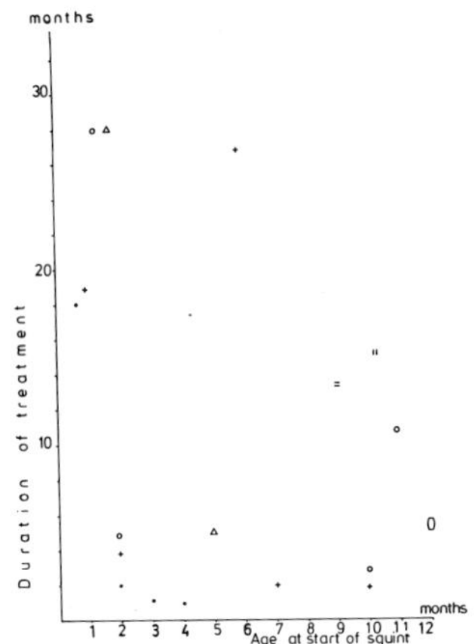

Figure 7. Duration of treatment (until straight for distance/near) and age of onset of 18 "congenital" strabismic cases are illustrated. There is seemingly no causal relation between these.

The formula of a hyperbole shows the resistance arising quickly during the interval between the onset of strabismus and the start of therapy, especially if the onset was at an early age. It is similar to a "learning curve" demonstrating the anomaly as an adaptation of the brain to the strabismic angle.

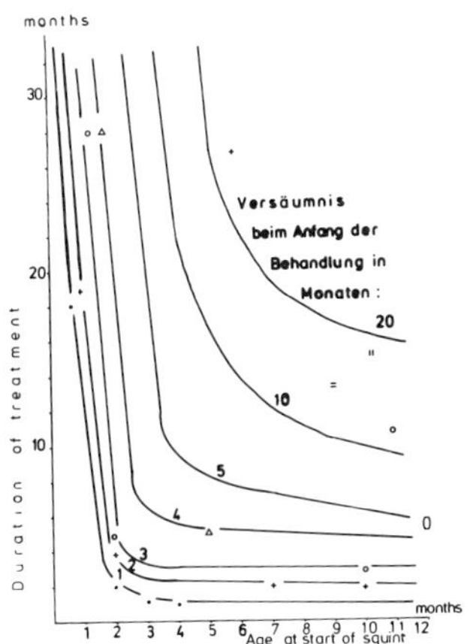

Figure 8. The relation between the time factors of the onset of strabismus and duration of necessary treatment are obvious if we connect with continuous lines the cases which had the same delay of treatment.

As for terminology: My proposal is to call anomalous retinal correspondence (ARC) adapted retinal correspondence (ARC) and non-adapted retinal correspondence (NRC).

In all our cases, the adjustment of the brain to the deviation was the cause of the resistance. If the necessary flexibility of the brain decreased, the strabismic position was stabilized, and the readjustment was no longer possible. Such cases are not analyzed in this paper.

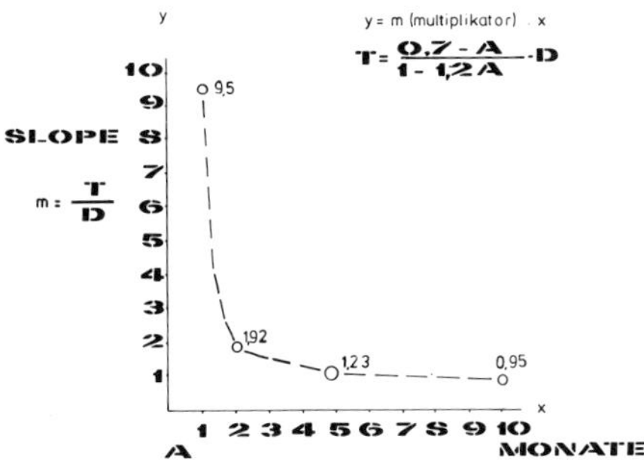

Figure 9. The equation of a hyperbole contains the time factors of age at onset (A), delay (D) and therapy duration (T) until the eyes regained parallelity.

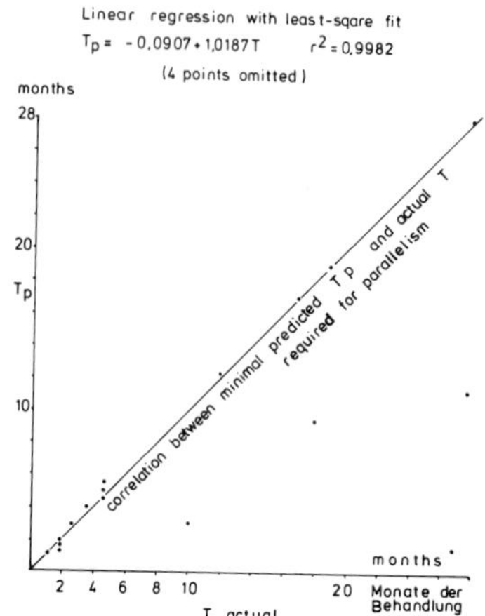

Figure 10. Good correlation between the predicted and required duration of treatment until bifoveal eye position. Four cases are omitted, because of intermittent wearing of the glasses the duration of the treatment was longer than the necessary minimal time.

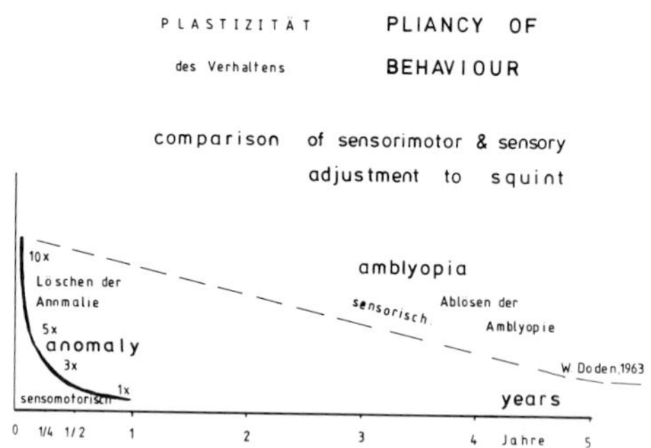

Figure 11. Different speeds of sensorimotor and sensory adaptations to strabismus.

DISCUSSION

We were able to show the range of growth of sensorimotor anomaly which arose quickly at an early age, as the cause of resistance to therapy.

In all "congenital" strabismus cases, we assume a decrease of plasticity to the adjustment by the brain. The angle of strabismus could not be reduced immediately but further adaptation was stopped immediately.

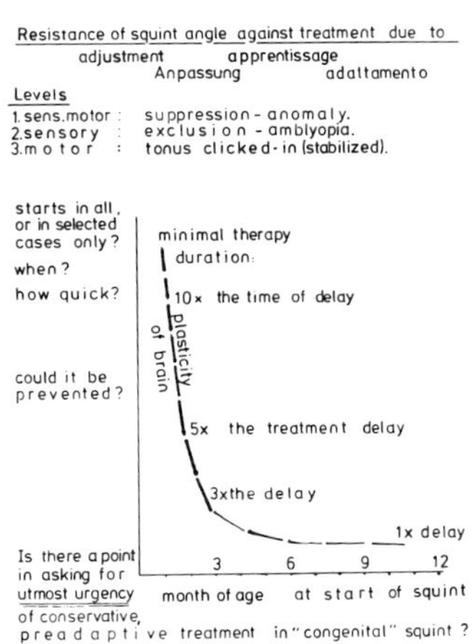

Figure 12. Decrease of plasticity of adaptive behavior is showed to be important in early strabismus.

A 4 month interval between the onset of strabismus and the start of treatment can cause irreversibility of adjustment (anomaly) by the prompt decrease of behavioral flexibility.

The reversal of amblyopia is easier than reduction of the strabismus. The decrease of sensorimotor plasticity (responsible for anomaly) is quicker than the plasticity for sensory adaptations of that occurring in amblyopia. The treatment of amblyopia is therefore not as demanding in respect to early antiadaptive treatment.

To understand the relations between the impulse pattern of the muscle tonus and the anatomic features emanating without fusional control, we can examine the baby during the first trimester of life as it learns to process the wealth of visual information. We can study the bifoveation during first weeks of life as the divergent anatomic position of the neonates is corrected by a compensation in the tonus impulses of the muscles.(6-8) The eye-hand coordination starts during the second and third months of life, stimulating more regular convergence and accommodation impulses. The first cases of intermittent strabismus can be observed at this age. This may be proof that fusion is present at this age. Fusion development is extremely sensitive to disturbances. Our new cases are more frequently intermittent strabismus. The behavior pattern is less stabilized than in babies referred at a later age for examination.

We did not establish the interval necessary to prevent successful treatment of congenital strabismus. When the immediate treatment of all strabismic babies becomes the routine for everyday practice, then the critical inverval may be established.

We hope this paper may lead some strabismologists to consider early medical treatment in some of the congenital strabismic cases which would usually be sent for surgery.

Strabismologists interested in the medical treatment of strabismic babies should correspond with each other. Such experiences and results should be circulated without delay to promote and establish early medical treatments. Further, the deterioration of accommodative esotropia to a nonaccommodative one that requires surgery means the failure of anti-adaptive measures. Sensorimotor adjustment (anomaly) can prevent the disappearance of the angle with glasses only. An "aggressive anti-accommodative therapy" as Baker and Parks employed in their 21 cases(1) is not enough because anti-adaptive treatment in form of binasal segments is also needed.

REFERENCES

1. Baker J, Parks M: Early on-set accommodative esotropia. Am J Ophthalmol 90:11-18, 1980.

2. Doden W: Stellungsanomalien und Motilitatsstorungen in Axenfeld: Lehrbuch und Atlas der Augenheilkunde. p. 134, Fischer, Stuttgart, 1963.

3. Bagolini B: Part II. Sensorio-motorial anomalies in strabismus (anomalous movements). Doc Ophthalmol 41:23-41, 1976.

4. Rethy I, Gal Z: Results and principles of a new method of optical correction of hypermetropia in cases of esotropia. Acta Ophthalmol 46:757-766, 1968.

5. Rethy S: Hologram zum Nachweis der Suppression und deren Anderungen. Der Augenspiegel 147:28, 1982.

6. Rethy S, Gal S: Motor tonus adaptation in squint. Doc Ophthalmol 32:101, 1982.

7. Rethy I: Development of the simultaneous fixation from the divergent anatomic eye-position of the neonate. J Pediatric Ophthalmol 6:92-96, 1969.

8. Rethy I: Congenital esotropia. Ann Ophthalmol 2:288-292, 1970.

A TEST FOR PREDICTING THE EFFECTIVENESS OF PENALIZATION ON AMBLYOPIA

K. W. Wright and D. L. Guyton

ABSTRACT

Penalization therapy is effective in treating in some but not all amblyopia. To help predict which children would benefit from penalization therapy before starting treatment, penalization conditions were simulated and fixation preference was evaluated to determine if fixation switched to the amblyopic eye. In "straight-eyed" children fixation preference was examined using 10 prism diopters of vertical dissociation. We prospectively studied 15 hyperopic children with moderate to dense (20/200) amblyopia. Penalization in both the pretreatment testing and during actual therapy consisted of cycloplegia of the uncorrected sound eye while the amblyopic eye received full optical correction. Eleven of the 15 patients switched fixation to the amblyopic eye during in-office penalization testing, and in all 11 cases amblyopia improved significantly with penalization treatment. Of 4 children who did not switch fixation, 3 failed to improve despite having better visual acuity in the amblyopic eye while penalized. Thus, fixation preference testing under penalized conditions proved to be a valuable predictor of the effectiveness of penalization therapy.

INTRODUCTION

Penalization of the non-amblyopic eye with cycloplegia has proven to be an effective method for the treatment of some but not all functional amblyopia.(1-7) Penalization treatment is based upon the principle of blurring the vision of the sound eye in order to encourage the use of the amblyopic eye. Unfortunately, a previous record of inconsistent results has plagued the use of penalization therapy, discouraging most clinicians from its use. Many authorities now restrict the use of penalization to a second choice treatment in mild amblyopia, or for maintaining vision obtained through previous occlusion therapy.(2,3,8)

The problem has been to identify those children who could benefit from penalization therapy, and to eliminate those who, after a lengthy treatment period, would end up as

STRABISMUS II
ISBN 0-8089-1424-3

penalization failures, only to require further treatment with patching. In addressing this problem, the ophthalmic literature has stressed three major predictive factors for successful cycloplegic penalization: (1) penalization should decrease visual acuity in the second eye below that of the amblyopic eye at least at near, (2) the hyperopia should be at least four to six diopters, and (3) the amblyopia should be mild, i.e., 20/80 or better.(2,3) Even with the use of these guidelines in selecting appropriate treatment groups, results from penalization continue to be less predictable than with patching. Improvement has been satisfactory in approximately 50-70% of children treated with penalization.(2,3)

Despite these inconsistent and variable results, interest in penalization continues primarily because of its many advantages over standard patching techniques. With cycloplegic penalization there is no worry about peeking around the patch, and cooperation in the hyperactive or problem child usually is excellent.

Cosmetic appearance of the child undergoing penalization therapy essentially is normal, thus eliminating the social stigma associated with patching therapy. Skin sensitivities to patches can also be avoided with penalization treatment. Penalization therapy often is more readily accepted by both the child and the parent, leading to improved doctor-patient rapport, and to better patient compliance.(2,3)

In the present study, we introduce a method for predicting which children will benefit from penalization, thus eliminating much of the uncertainty which has previously been associated with penalization treatment.

SUBJECTS AND METHODS

We prospectively studied penalizaton therapy in 15 hyperopic children with moderate (16/30 with Allen cards) to severe (20/200) amblyopia (Fig 1,2). Thirteen of these 15 children had recent unsuccessful patching therapy and were referred to our study as patching failures. Reasons for patching failure included behavioral problems, with 12 children removing the patch, and skin irritation to the patches of one child. Before starting penalization treatment, each child received a full ophthalmic examination including cyclopentolate 1% refraction. Visual acuity measurements were taken with linear Snellen letters or a linear E game in 8 children, and with Allen picture cards in

5 additional children. Binocular fixation patterns were determined on all patients including 2 children unable to give subjective visual acuities. In these 2 children binocular fixation patterns were used to determine and monitor the presence of amblyopia. Patients with straight eyes or deviations of less than 10 prism diopters were examined with the 10 prism diopter fixation test,(10) performed by placing a 10 diopter prism over one eye to induce a vertical deviation, thereby dissociating the eyes. Once vertically dissociated, binocular fixation patterns were determined in the usual manner. Patients who show strong fixation preference for one eye (i.e. "will not hold fixation" with the non-preferred eye for at least 4 seconds, or through a blink, or through smooth pursuit), are considered to be amblyopic. Those who spontaneously "alternate fixation" between one eye and the other, or "hold fixation well" with the nonpreferred eye, are considered not to have amblyopia.(10) All 15 patients in our study had pretreatment binocular fixation patterns of "will not hold fixation with the amblyopic eye."

In addition to a routine ophthalmic examination, each patient was given a pretreatment in-office test of penalization to determine the immediate effect of penalization conditions on fixation preference and visual acuity. Penalization test conditions consisted of using cyclopentolate 1% of the uncorrected sound eye while the amblyopic eye was given full optical correction. In one patient with mild hyperopia (patient #2), the blur from cycloplegic penalization was increased by placing a -2.00D lens over the cyclopleged sound eye. Only those patients who under penalization test conditions demonstrated a decrease in visual acuity in the amblyopic eye to equal or below the sound eye were considered as reasonable penalization candidates and entered into our study. While under penalization test conditions, the fixation preference was evaluated to determine if penalization of the sound eye would cause a switch in fixation preference to the amblyopic eye. Fixation preference was determined both at distance and near using only accommodative targets such as finger puppets, wiggle pictures, and cartoon movies. In children without manifest deivations, a 10 diopter prism was used to induce a vertical deviation and dissociate the eyes, thus allowing determination of fixation preference.

Actual penalization therapy closely matched the in-office testing conditions. Therapy consisted of daily

Atropine 1% or 1/2% for cycloplegia of the uncorrected sound eye and full optical correction without cycloplegia for the amblyopic eye. The one patient given the pretreatment penalization test with a -2.00D lens over the cyclopleged sound eye was also treated in a similar manner by prescribing a -2.00D lens for the atropinized sound eye. Penalization therapy was continued in all of these non-responding patients for at least 12 continuous weeks. If no improvement in either visual acuity or binocular fixation patterns could be detected by that time, penalization therapy was discontinued.

RESULTS OF THERAPY

Of the 15 patients studied, 12 showed dramatic improvement after penalization therapy, with binocular fixation patterns changing from "will not hold" fixation with the amblyopic eye to "holds well" or "alternates freely" (Fig 1). Confirmation of this improvement was obtained for the 10 children in this group who could respond reliably to visual acuity testing. Vision improved in all 10 children, becoming equal to, or within one line of the vision in the sound eye (Fig 1, 3). Improvement in these 10 children ranged from approximately 3 to 5 lines after a treatment period of 2 to 5 months. The remaining 3 patients studied showed no improvement in binocular fixation patterns or in visual acuity after a minimum of 12 weeks of constant penalization therapy (Fig 2,4).

ANALYSIS OF PREDICTIVE FACTORS

In order to identify those factors which are most reliable for predicting successful penalization therapy, we correlated results with the following factors: (1) the success rate of the penalization test conditions to cause an immediate switch in fixation preference to the amblyopic eye, (2) the success rate of penalization test conditions to decrease visual acuity in the sound eye below that of the amblyopic eye at least at near, (3) the degree of hyperopia present, and (4) the severity of the amblyopia.

1. Fixation Patterns Under Penalization Test Conditions. During penalization test conditions, 11 of the 15 children demonstrated an immediate switch in fixation preference from the sound eye to the amblyopic eye and all 11 children showed marked improvement with penalization treatment. Ten of the 11 children who switched fixation during penalization testing gave reliable pre- and post-treatment visual acuities; their improvement is charted in Figure 3.

IMPROVED WITH PENALIZATION

Age Years	Type of Amblyopia	Pre Rx VA	Pre Rx Fix	Post Rx VA	Post Rx Fix	Ref	Penalization test ΔVA	Penalization test ΔFix
1. 1 8/12	Strab. ET	N.O.	WNH	N.O.	ALT	+2.50	N.O.	D- N-
2. 3 2/12	Part. Cataract	18/30[A] 5/30	WNH	18/30[A] 15/30	HW	+2.00	N.O.	D- N+
3. 3 3/12	Strab. Et	18/30[A] 8/30	WNH	17/30[A] 16/30	ALT	+7.50	N.O.	D+ N+
4. 3 11/12	Strab. XT	20/30[A] 16/30	WNH	19/30[A] 20/30	HW	+2.00	N.O.	D+ N+
5. 4 0/12	Strab. ET	20/30[A] 16/30	WNH	20/30[A] 20/30	HW	+3.25	N.O.	D+ N+
6. 4 8/12	anisom.	20/30 20/80	WNH	20/30 20/40	HW	+3.50	D+ N+	D- N+
7. 4 9/12	Strab. XT	NO	WNH	NO	ALT	+3.25	NO	D+ N+
8. 5 4/12	Lat. Nyst. Strab. ET	18/30[A] 10/30	WNH	10/30[A] 18/30OU 14/30	HW	+4.00	D N=	D+ N+
9. 6 0/12	Strab. ET	20/70 20/25	WNH	20/30 20/25	ALT	+6.25	D+ N+	D+ N+
10. 6 1/12	Strab. ET	20/100 20/40	WNH	20/50 20/40	ALT	+5.25	D= N+	D- N+
11. 6 2/12	Strab. ET	20/30 20/80	WNH	20/30 20/40	HW	+4.75	D+ N+	D+ N+
12. 6 9/12	anisom.	20/200 20/40	WNH	20/50 20/50	HW	+4.75	D+ N+	D+ N+

NO IMPROVEMENT WITH PENALIZATION

Age Years	Type of Amblyopia	Pre Rx VA	Pre Rx Fix	Post Rx VA	Post Rx Fix	Ref	Penalization test ΔVA	Penalization test ΔFix
1. 6 0/12	Strab. ET	20/100 20/40	WNH	20/100 20/50	WNH	+5.50	D= N+	D- N-
2. 6 3 12	Strab. ET	20/20 20/200	WNH	20/30 20/200	WNH	+4.25	D= N+	D- N-
3. 8 7 12	Strab. ET	20/30 20/50	WNH	20/30 20/50	WNH	+4.75	D+ N+	D- N-

Figures 1 and 2. Summary of 15 patients studied; 12 improved and 3 remained unchanged after penalization therapy.

"VA" = visual acuity with linear letters of "E" game; "A" indicates Allen picture cards were used.

"Fix" = Binocular fixation patterns; "Alt" = Alternates fixation between fellow eyes; "HW" = Holds fixation well with either eye; "WNH" = Will not hold fixation with amblyopic eye.

<u>Penalization test</u>: "pdp VA" and "pdp Fix" indicates changes in VA advantage and fixation preference after the penalization test. "D" = Distance; "N" = Near; "+" = a change giving the amblyopic eye either VA advantage or fixation preference; "-" = sound eye retains VA advantage or fixation preference; and "=" means VA is equal in both eyes.

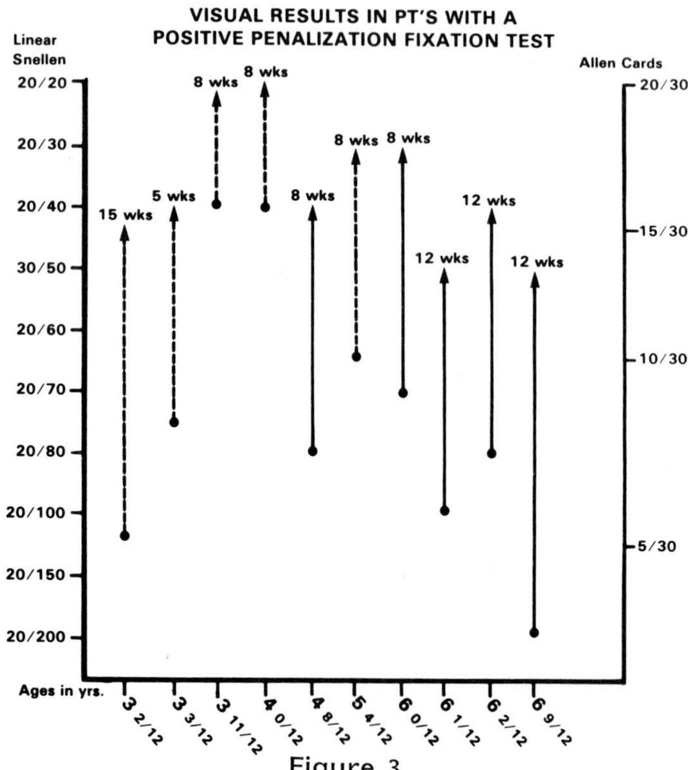

Figure 3

Of the 4 children who did not switch fixation to the amblyopic eye under test conditions, only 1 switched fixation during treatment. The other 3 who did not switch fixation under test conditions remained unchanged in both vision and fixation patterns after penalization treatment (Fig 2,4).

2. Visual Acuity Under Penalization Test Conditions. Visual acuity under penalization test conditions were obtained in 9 of the 15 children studied. In 8 of these 9 children penalization test conditions caused a decrease in visual acuity of the sound eye below the level of the amblyopic eye, at least at near, thus changing the visual acuity advantage to the amblyopic eye. Despite having better vision in the amblyopic eye under penalization test conditions, 3 of these 8 children did not switch fixation to the amblyopic eye, and all 3 ended up as penalization failures showing no visual improvement or change in fixation after prolonged penalization treatment.

3. Degree of Hyperopia. Four of the 15 children studied had high hyperopia (+5.00 to +7.50) with the remaining 11 children showing moderate hyperopia (+2.00 to +4.75). Three of the 4 high hyperopic children showed improvement and 9 of the 11 children with moderate hyperopia also improved. Interestingly, 6 of the 11 children who improved with penalization therapy only had +2.00 to +3.50 diopters of hyperopia.

4. Severity of Amblyopia. Thirteen of the 15 children studied could give visual acuity measurements both pre- and post-treatment. Eight of the 13 children originally showed dense amblyopia, equivalent to 20/80 to 20/200. Six of the 8 children with dense amblyopia improved after penalization therapy, and 2 remained as penalization failures. Of 5 children with more moderate amblyopia equivalent to 20/50 to 20/70, 4 improved and 1 showed no improvement.

DISCUSSION

We found fixation preference testing under simulated penalization conditions to be useful in identifying those children who would successfully respond to penalization therapy. Our findings suggest that if fixation preference switches to the amblyopic eye under penalization test conditions, then penalization therapy will be successful in treating amblyopia. On the other hand, if penalization test conditions do not provoke a change in fixation preference to the amblyopic eye than it is unlikely that penalization therapy will improve the amblyopia. An immediate switch in fixation preference to the amblyopic eye for both distance and near is the best insurance for improvement with penalization since the amblyopic eye will be constantly stimulated. Improvement can also be achieved, however, when fixation has changed to the amblyopic eye only at near. In fact, 3 of our patients did improve with penalization even though they initially changed fixation to the amblyopic eye only at near (Fig 1). We did see 1 child who continued to fixate with the sound eye during cyclopentolate penalization testing, but after one month of Atropine penalization therapy showed a switch in fixation preference to the amblyopic eye. This young child was uncooperative both in taking the cyclopentolate drops and in sitting still for the examination. The reason for the delayed switch in fixation preference in this child remains an enigma, but may be due to inadequate cycloplegia during testing. Our experience parallels that of others, indicating that daily Atropine

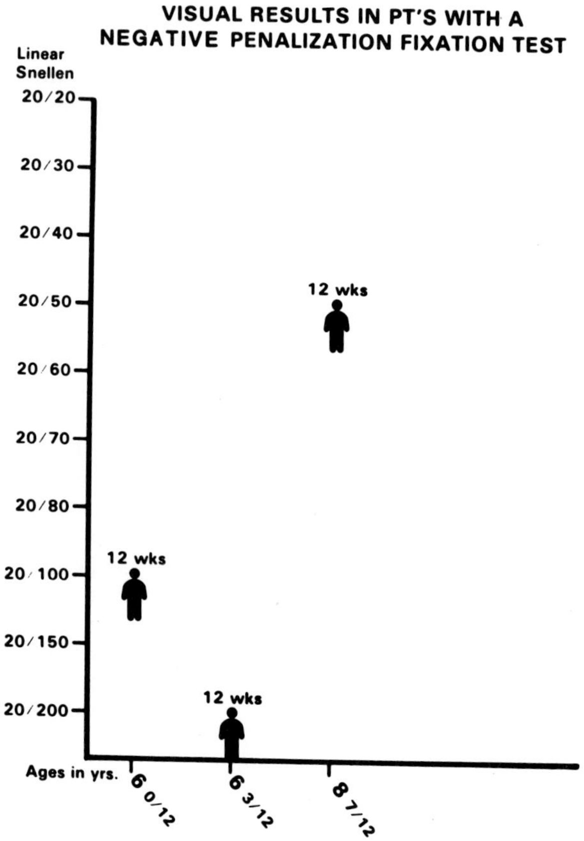

VISUAL RESULTS IN PT'S WITH A NEGATIVE PENALIZATION FIXATION TEST

Linear Snellen

20/20

20/30

20/40

20/50

20/60

20/70

20/80

20/100

20/150

20/200

12 wks

12 wks

12 wks

Ages in yrs.

6 0/12

6 3/12

8 7/12

Figure 4

drops are necessary to ensure complete cycloplegia during penalization therapy.(1,3) It is important not to depend on the presence of a dilated unreactive pupil as evidence for complete cycloplegia.(3,9)

One might speculate that the changes in visual acuity under penalization test conditions would give the same predictive information as fixation preference testing in determining if a child would improve with penalization therapy. That is, if penalization test conditions cause a decrease in visual acuity of the sound eye below the level of the amblyopic eye, then fixation preference would necessarily switch to the better seeing amblyopic eye, and vision would improve with penalization therapy. We found this not be the case as 3 children who had better visual acuity in the amblyopia eye under penalization test conditions failed to switch fixation preference to the amblyopic eye. These 3 children who continued to fixate with the penalized sound eye failed to show any improvement after prolonged penalization therapy. Additionally, 1 patient who had equal visual acuity under penalization test conditions switched fixation preference to the amblyopic eye and improved with penalization therapy. Thus, changes in visual acuity advantage do not always parallel changes in fixation preference. It is noteworthy that in treating amblyopia our goal is not simply to blur the vision of the sound eye, but to change fixation to the amblyopic eye. Patching accomplishes this goal effectively by totally shutting off the vision of the sound eye. Blurring of the sound eye with penalization also can work with the same effectiveness as patching if fixation has changed to the amblyopic eye. It makes little sense to send children out on penalization therapy if they continue to fixate with the blurred sound eye.

Hyperopia is an important prerequisite for successful penalization therapy, but we found that the degree of hyperopia necessary for improvement is less than has previously been reported.(2,4) In patients with mild degrees of hyperopia we have found "over minusing" the cyclopleged sound eye to be effective in increasing the blurring effort of the cycloplegia. The amount of minus lens necessary is determined by increasing the minus lens power over the cyclopleged sound eye until fixation preference switches to the amblyopic eye at least at near, and preferably for distance and near.

Another noteworthy finding in our study was that

penalization therapy was successful in treating even dense amblyopia of 20/200 as long as fixation preference switched to the amblyopic eye.

Our complications with penalization therapy were minimal. One child developed a skin flush to the Atropine drops which was effectively treated by reducing the Atropine concentration by half. Reverse or penalization induced amblyopia(11) occurred in 3 of the children studied. These children were treated by replacing the proper optical correction on the sound eye and by stoping the Atropine drops. In each case, vision promptly returned to pre-treatment levels (Fig 5).

REVERSE AMBLYOPIA

Ages	Pre Rx VA	Lowest VA	Last VA
3 2/12	18/30	5/30	18/30
3 3/12	18/30	14/30	17/30
4 0/12	20/30	10/30	20/30

Figure 5

As to the use of penalization as a first treatment in amblyopia, we believe that this should be individualized. An important criteria for starting penalization therapy is whether fixation preference switches to the amblyopic eye under penalization test conditions.

REFERENCES

1. Gregersen E, Pontoppidan M, Rindziunski E: Optic and drug penalization and favouring in the treatment of squint amblyopia. Acta Ophthalmol 52:60-66, 1974.

2. von Noorden GK, Milam JB: Penalization in the treatment of amblyopia. Am J Ophthalmol 88:511-518, 1979.

3. McKenney S, Byers M: Aspects and results of penalization treatment. Am Orthop J 25:85-89, 1975.

4. Johnson DS, Antuna J: Atropine and miotics for treatment of amblyopia. Am J Ophthalmol 60:889-891, 1965.

5. Pouliquen P: Zum problem der penalization. Klin Mbl Augenheilk 161:130-139, 1972.

6. Cibis L: Penalization, treatment of ARC and amblyopia. Am Orthop J 25:79-84, 1975.

7. Haase W: Experiences with penalization therapy in Moore S, Mein S, Stockbridge L (eds.): Present and Future. Stratton Intercontinental Medical Book Corp., 1976, pp. 105-111.

8. Flynn JT, Cassady, JC: Current trends in amblyopia therapy. Ophthalmol 85:428-450, May 1978.

9. Thompson, HS: The Pupil, Chapter 12, in Moses RA (ed.): 1981, pp. 326-356, Adler's Physiology of the Eye, C.V. Mosby Co.

10. Wright KW, Walonker F, Edelman P: 10-diopter fixation test for amblyopia. Arch Ophthalmol 99:1242-1246, 1981.

11. von Noorden GK: Amblyopia caused by unilateral atropinization. Ophthalmology 88:131-133, Feb 1981.

DISCUSSION BY SHINOBU AWAYA

I think that the penalization is essentially a kind of "mild or partial" occlusion of the good eye. Therefore, it is unlikely to cause an occlusion amblyopia of the good eye, so long as we keenly check up the vision of both eyes. However, it will do no use if it is too mild. Thus, it is most important to predict which children would benefit from the penalization therapy. In this sense Dr. Wright's paper is very helpful in predicting the possible effect of penalization. However, as to the successful results in their subjects, those 11 cases of the 15 cases which were hyperopic, amblyopia could have been successfully cured also by the sound eye occlusion, for the amblyopia of this category is usually very mild and has no eccentric fixation and could be easily cured, so long as the sound eye occlusion can be accomplished. For the children over five years of age the occlusion of the sound eye is not matter of great danger, so long as we check their visual acuity or ocular deviations of both eyes in the course of treatment. Therefore, a criterion for the choice is whether children can accept the sound eye occlusion or not.

I personally think the total sound eye occlusion is most effective and relatively safe for the treatment of amblyopia, so long as the visual acuity of both occluded and non-occluded eye is carefully checked up. The occurrence of occlusion amblyopia is likely to be rare and it is mild and curable even if it should occur. It is not right to have an over-exaggerated concern for the reduction of visual acuity of the occluded eye and to abandon the sound eye occlusion for the treatment of amblyopia. The only concern or the greatest obstacle in performing the sound eye patch in children is a phychological rejection or physiological skin irritation. In such cases, I would compromise and do penalization for the treatment of amblyopia.

One question remains. How good is the penalization for the amblyopic case with latent nystagmus which may be manifest by the conventional occlusion?

A CONTROLLED STUDY COMPARING CAM TREATMENT TO OCCLUSION THERAPY

K. G. Nyman, G. Singh
A. Rydberg and M. Fornander

ABSTRACT

We compared two groups of children (ages 4 - 6-1/2) randomly chosen and consisting of 25 children to be treated with the CAM-method and 25 children with occlusion. The parameter of comparison was distant visual acuity as measured with Snellen E chart. The children were totally untreated before and had retinoscopy after atropiniation. Those who had significant refraction errors were prescribed glasses with full correction. Only those who did not improve the visual acuity after having worn their glasses for two months were then randomly placed in the groups.

After the treatment the final visual acuities were measured by two colleagues who did not know which treatment the patient had received and who did not have access to the patients' records. No significant difference was found between the two methods as regards mean improvement. In both groups, 80% of the children showed an improvement of two lines or more. The conclusion is that CAM-treatment for anisometropic amblyopia is not worse than occlusion.

INTRODUCTION

The treatment of amblyopia is centuries old. A systematic description of occlusion therapy was provided by Leclerc(1) in 1743 and to this day the method by and large has remained unchanged. Although occlusion often leads to beneficial results,(2-4) it is frequently unacceptable to the child and frustrating for the patient. When occlusion has failed other methods(5-9) have been tried. Dazzling or after-image stimulation of the foveola requires active cooperation by the child and therefore is often applied in a late stage of the visually immature period.(7) The success rate is poor. Penalization, another alternative, works best in cases of amblyopia combined with hyperopia and/or nystagmus.(10)

STRABISMUS II
ISBN 0-8089-1424-3

In one of their early papers, Hubel and Wiesel(11) showed that cell clusters in the visual cortex are present that only respond to rectangular stimuli with a specific orientation. Different clusters respond to different angles of orientation. This forms the basis of the latest addition to the amblyopia therapy arsenal--the CAM stimulator. When Banks et al(12a,b) in 1978 reported improvement in 38 of 40 cases, using the CAM stimulator the method seemed promising. This led us to initiate this study in which CAM is compared to occlusion using equally large randomly allocated groups. Since then other authors(13,14) have reported that CAM is not only as efficient as occlusion but also produces results sooner and therefore should be the treatment of choice.

METHODS AND SUBJECTS

Subjects

Children between 4 and 6-1/2 years, who as part of the general health program (this involves virtually all children in the age group) had an eye check up at pediatric care centers in the northern part of Greater Stockholm between August 1978 and April 1981, constitute the population. Children who showed a difference of at least 2 lines in distant visual acuity between the two eyes (as measured by Snellen E chart with decimal steps) provided the weakest eye did not have a v.a. better than 0.7 were considered to have amblyopia. These subjects were referred to our clinic.

Examination

A complete orthoptic assessment, cycloplegic refraction (Atropine topically for 3 days) and inspection of ocular media and fundus were made. Whenever necessary (Hyperopia > 1D, Myopia > 0.5D, and Astigmatism > 0.5D) full corrective glasses were provided. After these glasses had been worn for eight weeks, the subjects were given a new assessment including visual acuity. Those who no longer were amblyopic as defined above were excluded from the study. The remaining 50 subjects were randomly allocated to occlusion and CAM groups, respectively, consisting of 25 subjects each.

Occlusion therapy

Occlusion therapy consisted of either total occlusion of Einschleich dimmage (Manuf: Ruser). In cases of tropia the best eye was occluded for five days alternated by the amblyopic eye for two. With Heterophoria or Orthophoria,

Einschleich, corresponding to a visual acuity of 0.2 less than that of the amblyopic eye was worn continuously in front of the best eye.

CAM therapy

The CAM vision stimulator marketed by Clement Clark was used. The amblyopic eye - the other eye being occluded only during treatment - was presented plates with black and white gratings starting with those of the highest constrast and the child was asked to identify the correct orientation. The plate of the least contrast that was correctly identified and the two next of higher contrast were used in the CAM stimulator. Stimulation by three plates took approximately seven minutes. The number of treatments given varied between five and ten.

Improvement

The criterion was that the visual acuity in the treated eye had to improve by at least two lines on Snellen chart.

RESULTS

Tables 1-5 below presents the distribution of certain variables in the CAM and occlusion groups respectively.

TABLE 1

Distribution of degree of strabismus in the CAM and Occlusion groups prior to treatment.

	CAM No of subj	rel freq %	Occl No of subj	rel freq %
No strabismus	6	24	9	36
$<5°$	4	16	7	28
$>5°$	3	12	2	8
Phoria	12	48	7	28
	25	100	25	100

MANN - WHITNEY U test gives Z = 1.52 P 0.0643

There is no significant difference between the two groups.

TABLE 2

Distribution of type of deviation in the CAM and Occlusion groups prior to treatment.

	No of subj	
	CAM	Occl
Exo	10	7
Eso	9	9
Ortho	6	9
	25	25

TABLE 3

Distribution of refractive errors in CAM and Occlusion groups prior to treatment.

	No of subj	
	CAM	Occl
Hyperop, astigmat	17	17
Hyperop	6	6
Astigmat	1	2
Myop	1	
	25	25

TABLE 4

Distribution of Bagolini striated glass test in CAM and Occlusion groups prior to treatment.

	CAM No of subj	rel freq %	Occl No of subj	rel freq %
Positive	21	84	24	96
Non positive	4	16	1	4
	25	100	25	100

TABLE 5

Distribution of crowding phenomenon in CAM and Occlusion groups prior to treatment.

	CAM No of subj	rel freq %	Occl No of subj	rel freq %
Present	4	16	2	8
Absent	19	76	17	68

TABLE 6

Mean and standard deviation for distant visual acuity in CAM and Occlusion groups prior to treatment.

	Mean	S.D.
CAM	0.3960	0.1485
Occl	0.4348	0.1584

As can been from tables above the two groups are comparable regarding a number of relevant variables. Tables 7 and 8 show the improvement in visual acuity in the two groups provided it consisted of 2 lines or more on Snellen E chart.

TABLE 7

Improvement in visual acuity in the CAM group after treatment.

Improvement in no of lines	freq	rel freq %
2	5	26.3
3	10	52.6
4	2	10.5
5	1	5.3
6	1	5.3
	19	100.0

Mean 3.105
S.D. 1.049

TABLE 8

Improvement in visual acuity in the Occlusion group after treatment.

Improvement in no of lines	freq	rel freq %
2	6	30
3	6	30
4	6	30
5	1	5
7	1	5
	20	100

Mean 3.30
S.D. 1.26

TABLE 9

Improvement in visual acuity in Occlusion and CAM groups after treatment.

Therapy	Improvement less than 2 lines	at least 2 lines	number of subjects
CAM	6	19	25
Occl	5	20	25

Fishers exact probability test gives a P value of 0.50. MANN WHITNEY test gives the same results.

CONCLUSIONS AND DISCUSSION

The main object of this study was to compare occlusion treatment to CAM stimulation regarding the parameter of distant visual acuity. We have not been able to demonstrate any significant difference. By both methods an improvement of at least two lines on the Snellen chart was achieved in 80% of cases. Regarding CAM it has not been established that gratings are responsible for the visual improvement. Equally good results using grey discs instead of gratings have been reported.(16) It may well be that the combination of occlusion and near work requiring visual concentration is responsible for the improvement.(15)

We subclassified our material according to the type of amblyopia anisometropic, strabismic and stimulus deprivation. The anisometropic group was by far the largest (13 CAM and 12 occlusion) thus not allowing valid conclusions about differences in improvement in the other subgroups. However, the distribution in the CAM and the occlusion groups were similar.

A point of practical interest is that a number of parents found it inconvenient to take time off from their work to accompany the child to our clinic for CAM stimulation twice a week. Some even asked for a switch over to occlusion but were persuaded against it until at least five sessions were completed.

Summing it up we feel that CAM is a useful alternative where occlusion cannot be used.

ACKNOWLEDGEMENTS

This paper was supported by a grant from Carmen and Bertil Regners fund for forskning inom omradet ogonsjukdomar, Stockholm.

REFERENCES

1. Buffon Geoges Louis Le Clerc, Compte: Sur le cause de strabisme on les yeux louches, Histoire de L' academie Royale des sciences avec les memoires mathematique et physique, 1743 pp 231-238 (mem).

2. Mackensen G, Kroner B, Postic G, Kelock W: Untersuchen zum Problem der excentrischen Fixation. Doc Ophthalmol 23:221-262, 1967.

3. Haase W: Worth and unworth of occlusion therapy in the treatment of squint. Muench Med Wochenschr 120(4):99-102, 1978.

4. Verronneau-Troutman S: Conventional occlusion vs. pleoptics in the treatment of amblyopia. Am J Ophthalmol 78:117-120, 1974.

5. Comberg W: Ein Gerat zur Uebung des Zentralen Sehens bei funktioneller Schwachsichtigkeit. Ber Deutsch Ophthalmolog Ges 51:441-443, 1936.

6. Bangerter A: Behandlung der Amblyopie. Ophthalmologica 111:220, 1946.

7. Cuppers C: Moderne Schielbehandlung. Klin Mbl Augenheil 129:579-604, 1956.

8. Bangerter A: Orthoptische Behandlung Des Begleitschielens. Pleoptik (Monokulare Orthoptik). Proceedings of the XVIII Concilium Ophthalmologicum, Bruxelles, Imprimerie Medicale Et Scientifique, S.A., 1959.

9. Schmidt D, Stapp M: Uber die Wirkungen der Euthskop und Okklusionsbehandlung beim Konvergenzschielen. Klin Mbl Augenheil 171:105-117, 1977.

10. Burian H, von Noorden GK: Binocular Vision and Ocular Motility, St. Louis, C.V. Mosby, 1980.

11. Hubel DH, Wiesel TN: Receptive fields, binocular interaction and functional architecture in the cat's visual cortex. J Phyiol (Lond) 160:106-154, 1962.

12a. Banks RV, Campbell FW, Hess R, Watson PG: A new treatment for amblyopia. Br Orthopt J 35:1-12, 1978.

12b. Campbell FW, Hess RF, Watson PG, Banks R: Preliminary results of physiologically based treatment of amblyopia. Br J Ophthalmol 62:748-755, 1978.

13. Willshaw HE, Malmheden A, Clarke J, Williams A and Dean L: Experience with CAM vision stimulator: preliminary report. Br J Ophthalmol 64:339-341, 1980.

14. Sullivan GD, Fallowfield LJ: A controlled test of the CAM treatment for amblyopia. Br Orthopt J 37:47-55, 1980.

15. Linke B: Erfahrungen mit der Amblyopibehandlung mit dem Campbell-Stimulator. In: Freigang M. (ed.). Arbeitskreis Schielen, Wiesbaden 1979, BVA Publikationen 12:67-73, 1980.

16. Keith CG, Howell ER, Mitchell DE, Smith S: Clinical trial of the use of rotating grating patterns in the treatment of amblyopia. Br J Ophthalmol 64:597-606, 1980.

DISCUSSION BY SHINOBU AWAYA

I would like to comment Dr. Nyman's paper on the CAM treatment. Since Banks, Campbell, Watson and others reported on CAM, there have been many papers in pros and cons regarding the effectiveness of this new treatment. Thus, it is a good paper to get a final conclusion for the validity of this method with the statistic analysis made without any bias in dealing with patients in the entire course of treatment. Dr. Nyman's paper showed that no statistic difference between the two methods; the CAM treatment and the conventional sound eye occlusion. His meticulous way of analyzing their data from several parameters was very acceptable, though the total number of the cases studied was not large enough and the subjects were only anisometropic amblyopes.

I have had almost no personal experience with the CAM, but I have my impression that the CAM treatment could give a slight recovery of linear visual acuity. In other words, the linear E acuity, which is worse than the single E acuity before the treatment, may reach the level of the single E acuity which has been already obtained before the treatment.

Dr. Lennerstrand from Sweden reported essentially the same results with the CAM treatment. That is, he found almost no difference between the results by the conventional sound eye occlusion and those by the CAM treatment, not only in cases of anisometropic amblyopia but also in cases of strabismic amblyopia. Dr. France talked on the same subject in the poster session yesterday, and he could scarcely get the effect of the rotating stimulus, but the effect, if any, may be due to the exercises of the amblyopic eye for near fixation. Dr. Nyman was right, however, when he said that the CAM treatment was "not worse" than the conventional occlusion.

I personally think that the conventional occlusion is effective enough, if it can be performed, for the visual stimuli in the daily circumstances have essentially all meridians and stimulate the visual system for all meridians without any rotating stripes. Just like the penalization, the CAM treatment may be a treatment of choice, if the long-term sound eye occlusion cannot be performed for any reason.

Here, my question is: By which way was visual acuity measured before and after the treatment? Do you expect any change in the level of contrast acuity or spatial frequency acuity after the CAM treatment, although no seemingly significant change was encountered in the level of the conventional measurement of visual acuity?

KIDS VERSUS KITTENS
OR IS A LONG TERM CONSTANT OCCLUSION DANGEROUS?

J.B. Weiss

ABSTRACT

Occlusion is the best treatment for strabismic amblyopia. Constant occlusion can be maintained for long periods of time; after such long term constant occlusion (LTCO), reverse amblyopia of the patched eye can be avoided with the Boulad technique of desocclusion. This technique of desocclusion consists of allowing the patched eye to see only during short periods of time, then to gradually increase the time of desocclusion. With this method, even when constant occlusion has been maintained for long periods, all reverse amblyopias have been cured, and the visual acuity of the patched eye restored to 20/20. The curve of the maximum duration of the LTCO for diffeent ages is given.

INTRODUCTION

Javal showed that strabismic amblyopia is functional and that it could be cured in most cases by a long term constant occlusion (LTCO). For some children he prescribed occlusion of several years (1). But as occlusion is troublesome for the ophthalmologists and/or the family, the search of a miraculous not occlusive treatment (NOT) has continued and/or for a scientific pretext not to occlude. Even in the time of Javal, amblyopia was said by many to be organic.

When starting training in ophthalmology, I was not allowed to occlude eccentric fixation, as Cuppers and Bangerter had said that with such treatment eccentric fixation would be reinforced. The child was supposed to wait until the age of 5 to 6, for pleoptic treatment.

More recently, the experiments of Hubel and Wiesel on kittens have been interpreted by some ophthalmologists as a reason not to occlude. And by coincidence, Campbell, another well known physiologists, patented his CAM. Faithfully, we tried extensively to cure our patients with rotating patterns. And to give them all their chances, we gave them apparati for training at home every day for 3 months or more. The statistical study of our results was easy to do, as in 60 cases of previously treated amblyopia we did not have a single case with a significant improvement of the visual acuity.

STRABISMUS II
ISBN 0-8089-1424-3

For 6 years, we have also tried the treatment of amblyopia on young babies by the method of sector occluders. Our results do not support this NOT. When there is only a dominant eye, the sectors can induce an alternating fixation, but if ambloypia is deep, the sector method is ineffective. In such a case, only a constant occlusion can restore a normal visual acuity to the amblyopic eye.

In 1982, my opinion is clear. In all cases, constant occlusion is the shortest and the most efficient treatment of amblyopia. Other treatments cause a loss of time and/or money.

Is a LTCD a dangerous method? How long can we occlude without danger? How can we avoid occlusion amblyopia of the sound eye? These are the real questions we should try to answer. And as kids are different from kittens, the best way to know is to occlude babies and kids and to collaborate with clinical experimentation.

Technique of Constant Occlusion Followed by a Desocclusion

The occlusion is constant; the patch on the sound eye is removed every two days, in darkness. The child is never allowed to see with the sound eye. This constant occlusion is maintained until: the VA is equal or greater than 20/40, or a baby's fixation of the amblyopic eye seems good, or when the case is judged not curable.

During this constant occlusion, the VA or the fixation of the occluded eye is never checked by the ophthalmologist or the orthoptist.

At the end of the LTCD, we check the fixation and the VA of the second eye in a dimly lighted room. If the VA is of 20/20, we switch to an alternated occlusion. But when the fixation of the patched eye is not steady and/or the VA is reduced, as the alternated occlusion could produce a permanent amblyopia of the patched eye we practice a progressive desocclusion, as described by Boulad.(3)

DESOCCLUSION

The occlusion of the sound eye is maintained night and day. Both eyes are never allowed to see at the same time. But every day, for a short period of time, the amblyopic eye is closed, and the sound eye, is allowed to see in a dimly lighted room. At the beginning, the duration of this desocclusion is of 5 minutes; and this duration is progressively increased, until the parents tell us that the child seems to see normally. Then, and only then do we check again the VA of this eye. In some of our cases, the desocclusion lasted several months.

With this technique, all our cases of reverse amblyopia have been successfully cured. So, now, we have no fear of the LTCD. LTCD has been well accepted by children. But in a few cases, after six months of permanent occlusion, the mother showed a depressive mood.

RESULTS

The duration of the constant occlusion ranged from a week to 14 months, depending on the age of the child and the deepness of the amblyopia. The important figure is the maximum duration of the LTCD for a given age maintained without producing a definitive reverse amblyopia. Bouland has given her results. From our clinical experience, we are able to confirm her results for children between 2 and 8 years old, and to complete the curve under the age of 2.

Recently, Kushner(3) reported cases of functional amblyopia associated with organic lesions which he treated by LTCD. (See case no. 12.). He did not produce reverse amblyopia.

COMMENTS

1. Permanent occlusion is the fastest and most efficient treatment of amblyopia. LTCD is not dangerous if it is followed by a progressive desocclusion as described by Boulad.

2. The curve of the maximum duration of a LTPD versus the age of the child should be established by a collaborative clinical experimentation, especially under the age of two.

3. Physiologists should study and use the Boulad desocclusion method to cure their occluded kitten.

4. When a new NOT is presented, the only question we should ask the author is the following: "Is your treatment faster than plain occlusion?" Till now, the answer has always been: "No."

REFERENCES

1. Javal E: Manuel du Strabisme. Paris, Masson, 1896, p. 233.

2. Boulad MTh: Amblyopies. Occlusion totale. Mode de desocclusion. J Fr Orthopt 10:115, 1978.

3. Kushner BJ: Functional amblyopia associated with organic ocular disease. Am J Ophthalmol 91:39-45, 1981. (See case 12)

DISCUSSION BY SHINOBU AWAYA

I think Dr. Weiss's paper raises two points for discussion. First, I can understand the possibility of occurrence of amblyopia when he mentioned that at the age of six months, the occlusion of one eye only for one week was likely to have caused deprivation amblyopia, and such a long-term occlusion as ten months may have caused deleterious damage to the visual system and developed amblyopia even at the age of six years as reported by Dr. Weiss. In kittens and monkeys, according to several investigators, as Wiesel, Hubel, von Noorden, and others, it lasts up to the third or fifth month of life. According to Wiesel, this does not sharply terminate but it lingers in a waning down-slope up to the end of the second year, beyond which time no electrophysiological changes are encountered. We found the same in humans, over 150 cases of deprivation amblyopia caused by monocular visual deprivation of various durations and at various times of onset. The sensitivity is likely to be less marked in the first month and to become highest between the 3rd and 24th month; and, thereafter, it declines in the waning slope which continues up to the end of the 8th year of life.

The causative effect for the development of amblyopia is partially the multiplication of the extent of sensitivity and the length of causative occlusion. Therefore, in order to study the length of the critical period, we need to collect and accummulate as many cases as possible and do a retrospective analysis. I agree with him that we should not have over-concern about the possible reduction of visual acuity of the sound eye by the occlusion. We should not abandon this good and effective method of sound eye occlusion for the treatment of amblyopia because of too much fear for the occlusion amblyopia. Generally, it is not dangerous to patch the good eye when there is a big difference in visual acuity between the two eyes. However, it is dangerous to patch one eye when both eyes are equal and immature.

Secondly, I cannot agree with him in that he claims that a permanent occlusion is harmless, so long as he terminates this permanent occlusion by the method of "desocclusion". He said, "Upon the termination of the permanent occlusion, we should not patch the other eye, for the alternate occlusion is very dangerous, and thus, we should expose the so far occluded good eye to the light stimulus gradually from the dim to the bright light." I personally think it is hardly possible to get recovery from the decreased visual acuity of the so far good eye only by exposing it to the light stimulus but not to the pattern stimulus, for it is the deprivation not from light stimulus but from pattern stimulus that causes deprivation amblyopia. Therefore, we need to expose the so far occluded and possible deteriorated eye to the pattern stimulus, but not to the light stimulus, for the treatment of the occlusion amblyopia. We should always be careful not to give any "permanent occlusion" to the good eye as the treatment of amblyopia. We should always remember that the cross-patching effect can occur within the sensitive period.

PATTERN REVERSAL VISUAL EVOKED POTENTIALS IN CONGENITAL ESOTROPIA

A.O. Ciancia, H. Garcia, and A. Cammarota

ABSTRACT

The data shows the following aspects of the visual acuity and the pattern reversal-visual evoked potentials (PR-VEP) in congenital esotropia.

1. Facilitation and partial summation appear to be a rule under binocular stimulation in these cases.

2. Twenty-five percent of the patients lost the VEP in monocular conditions and half of them recovered the VEP when the eye was put in adduction.

3. In spite of the fact that nystagmus could be one cause for the loss of the monocular VEP, there seems to be some other mechanism involved, since there is no correlation between latencies or amplitudes of the VEP and frequency or amplitude of nystagmus.

4. The concept that cortical organization with regard to stereopsis could be of importance for the binocular facilitation in normal subjects is hard to apply in the bilateral limitation of abduction (BLA), since stereopsis was not present in these cases. However, in the BLA, the same cortical organization could play a role of mechanism either independent or complementary to stereopsis.

5. In BLA, the mechanisms that alter the monocular vision are apparently not necessarily correlated with those producing nystagmus, at least in some patients.

VEP obtained by alternating checkerboard patterns is the best objective test and the only one permitting correlations of some experimental electrophysiological findings with clinical ophthalmology.1-3 The procedure has found considerable acceptance and it has been outstanding as an objective test for infantile visual diseases.

STRABISMUS II
ISBN 0-8089-1424-3

In the present work, 20 patients suffering from congenital esotropia in a form defined by one of the authors (ADC) as bilateral limitation of abduction (BLA)4 were studied.

The prominent signs of the affection are: esotropia, torticollis, alternating hyperphoria, latent nystagmus and in many cases, a monocular amlyopia of a diverse degree.

Two facts were found to be of particular interest in these cases: 1). The visual acuity tests showed that binocular visual acuity was often much better than monocular, even considering the best eye. 2). The latent nystagmus, only significant in monocular conditions, when measured by electroculographic (EOG) studies, showed differences in frequency and amplitude that potentially could affect the monocular visual acuity (VA). The aim of this reseach was to evaluate the PR-VEP and to correlate its amplitude and latency in binocular and monocular conditions with the visual acuity and the amplitude and frequency of the nystagmus. In addition, possible cortical mechanisms that could be involved in these process are considered.

MATERIALS AND METHODS

A total of twenty patients of both sexes were studied. Eighteen were children 4 to 12 years old, two were teenagers of 17. Their VA was tested by means of the Snellen chart and expressed in decimals. In all cases measurements were made in each eye independently and in both eyes simultaneously.

The PR-VEP studies were performed with a Nicolet CA 1000 biological computer system. The image was emitted by a TV monitor with a reversal frequency of 1.8/sec. The screen displays 15 x 15 mm squares at a high contrast (0.8).

All patients were comfortably seated, facing the TV set, at a distance of one meter from the screen. Fifty to 100 stimuli were produced, and the total number was regulated according to the degree of attention of the subject during the procedure.

In all cases double measurements were obtained with binocular vision and with monocular vision; under the following conditions: with the fixing eye in primary positions and with the fixing eye in adduction.

The eye position was maintained with a simultaneous

rotation of the head, held in the necessary angle so as to keep the eye in the direction of the TV monitor. The adduction usually produces a blockage of the nystagmus, and changes in the VEP can be recorded.

The EOG tracings of the nystagmus were recorded in a Berger NG 104 nystagmography unit with the published technique.5

Table 1

ET - BLA - 20 PATIENTS
VISUAL ACUITY

PATIENT	SEX	YEARS	R.E.	L.E.	BOTH EYES
1. MA	F	5	5/10	4/10	6/10
2. ML	F	17	1/10	5/10	6/10
3. MG	F	7	5/10	6/10	6/10
4. AK	F	8	1/10	1/10	5/10
5. MG	M	10	6/10	10/10	10/10
6. NB	F	8	6/10	7/10	10/10
7. JP	M	5	5/10	5/10	7/10
8. PM	M	6	3/10	3/10	4/10
9. FB	M	5	1/10	2/10	6/10
10. FN	M	5	6/10	6/10	6/10
11. EP	F	9	4/10	7/10	9/10
12. RP	F	6	1/10	3/10	3/10
13. MS	F	7	2/10	1/10	5/10
14. IR	F	5	6/10	1/10	6/10
15. GS	M	5	2/10	1/10	7/10
16. ML	F	13	4/10	1/10	9/10
17. PD	F	17	9/10	10/10	10/10
18. BL	F	5	2/10	4/10	5/10
19. MR	F	9	5/10	3/10	8/10
20. MB	F	4	1/20	3/10	4/10

Table 1 indicates the age and the sex of each patient. The VA is expressed in decimals. The binocular VA and 10/10 in patients 5, 6 and 17, and cases 5 and 17 presented 10/10 also in one eye. Six cases showed substantially better VA with both eyes than with each eye individually.

Table 2

ET - BLA - 20 PATIENTS
VISUAL ACUITY

	10/10	9/10	8/10	7/10	6/10	5/10	4/10	3/10	2/10	1/10
BOTH EYES	3	2	1	2	6	3	2	1	-	-
RIGHT EYE	-	1	-	-	4	4	2	1	3	5
LEFT EYE	2	-	-	2	2	2	2	4	1	5

Table 2 shows the distribution of VA in the different clinical conditions, between 10/10 and 1/10, for both eyes, and for each one individually. It is noteworthy that 14 patients showed 6/10 or better with binocular vision, while that range of VA was reached only by 5 patients with RE and 6 with LE.

Table 3

ET - BLA - 20 PATIENTS
DIFFERENCE IN V.A. (Δ)

Δ/10	BETWEEN BOTH EYES - BEST EYE	BETWEEN BEST EYE - POOR EYE
0	6	4
1	5	7
2	2	4
3	3	2
4	2	2
5	2	1

Differences in VA between both eyes simultaneously and the best eye, and the best eye and the poorer eye, are expressed in Table 3. No difference in VA was found between the best eye and in binocular vision in 6 patients, while 14 patients showed difference between 1/10 and 5/0. The difference between the better and the poorer eye was found to be equal to zero in 4 patients, 1/10 in 7 patients and between 2/10 and 5/10 in the remaining 9 patients.

PR-VEP

Two parameters were measured: the amplitudes and the latencies. The amplitudes showed considerable differences among patients. They ran between 2.00 uV (case 12) and 19 uV (Case 10). The data was classified according to the criteria of Apkarian et al6, in which the maximum ratio for binocular versus monocular VEP amplitude is called facilitation and the minimum, inhibition. Intermediate stages are summation, partial summation and zero summation.

Table 4 ET - BLA - 20 PATIENTS
PATTERN - V.E.P. - AMPLITUDES

PAT.	SEX	R.E. (PP)	L.E. (PP)	BOTH EYES	R.E. (AD)	L.E. (AD)
1MA	F	3.00	NEG.	3.9	3.2	3.2
2ML	F	1.8	1.9	4.2	NEG.	1.5
3MG	F	8.00	7.00	16.2	2.8	10.00
4AK	F	NEG.	NEG.	3.00	NEG.	NEG.
5MG	M	2.5	2.2	4.50	NEG.	1.00
6NB	F	NEG.	1.5	3.00	2.00	-
7JP	M	4.7	3.20	3.7	3.00	4.6
8PM	M	1.8	3.2	2.8	2.0	3.00
9FB	M	NEG.	NEG.	3.5	3.3	3.4
10FN	M	11.5	10.00	19.00	19.0	19.0
11EP	F	3.00	4.7	11.4	3.00	3.00
12RP	F	NEG.	1.5	2.00	NEG.	1.00
13MS	F	NEG.	NEG.	8.00	3.8	1.8
14IR	F	1.00	1.00	5.00	5.00	5.00
15GS	M	3.00	NEG.	6.00	6.00	6.00
16ML	F	NEG.	NEG.	3.6	NEG.	NEG.
17PD	F	4.00	2.00	4.00	NEG.	NEG.
18BL	F	2.8	NEG.	3.2	2.9	3.0
19MR	F	NEG.	NEG.	2.5	NEG.	1.00
20MB	F	2.8	NEG.	3.2	2.9	3.0

In Table 4, amplitudes of the VEP are expressed, under binocular and monocular conditions, in primary position and in adduction, since this last condition is the one in which patients usually developed better VEP. In this context, 8 patients showed facilitation, 7 partial summation, 4 zero summation, and 1 showed summation. In brief, 15 over 20 patients showed a high degree of difference in favor of binocular over monocular VEP. Only two patients did not develop VEP in monocular conditions with either eye regardless of the eye position. An example of this type can be observed in Figure 1. In these cases the facilitation can be considered maximal. On the other hand, no simple correlation could be established between amplitude of the potential and visual acuity under binocular conditions.

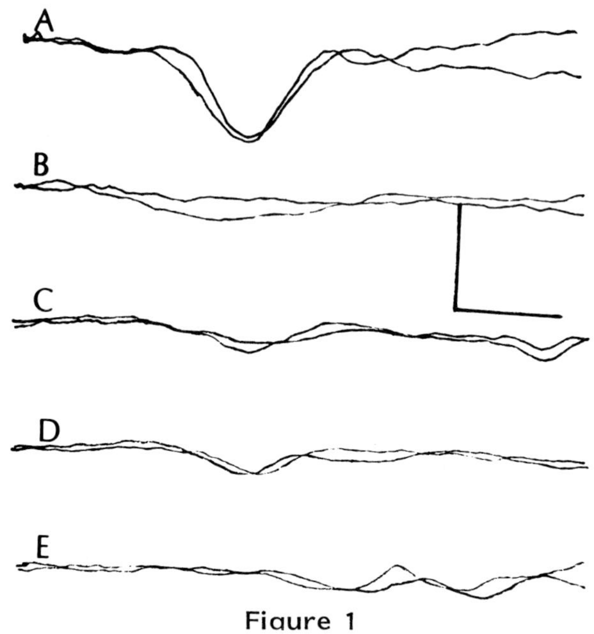

Figure 1

The other parameter to be measured in the VEP is the latency. The latencies to the maximal positive peak (P100) of the VEP are shown in Table 5. The most prolonged latency for binocular test was 116.5 msec (case 5) and the minimal 91.00 msec (case 9). When the VEP was tested in monocular vision, patients 1, 6, 12, 15 and 20 developed VEP in primary position with one eye but not with the other, while in cases 4, 9, 13, and 19, it was not apparent as to which was the fixating eye.

ET - BLA - 20 PAIIENTS
PATTERN-V.E.P. - LATENCY P 100

PAT.	SEX	R.E. (PP)	L.E. (PP)	BOIH EYES	R.E. (AD)	L.E. (AD)
1.MA	F	85.5	NEG.	99.7	93.6	106.8
2.ML	F	128.7	112.5	106.7	NEG.	111.6
3.MG	F	98.2	100.5	101.0	93.0	100.0
4.AK	F	NEG.	NEG.	98.5	NEG.	NEG.
5.MG	M	130.25	115.5	116.5	NEG.	129.0
6.NB	F	NEG.	98.75	97.05	115.0	98.00
7.JP	M	117.75	104.2	108	107.5	93.7
8.PM	M	115.8	111.50	110	114.00	96.0
9.FB	M	NEG.	NEG.	91.00	96.00	95.00
10FN	M	95.25	95.5	95.00	95.00	95.00
11EP	F	127.25	125.00	115.5	128.7	123.00
12RP	F	NEG.	120.00	117.0	NEG.	122.00
13MS	F	NEG.	NEG.	110.5	112.0	122.2
14IR	F	105	108	110.5	110.5	110.5
15GS	M	118.00	NEG.	106.00	106.00	106.00
16ML	F	NEG.	NEG.	108	NEG.	NEG.
17PD	F	104.75	107.5	98.00	NEG.	NEG.
18BL	F	100.5	99.75	100.00	100	99.0
19MR	F	NEG.	NEG.	115.25	NEG.	114.0
20MB	F	97.78	NEG.	92.5	98.00	100.00

Table 5

In those cases where only one eye failed to produce VEP, it developed when the eye was in adduction. Out of five cases that showed no potential with monocular fixation in primary position, 3 developed the VEP when the eye was in adduction (Fig 2). In the other cases, the VEP showed the following variations: 10 patients had an increase of the latencies to P100 which ranged from a minimum in case 10, where the increase changed from 95.0 to 95.25 msec, to a maximum as in case 5 that presented a difference of 13.5 msec.

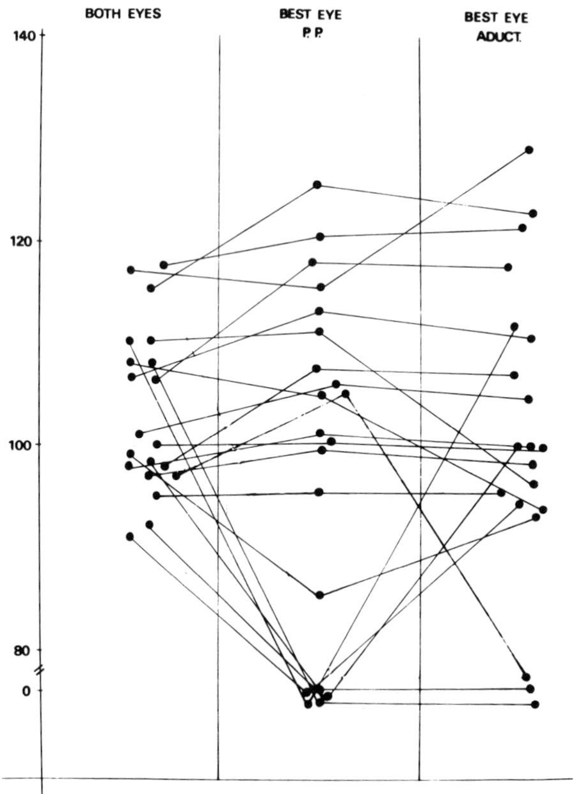

Figure 2

Nystagmus

Nystagmus was manifest clearly during monocular fixation. This type of nystagmus showed significant variations, as it is shown in Table 6. This variation was relevant in amplitudes as well as in frequencies. In all cases nystagmus showed the features of the BLA type.7 A maximal amplitude of 5o was observed in only one case, but in general they were in the order of 1o. Frequencies ran between 0.5/sec and 5/sec. Although nystagmus seemed to be a simple cause of deficit of monocular VA, no acceptable correlation was found between the latency to the P100 peak and amplitudes (Fig 3) or frequency (Fig 4) of nystagmus.

ET - BLA - 20 PATIENTS
NIGSTAGMUS

PATIENT	R.E. FREQ. AMP.	L.E. FREQ. AMP.
1. MA	0.5/SEC. 1°	4/SEC. 2°
2. ML	NEG.	1/SEC. 1°
3. MG	NEG.	NEG.
4. AK	5/SEC. 4°	4/SEC. 4°
5. MG	3/SEC. 1°	4/SEC. 3°
6. NB	3/SEC. 1°	3/SEC. 1°
7. JP	1/SEC. 1°	1/SEC. 1°
8. PM	-	-
9. FB	5/SEC. 1°	5/SEC. 1°
10. FN	1/SEC. 1°	1/SEC. 1°
11. EP	1/SEC. -	1/SEC. -
12. RP	3/SEC. 1°	3/SEC. 1°
13. MS	2/SEC. 3°	2/SEC. 4°
14. IR	4/SEC. 1°	3/SEC. 1°
15. GS	3/SEC. 5°	3/SEC. 5°
16. ML	1/SEC. 1°	3/SEC. 3°
17. PD	1/SEC. -	1/SEC. N
18. BL	3/SEC. 1°	3/SEC. 1°
19. MR	3/SEC. 1°	3/SEC. 1°
20. MB	-	-

Table 6

Special attention was paid to the nystagmus affect in those cases in which a substantial difference was found between binocular and monocular VA (cases 9, 13, 16, and 19). In these cases only one patient showed considerable amplitude variations. Frequency was high in one case only. Of particular interest is the fact that case 5 showed better VA in the left eye (10/10) which curiously enough was the one presenting higher frequency and amplitude as compared with its fellow eye, in addition to having shorter latency to the P100.

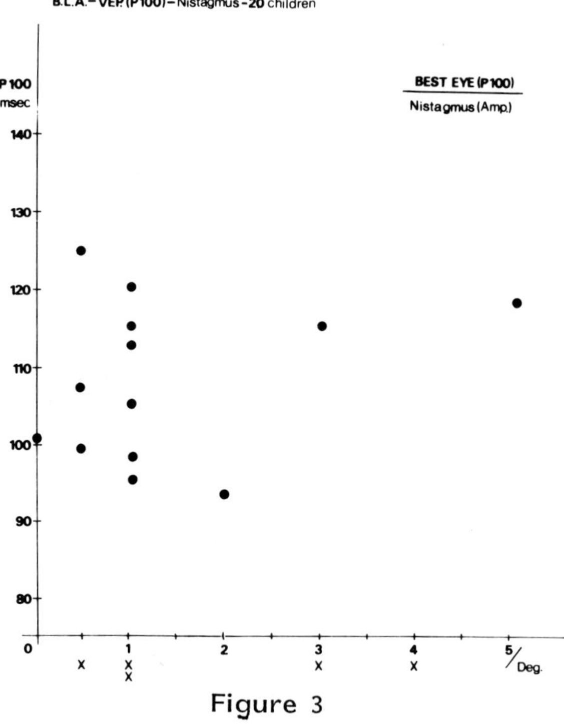

Figure 3

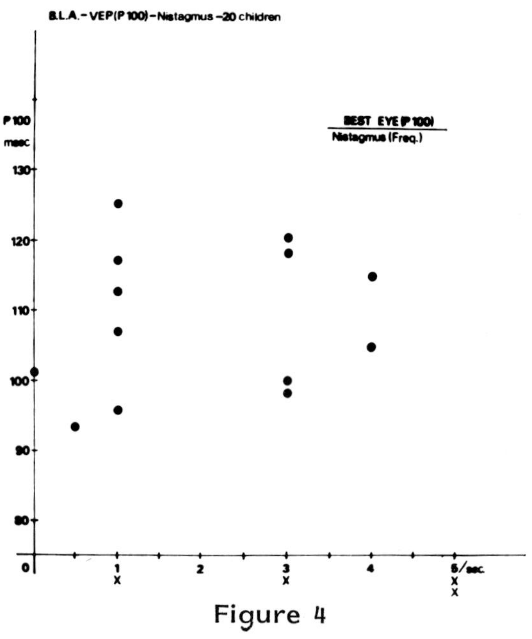

Figure 4

REFERENCES

1. Arden GB, Bernard WM, Mushin AS: Visually evoked responses in amblyopia. Br J Ophthalmol 58:183-192, 1974.

2. Lennerstrand G: Binocular interaction studied with visual evoked responses (VER) in humans with normal or impaired binocular vision. Acta Ophthalmol 56:628-637, 1978.

3. Campos EC: Evaluation of binocularity by means of visual evoked responses. Proc CESS Symposium, Florence, 1982.

4. Ciancia AO: La esotropia con limitacion bilateral de abduccion en el lactante. Archivo de Oftalmologia, Buenos Aires, 37:207-211, 1962.

5. Ciancia AO, Melek N, Garcia H: Los movimientos de sacudida, fijacion y persecusion en los strabismos no paraliticos. Archivos de Oftalmologia, Buenos Aires, 51:73-80, 1976.

6. Apkarian PA, Nakayama K, Tyler CW: Binocularity in the human visual evoked potentials: facilitation, summation and suppression. Electroencephalogr Clin Neurophysiol 51:32-48, 1981.

7. Melek N: El nistagmus en la esotropia con limitacion bilateral de la abduccion, in Souza-Dias C, Vesugi CF, Rangel, CF (eds): Anais do V Congresso do Conselho Latino-Americano de Estrabismo (CLADE), Guaruya, Brazil, 1976, p. 27-31, 1976.

DISCUSSION BY SHINOBU AWAYA

Dr. Ciancia´s paper is interesting and important for the electrophysiological analysis of the Ciancia syndrome, especially for elucidating a binocular input-output mechanism through VEP and EOG. It is interesting that monocular VEP did not appear in either eye even in cases where nystagmus was demonstrated only in one eye and good visual acuity in either eye.

My question is: What was the status of "accommodation" in these cases? Is there any possibility of the following interpretation for the results of your experiments? When nystagmus occurs, it causes the pattern image to be blurry and extinguishes VEP and when nystagmus does not occur, the convergence-induced accommodation causes defocusing the pattern image and results in extinct VEP?

RECURRENT ESOTROPIA FOLLOWING EARLY SUCCESSFUL SURGICAL CORRECTION OF CONGENITAL ESOTROPIA

D. A. Freeley, L. B. Nelson, and J. H. Calhoun

ABSTRACT

This study used a group of congenital esotropes who had an adequate surgical alignment prior to 18 months of age, to determine how many of them would redevelop esotropia. In the group that redeveloped the condition, a high percentage of the esotropia was accommodative in nature and was therefore able to be corrected with spectacles. Both the initial refractive error and changes in refractive error were noted to be significant. The study emphasizes the importance of monitoring the refractive state continuously, especially in children with subnormal fusion.

INTRODUCTION

It is well-known that children with congenital esotropia go on to manifest many other disorders, despite successful surgical alignment of the deviation and no matter at what age surgery occurs. These problems include: overaction of inferior oblique muscles, dissociated vertical deviations (DVD), nystagmus, amblyopia, exotropia, and esotropia. The incidence of most of these disorders has been addressed in several studies.(1-3) It has been our clinical impression that esotropia, and more specifically accommodative esotropia, is a frequent sequela to successful surgical alignment of congenital esotropia. The purpose of this article is to review a selected group, infants with congenital esotropia who had achieved successful surgical alignment of their congenital esotropia prior to 18 months of age, in order to ascertain the frequency and nature of subsequent esotropia.

MATERIALS AND METHODS

We analyzed retrospectively all cases of congenital esotropia operated on at Wills Eye Hospital from 1976 through 1980. Criteria for patient selection included (1) diagnosis of congenital esotropia prior to 6 months of age, (2) surgical alignment within 10 prism diopters prior to 18 months of age, (3) a minimum of 6 months follow-up, and (4) adequate data in the patient's chart. Any patient with neurologic abnormalities or mental retardation was excluded. No consideration was given to the type or amount of surgery

STRABISMUS II
ISBN 0-8089-1424-3

performed, and patients in the study had from one to three surgical procedures. Of more than 200 patients who were operated on during this period for congenital esotropia, 83 met criteria for inclusion in this study. Charts were analyzed for the following data: (1) age of presentation, (2) initial deviation, (3) initial refractive error, (4) age when eyes aligned, (5) amount of subsequent esotropia, (6) amount of time between successful alignment and subsequent esotropia, and (7) change in refractive-error results.

RESULTS

Twenty-three of the 83 patients developed a subsequent esotropia (Table 1). The average age of presentation of the congenital esotropia of these patients was 7.8 months, although existence of esotropia was confirmed in all patients prior to 6 months of age by photography, unequivocal history or pediatric observations. The initial deviation averaged 45 diopters (range 30 to 70). The initial refractive error averaged +1.50 (range -1.00 to +5.00). Several patients had spectacles prescribed for their hyperopia, however, non had any response. These figures conform to the typical congenital esotrope. The average age at which these children's eyes were aligned successfully to within 10 prism diopters was 10.5 months (range 4 through 17 months). The average time until subsequent development of esotropia was 14 months (range 4 through 39 months). The average amount of deviation of the subsequent esotropia was 24.5 diopters (range 12 through 40). The average refraction at the last visit of these patients was +2.6 diopters (range +.50 to +5.00). In 18 of the patients, glasses were prescribed to correct hyperopia; in 14 of these a satisfactory alignment was achieved, thus establishing their esotropia as accommodative in nature. Patient No. 18 was given glasses. However, the prescription was based on the initial refraction, which was more than a year old, and this patient may well have had more hyperopia. Five patients had surgery as therapy for the subsequent esotropia without any attempt at spectacle correction; several of them deserve note. Patient No. 2 had a refraction of +2.00 but glasses were not attempted. In patient No. 17, who had a refraction of +3.50, no glasses were given either. There is a good possibility that either or both of these patients would have had altered or zero angle of deviation if correction with glasses had been attempted. In addition, patient No. 3 did not have a current refraction and may well have increased his hyperopia in the year and a half since his initial refraction. The 23 patients who developed esotropia represent an incidence of 28% of the total group. The patients who were diagnosed definitively as having accommodative esotropia by their response to spectacles represent 61% of the subgroup. If the four additional patients who either were not given glasses or who were given what may have been an inadequate spectacle correction were added to the group of accommodative esotropes, the percentage would rise to 78%. A special note should be made that the average refractive error increased by more than a diopter of hyperopia in these patients. A longer follow-up may well have produced more esotropia; therefore, the true incidence of subsequent esotropia is probably higher than 28%.

COMMENTS

Over the past few decades, there have been several excellent studies analyzing the results of treatment of congenital esotropia. Although the controversy about when to operate on these children is not over, most authorities seem to agree that 2 years of age is the upper limit for achieving a high degree of binocularity. Although the incidence of DVD, overacting inferior oblique muscles, and nystagmus has been reported in various papers, no specific incidence of subsequent accommodative or nonaccommodative esotropia has been reported. In a 1966 study, Ing and associates analyzed a group of patients who had undergone early surgery.(3) They found that 34% had residual esotropia of more than 10 prism diopters and noted that three of the cases were accommodative. It is not stated whether these patients ever acquired satisfactory alignment or whether their esotropias occurred after a satisfactory alignment had been achieved with surgery. Several reports have addressed the fact that postoperative miotics and spectacles are necessary in a high percentage of cases. Foster and colleagues, in describing 34 patients, reported that many patients used glasses, but apparently they were eith prism or minus lenses.(4) Hiles and coworkers, in a study on early bimedial rectus recession, reported that 94% needed some sort of medical therapy in the way of miotics or spectacles postoperatively.(2) They state that the glasses were used to improve visual acuity, myopia, and astigmatism and that miotics were used for abnormal distance/near relationships. They did not make direct mention of what percentage of their patients were accommodative esotropes.

Current studies indicate that approximately 40% to 60% of congenital esotropes, if operated on early, go on to develop the monofixation syndrome described by Parks.(5-7)

Because of the normal fusional vergences that are present in the monofixational syndrome, most of these children should have a fairly stable ocular alignment throughout their lives. The remaining children are not so fortunate. In them, binocularity ranges from poor to nonexistent, and a wide range of change in their alignment over the years may be expected. Hyperopia of moderate to high degree (+2 diopters or more) is prevalent in this age group. The accommodative convergence stimulated by the accommodation required for a clear retinal image requires an intact fusional divergence mechanism to maintain proper eye alignment. The less the binocular fusion, the smaller the fusional divergence the child will possess. Thus, any child with poor fusion as a consequence of congenital esotropia, who has any more than a minimal amount of hyperopia, would be at great risk to develop a subsequent esodeviation. Our statistics seem compatible with this concept. The results emphasize the importance of considering an accommodative cause of any subsequent esotropia in these patients. The results also point out that an attempt to correct, with spectacles, any hyperopia in excess of 1.5 diiopters is warranted before turning to repeat surgery. We suggest that it is imperative to have a current cycloplegic refraction on which to base the prescription. As Brown has shown, hyperopia in children increases until the age of about 7 years, so the cycloplegic refraction at 1 year of age may not represent the true refractive state when the patient returns with a recurrent esotropia later in life.

ACKNOWLEDGEMENTS

This work was made possible in part by a grant from Fight for Sight, Inc. of New York to the Fight for Sight Children's Eye Center of Wills Eye Hospital and by the Research Division, Wills Eye Hospital, Philadelphia, PA.

REFERENCES

1. Ing MR: Early surgical alignment for congenital esotropia. Trans Am Ophthalmol Soc 1981; 79:625-663.

2. Hiles DA, Watson BA, Biglan AW: Characteristics of infantile estropia following early bimedial rectus recession. Arch Ophthalmol 1980; 98:697-703.

3. Ing MR, Costenbader FD, Parks MM, Albert DG: Early surgery for congenital esotropia. Am J Ophthalmol 1966; 61:1419-1427.

4. Foster RS, Paul TO, Jampolsky A: Management of infantile esotropia. Am J Ophthalmol 1976; 82:291-299.

5. Vazquez RB, Calhoun JH, Harley RD: Development of monofixation syndrome in congenital esotropia. J Pediatr Ophthalmol Strabismus 1981; 18:42-44.

6. Taylor DM: Is congenital esotropia functionally curable? Trans Am Ophthalmol Soc 1972; 70:529-576.

7. Parks MM: The monofixation syndrome. Trans Am Ophthalmol Soc 1969; 67:609-657.

8. Brown EVL: Net average yearly changes in refraction of atropinized eyes from birth to beyond middle life. Arch Ophthalmol 1938; 19:719-733.

DETERIORATED ACCOMMODATIVE ESOTROPIA

T. Nakagawa

ABSTRACT

Twenty-six cases of fully accommodative esotropia as reported which deteriorated into partially accommodative esotropia or microtropia. Twelve of them maintained either orthophoria or esophoria under ten prism diopters at distant fixation for three to six months. The rest of them maintained for seven months to five years, averaging 14.5 months after wearing glasses. After the accommodative period, esotropia recurred either following occlusion, after changing to undercorrected glasses, following the development of high AC/A ratio, or for no apparent cause.

Once the fusion was not maintained, the patients never responded to further nonsurgical treatment of refractive corrections or the instillation of miotics.

The final results revealed that 65% had microtropia and 35% had orthophoria or heterophoria for distance. However, most had suppression scotoma and poor stereopsis. Only two cases had bifoveal fusion for distant and near fixation.

We assume that the primary microtropia was masked under accommodative esotropia and it became apparent after the successful management of the accommodative element.

INTRODUCTION

Deterioration of what was initially pure accommodative esotropia has seldom been described. This paper reports the clinical characteristics of twenty-six deteriorated accommodative esotropes. Deterioration began after a prolonged period of fusion. Partially accommodative esotropia or microtropia developed. The clinical course and causes of deterioration are discussed.

MATERIALS AND METHODS

Twenty-six cases of accommodative esotropia included twelve males and fourteen females.

STRABISMUS II
ISBN 0-8089-1424-3

The patients' average age at the first visit was three years, four months (Fig 1). They ranged from four patients of one year, six of two years, and the remainder (62%) at three or more years.

Onset of Deteriorated Accommodative Esotropia

Onset / Cares	under 12months	1 y・o	2 y・o	3 y・o・ or more	Average
Declared	4 17%	5 22%	7 30%	7 30%	24months
Confirmed	0%	4 15%	6 23%	16 62%	40months

Figure 1

Parents reported the onset of esotropia at the average age of twenty-four months, which was was sixteen months prior to the first visit to our clinic. Treatment started at the average age of forty months. Four cases had their onset before twelve months of age. In two cases, the onset was at four to six years of age. The observation period ranged from two years to over ten years. The average observation period was six years and two months.

In most cases, esotropia for distance disappeared within four weeks after starting to wear the full hyperopic correction (60%), within eight weeks (24%) and exceptional cases within several months.

Patients remained orthophoric or esophoric under ten prism diopters for distance and near fixation. These orthophoric periods lasted from three months to five years, averaging 14.5 months. Five of them remained phoric for one to three months, twelve for four to twelve months and nine for more than one year (Fig 2).

Period of orthophoria

month / case	1～3 Ms	4～6 Ms	7～12 Ms	13～24 Ms	25 Ms or more
Number %	5 19%	7 27%	5 19%	4 15%	5 19%
	19%	46%		34%	

Average : 14.5months

Figure 2

All patients were given the following tests when possible: visual acuity, atropine refraction, fundus examination, visuscope, cover test, alternate prism cover test (PCT) and simultaneous PCT, synoptophore, four prism diopter base out test, Bagolini striated glasses, after image and the Titmus stereo test.

RESULTS

Clinical characteristics of this group were, as follows:

1. Initial deviation: Most cases had esodeviation under forty prism diopters. Distant deviation could not be mesured in eleven cases. Three cases had a high AC/A ratio.

2. Deviation at recurrence (Fig 3): Fifty percent of the cases had deviations for distance under ten prism diopters, six of which were intermittent. Eight cases (31%) had deviation between eleven and twenty prism diopters. Six cases had a mildly high AC/A ratio, five of which did not have a high AC/A on the first visit. On the last visit, only one case had a high AC/A ratio. The largest group had esodeviation under ten prism diopters, 38% for distance and 50% for near.

Figure 3

Recurrent deviation

	for distance	for near
Exotropia	1 (4%)	1 (4%)
Uncertain	3 (12%)	0 (0%)
Eso 1～10△	13 (50%)	5 (19%)
Eso 11～20△	8 (31%)	12 (46%)
Eso 21～30△	1 (4%)	7 (27%)
Eso 31～60△	0 (0%)	1 (4%)

3. Preoperative deviation (Fig 4): Fourteen cases underwent surgery. Preoperative deviations were greater than eleven prism diopters in 93% of cases. The largest group had deviations of between eleven and twenty prism diopters.

Figure 4

Preoperative deviation for distance

Esodeviation	Number of cases
0～10△	1 (7%)
11～20△	7 (50%)
21～30△	4 (29%)
31△～	2 (14%)

14 surgical cases (54%)

4. Final deviation (Fig 5): Seventeen cases (65% had constant tropia for distance and near fixation. Deviations seldom exceeded ten prism diopters. Orthophoria and heterophoria were seen in seven cases for both distant and near fixation. However, there were only two cases of bifoveal fusion for distant and near which did not have suppression scotoma and excellent stereopsis (50" or more).

Figure 5

Final motor alignment for distance

	Number
orthophoria	8
ET 2～10P.D.	10
ET 12～16P.D.	3
Exo 6P.D. or less (XT, X)	3
HT 3P.D. or less	2

5. Accompaning abnormalities: Seventeen cases (65%) had inferior oblique overaction (IOOA) (15%), superior oblique overaction (SOOA) (4%), hypertropia (15%) and high AC/A ratio (31%) in the course of the disease. Mild hypertropia (two eight prism diopters) was observed in four cases, two of which were accompanied by minimal esotropia.

6. Refraction (Fig 6): Seventy percent of the cases had moderate to high hypertropia. Only 12% had hyperopia of less than two diopters. Astigmatism or anisometropia was observed in two cases respectively.

Refraction

	Number of cases
0~ +2.0 D	3 (12%)
+2.1~+4.0 D	5 (19%)
+4.1~+6.0 D	12 (46%)
+6.1~+8.0 D	6 (23%)
Astigmatismus over 2D	1 (4%)
Anisometropia over 2D	1 (4%)

Figure 6

7. Visual acuity of amblyopic eye (Fig 7): Fifty-eight percent of the cases had visual acuity of less than 0.3 when the first visual acuity test was taken. Half of the cases had amblyopia with VA 0.3 or less and another half 0.4 to 0.6 when esotropia recurred. On the last visit, 15% of cases had visual acuity of less than 0.3 and 15% 0.4 to 0.7.

Visual acuity of amblyopic eye

V·A	~0.1	0.2 ~0.3	0.4 ~0.7	0.8 ~0.9	1.0~	undetermined
First visit	5	10	7	1	2	1
	58%		27%	12%		
Final visit	1	3	4	6	11	1
	15%		15%	65%		

Figure 7

8. Fusion range: Most had fairly good fusion. Only 12% had no range on the synoptoscore.

9. Fixation: Foveal fixation was observed in fourteen cases (54%) which was twice those with parafoveal fixation. Peripheral and macular fixation were seen in 12% of the cases.

10. Retinal correspondence: Nearly 70% had normal retinal correspondence (NRC) and the rest had harmonious abnormal retinal correspondence (ARC) except one undetermined case. Retinal correspondence was tested by afterimage, Bagolini striated glasses and synoptosphore. The results among these tests agreed in all of our cases.

11. Stereopsis (Fig 8): Titmus circles were used to measure stereopsis. Half of the cases had stereopsis better

than 200". However, only two cases had stereopsis better than 50" and those had no suppression scotoma by the four prism base-out test for distant and near.

Stereopsis at the final visit

	Number of cases
None	1 (4%)
Fly (+)	4 (15%)
800"~400"	9 (35%)
200"~140"	9 (35%)
80"~ 40"	3 (12%)

(Titmus)

Figure 8

DISCUSSION

The onset of accommodative esotropia usually occurs between the ages of one and three years. Since binocularity develops to some extent before the onset of esotropia, the prognosis for binocular function is thought to be excellent for the full accommodative esotrope.

Twenty-six cases in this report, coincided to the criteria of accommodative esotropia defined by Burian1, Fletcher and et al2 in its initial stage. These cases reponded well to the full hyperopic cycloplegic correction. Initial deviations could be reduced to within ten prism diopters of esophoria or orthophoria when wearing spectacles or instilling miotics.

Deterioration of accommodative esotropia begain an average of 14.5 months after initial treatment and ranged from three months and to several years. They deteriorated into microtropia (58%) or partially accommodative esotropia (42%) in spite of further adequate anti-accommodative therapy. Fourteen cases underwent surgery to eliminate esotropia. The final examination revealed that the alignment for distance was orthophoria in 30%, and the remainder were microtropic.

Most had central suppression scotoma and poor stereopsis. Only two cases had bifoveal fusion both for distance and near. The reasons were obscure why the initial satisfactory fusion broke down and heterotropia recurred.

Shortly prior to the recurrence of heterotropia, seven cases had been prescribed undercorrected glasses, five cases had started occlusion, four cases had developed a high AC/As and one case had had both changed glasses and developed a high AC/A. Nine cases had no apparent cause (Fig 9).

ASSUMED CAUSES OF RECURRENCE

1. CHANGE TO UNDERCORRECTED GLASSES	7CASES
2. OCCLUSION	5CASES
3. HIGH AC/A	5CASES
4. (1+3)	1CASE
TOTAL	18CASES
17/26	(69%)

Figure 9

Manley3,4 reported the deterioration rate to be directly related to the severity of the high AC/A. However in our series, only nineteen percent of cases seemed to be related to the high AC/A.

When esotropia recurred, half of the cases had amblyopia with a VA of 0.3 or less and the other half, 0.4 to 0.7. The amblyopias were obstacles to further development of normal bifoveal fusion.

Eleven cases had partially accommodative esotropia in the course of the disease. These cases are supposed to have an abnormal fusional mechanism. Peripheral fusion was delicate and was easily disrupted by sensory obstacles, and bifoveal fusion was originally defective so that an apparently satisfactory alignment deteriorated into partial accommodative esotropia or microtropia.

Partial accommodative esotropia is defined as having residual esotropia after anti-accommodative therapy. It is never a phoria for a prolonged period of time. Cases reported in this paper seem to fit between an accommodative ET and a partial accommodative ET classification.

In conclusion, we believe deteriorated accommodative esotropia was originally a combination of microtropia and accommodative esotropia. Initially it seems to respond satisfactorily to the anti-accommodative therapy, however, it deteriorates into an irreversible esotropia once the fusional mechanism is broken by undercorrected glasses, occlusion and/or a high AC/A. Finally microtropia appears (Fig 10).

Figure 10

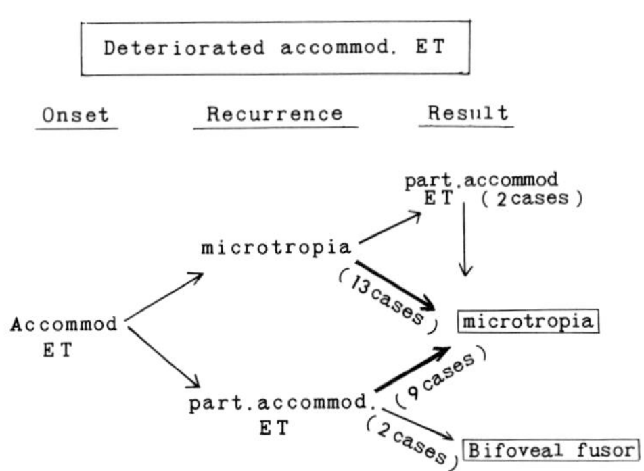

REFERENCES

1. Burian HM et al: Binocular Vision and Ocular Motility. St. Louis, CV Mosby Co, 1974.

2. Fletcher MC, Silverman SJ: Strabismus, Part I. A summary of 1,110 consecutive cases. Am J Ophthalmol 61:86-94, 1966.

3. Manley DR: Symposium on Horizontal Ocular Deviations. St. Louis, CV Mosby Co, 1971.

4. Parks MM: Management of acquired esotropia. Br J Ophthalmol 58:240-247, 1974.

DECOMPENSATED STRABISMUS

R.L. Hiatt

ABSTRACT

This paper reviews the decompensated strabismus in which fusion deteriorates and a phoria become a tropia, usually in adult life and usually with the onset of diplopia. Long standing paresis of the fourth cranial nerve is the most common etiology with deteriorated exotropia second and deteriorated esotropia being third. Recognition of this entity can prevent a costly and unnecessary workup to rule out a serious nervous system disorder. The treatment is usually surgical and the results are good. Forty-seven cases of decompensated strabismus are reviewed, including the physical findings, sensory study evaluations, management and results.

INTRODUCTION

In the spectrum of strabismus, a group of patients can be studied as an entity because they have certain factors in common. The purpose of this paper is to review an unusual group of strabismus patients in which a phoria deteriorates into a tropia, usually in adult life, with the onset of diplopia. The fourth cranial nerve is most commonly involved, with deteriorated exotropia second and deteriorated esotropia being third. The diagnosis, treatment and follow-up will be described along with the case histories of illustrative patients.

The title of Decompensated Strabismus indicates what may happen in these patients in that they had some degree of fusion and binocularity but were unable to maintain it when antagonistic factors come into play, and therefore they "decompensate." It is important to differentiate this group from true acquired strabismus in which diplopia is also a presenting sign and may herald central nervous system disease. Decompensated strabismus is seen in the general practice of ophthalmology, but particularly in a practice which involves a large number of children and adult strabismus.

STRABISMUS II
ISBN 0-8089-1424-3

BACKGROUND

Some forms of strabismus are related to decompensation. In cyclic esotropia the eyes are straight with normal binocular function with fusion and stereopsis, but on other days the deviation is present up to 35o and poor binocular function because of suppression and no diplopia.1 This illustrates a type of intermittent decompensation that can exist. In occasional or intermittent strabismus, the full deviation can be ascertained with the cover test. This is not true with cyclic esotropia.

We could ask: What happens to patients who give up binocularity and decompensate and why does this occur? Lyle states that there are certain factors favorable for the restoration of binocular vision once it is lost.2

1. The sudden and late onset
2. The short duration
3. Intermittency
4. Normal retinal correspondence
5. Fusion demonstrated
6. Accommodative characteristics
7. Good visual acuity in each eye

He further states that it is rare for diplopia to occur after an operation provided supression has not been overcome by orthoptic treatment.3 He points to the evidence which characterizes the absence of fusion.4

1. With the synoptophore we can determine:
    a. Inability to superimpose fusion slides correctly
    b. Inability to maintain a range of fusion
    c. Inability to maintain a range of fusion on side movements
    d. Fusion attempted at an angle greater than the angle of deviation
    e. Fusion attempted with a small variable degree of vertical error and inability to appreciate stereoscopic vision with even the simplest of tests

2. Diplopia testing:
    a. Anomolous projection. As a convergent strabismus with increased diplopia with images closer than consistent with the objective angle.
    b. The ability to recognize diplopia but the inability to see single even with prisms.

c. Partial correction of the deviation by prisms may elicit diplopia. This would suggest that similar state of affairs might result following the reduction of a convergent deviation by operation.

3. Prism Vergence Test: No fusion range is available when the deviation is corrected.

These three groups of tests: the synoptophore, the diplopia test, and the prism vergence test can be used to predict those patients who will probably have average fusion once treatment has begun for an adult onset strabismus whether it be acquired or of the decompensated variety. He points out further that the degree of diplopia depends upon:5

1. The reserve neuro-muscular power

2. The strength or desire for binocular vision and this depends on:
   a. Ill health
   b. Ocular fatigue
   c. Mental health status
   d. Occupation, such as clerks and drivers
   e. Advancing age

The symptoms one gets are headaches, difficulty in focusing eyes, photophobia, and blurring of print.

On the other hand, intermittent diplopia may occur in which the patient has difficulty judging the position of a ball at games, in carrying out precision tool work, in estimating the distance he is from the ground, or in ocular fatigue with stereoscopic devices as the microscope.

Burin states that acute strabismus may occur after artificial interruption of binocular vision and that temporary occlusion of one eye may, in certain cases even with no history of disturbance of binocular vision, result in diplopia.6 This is a precipitating cause of decompensation in strabismus.

Fink states that a great fusional amplitude allows large deviations to remain latent.7 Hyperphoria in the primary position may be replaced by hypertropia when the eyes are moved into the sphere of action of a defective muscle. He further states that the phoria may be intermittent, but break with conditions of physical and mental fatigue, illness, emotional stress, or moderately close work.

It can be seen tht decompensated strabismus is built on certain definitely known physiological principles which center around the fusion mechanism and ability or inability to cope with stress.

METHODS AND MATERIALS

The records for the past nine years in my private office and in the clinics of the University of Tennessee Center for the Health Sciences were screened for patients who demonstrated the characteristics of decompensated strabismus. They were categorized according to age, sex, occupation, the presence of diplopia, visual acuity, deviation, the presence of fusion, the treatment, and the final result. (See Table I.) Seven cases were selected for particular emphasis.

RESULTS

Age: The age ranged from seven to 68 with the mean being 31.

Sex: 28 males and 19 females

Occupation: The occupations were as follows:

- professional - 8
- business - 10
- technical - 4
- workers - 8
- students - 11
- others - 6

Diplopia: Diplopia was present in all but 1 of the 47 patients at least in some direction of gaze.

Visual Acuity: Visual acuity was 20/20 in most cases. The lowest visual acuity recorded was 24/40 in one eye. A normal visual acitty, defined as 20/25 or better, was present in 41 of the 47 patients.

Head Position: The head position was abnormal in 30 of the 47 patients.

Deviation: The deviation revealed an IV cranial nerve palsy in 25, exotropia in 11, esotropia in 10, and a other than that caused by IV cranial nerve palsy, in one.

Fusion: All patients, except one were able to fuse with or without prisms in some direction, and were able to demonstrate fusion on the Worth lights either at distance or near or on the Titmus fly test in at lease one direction of gaze.

Treatment: Treatment was surgical in 41 patients and was recommended in two others but not performed. Four patients of the 47 had prism treatment, although others had prism treatment in the past. One patient had orthoptic exercises. There were no patients that had medical treatment or patching.

Results: There was marked improvement, defined as the absence of conscious diplopia and a deviation of less than 4 prism diopters in any direction in 26 of the 47 patients. There was improvement in another 17. There was no patient in which there was no change other than the two patients who refused surgical intervention and no patient was made worse.

EXAMPLES

Case #1 was a 51-year-old white male whose chief complaint was that prism glasses weren't controlling his eyes. He was a university professor who began to have diplopia twenty years before and had eye exercises 27 years before that. At age 19, he broke his neck and glasses were given after this. His present glasses were O.D. +2.75-.25 x 90o with 6 prism diopters base down and O.S. +2.50 sphere, with 6 prism diopters base up. His corrected vision was O.D. 20/25-1 and O.S. 20/15-1. His deviation measured 25 prism diopters RHT in the primary position and 35 RHT in left gaze. He fused the Worth 4-Dot at distance with 17 prism diopters base down O.D. On the Troposcope, he fused both grades I and II targets with 3 prism diopters B.O. with 8 prism diopters of left hypotropia corrected, but could not maintain fusion. Treatment was a recession of the right inferior oblique of 10 mm, with a residual of 4 RHT and 1.5 degrees of excyclotorsion. He was happy.

Case #2 was a 29-year-old white male who was a salesman and a pilot. His symptoms included diplopia, more noticeable

	Name	Age	Sex	Occupation	Diplopia	VA(cc/sc)
1.	L.T.	33	F	self-structural detailing comp.	Yes	(cc)20/20-2 20/15-2
2.	N.D.	27	F	nursing home administrator	Yes	(cc)20/80, 20/20
3.	E.P.	59	M	professor	Yes	(cc)20/25-1 20/15-1
4.	S.S.	16	M	student	Yes	(sc)20/25, 20/20+1
5.	S.S.	25	M	dental student	Yes	(sc)20/15, 20/20-3
6.	K.R.	28	F	manager	Yes	(cc)20/25, 20/30+3
7.	E.T.	29	F	hospital clerk	Yes	(sc)20/20, 20/20
8.	M.A.	29	M	salesman	Yes	(sc)20/20, 20/20
9.	J.J.	15	F	student	Yes	(sc)20/20, 20/20
10.	S.M.	32	F	sales manager	Yes	(cc)20/20, 20/20
11.	C.B.	68	M	retired veteran	Yes	(sc)20/20, 20/20
12.	P.T.	20	M	unemployed veteran	Yes	(cc)20/15, 20/400
13.	R.M.	49	M	unemployed veteran	Yes	(cc)20/25, 20/25
14.	W.T.	60	M	retired veteran	Yes	(sc)20/20, 20/15
15.	D.M.	35	M	salesman	Yes	(cc)20/15, 20/15-1

Head Position Deviation	Fusion with Worth 4-Dot	Treatment	Results
Decompensated X(T)	Fusion (D&N)	R&R to OD (7mm)	total fusion
LH(T) c̄ poor control	c̄ prism glasses	LIO recession (8mm)	stereopsis
RHT c̄ poor control	c̄ prism glasses	RIO recession (10-mm)	residual R. hyper
R Head tilt c̄ LH(T) & E(T)	Fusion (D&N)	LIO recession (10mm)	no head tilt
R head tilt c̄ LHT	Fusion (D&N)	LIO recession (10mm)	residual LH in R gaze
XT fixing c̄ OD ET fixing c̄ OS	Briefly (D&N)	LLR recession (7mm) c̄ inf displace (2mm)	Cosmetically good
R head tilt c̄ LH(T) 2° excyclotorsion (OS)	Fusion (D&N)	LIO recession (7mm)	slight LH in R gaze
RHT in L gaze 3° excyclotorsion (OD)	Fusion (D&N)	RIO recession (10mm)	total fusion
RH(T) c̄ 5° ex-cyclotorsion (OD)	only at near	RIO recession (10mm)	residual RH - no torsion
Residual small angle ET	only at near	LMR recession (4mm)	total fusion
Large angle XT who decompensated	Briefly	LSR recession (4mm) RLR recess (8mm) RMR resect (10mm)	residual XT c̄ fusion
LET at near	only at distance	none, since pt is ortho at D	old acc. ET c̄ fusion
Decompensated XT at distance	only at near	Medically treat Bleph, then R&R to OS	Good
RH(T) worse in L gaze	Briefly	None	Pt had Cerebral Vascular Emboli
R head tilt c̄ LH(T) & X(T) at near	Yes, with effort	LIO recession (10mm)	Good

	Name	Age	Sex	Occupation	Diplopia	VA(cc/sc)
16.	C.B.	16	M	student	Yes	(sc)20/20, 20/15
17.	S.L.	35	M	Dentist	Yes	(sc)20/15, 20/15
18.	E.S.	50	F	homemaker	Yes	(cc)20/25, 20/30
19.	T.N.	21	M	engineering student	Yes	(sc)20/25, 20/70
20.	M.A.	28	F	secretary	Yes	(sc)20/20, 20/20
21.	D.C.	55	F	plant manager	Yes	(cc)20/25, 20/25
22.	J.P.	38	F	homemaker	Yes	(cc)20/15, 20/15
23.	K.P.	24	M	factory operator	Yes	(sc)20/20, 20/15
24.	C.S.	14	M	student	Yes	(sc)20/15, 20/15
25.	D.M.	31	M	hospital employee	Yes	(sc)20/20, 20/20
26.	S.M.	10	M	student	Yes	(sc)20/20, 20/20
27.	S.W.	23	M	U.S. Coast Guard	Yes	(sc)20/15, 20/15
28.	T.M.	8	F	student	Yes	(sc)20/70-2 20/20
29.	E.J.	32	F	teacher	Yes	(cc)20/15, 20/15
30.	P.S.	32	F	bank teller	Yes	(sc)20/20, 20/20
31.	M.K.	37	F	physical therapist	Yes	(sc)20/20, 20/25

Head Position Deviation	Fusion with Worth 4-Dot	Treatment	Results
LH(T) c X(T)	Diplopia at distance	Orthoptic exercises & prisms	Fusion has improved
Decompensated large angle X(T)	only at near	Re-recess LLR resect RMR, resect LMR	Fusion
Decompensated X(T) c̄ LSO palsy	Diplopia at D&N	LMR resection	Total fusion
R̲ face turn c̄ E(T)	only at near	LLR recess LIO recess R&R to OS	Total fusion
Decompensated large angle XT c̄ LH	only at near	Recession LR (7.5mm) OU	Residual X
Double hyper c̄ X(T) OA IO(OU)	only at near	Tuck SO (OU)	3° excyclo (OD) 4° excyclo (OS)
R̲ head tilt c̄ LH(T)	Fusion (D&N)	LIO recession (10mm)	Total fusion
LH(T) c̄ X(T)	Briefly	Recess LSR (4mm) resect LIR (5mm)	Good
R head tilt c̄ LH(T) in R gaze	Fusion (D&N)	LIO recession (10mm)	Total fusion
Consecutive X(T) who has ARC & NRC	Homonyomous & Heteronomous	Surgery recommended	---
Ptosis OD altern ET	Fusion c̄ 40 BO at D&N	Repair lacr appar OD, bime rectus reces 3mm	Total fusion
X(T) with poor control	Fusion (D&N)	Recession LLR (7.5mm)	Good
Acquired ET	Uncrossed diplopia (D&N)	Recession MR (OU) (5mm)	Total fusion
Normal/12 X(T)	Alt. (D) Fused (N)	Recession LLR (6mm)	Total fusion
R head tilt 8 LHT c̄ 5° cyclo. OS	Fused c̄ vert. prism	Recession LIO (8mm)	Total fusion
L head tilt 25 RH(T)	Fused c̄ prism (D) fused (N)	Recession RIO (8mm) tuck RSO (10mm)	Residual RH

	Name	Age	Sex	Occupation	Diplopia	VA(cc/sc)
32.	J.R.	24	F	owner, health spa	Yes	(cc)20/15, 20/20
33.	T.M.	39	M	retired Marine Corps	Yes	(sc)20/20, 20/20
34.	L.R.	30	M	medical student	Yes	(sc)20/20, 20/20
35.	J.G.	52	F	executive	Yes	(cc)20/25-1 20/30-2
36.	M.D.	12	M	student	Yes	20/20 20/50
37.	LCB	59	M	carman	Yes	20/20 20/20
38.	D.P.	32	M	farmer	Yes	20/20 20/20
39.	B.D.	40	F	dental assistant	Yes	20/20 20/20
40.	T.H.	18	M	student	occasional	20/30 20/20
41.	B.B.	16	M	student	Yes	20/20 20/20
42.	G.C.	31	M	factory worker	Yes	20/20 20/20
43.	A.K.	11	F	student	Yes	20/20 20/20
44.	H.D.	50	M	insurance broker	Yes	20/20 20/25
45.	A.B.	32	F	physician	Yes	20/20 20/20
46.	J.H.	31	M	chemist	Yes	20/20 20/20
47.	B.D.	7	M	student	Yes	20/20 20/20

Head Position Deviation	Fusion with Worth 4-Dot	Treatment	Results
L head tilt c̄ face turn/18 LHT c̄ +3 OA RSO	Fused only at near	Recession LSO (4.5mm)	Residual LHT
L head tilt/25 RHT	Fused only at near	Recess RIO (8mm) RSR recess (2mm)	4 RH c̄ +1 OA RIO
Deteriorated X(T) 40 X(T)	Alt. (D) Fused (N)	Recession LR (OU) (8mm)	Total fusion
R head tilt (had prism glasses) 6 LHT OD 4ΔB↑ OS 1ΔB↓	Fused (D&N)	Recommended recession LIO (6mm)	
Lt. ET = 20 straight	Fusion with prism	Recession LMR	Good
Head lt. RHT = 10	fuse rt.	Recess RSR 4 3 p.d. base down	Good
LHT = 10 rt. head tilt	fuse lt.	Recession LIO	Good
Alt. ET = 10	fuse	Recession LMR 4 and prism	Excellent
RHT = 16 head tilt left	fleeting	None	---
RHT = 5 head tilt left	fuse	Recess RSR 4.5 Recess RIO 8.0	Good
LHT = 10 head tilt rt.	fuse left	Recession LIO 10	Excellent
RHT = 8 head tilt left	fuse rt.	Recession LIO 8	Excellent
ET = 20 head turn left	fuse rt.	None	---
LHT = 15 head tilt rt.	fuse lt.	Recession LIO 8	Good
ET = 20	fuse rt.	Recession LMR 6	Good
ET = 30	fuse	Recession RMR 4.0 Recession LMR 4.0	Excellent

in left gaze with onset at age 17. His uncorrected vision was O.D. 20/20+3, O.S. 20/20-1. The primary deviation measured 5 diopters of RHT, worse in left gaze, with 3 degrees of excyclotorsion O.D. He could fuse the 4-Dot at distance and at near. His stereopsis was excellent. On the troposcope, he fused grades I and II targets between 5-8 prism diopters B.O. with 2 prism diopters of left hypotropia corrected. He "broke" fusion easily. A recession of the right inferior oblique of 10 mm was done with disappearance of symptoms.

Case #3 was a 24-year-old male dental student. His chief complaint was diplopia, worse on right gaze. His lenses were O.D. +.25 sphere with 1.5 prism diopters base up to at 90o and O.S. +.25 sphere with 1.5 prism diopters base down at 90o with vision of O.D. 20/15 and O.S. 20/20+3. A right head tilt was noted. The deviation measured 20 prism diopters of L.H.T. He fused the 4-Dot at distance and at near with his head slightly tilted. On the troposcope he fused both grades I and II targets with from 2-4 prism diopters L.H. with 8 prism diopters base out and with 5o of excylcotorsion in the left eye. His surgery consisted of a recession of the left inferior oblique by 10 mm. Postoperatively, he had 6 prism diopters of L.H., in extreme right gaze but 0 in primary.

Case #4 was a 35-year-old white male dentist who complained of intermittent diplopia which progressively worsened. A large exotropia was present. At age 19, he had surgery for his X(T) with a LR recession O.U. The vision was O.D. 20/15, O.S. 20/15 uncorrected. His deviation measured 40 prism diopters X(T) with 3 prism diopters L.H. (T) and at near from 0-27 X(T) with an L.H. (T). He fused the 4-Dot at distance at near with effort. His stereo was 9/9 with the Titmus series. On the synoptophore, he fused both grades I and II targets at the zero setting. His amplitudes were, convergence +35/+39, divergence -38/-30. Both medial recti were resected 8 mm. Postoperatively diplopia was absent and he was orthophoric and extremely happy.

Case #5, a 10-year-old black female, gave a history of "being bitten by an insect" on the RLL four weeks prior to appointment. She developed cellulitis, conjunctivitis, and corneal edema. Neosporin drops and Ampillicin were prescribed. One week latter she exhibited interstitial keratitis and was then given homatropine (5%) and decadron (1%) topically. The vision was OD 20/50+2, and OS 20/30. After two weeks of using homatropine, she developed a constant right esotropia with a sudden onset of diplopia. Ductions showed that she could abduct the right eye well. The impression was that this child had a latent esophoria that was made manifest by blurred vision in the right eye, so the two medications were discontinued.

Later the next week, the vision had returned to OD 20/30 and OS 20/25. The refraction was -1.25-1.75x180o (OU). The right esotropia persisted along with the diplopia and measured 45 prism diopters in all directions of gaze. The 4-Dot test showed suppression of the OD at distance and uncrossed diplopia at near.

On the synoptophore, grade I fusion was appreciated at the objective angle. Surgery was recommended for this acquired ET which consisted of a bimedial recession of 5 mm.

Four days post-op, the eyes appeared straight. Diplopia disappeared, but with the 4-Dot, at distance, she still showed a residual uncrossed diplopia. Prism measurements revealed 8E at distance, and orthophoria at near. Stereopsis was 4/9 circles from the Titmus series. On the synoptophore this patient subjectively fused grades I & II slides at the 0 setting with amplitudes within normal limits.

Case #6, a 12-year-old boy, had kerato conjunctivitis in the left eye caused by chicken pox and developed a severe iritis and subsequent esotropia of 15 prism diopters. The iritis resulted in a cataract which necessitated a cataract extraction and the corneal opacity required a corneal transplant. The esotropia increased to 20 prism diopters with double vision. He had diplopia when a contact lens was placed before the eye; however, the visual acuity was 20/50 with the lens. Fusion could be obtained with the 4 Dot test with 20 prism diopters base out. Recession of the left medial rectus on an adjustable suture resulted in a realignment of the eyes and a disappearance of the diplopia.

Case #7, a 7-year-old boy, had a corneal abrasion from a tree limb. He was treated by a local ophthalmologist with antibiotics and a patch for three days. On removal of the patch, thirty prism diopters of esotropia was discovered with constant diplopia and 20/20 vision. A trial of glasses, miotics, and a patch gave no change in the deviation. Fusion could be obtained with the 4 Dot test with 30 prism diopters base. Recessions of the medial rectus muscles of 4 mm in each eye resulted in fusion and single vision.

DISCUSSION

Decompensated strabismus has been found to be more common in IV cranial nerve palsy than with any other condition. However, it does occur in exophoria, esophoria, and hyperphorias. Secondly, it nearly always occurs in adults. Often a history can be obtained of strabismus in youth which might have been trated with glasses, orthoptics or just left alone. The vision is usually good, but abnormal head positions are common. These patients demonstrate a wide but weak fusion range. I agree with Lyle that the fusional ability is of paramount importance in managing of these problems. The vertical fusion range, rather than being in the six to eight, may be in the range of 15 prism diopters. The patients are highly motivated and are characterized as being achieving, elite and from precision occupations. This may mean that there are many more patients with this condition, but because of their lack of demand for binocularity or the lack of demanding use of the eyes to produce symptoms, they fail to seek treatment. Gradual "occlusion" of vision in one eye, as with a cataract, may cause deviation (usually exotropia) by allowing the overlying tendency to become manifest. One unusual precipitating cause is that of temporary occlusion which interrupts binocular vision. The patients complain of either diplopia or confused vision in one field of gaze as the chief presenting problem. We cannot over estimate the prognostic significance of the ability or inability to fuse when prisms are placed before the eyes to compensate for the deviation. The treatment is often surgical, although glasses and prisms can be helpful in selected patients, as well as orthoptic exercises. Whatever treatment is done. The patients respond well not only because the condition is treatable, but the patients are usually highly motivated.

CONCLUSIONS

The condition of decompensated strabismus is fairly common in a large practice involving mainly strabismus. It must be distinguished from adult onset, acquired strabismus of a more serious nature, such as that caused by central nervous system disease. Careful history, examination, and particularly sensory evaluation, can help one to infer a conclusion that is usually correct without subjecting the patient to extensive consultations and tests. The treatment is usually surgical and results are good. One should not try to overtreat these patients, but merely to improve them.

ACKNOWLEDGEMENTS

We would like to acknowledge the help and assistance of Janet Johnson. Supported by the Ophthalmology Education Fund, Department of Ophthalmology, University of Tennessee College of Medicine.

REFERENCES

1. Duke-Elder S: Systems of Ophthalmology, Volume VI, Ocular Motility and Strabismus. St. Louis, The CV Mosby Co., 1973, p. 612.

2. Lyle JK and Wybar K: Practical Orthoptics in the Treatment of Squint, V Edition. Charles C. Thomas, publishers, Ltd., Lewis & Co., Ltd., Glasco, 1967, p. 383.

3. Ibid, p. 384.

4. Ibid, p. 388.

5. Ibid, p. 424-434.

6. Burian H and von Noorden GK: Binocular Vision and Ocular Motility, St. Louis, CV Mosby Co., 1977, p. 385.

7. Fink W: Surgery of the Oblique Muscles of the Eye. St Louis, CV Mosby Co., 1951, p. 164.

LATENCY (P_2) OF THE TRANSIENT RESPONSE (VECP) IN DIFFERENT TYPES OF AMBLYOPIA

W. Haase and H. Goossens

ABSTRACT

Visually evoked cortical potentials were stimulated by a TV-screen-checkerboard reversal pattern consisting of 2 Hz, 7 degrees x 9 degrees field with squares of 30' arc, 90% contrast. This pattern induced a good response which was reproducible in visually normal individuals over a period of 12 months. Patients with squint-amblyopia (n = 15) who were emmetropic, or only slightly ametropic up to ± 2.25 sph, were not significantly different from the normal control group (n = 18). P_2-latency of the control group were (mean) 113 msec (SD = standard deviation nondominant eye 4.3). In strabismic amblyopia the P_2-latency was (mean) 119 msec, SD 8.0 (amblyopic eye). In comparison to these results, patients with parallel eyes but unilateral or bilateral refractive amblyopia due displayed a prolonged P_2-latency. Mean latency (n = 19; ametropia > 3 D) was 141 msec, SD 23.3. The VECPs were recorded in patients wearing their correction. The possible causes of the results are discussed.

INTRODUCTION

The majority of visually evoked cortical potentials (VECP) investigations in amblyopia are concerned with the amplitude of the response due to the type of the stimulus-steady-state VECP. On the other hand, it is well known that in some patients with amblyopia P2-latency is delayed. As far as we know there is no report in the literature to correlate the type of amblyopia and the P2-latency.

The purpose of this paper is to report the 60 cases of amblyopia we examined who were between 4 years and 45 years old, with the majority between 6 and 12 years.

METHOD

Stimulation was by checkerboard reversal pattern on tV-screen. STimulus frequency was 2 Hz, the whole field size 9 x 7 degrees, single field size 30 minutes of arc. The contrast between bright and dark fields was 92%. 100 summations were done.

STRABISMUS II
ISBN 0-8089-1424-3

SUBJECTS

Group I: Twenty-nine persons between 18 and 49 years old, emmetropic or wearing glasses for years. Ametropia was limited up to +/-2.25 diopters. Normal monocular and binocular functions were present.

Group II: Sixty patients who suffered from amblyopia of one or both eyes.

We classified the amblyopes into 3 groups:

1. Pure strabismic amblyopia: esotropia or exotropia (n=18) limit of ametropia +/-2.25 diopters (corrected), 5 cases with eccentric fixation of the amblyopic eye.

2. Form deprivation amblyopia due to ametropia (n=19) of +/-3 diopters or more, or anisometropia greater than 1 diopter. Parallel eyes. Three cases had monocular eccentric fixation.

3. Mixed form = strabismic and ametropic amblyopia (n=23) amblyopia. Five cases had monocular eccentric fixation.

RESULTS

Twenty-nine visually normal persons had an inter-individual spread of P2-latency from 102 to 121 milliseconds. The mean of all persons was 114.3 ms for the dominant eye, 113.8 ms on non-dominant eye (figures 1 and 2). The intra-individual fluctuation of 2 normal persons over a period of 12 months was less than +/-3.0 ms.

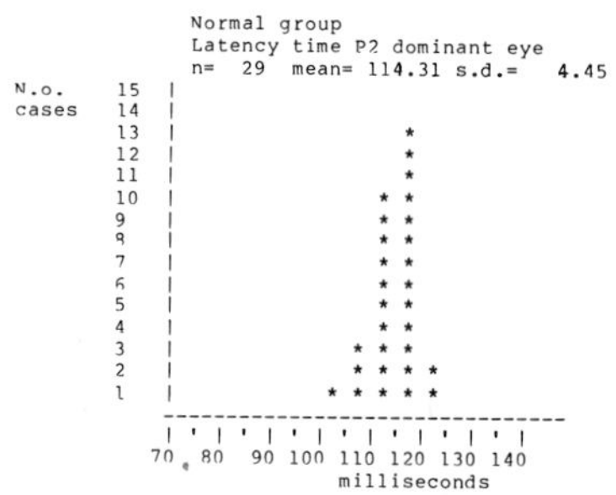

Figure 1.

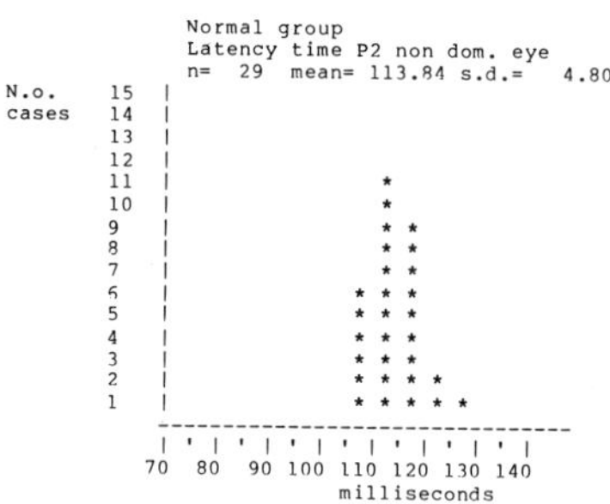

Figure 2.

The responses in the strabismic amblyopia group did not differ significantly from that of the normal population. P2-latency of the amblyopic eye scattered from 101 to 134 ms, mean 116.8 ms. 117.2 ms was for the dominant eye (figures 3 and 4).

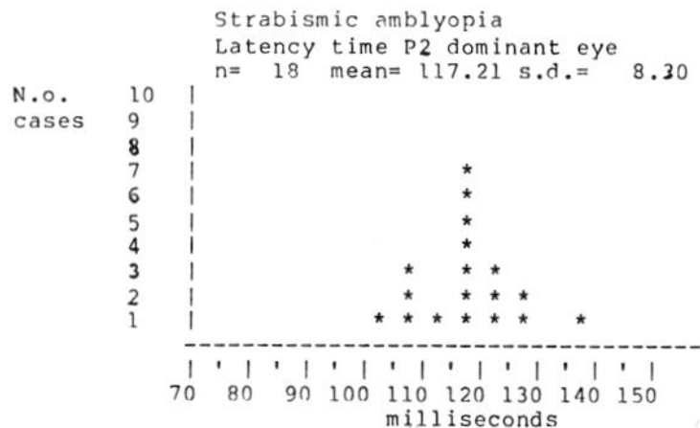

Figure 3.

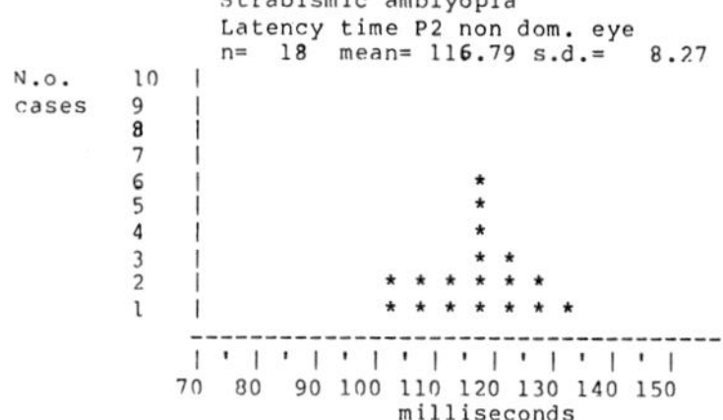

Figure 4.

In ametropic amblyopia, the P2-latency of the amblyopic or the more amblyopic eye scattered inter-individually from 112 ms to 195 ms, mean 143.9 ms. P2 of the dominangt eye was distributed between 105 ms and 150 ms, mean 127.6 ms (figure 5 and 6).

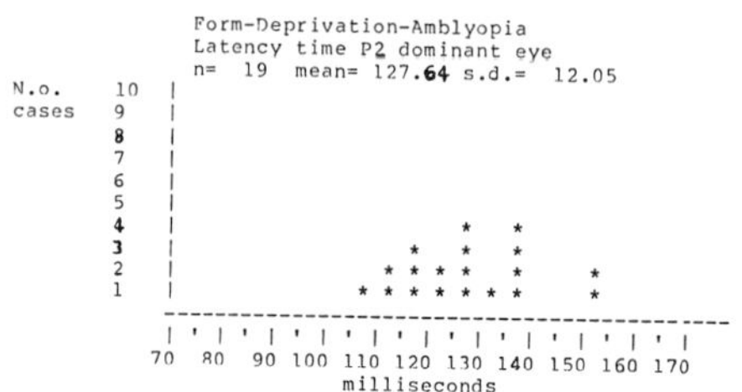

Figure 5.

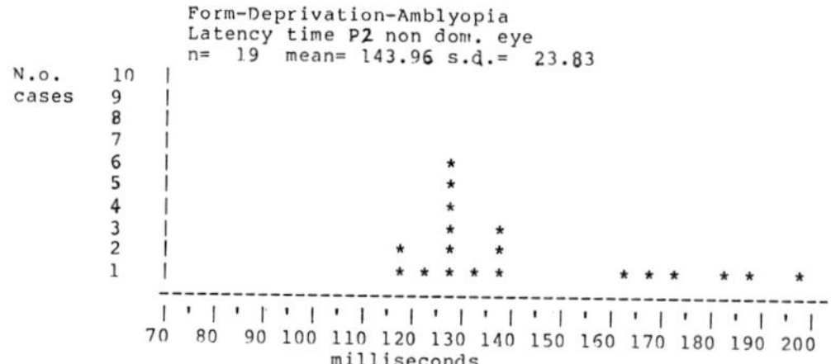

Figure 6.

In so-called mixed amblyopia - strabismics who were also ametropic the P2-latency was between 110 ms to 170 ms, mean 125.7 ms on the amblyopic side, 100 ms to 135 ms on the better viewing eye, mean 123.3 ms (figures 7 and 8).

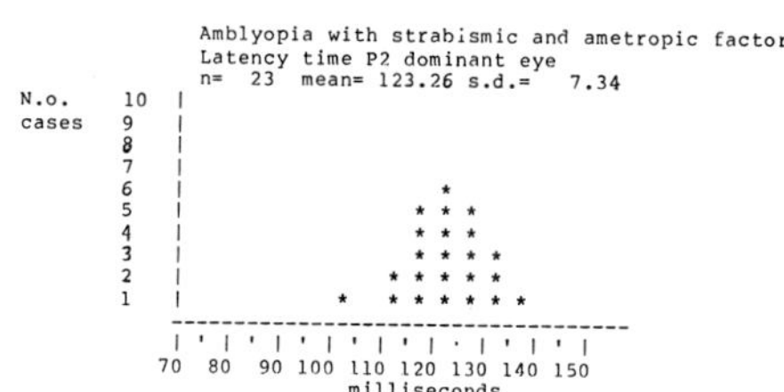

Figure 7.

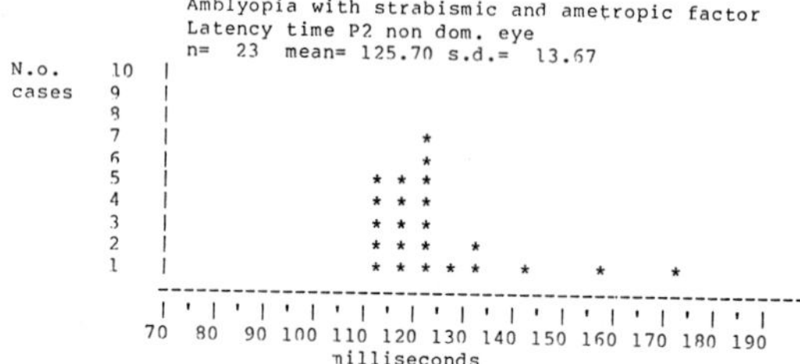

Figure 8.

DISCUSSION

In comparison to the cortical response of visually normal subjects, we define the delay of the Ps-latency by the following two criteria:

1. P2-latency above normal mean (114 ms) plus 3x standard-deviation (4.4 x 3) = 127.5 ms.

2. The maximal difference between the two eyes among our normal 29 subjects was 5 ms. The mean of the difference of two normal eyes plus the 3 x standard-deviation was 10 ms. A larger difference is suspected to be pathologic.

Table 1: Number of Patients with Delayed P2-Latency in the Different Groups of Amblyopia

	Normals N = 29	Squint-amblyopia N = 18	Ametropic-amblyopia N = 19	Mixed form N = 23
Crit.1 P2 Lat. >128ms	-	2	12	6
Crit.2 Diff.> 10 ms	-	1	11	8
Crit. 1+2	-	3	14	11

According to these criteria the majority (74%) of the patients who suffered from ametropic or anisometropic amblyopia showed P2-latency above the normal range, while in cases of strabismic amblyopia this finding is exceptional (Table 1). Why do not all of the patients with ametropic amblyopia exhibit this increased P2-latency? The follow-up of a few patients for a period of 1-2 years showed the effect of corect glasses. Within weeks or months of wearing the glasses, the P2-latency became shorter, but not normal in every case. An example is demonstrated by the diagrams (figures 9 and 10). At present we have only 6 cases of the ametropia group with normal P2-latency or moderate delay. Correct glasses had been order during pre-school age. The glasses had been worn for a minimal period of 2 years.

Delay of the P2-latency found in some cases with

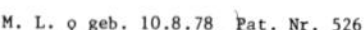

M. L. ♀ geb. 10.8.78 Pat. Nr. 526

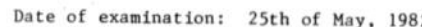

Date of examination: 25th of May, 1982

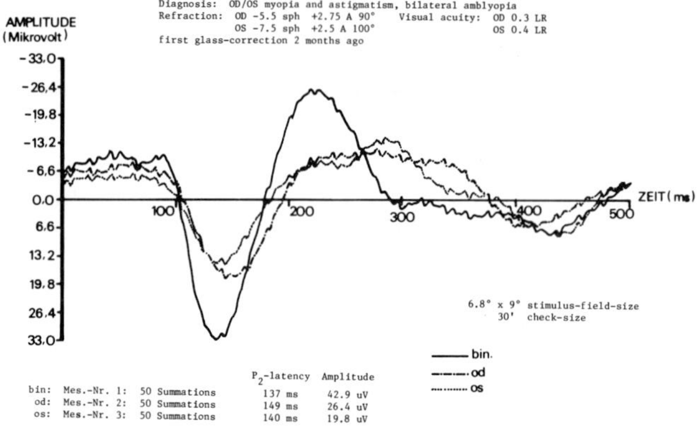

Figure 9.

M. L. ♀ geb. 10.8.78 Pat. Nr. 526 Date of examination: 23rd of August, 1982

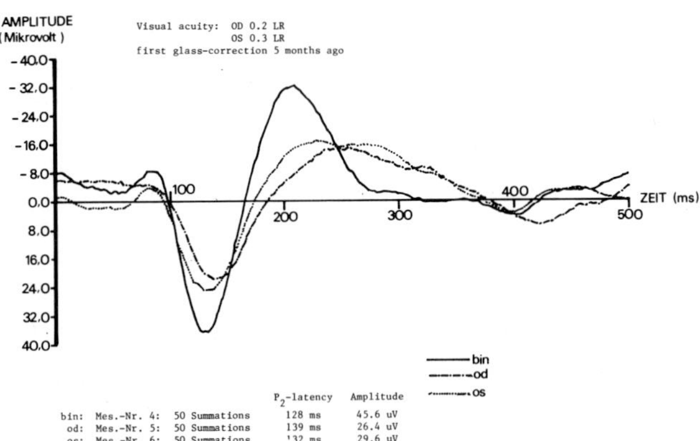

Figure 10.

amblyopia has been reported by several authors.(1,2,3) Awaya and co-workers found the phenomenon in cases of deprivation-amblyopia.(4) Barnard and Arden found it as an effect of occlusion therapy on the occluded eye.(5)

In pure strabismic amblyopia the scotoma is restricted to a small area on and near the fovea. The larger area of the central visual field shows a normal perimetric pattern. In comparison to strabimic amblyopia, in ametropic or anisometropic amblyopia, the reduced form transmission applies to the whole visual field and especially to its central part. The number of elements which perceive small stimulus-size-pattern is reduced. This lowers the amplitude of the response and P2-latency increases. Measurements by smaller and larger stimulus-sizes seem to confirm this. P2-latency, measured by single field-size of 60' or 120' of arc shows a shorter latency than with 30' size.

SUMMARY

The VECP-examination of different groups of amblyopia, who had been clinically classified showed the following results: P2-latency was normal in cases of pure strabismic amblyopia. An increased P2-latency was found in the majority of the cases who suffered from ametropic or anisometropic amblyopia. The authors assume that this phenomenon is due to a moderate form-deprivation-effect in the ametropic group.

REFERENCES

1. Wanger P and Nilsson BY: Visual evoked responses to pattern reversal stimulation in patients with amblyopia and/or defective binocular functions. Acta Ophthalmologica 56:617-627, 1978.

2. Wanger P and Persson HE: Visual evoked responses to pattern-reversal in childhood amblyopia. Acta Ophthalmologica 58:697-706, 1980.

3. Mayles WPM and Mulholland WV: The response to pattern-reversal in amblyopia. Evoked potentials, Baltimore, MD, in Colin Barber, (ed.): University Park press, 1980, p. 243-249.

4. Awaya S, Miyake Y, Imaizumi Y, Shoise Y, Kanda and Komuro K: Amblyopia in man, suggestive of stimulus deprivation amblyopia. Jpn J Ophthalmol 17:69-82, 1973.

5. Barnard WM, Arden GB: Changes in the visually evoked response during and after occlusion therapy, in Mein J, Moore S (eds): Transactions of the Fourth International Orthoptic Congress, Bern, Switzerland, Sept. 3-9, 1979. London, Henry Kimpton, 1979, p. 81-83.

PRELIMINARY RESULTS OF TREATMENTS OF HIGH AC/A WITH MEDIAL RECTUS RECESSION

T.A. Zak

ABSTRACT

Twenty-five children between age 3 and 12 years who manifested the following were treated with a 5.5 mm recession of one medial rectus: equal vision O.U., orthophoric at distance with esotropia of 12 to 30 prism diopters at near, wearing maximum hyperopic correction, no previous surgery, normal ocular and neurologic status, and refusal or intolerance of bifocal correction. An average follow-up of 12 months was available. In the first group: (12 - 18 prism diopters ET') seven were orthophoric at near, and three were 2 - 5 prism diopters E'. In the second group: (20 - 25 prism diopters ET') three were orthophoric at near, three were 2 - 5 prism diopters E', three were 5 - 10 prism diopters E', and one was 12 prism diopters E'. In the third group (over 25 prism diopters ET') one was 2 - 5 prism diopters E', and one was 6 - 10 prism diopters E', and three were 11 15 prism diopters E(T)'. Of the 25 patients, 22 showed no shift at distance, and three measured 5 - 10 exophoria. No serious complications were encountered.

In this highly selected group of patients, single medial rectus recession appears to be a safe, effective means of correcting high accommodative convergence to accommodation AC/A ratio of less than 25 prism diopters. Longer followup will be required to establish the long term efficacy.

INTRODUCTION

The treatment of high AC/A in children has usually been approached with bifocals(1,2) and/or miotic therapy.(3) However, relatively little has been reported on the efficacy of such treatment. Parks and Manley(4) reported that the risk of deterioration into a nonaccommodative esotropia increased as the AC/A increased. Von Noorden, Morris, and Edelman(5) reported that the highest AC/A children responded best to bifocal therapy, and that 53 of 84 patients were not good responders to bifocal therapy, either because of deterioration or total dependence upon bifocals. Von Noorden et al(5) reported that treatment of such patients with

STRABISMUS II
ISBN 0-8089-1424-3

bimedial recessions was encouraging, but no details were given.

In 1958, Parks(6) reported the effect of medial rectus recession upon the AC/A in patients with esotropia. In 74 patients who averaged 18 prism diopters ET, 50 prism diopters ET', the near deviation was decreased to 25 prism diopters ET' following a recession of 4.5 mm upon one medial rectus. However, Parks stressed that only patients with deviation at distance should receive such surgery, fearing that otherwise postoperative exotropia would result. Parks(7) additionally observed that children with a high AC/A had less exo-shift at distance that normal AC/A patients with bimedial recession.

Sheppard, Panton, and Smith(8) reported an average exo-shift of 4 to 6 prism diopters from 4.0 mm single medial rectus recess in 55 patients with esotropia and normal AC/A's with greater response at near only in those patients without suppression.

Pollard and Manley(9) reported an average exo-shift of 11.3 prism diopters at distance and 10.7 prism diopters at near following 5.0 mm unilateral medical rectus recession in a group averaging 16 prism diopters ET at distance and near.

One group of patients that has been largely ignored has been the high AC/A children who fail to comply with therapy. Obviously, bifocals and/or miotics are of no value if not used, and to neglect this group is likely to result in deterioration into constant nonaccommodative esotropias. Additionally the cosmetic and psychologically significance should not be underestimated.

Recession of a single medial rectus in such non-compliant children would appear to be a possible means of surgical treatment; since greatest effect would be anticipated at near; and the risk of consecutive distance exotropia would appear small. This paper presents the results of such surgery in 25 patients.

METHOD

Twenty-five children with a high AC/A, between the ages of 3 to 12 years, and who were failures with conventional bifocal or miotic therapy, and who met the following criteria were treated with a 5.5 mm recession of one medial rectus muscle:

1. Wearing full refractive correction, verified by atropine refraction x 2
2. Equal vision O.U.
3. No previous surgery
4. Normal ocular/neurologic status
5. Orthophoria at distance
6. Esotropia at near (12 - 30 prism diopters ET')
7. 10 prism diopters or more fusional convergence at distance, measured by Risley prism

The records of the orthoptic clinic were screened to identify such patients, and out of 53 patients, 18 were suitable candidates and desired surgery, 7 other patients were from the author's practice. The author personally performed all measurements and surgery. Table 1 lists the reasons for failure of the conventional therapy.

TABLE 1. Reasons for Failure with Bifocals/Miotics

Parents	1.	Cost	- 5
	2.	Appearance	- 2
	3.	Cooperation	- 5
Children	1.	Noncompliance	- 7
	2.	Failure to wean	- 6

A simple 5.5 mm recession of one medial rectus muscle via a limbus incision without conjunctival recession was performed in each case.

All measurements were made with 20/20 targets at 6 m and 0.33 m, using the prism cover test and/or alternate prism cover test, and 4 prism diopters base out test.

RESULTS

Table 2 displays the pre and postoperative data for each patient. All measurements were performed with the full refractive correction. For purposes of discussion, the patients are divided into three groups.

Table 2: Results

Patient	Age (Yrs)	Initial ET (Prism Diopters)	Refraction	Post-Op Alignment (Prism Diopters)
1	12	12	+1.5	0 (6 X)
2	5	14	+2.0	2 E'
3	4	14	+1.0	0
4	6	16	Plano	0
5	3	16	-0.5	0
6	5	16	+3.0	0
7	7	16	+2.5	0
8	6	16	+1.75	0 (6 X)
9	4	18	+2.25	2 E'
10	8	18	+1.25	4 E'
11	10	20	+1.5	0 (4 X)
12	6	20	-0.5	0 (8 X)
13	4	20	-0.75	0
14	5	22	+2.0	6 E'
15	11	22	+1.75	4 E'
16	7	22	+0.75	8 E'
17	3	22	+2.25	0
18	12	25	-1.00	12 E'
19	8	25	+1.25	2 E'
20	10	25	+2.00	8 E'
21	8	27	+0.75	2 E'
22	6	30	+2.00	15 E(T)'
23	10	30	+1.50	12 E(T)'
24	5	30	+2.75	8 E'
25	7	35	+3.00	15 E(T)'

Group I - 10 measured from 12 prism diopters ET' to 18 prism diopter ET'. All were aligned to less than 5 prism diopters E'. All patients except #6 and 9 remained esophoric even without spectacles. Patient #8 was orthophoric at distance and 4 prism diopters E' without correction; and patient #1 was orthophoric at distance and 2 prism diopters E' without Rx.

Group II - 20 measured from 20 prism diopters ET' to 25 prism diopters ET'. Only three of those patients became orthophoric, three became small esophorias (2 to 4 prism diopters E'), three became moderate esophorias (6 to 8 prism diopters E'), and one (#10) became a 12 prism diopters E', decreasing to 4 prism diopter s E' without the -1.00 Rx. Patients, #14, 17, and 20 required the spectacle Rx to maintain esophoria.

Group III - Patients 21 - 25 measured from 27 to 35 prism diopters ET'. No patients became orthophoric, one patient had a small esophoria (2 prism diopters E'), one a moderate esophoria (8 prism diopters E'), and three remained intermittent esotropes (12 - 15 E(T)'). Patient #24 required the spectacle Rx to remain esophoric. Patients 22 and 25 retained 10 prism diopters of fusional convergence at distance, and six months after initial surgery received a 5.5 mm recession of the contralateral medial rectus. Patient #22 became orthophoric with spectacle Rx, patient #25 measured 4 prism diopters E' without spectacle Rx.

A minimum followup of 12 months was obtained on each patient and no deterioration of results were observed.

Only three patients became exophoric at distance. Two of these were converted to orthophoria by withdrawing the distance correction. The third patient was over-minused by -1.00 diopters and became 4 prism diopters E', 2 prism diopters X. No serious complications were encountered.

Two subjective parameters were also considered. The teachers of 20 patients were contacted to evaluate any change in school performance. Twelve patients were felt to have substantially improved in reading and writing skills, four others improved grades in all subjects, and four were unchanged.

Twenty of the patient's parents were fully satisfied. Five were unhappy with the need for continuing spectacle wear, but were complying after one year.

No significant lateral incomitance was encountered.

All patients demonstrated stereopsis at near, ranging from 40 to 300 seconds of arc on the Titmus test.

DISCUSSION

The ideal treatment for a high AC/A would encompass a simple, safe modality requiring minimal effort on the part of child or parent, permanent restoration of the AC/A to the normal range without spectacles or drops, and no deleterious effects on ocular motility or distance alignment.

Although spectacles and bifocals certainly are efficacious, they require continuing compliance on the part of child and parent, often fail to maintain alignment due to deterioration, and frequently must be abandoned to subsequent surgery. Not all patients can be successfully weaned, and the cost of repeated follow-up visits, replacing broken bifocals, etc., is becoming prohibitive. The indigent patient in the future may find medicaid providers unwilling to cover all of these expenses, which is likely to decrease compliance further.

Most studies of bifocal therapy are inherently biased, since the noncompliers or dropouts are automatically excluded by virture of failing to qualify for minimum follow-up criteria. A single medial rectus recession would appear to be an effective treatment for high AC/A patients with less than 25 prism diopters ET's. All of these patients were converted to esophoria or orthophoria at near, with most patients able to abandon spectacles.

The average exo-shift was 17 prism diopters at near, and 1 prism diopters at distance. The near shift ranged from 12 to 25 prism diopters, and did not appear to be related to age. A larger shift was encountered in those patients with larger deviation, averaging 15 prism diopters in patients <18 prism diopters ET', 18 prism diopters in patient 20 - 25 prism diopters ET', and 20 prism diopters in patients over 25 prism diopters ET'.

For patients over 25 prism diopters ET', single medial rectus recession would appear to be less effective, since only 4 of 8 were converted to esophorias. It would appear that in these patients, late recession of the contralateral medial rectus may be necessary to achieve alignment. Since recovery of the distance covergence amplitudes was observed, this would not appear to be likely to cause consecutive exotropia. Bimedial recessions might be another alternative, but might overwhelm the distance convergence amplitudes.

It must be emphasized that only a relatively short followup (one year to 18 months was obtained, thus this is only a preliminary report. From the good fusional characteristics and amplitudes, no significant change in results is anticipated, however, this should be documented.

In addition, this paper does not advocate substituting surgery for bifocals, but rather suggests it as an alternative when bifocals are not accepted.

Meticulous attention to measurements with maximal

accommodative stimuli cannot be overemphasized. If a child who is 35 prism diopters ET' is measured improperly, a lesser esotropia may be found, and disappointing results obtained. Similarly, if a distance esotropia is undetected, undercorrections may be likely and bimedial recessions would be preferable.

It should be noted that an extremely select group of patients received surgery. Equal vision and normal binocular vision at distance with good distance convergence amplitudes were required. Poorer results might be anticipated when amblyopia and abnormal retinal correspondence are present. #

It is usually distasteful for physicians to consider compliance failures, and von Noorden's study suggest that even good compliance is not always rewarded with eventual cure. Hopefully, further studies will assist in deveoping a more encompassing approach to children with high AC/A's.

REFERENCES

1. Burian HM: Use of bifocal spectacles in the treatment of accommodative esotropia. Br Orthopt J 13:3-6, 1956.

2. Parks MM: Ocular motility and strabismus. Hagerstown, Harper and Row, 1975, p. 100.

3. Goldstein JH: The role of miotics in strabismus. Surv Ophthalmol 13:31-46, 1968.

4. Manley DE, Parks MM: Ocular motility and strabismus. Hagerstown, Harper and Row, 1975, p. 103.

5. von Noorden GK, Morris J, Edelman P: Efficacy of bifocals in the treatment of accommodative esotropia. Am J Ophthalmol 85:830-834, 1978.

6. Parks MM: Abnormal accommodative convergence in squint. Arch Ophthalmol 59:364-380, 1958.

7. Parks MM: Ocular motility and strabismus. Hagerstown, Harper and Row, 1975, p. 103.

8. Sheppard RW, Panton CM, Smith DR: The single horizontal muscle recession operation. Can J Ophthalmol 8:68-74, 1973.

9. Pollard ZF, Manley D: Unilateral medial rectus recession for small angle esotropia. Arch Ophthalmol 94:780-781, 1976.

AN EVALUATION OF ACCOMMODATIVE ESTROPIAS

M. L. Mazow, L. C. Kaldis, and T. C. Prager

ABSTRACT

Accommodative esotropia, divided into high and low accommodative convergence to accommodation ratio (AC/A), has always been a most gratifying and treatable esotropia, if diagnosed and managed at an early enough age. Both from a cosmetic and a functional standpoint, accommodative esotropias have been considered marked successes and only infrequently is surgery encountered in order to eliminate the strabismus that is recalcitrant to medical therapy.

This paper evaluates accomodative esotropias, as to how the age of onset is related to the age of initiation of treatment. The development of binocularity and bifoveality, in relationship to the age of onset of the disease and with relationship of the initiation of therapy from the time of onset, is studied to determine if, indeed the sooner the treatment, the better the binocuar vision development. Seventy-five selected accommodative esotropia patients were evaluated to determine the above relationships. The results of binocular vision related to age of onset, as well as time interval between onset and treatment, is discussed and predictabilities of binocularity are covered.

INTRODUCTION

The prognosis for binocularity in children with accomodative esotropia is difficult to study. Parents often get confused about the goals of therapy which may include glasses, miotic drops, patching, and surgery. Predicting their child's potential for fusion has been impossible. However, it seems logical that the longer the child's eyes are properly aligned, the better the prognosis after treatment. Thus, the older the child at the onset of the deviation, and the shorter the time interval between this and initiating proper treatment, might correlate with good final stereopsis. Likewise, the longer a deviation is present, the more ingrained a suppression scotoma might become. We undertook this retrospective study to explore this hypothesis.

STRABISMUS II
ISBN 0-8089-1424-3

MATERIALS AND METHODS

Seventy-six patients with accommodative esotropia were included in the study if the following requisites were met:

(1) Parents could give a good history of age of onset, and the interval between onset and beginning treatment.
(2) Patients could respond to the sensory tests reliably. All patients were at least 5 years old.

The following tests were done.

(1) Visual acuity - Snellen, HOTV, E-game
(2) Cycloplegic refraction
(3) Motility evaluation- prism -uncover, alternate cover at 20 feet and 14 inches, with and without glasses, above and through the bifocal add, if present.
(4) Stereo tests - Titmus, Randot, TNO, Distance vectograph
(5) Worth-4-dot - Checked at distance and near with peripheral and foveal targets.
(6) Bagolini Striated Lenses
(7) Synoptophore if no steropsis present

All sensory tests were done while the patient was wearing full optical correction by either the orthoptists or the ophthalmologist in the same office.

Patients were subdivided into low or high AC/A as dependent on the near deviation change with a bifocal add.

RESULTS

Both low and high AC/A's had an age of onset varying from less than six months to as late as nine years. The majority in each type had an age of onset between two and six years. The interval between onset and institution of therapy varied and was not correlatable with development of: 1) good equal visual acuity or amblyopia and 2) good binocular (bifovealar) stereoacuity. The chance alone of development was around 20:100.

Equal numbers of monofixation syndrome occurred regardless of age of onset, interval between onset, therapy, and age of institution of therapy.

The positive findings in this study were as followed. As mentioned in the methods, the high and low AC/A's were matched, to give more meaningful answers. In both groups the visual acuity results even in the worse eye was excellent with therapy. 37 of 38 (97.4%) of the patients had a visual acuity of 20/40 or better. This was in the high AC/A group as well as the low AC/A group.

Stereoacuity comparisons in each group varied. Thirty seconds or better was considered to be an excellent acuity. 50 to 80 seconds is good but this including some monofixations, 100 seconds or greater was considered to be poor. 10 of 38 patients (26.3%) of the low AC/A group had 30 seconds or better while only 3 of 38 patients (7.9%) of the high AC/A group had such acuity. Fifty percent of the low AC/A group, 19 of 38 patients had 80 seconds or better, and 8 of 38 patients (23.7%) had acuity between 80 seconds and 30 seconds. In the high AC/A group (26.3%) 10 of 38 patients had acuity better than 80 seconds and (17.4%), 7 of 38 patients had acuity between 80 seconds and 30 seconds of arc.

Twenty eight of thirty eight patients (74.7) of the high AC/A group had stereoacuity of 100 seconds of greater compared to 19 of 38 of the low AC/A group. Of interest is that both groups had acuity of 400 seconds or less in a similar number. In the low AC/A group 13 of 38 (34.2%) and in the high AC/A group 16 of 38 (42.1%) had poor stereoacuity.

DISCUSSION

Pratt-Johnson et al. studied prospectively 50 patients with accommodative esotropia and found 24% had no fusion. He was unable to correlate this endresult with the age of onset or the time interval between this and seeking medical advice. Fifty-two percent had peripheral fusion and stereo, and 24% had 60 seconds arc or better stereopsis. In our study, 17 of the 76 total patients (22.5%) never achieved stereopsis although some degree of fusion on synoptophore was present. There appears to be no correlation of stereopsis to the age of onset of the deviation or to the duration of the deviation. A parent's history can be frought with misleading information. Also the deviation is often intermittent and perhaps are not noted until a later age. Some of the children may have been monofixation syndromes that had fusional control breakdown and who never had potential for better than 60 sec. arc stereopsis.

Although the AC/A groups differed in refraction and

deviation measurements, the final results in binocular function did not differ significantly.

REFERENCES

1. Chamberlain W: The significance of the monofixation syndrome. J Pediatr Ophthalmol 10:252-255, 1973.

2. Parks MM: Monofixation Syndrome: A frequent end stage of strabismus surgery. Trans Am Acad Ophthalmol Otolaryngol 79:733-735, 1975.

3. Pratt-Johnson JA, Barlow JM: Stereoacuity and fusional amplitude in foveal suppression. Can J Ophthalmol 10:56-60, 1975.

4. Pratt-Johnson JA, Barlow JM: Binocular function and acquired esotropia. Am Orthopt J 23:52-59, 1973.

5. Pollard ZF: Accomodative esotropia during the first year of life. Arch Ophthalmol 94:1912-1913, 1976.

6. Baker JD, Parks MM: Early-onset accommodative esotropia. Am J Ophthalmol 90:11-18, 1980.

7. Von Noorden GK, Morris J, Edelman P: Efficacy of bifocals in the treatment of accomodative esotropia. Am J Ophthalmol 85:830-834, 1978.

8. Hohmann A, Creutzfeldt OD:Squint and the development of binocularity in humans. Nature 254:613-614, 1975.

9. Bishop PO: Stereopsis and fusion. Trans Ophthalmol Soc NZ 26:17-27, 1974.

10. Cassin B, Beecham B, Friedberg K: Stereoacuity, fusional amplitudes, and AC/A ratio in accomodative esotropia. Am Orthopt J 26:60-64, 1976.

11. Pigassou R: 'Entente cordiale' in the early treatment of squint. Br J Ophthalmol 61:16-22, 1977.

12. Simons K: A comparison of the Frisby, Random-Dot-E, TNO, and Randot Circles stereotests in screening and office use. Arch Ophthalmol 99:446-452, 1981.

DISCUSSION BY T. K. LYLE

Accommodative esodeviation is observed in either of two contexts: (1) refractive (and solely attributable to excessive hypermetropia) and a normally linked accommodative convergence; and (2) non-refractive (and associated with modest hypermetropia) and an abnormal convergence mechanism.

A characteristic of accommodative esodeviation is the frequent presence of a non-accommodative component as well. Progress to this state has been referred to as "deterioration" which is often not complete and there is often a partial retention of the original accommodative component. This change has been attributed to contracture of the medial recti or of surrounding tissues. Proper case management is essential by means of adequate cycloplegic refraction and full correction of hypermetropia.

It is common knowledge that childhood refractive errors often undergo sizeable changes--particularly in the case of hypermetropia, indicating that patients with accommodative esodeviation should be refracted at frequent intervals and especially when their state of control is precarious; and for this reason many experienced ophthalmologists prefer to use atropine in cycloplegic refraction.

In a review of the records of patients in his practice Raab found that 193 were identified as having presented initially with pure accommodative esodeviation, but 32 (17%) subsequently developed a non-accommodative component.

Based on the prevalence of normal AC/A ratios as estimated by comparison of distance and near heterophorias 13 of 102 (13%) of those with a normal and 19 of 91 (21%) of those with a high AC/A ratio showed deterioration. This difference was not significant. Hypermetropia at first examination and at age of deterioration was similar for both AC/A groups.

In 18 of the 32 "deteriorated" cases, there were changes in hypermetropia prior to the age of 7 years. In these 36 eyes hypermetropia showed an increase of +0.22 to +0.26 D per year.

These observations suggest that deterioration in accommodative esodeviation cannot be attributed solely to a high AC/A ratio nor to large increases in hypermetropia.

THE USE OF EXTENDED-WEAR CONTACT LENSES IN THE TREATMENT OF ACCOMMODATIVE ESOTROPIA

C. Calcutt, B. Holland and B. Mathalone

ABSTRACT

A series of twenty cases has been reviewed where extended- wear contact lenses have replaced the spectacle correction in children with accomodative esotropia. Follow-up revealed a generally good tolerance of the lenses while no patient experienced a deterioration in the maintenance of binocular single vision (BSV) with the contact lenses compared with the glasses. The necessity for careful selection of children was underlined by the fact that seven cases discontinued lens wear in the early stages of the project. Thirteen patients wore their lenses for a period of three months, and only two of these demonstrated an intermittent deviation at near, compared with the nine who had had an intermittent or constant esotropia at near with the spectacle correction. Eight cases have worn their contact lenses for periods of six months or more, and all have maintained comfortable BSV with the lenses. Further research into the effects of extended-wear lenses in accommodative esotropia with convergence excess is warranted.

INTRODUCTION

The main reason for the failure of optical and orthoptic therapy in the treatment of accommodative esotropia is poor toleration of the spectacle correction, which may result in gradual decompensation of the esophoria. Surgery may become necessary to restore binocularity or may be attempted in an effort to eliminate the accommodative element and thus dispose of the glasses. The purpose of this study was to discover the effect of contact lenses on the accommodative types of esotropia, and to decide whether this method of therapy might form a useful adjunct tc available methods of treatment.

Criteria for inclusion in the study:

1. Age: The upper age limit was eight years, although the original intention had been to exclude children over the age of five years. This rule was modified before the start of the project in order to include as many patients as possible in the series.

STRABISMUS II
ISBN 0-8089-1424-3

2. Refractive Error: No parameters were set with regard to hypermetropic error, nor was a limit set on anisometropia. Only small amounts of astigmatism were acceptable due to the choice of extended-wear soft lenses for the study.

3. State of the deviation: Patients with a demonstrable esophoria for distance, or near and distance with single focus or bifocal spectacles, and esotropia without the glasses were selected provided that there was no evidence of amblyopia. Previous surgical, orthoptic, miotic and oiptical therapy were considered irrelevant if there was a manifest strabismus still present without spectacles, or on accommodation with glasses.

4. Motivation: Contact lens tolerance in any patient is reliant upon the desire to dispose of the spectacles, and every parent had this explained to them.

5. Hygiene: Families where we suspected low standards of hygiene or lack of intelligence were excluded from the study.

Selection of Cases: A total of 25 children from three centers were considered to fullfill the criteria for inclusion in the series. Five cases were exlcuded from the study due to difficulties in insertion of the lenses, or objections from the parents. Insertion of the lenses under anesthesia was not considered satisfactory to the project. Twenty children wore their lenses over a minimum of two months.

METHODS AND MATERIALS

All the children were fitted with Sauflon 77 extended-wear soft lenses on the basis of a large diameter with approximately 2mm. scleral touch, and as flat a fit to the cornea as tolerable from the position of satisfactory centering, comfort and the maintenance of corneal integrity. The average fit was 1mm. flatter than the keratometry reading in the flattest meridian. Large diameter lenses were used with the small lid apertures to reduce the possibility of loss or displacement during wear. 0.9% BP Saline was used night and morning as a irrigation agent. Continuous wearing periods varied from three months to three days without removal with an average of two weeks, at which time the lenses were removed, usually by the parents, cleaned with a surface cleaner and boiled in 0.9% BP Saline. This regime was also observed if one or both lenses were inadvertently removed by the child. Each child had a spare set of lenses to ensure constant wear, if one set was removed for cleaning. Lost lenses were replaced immediately, so that no child was without two pairs of lenses.

RESULTS

Each child was examined at weekly intervals for the first month to establish the effect of the lenses on the accommodative esotropia, and the fitting and tolerance of the lenses. Two months after the lenses were originally inserted, the situation was re-assessed. A total of seven cases did not continue with the lenses, despite the fact that in each case BSV had been judged to be present with the lenses in situ, and the parents reported an improvement in the child's behaviour patterns. However, the lenses had been worn only for short periods, the parents felt unable to cope with the cleaning and insertion regime, and the patients reverted to the use of spectacles.

Follow-up at three months after Contact Lens Insertion

Thirteen children have worn their contact lenses for three months or more. Before contact lens trial all cases demonstrated fully accommodative esotropia (Table 1) while four had esotropia with convergence excess, which had failed

Table 1
Pre-Contact Lens Data

Case	Age	Sex	Diagnosis	Spectacle Correction R.E.	L.E.
1	4	F	Fully Accomodative	+1.50 +1.00	+2.00 +1.00
2	3	F	Convergence Excess	+3.50	+4.00
3	4	M	Fully Accommodative	+1.50	+1.50
4	3	M	Fully Accommodative	+2.50	+2.25
5	8	F	Convergence Excess	+1.25	+1.25
6	7	F	Fully Accommodative	+2.50	+4.00
7	8	F	Fully Accommodative	+4.00	+4.50
8	3	F	Fully Accommodative	+3.00	+3.00
9	3	M	Fully Accommodative	+4.00	+4.00
10	7	F	Convergence Excess	+5.50	+4.50
11	4	M	Fully Accommodative	+2.00	+2.00
12	7	F	Convergence Excess	+3.00	+3.00
13	4	F	Fully Accommodative 'V' Pattern	+3.50	+4.00

to improve with miotics in cases 2, 5, and 12. Case 5 was wearing a near addition of +2.0 o.u. in bifocals prior to contact lens trial. The binocular state with contact lenses in situ (Table 2) shows that in each case there had been an improvement in the control of the deviation compared with the spectacle correction. Cases 2, 3 and 5 needed a small increase in their hypermetropic corrections to establish comfortable BSV on accommodation, but this has been attained without reducing the distance visual acuity beyond 6/9 in either eye. Case 10 continued to produce an intermittent esotropia at near with suppression of the eye, but before a trial increase in lenses and occlusion could be attempted, the lenses were discontinued. Case 13 also showed a tendency to an intermittent deviation at near but this was attributed to the presence of the associated 'V' pattern.

Follow-up at six months

Eight patients have now worn their lenses for periods in excess of six months. Cases 2 and 5, who had convergence excess type of esotropia, demonstrate good binocular visual acuity at near and distance, (Table 3), while patient 7 is tolerating a reduced correction well, a situation we were not able to achieve while she was wearing glasses Progressive weakening of the lenses by 0.25 D.S. is envisaged, when the strength of the binocular vision can be assessed accurately in each case. Four of the children are still too young for reliable subjective testing.

Table 2
State of Deviation at 3 Months Contact Lens Wear

	Glasses		C C.L.S.		
Case	Near	Distance	Near	Distance	Comments
1	E(T)	E	E	E	Corneal abrasion
2	ET	E	E	E	CL Inc to +4.0 +4.50
3	E	E	E	E	CL Inc to +2.0 R&L
4	E	E	E	E	
5	ET	E	E	E	CL Inc to +1.75 R&L
6	E	E	E	E	Loses CLs ++
7	E	E	E	E	
8	E(T)	E	E	E	Corneal abrasion
9	E(T)	E	E	E	
10	ET	E	E(T)	E	
11	E(T)	E	E	E	Conjunctivitis
12	ET	E	E	E	Conjunctivitis
13	E(T)	E	E(T)	E	

Table 3
Deviation at 6 Months C.L. Wear

Case	Deviation		BVA		Comments
	Near	Distance	Near	Distance	
2	E	E	6/12	6/12	Aged 3
3	E	E	6/9	6/9	Aged 5
4	E	E	6/6	6/12	Aged 3
5	E	E	6/6	6/5	
7	E	E	6/6	6/9	Now has 0.50 D.S. less
9	E	E			
11	E	E			
13	E	E			

Discontinuation of lenses

Five of the children ceased wearing contact lenses between the three and six month follow-up periods. (Table 4). Corneal abrasions, persistent conjunctivitis and domestic difficulties were the reasons for the failures at this stage. These difficulties seem unavoidable, although it must be noted that two requests for further trials have been received, in one case the mother is hoping for both children to be included in the series. The patients who ceased wearing their lenses at this stage contrast sharply with those who discontinued contact lenses in the early part of the project, these cases failing due to poor selection of child and family. The necessity for careful selection of suitable cases became more apparent as the project proceeded.

Table 4
Causes of Failure

Case	Reason for Discontinuation	Comment
1	Corneal abrasion	Further trial requested, also for sister
6	Lack of cooperation, conjunctivitis	Child now happy with glasses
8	Corneal abrasion X 2	Further trial requested
10	Domestic difficulties	ET at near again with glasses
12	Corneal abrasion, domestic difficulties	Now ET at near with glasses again

DISCUSSION

Chavasse (1939) stated "It seems highly probable that if glasses were given to an infant immediately, and as a matter of extreme urgency at the first momentary glide of the eye, the problem of accommodational squint ... would disappear. Operations would not be necessary." It is generallly accepted that the adequate and early correction of errors of refraction may obviate the necessity for operative intervention in accommodative esotropia, but that successful treatment is dependent upon the constant use of the spectacles. This is rarely achieved, but the insertion of extended-wear contact lenses, correcting the hypermetropia during all waking hours should provide the optimum solution if the lenses have the same effect on the accommodative element of the strabismus as does the wearing of spectacles. In the children we have studied, no case showed deterioration with contact lenses as opposed to glasses and the majority were considerably improved while the lenses were in situ. Since our preliminary task was to discover the effect of contact lenses on accommodative esotropia, the results were good and we were delighted that Murray (1982) is experiencing similiar success with daily wear lenses in accommodative esotropia. This achieve- ment leads us to suggest that extended-wear lenses can be used as an alternative to spectacles in the therapy of fully accommo- dative esotropia, particularly where there is a tolerance problem with the glasses. The success with the two children with convergence excess esotropia must be further investigated before conclusions are drawn regarding the use of the lenses with this type of strabismus. It was unfortunate that the two other cases with convergence excess withdrew from the project, having demonstrated that at short-term follow-up there was definite improvement from the situation with the spectacle correction.

ACKNOWLEDGEMENTS

The project has been supported by a research grant from South West Thames Regional Health Authority of Department of Health and Social Security. Janet Mynors and Daphne Marshall have assisted with the selection and monitoring of the cases, while Barry Holland has fitted all the lenses and advised on the wearing periods and hygiene regime. The children and their parents who agreed to take part in the project have given us full co-operation. To them all go our grateful thanks for their help and support.

REFERENCES

1. Chavasse FB: Worth's squint or the binocular reflexes and the treatment of strabismus. 7th Edition, Philadelphia, P Blakiston's Son Co, 1939.

2. Murray T: (1982) Personal Communication.

DISCUSSION BY T. K. LYLE

This paper was one of great interest. Fifteen children, between the ages of 2 1/2 and 8 years diagnosed as having a fully accommodative esotropia, were under observation in the orthoptic clinic at the Royal Eye Unit at Kingston Hospital, Surrey, England, for a minimum period of six months. All cases had an esotropia without glasses; but with full spectacle correction, there was a demonstrable esophoria with rapid recovery.

Extended-wear contact lenses (Sauflon 77 soft lens) were made for each patient to correct an amount of hypermetropia similar to the spectacle correction.

The tolerance of extended lens wear was good. Each child had spare lenses so that a lost contact lens could be replaced immediately. Only one child refused to allow the lenses to be inserted; and in two cases, the lenses set up redness and slight inflammation and were only used for a short period. But in 14 cases comfortable binocular single vision was maintained with the lenses in situ. Each patient was monitored at fortnightly intervals and the periods of wear varied from 48 hours to 3 months.

As a result of this preliminary study, it is now planned to use extended-wear contact lenses for a much larger number of children and to follow them up for a much longer period.

The most important preliminary is to talk to the parents and make sure that they have a high standard of hygiene in the house and do not lack intelligence and cooperation, for they have to deal with the cleaning and manipulation of the contact lenses. Also, there should be a desire to dispense with spectacles.

THE SURGICAL TREATMENT OF COMBINED-MECHANISM ACCOMMODATIVE ESOTROPIA

D. Mittelman

ABSTRACT

Forty patients with accommodative esotropia, whose eyes were straight for distance with their full hypermetropic spectacle correction but still esotropic on near fixation, underwent a 5mm recession of a single medial rectus muscle. In 24 patients (60%), this residual near esotropia was eliminated. The mean cycloplegic refraction in these patients, followed for greater than five years, decreased 19 diopters. Fifteen patients maintained a persistent near esotropia following surgery, while one patient became esotropic. The reduction in the mean cycloplegic refraction in these patients was only 0.6 diopters ($p<0.01$).

INTRODUCTION

In pure accommodative esotropia, full correction of the hypermetropic correction, as determined by cycloplegic refraction, will generally eliminate the deviation both for distant and near targets. However, in many patients, if the accommodative convergence/accommodation ratio (AC/A) is higher than normal, the eyes may be straight for distance, but an esotropia will persist at near fixation. I have termed this condition combined-mechanism accommodative esotropia either pharmacologically by prescribing miotics to alter the abnormal AC/A or by using bifocals to alter the refractive state. It is the purpose of this report to review the results of performing a 5mm recession of a single medial rectus muscle to correct the residual near esotropia in forty consecutive patients.

MATERIALS AND METHODS

The age of the patients at that time of onset of the esotropia varied from birth to five years, with an average age of two years. Surgery was performed when the patients were between three and 17 years with a mean age of 6 1/2. All the patients had at least 2 diopters of hypermetropia

STRABISMUS II
ISBN 0-8089-1424-3

pre-operatively with a mean spherical equivalent refractive error of +4.3D as determined by cycloplegic refraction utilizing topical 1% atropine sulfate solution. Any amblyopia had been previously treated and the visual acuity measured at least 20/30 in each eye at the time of surgery. The deviation measured less than 10 prism diopters eso in the distance and between 12 to 35 prism diopters at near to an accommodative target in all patients with their full hypermetropic spectacle correction in place.

A 5mm recession of one medial rectus muscle was performed in each patient. Arbitrarily, this was done on either the eye that habitually turned in or the eye that had been amblyopic previously. Follow-up ranged from 2 years to 11 years with a mean of 7 years.

RESULTS

In 24 patients (60%), the near esotropia was eliminated following surgery without any significant effect on the deviation for distance. One patient became esotropic, while the remaining 15 patients (38%) maintained a near esotropia to an accommodative target (see table). The average cycloplegic refraction, in those patients who were followed for more than five years and who were corrected by the procedure, reduced by an average of 1.9 diopters, thus eliminating the need for glasses in nine patients.

DISCUSSION

In pure accommodative esotropia, if the AC/A ratio is normal, full correction of any hypermetropic refractive error should completely eliminate the deviation for distant and near targets. However if the AC/A is higher than normal, as commonly occurs in accommodative esotropia, the glasses may correct the deviation for distance, while an esotropia persists for near. Miotics, particularly long acting anticholinesterase inhibitors such as diisopropyl fluorophosphate (Floropryl, DFP), echothiphate iodide (Phospholine Iodide), and demecarium bromide (Humorsol) have been suggested for such patients. (1) These drugs stimulate the ciliary body, thus facilitating accommodation. Since less effort is required for accommodation, this results in less accommodative convergence and a reduction in the near esotropia in these patients. Because many adverse reactions accompany the use of these drugs, (2) prolonged treatment with these agents is frequently not advisable. Local side effects include severe eye irritation, headaches, dimness of the environment, blurred vision, "cysts" or nodules of the iris pigment epithelium at the pupillary margin, and less commonly, cataract formation and retinal detachment. Occasionally, there is enough absorption of the drug to produce systemic signs of cholinesterase inhibition such as sweating, nausea, abdominal cramping, vomitting, and diarrhea. In addition, topical application of these drugs can lower circulating cholinesterases such as serum pseudocholinesterase and erythrocyte cholinesterase. Since these enzymes are required for deactivation of succinylcholine, a drug commonly used to produce respiratory paralysis to facilitate general anesthesia, prolonged apnea may result should succinylcholine be inadvertently used in a patient regularly receiving anticholinesterase miotics.

Bifocals have also been suggested for those patients who are straight in the distance wearing their full cycloplegic correction, but still develop an esotropia when viewing a nearby accommodative target. However, because the bifocals are not necessary for vision, it is sometimes difficult to get children to look through the proper portion of the glasses. In addition, Breinin and co-workers (3) have suggested that theoretically total inhibition of a child's available accommodation represents a non-physiologic state which, following long term use, may induce irreversible weakness of the accommodative mechanism resulting in permanent reliance on spectacles for vision. Finally, because the reading segment must necessarily be large in children, (4) patients and their parents frequently find the cosmetic appearance of bifocals to be objectionable.

VonNoorden (5) studied the results of treatment with bifocals in a group of 84 patients who were essentially straight for distance but maintained a persistent esotropia for near fixation while wearing their full cycloplegic correction. By gradually reducing the power of the bifocals he was able to eliminate their use eventually in 31 patents (37%). Fourteen patients (17%) maintained a near esotropia however even with their bifocals and the largest group of 39 patients (46%) continued to require bifocals to maintain fusion for near targets. Because he felt the bifocals would become a cosmetic problem and possible interfere with athletic activities, VonNoorden suggested bilateral medial rectus muscle recessions in this latter group of patients when they reached their early teens to eliminate the near esotropia.

Parks (6) studied the effect of various treatment

Age of Onset	Age at Surgery	Pre-operative Deviation (Prism Diopters) Distance	Near	Pre-operative Refraction (Spherical Equivalent)
4½ y/o	7 y/o	ortho	20 BO	+4.2 D
4½ y/o	8 y/o	ortho	24 BO	+5.2 D
3 y/o	7 y/o	8 BO	35 BO	+5.3 D
3½ y/o	6 y/o	2 BO	20 BO	+4.3 D
2½ y/o	6 y/o	3 BO	15 BO	+6.3 D
3½ y/o	7 y/o	2 BO	15 BO	+2.3 D
2 y/o	6 y/o	2 BO	28 BO	+4.4 D
1 y/o	17 y/o	4 BO	32 BO	+4.1 D
2 y/o	9 y/o	ortho	22 BO	+2.0 D
3½ y/o	5 y/o	ortho	20 BO	+3.0 D
2½ y/o	5 y/o	8 BO	35 BO	+4.1 D
3 y/o	6 y/o	7 BO	15 BO	+6.0 D
2½ y/o	6 y/o	6 BO	20 BO	+4.4 D
2½ y/o	8 y/o	3 BO	25 BO	+3.4 D
4 y/o	11 y/o	5 BO	28 BO	+5.0 D
3½ y/o	6 y/o	6 BO	30 BO	+4.3 D
1½ y/o	6 y/o	ortho	18 BO	+2.6 D
5 y/o	8 y/o	2 BO	30 BO	+5.1 D
3 y/o	6 y/o	3 BO	25 BO	+3.6 D
2½ y/o	5 y/o	ortho	25 BO	+3.1 D
4 y/o	5 y/o	3 BO	30 BO	+6.6 D
3 m/o	14 y/o	ortho	18 BO	+3.3 D
2½ y/o	7 y/o	3 BO	23 BO	+5.4 D
2 y/o	6 y/o	ortho	17 BO	+2.8 D
2½ y/o	7 y/o	ortho	25 BO	+3.9 D
2 y/o	5 y/o	ortho	12 BO	+5.8 D
2 y/o	7 y/o	2 BO	15 BO	+3.5 D
2 y/o	5 y/o	3 BO	16 BO	+4.6 D
2 y/o	4 y/o	ortho	22 BO	+3.2 D
3 y/o	5 y/o	2 BO	27 BO	+4.5 D
3 y/o	5 y/o	ortho	15 BO	+3.8 D
6 m/o	4 y/o	4 BO	30 BO	+5.4 D
1 y/o	6 y/o	ortho	25 BO	+3.7 D
1½ y/o	3 y/o	10 BO	25 BO	+4.0 D
congenital	3 y/o	8 BO	35 BO	+4.9 D
1½ y/o	4 y/o	3 BO	30 BO	+4.7 D
1½ y/o	7 y/o	ortho	12 BO	+4.3 D
4 y/o	6 y/o	3 BO	24 BO	+5.6 D
3 m/o	4 y/o	ortho	18 BO	+4.5 D
1 y/o	3 y/o	ortho	26 BO	+4.8 D

Post-operative Deviation (Prism Diopter)		Post-operative Refraction (Spherical Equivalent)	Stereopsis	Follow-up (Years)
Distance	Near			
ortho	ortho	+2.4	+	8
ortho	8 BO	+5.1	-	3
4 BO	22 BO	+5.4	+	11
ortho	ortho	+3.1	+	11
ortho	ortho	+2.7	+	10
2 BO	12 BO	+1.5	-	2
ortho	15 BO	+4.1	+	4
3 BO	12 BO	+4.0	-	8
ortho	3 BO	+0.8	+	8
ortho	ortho	plano	+	7
5 BO	16 BO	+3.6	-	6
ortho	4 BO	+4.5	+	2
25 BI	30 BI	+3.8	+	10
3 BO	25 BO	+3.1	+	9
2 BO	25 BO	+5.0	+	3
5 BO	16 BO	+4.3	+	2
ortho	ortho	+0.3	+	11
3 BI	20 BO	+4.8	-	10
ortho	6 BO	+2.7	-	11
ortho	14 BO	+1.3	+	9
ortho	6 BO	+3.3	+	9
ortho	4 BO	+3.1	+	10
ortho	6 BO	+4.4	+	9
ortho	ortho	-0.5	+	9
4 BI	8 BO	+2.0	+	10
ortho	2 BO	+3.2	+	9
ortho	ortho	+2.1	+	5
3 BO	15 BO	+4.2	-	3
ortho	ortho	+1.5	+	6
2 BI	6 BO	+3.8	+	2
ortho	ortho	+2.8	+	4
2 BO	18 BO	+4.9	+	7
6 BI	5 BO	+2.9	-	7
2 BO	15 BO	+3.7	-	5
4 BO	20 BO	+4.7	-	2
2 BO	17 BO	+4.4	-	3
ortho	ortho	+2.9	-	8
2 BO	ortho	+3.3	+	11
ortho	ortho	+4.3	+	2
ortho	8 BO	+4.5	+	3

modalities on the AC/A and concluded that although bifocals do control the symptoms of abnormal AC/A in esotropia, neither bifocals nor dissociation exercises appreciably improve the abnormal AC/A. Miotics almost always normalized the AC/A while the drug was being used but the abnormal relationship returned to pretreatment levels upon cessation of therapy. Surgery however permanently improved the abnormal AC/A in the majority of patients thus treated, but Parks did not feel that an operation was justified unless a sizeable esodeviation existed at distance fixation for fear of producing a consecutive esotropia.

Separate studies by Albert and Lederman (7) and Rosenbaum, Jampolsky, and Scott (8) found, however, that the near esotropia associated with high AC/A can be safely corrected by bilateral medial rectus muscle recessions without fear of overcorrection at distance. Albert and Lederman did not feel that the long term results were significantly better than treatment with bifocals alone and thus did not recommend surgery for all such patients, while Rosenbaum, Jampolsky and Scott limited their surgery to patients with less than 3.75 diopters of hypermetropia.

Sears and Gruber (9), and Bateman and Parks (10) also reported that esotropic patients with high pre-operative AC/A's are likely to undergo normalization of this ratio after bilateral medial rectus recession.

As an alternate method of correction of the abnormal AC/A, a single medial rectus muscle was recessed 5mm in our group of 40 patients with combined mechanism accommodative esotropia. In 60%, the near deviation was either completely eliminated or changed to a small phoria, although on extreme downgaze several of the patients still had a small manifest esotropia. In order to enhance the divergence fusional amplitudes of these patients, the minimum plus lenses required to keep their eyes straight were prescribed. By doing this, the power of the glasses was reduced in most of the patients and was completely eliminated in nine patients. Interestingly, repeated refractions using cyclopentolate hydrochloride 1% (Cyclogyl) revealed a 1.9 diopter average decrease in the overall hypermetropia in those patients who were straightened by the procedure and who were followed for at least five years. This change did not occur in those patients who remained esotropic following the procedure and continued to wear their full hypermetropic correction. The average reduction in hyperopia of those patients followed for greater than five years in this group was only 0.5 D ($p<0.01$). One can speculate that this change in the refractive error occurred in those patients who were straightened by the procedure and no longer wore their full cycloplegic refraction because they allowed a much greater amplitude of accommodation than those patients who had a persistent near esotropia and still wore plus lenses.

Thus recession of a single medial rectus muscle appears to be a fairly safe, effective method for eliminating the near esotropia in those patients with accommodative esotropia who are straight for distance with their glasses but still esotropic at near. In addition, one-third of those patients who are straightened by this procedure will no longer require glasses of any sort. A substantial number of patients (38% in this study) will still be esotropic following this procedure, and it is hoped that these patients can be more easily managed by either bifocals or miotics.

REFERENCES

1. Abraham SV: The use of miotics in the treatment of convergent strabismus and anisometropia. Am J Ophthalmol 32:233-240, 1949.

2. Grant WM: Toxicology of the Eye. Springfield, Charles C. Thomas, 2nd ed, 1974, 706-718.

3. Breinin GM, Chin NB, Ripps H: A rationale for therapy of accommodative strabismus. Am J Ophthalmol 61:1030-1037, 1966.

4. Burian HM: Use of bifocal spectacles in the treatment of accommodative esotropia. Br Orthopt J 13:3-6, 1956.

5. von Noorden GK, Morris J, Eddman P: Efficacy of bifocals in the treatment of accommodative esotropia. Am J Ophthalmol 85:830-834, 1978.

6. Parks MM: Abnormal accommodative convergence in squint. Arch Ophthalmol 59:364-380, 1958.

7. Albert DG, Lederman ME: Abnormal distance-near esotropia. Doc Ophthalmol 34:27-36, 1973.

8. Rosenbaum AL, Jampolsky A, Scott AB: Bimedial recession in high AC/A esotropia. Arch Ophthalmol 91:251-253, 1974.

9. Sears M, Gruber D: The change in the stimulus AC/A ratio after surgery. Am J Ophthalmol 64:872-876, 1967.

10. Bateman JB, Parks MM: Clinical computer-assisted analysis of preoperative and postoperative accommodative convergence and accommodation relationships. Ophthalmology 88:1024-1030, 1981.

DISCUSSION BY T. K. LYLE

Forty patients are reported whose onset of accommodative esotropia was at the average age of two years. All patients had straight eyes for distance with their full hypermetropic spectacle correction, but they were still esotropic on near fixation because the AC/A ratio was higher than normal. He has termed this condition "combined mechanism accommodative esotropia".

He carried out a 5 mm recession of the medial rectus muscle of one eye only in all the 40 patients. Surgery was performed between the age of 3 and 17 years with a mean age of 6 1/2. Any amblyopia present had been treated and the visual acuity measured at least 20/30 in each eye. The deviation was less than 10 prism diopters eso for distance and between 12 and 35 prism diopters for near.

In 24 patients (60%) this residual "near esotropia" was eliminated and the mean cycloplegic refraction decreased by 1.9 diopters. The need for glasses was eliminated in nine patients.

In 15 patients the "near esotropia" was maintained and one patient became exotropic. The reduction in the mean cycloplegic refraction in these patients was only 0.6 diopters.

For those patients who are still esotropic for near despite the operation on one eye, surely a second operation of a similar nature on the other eye would be a sensible second stage.

DETERIORATION IN ACCOMMODATIVE ESODEVIATION

E. L. RAAB

ABSTRACT

Of 193 patients presenting initially with pure accommodative esodeviation, 32 (17%) subsequently developed a non-accommodative component.

Based on the prevalence of normal and high ratios accommodative convergence/accommodation (AC/A) as estimated by comparison of distance and near heterophorias, 13 of 102 (13%) of those with a normal, and 19 of 91 (21%) of those with a high AC/A showed deterioration. This difference was not significant ($p > .05$). Hypermetropia at first examination and age at deterioration were similar for both AC/A groups, as was the interval from reported onset to deterioration.

In 18 of the 32 deteriorated patients, it was possible to observe changes in hypermetropia occurring prior to age 7 years, the interval considered most important in the natural history of accommodative esodeviation. In these 36 eyes, hypermetropia showed an increase of $+0.22 \pm 0.26$ D (mean and S.D.) per year. The corresponding mean annual change for the largest reported study of children not selected for strabismus was +0.28D.

These observations suggest that deterioration in accommodative esodeviation cannot be attributed in most patients solely to the high AC/A nor to large increases in hypermetropia. Other likely contributing factors could not be identified in this series.

INTRODUCTION

Accommodative esodeviation is observed classically in either of two contexts; one, referred to as refractive and attributable to excessive hypermetropia and normally-linked accommodative convergence acting under this disadvantageous optical circumstance, and another termed nonrefractive and associated with modest hypermetropia and an abnormal convergence mechanism. (1-4) An infrequent entity similar to

STRABISMUS II
ISBN 0-8089-1424-3

nonrefractive accommodative esodeviation was identified by Costenbader (3) and labeled hypo-accommodative; its mechanism is the excessive focusing effort required for close viewing by an individual having a subnormal amplitude of accommodation.

A characteristic of accommodative esodeviation is the presence, in many cases, of a nonaccommodative component as well, i.e. some portion of the total crossing that does not respond to the reduction of accommodation effort. This change has been attributed to contracture of the medial recti or of surrounding tissues thought to be the result of sustained convergence, (1,5) such that they are no longer entirely capable of relaxing when accommodation is discouraged. Progress to this state has been referred to as "deterioration".

Deterioration is a frequent sequel in the untreated or inadequately treated patient, including those in whom hypermetropia progressively increases, such that treatment chronically lags behind need. However, it may occur also in patients diagnosed timely and initially responsive (2,4) despite careful management and close observation. This latter group has been thought to consist primarily of nonrefractive accommodative esodeviators. (6)

The aim of this study was to examine the role of factors thought to influence the natural course of accommodative esodeviation, and in particular the incidence of deterioration in cases showing each major etiologic factor.

MATERIALS AND METHODS

In a review of my practice, 287 patients were identified as having presented initially with pure accommodative esodeviation, i.e. their distance misalignment was reduceable to ten prism diopters or less by measures to relax accommodation. Of these, 193 had been followed longitudinally such that sufficient information for this study was available. All examinations were conducted personally by the author.

An accurate history of onset age was difficult to obtain due to imperfect recollection on the part of many parents. A best estimate based on all items in the history was made. In some cases, records of other ophthalmologists were available to establish age of onset and initial response to treatment; other data pertaining to previous refractions and to alignment were not utilized.

Measurements of binocular alignment were made in most cases by the prism and alternate cover method. Amblyopia persisting despite treatment which did not impair accurate fixation (a requirement for this method of measurement) was not used as grounds for exclusion. Light reflex measurements were relied on where prism and cover measurements could not be accomplished. Since small deviations or changes in alignment of ten prism diopters present difficulty in measurement by light reflex testing, even in these patients a brief cover test enabling at least an estimation of the size of the refixation shift usually was possible. The same efforts to control accommodation were made as for the prism and cover test.

Despite its limitations, the distance-near alignment comparison was designated the AC/A. A high AC/A was defined as an alignment at 33 cm more convergent by ten prism diopters than that at distance fixation, with the refractive error corrected. In patients examined several times, some fluctuations in these parameters occurred; in such cases the recorded contemporary impression was relied on in this retrospective study.

The refractive errors of these subjects were surveyed for changes in hypermetropia occurring over the first seven years of life. This age span encompasses the time of onset of the vast majority of accommodative esodeviations, and terminates at the expected peak of hypermetropia. (10-12) Clinically important changes in this measurement would be expected to occur in this interval. Serial cycloplegic refractions done over the longest possible time interval (of at least two years and not beyond the seventh birthday) for 18 of these subjects were available for analysis. The total spherical equivalent change of each eye was divided by the number of months in the interval and expressed as an annual change. Both eyes of each subject were observed. Most patients had one or more additional cycloplegic refractions within each one's own study interval and beyond.

TABLE I: ROUTINES FOR CYCLOPLEGIA

Agent(s)	Number of Instillations
Cyclopentolate 1 %	2
Cyclopentolate 1%*	1
Cyclopentolate 2%*	1

*Occasionally with tropicamide 1%

The cycloplegic routines were those listed in Table I. To this extent these comparisons of cycloplegic measurements are not strictly uniform. However, no data are included in which tropoicamide (MydriacilR) was the only cycloplegic agent used. The refraction findings were not obtained during, nor within several weeks of discontinuing, the use of anticholinesterase miotics.

Patients with ophthalmoscopically visible organic lesions or significant cornea or lens opacification precluding useful vision were eliminated. Additional criteria for rejection were major generalized neurologic or neuromuscular disorders, prominent congenital or other nystagmus, horizontal noncomitance due to paretic or restrictive causes, and prior surgery on the extraocular muscles. A or V pattern variations of the horizontal deviation were ignored, as was any vertical deviation not considered to be an element of a paretic or restrictive condition.

OBSERVATIONS

Of the 193 patients in this series, 32 (17%) showed deterioration and the appearance of at least a partial nonaccommodative component, at distance as well as at near (Table II). All 32 showed an increase in the distance deviation with accommodation controlled of more than ten prism diopters over their previous best position, irrespective of whether fusion had been lost.

TABLE II: DETERIORATION IN PATIENTS PRESENTING WITH PURE ACCOMMODATIVE ESODEVIATION

AC/A	Number of Patients	Number Deteriorated	Hypermetropia* (D)	Age* at Deterioration (mo)	Duration* From Onset (mo)
Normal	102	13 (13%)	$+3.32 \pm 1.68$**	81.62 ± 44.97	41.85 ± 36.81
			(+1.00 to +6.50)	(28 to 178)	(5 to 136)
High	91	19 (21%)	$+2.37 \pm 1.57$**	72.00 ± 22.48	45.95 ± 16.43
			(+0.87 to +6.75)	(24 to 111)	(21 to 75)
Total	193	32 (17%)			

*Mean $\pm$ S.D.

(range)

**Spherical equivalent of less ametropic eye

Based on the prevalence of AC/A prior to deterioration in all serially followed patients, 13 of 102 (13%) of those with a normal AC/A, and 19 of 91 (21%) of those with a high AC/A, showed deterioration. This difference is not significant ($p > .05$).

Thirteen patients had been classified prior to deterioration as having a normal AC/A; in two of these the AC/A had become abnormally high with the appearance of deterioration. Nineteen patients were originally among those in the high AC/A group; six of these had altered to a normal AC/A with deterioration and the increase in their distance misalignment. If classified according to the AC/A at the appearance of deterioration, 17 of 106 (16%) normal AC/A, and 15 of 87 (17%) high AC/A patients, deteriorated.

Hypermetropia, age at deterioration, and the duration from reported age of onset for each group are given. The differences are not significant (test).

TABLE III: Inferior Oblique Overaction and Dissociated Vertical Deviation in Deteriorated Accommodative Esodeviation

Deterioration	Number of Patients	Overaction I.O.	DVD
Present	32	11 (34%)	4 (13%)
Absent	161	22 (14%)	7 (4%)
Total	193	33 (17%)	11 (6%)

Overaction of one or both inferior obliques was present in 11 (34%), and dissociated vertical deviation (DVD) in 4 (13%) of cases showing deterioration; in the 161 cases remaining controlled, 22 (13%) and 7 (4%), respectively, showed these associated anomalies (Table III). For this small sample, the difference in the incidence of inferior oblique overaction was significant ($p < .01$). For DVD, the difference also was not significant ($p > .05$).

In the 18 subjects (36 eyes) conforming to the criteria for inclusion in the study of refraction changes prior to age seven years, hypermetropia showed an increase of +0.22 + 0.26 D per year (Table IV).

TABLE IV: Change in Hypermetropia to Age Seven Years In Patients with Deteriorated Accommodative Esodeviation

Number of Patients	18
Number of Eyes	36
Age* at First Refraction	28.95 + 14.35 mo
Observation Interval*	41.47 + 12.76 mo
Initial Refraction*	+2.95 + 1.46 D
Annual Change* in Hypermetropia**	+0.22 + 0.26 D (range -0.31 to +1.03 D)

*Mean + S.D.
**Spherical equivalent

DISCUSSION

Deterioration to nonaccommodative esotropia is a prominent and anticipated complication of accommodative esotropia. Manley and Parks6 cited an overall frequency of 20%, heavily weighted to the magnitude of the abnormal AC/A. Baker and Parks (7) noted an incidence of 48% deterioration in 21 infants presenting with pure accommodative strabismus. Folk (8) reported that 11% of intermittently esotropic children evolved to constancy. The 17% incidence reported here is within the range of these authors' pooled experiences.

Deterioration is said to occur almost exclusively in cases showing a high AC/A; (1,4,6) however my analysis shows that deterioration is not a characteristic of this group exclusively. The change from a normal to a high AC/A in two patients, and in the opposite direction in six, concurrent with their deterioration may illustrate the conceptual discrepancy between the distance-near comparison and the true AC/A ratio.

The normal and high AC/A groups were similar in their means and ranges of hypermetropia. The comparative incidences of inferior oblique overaction and DVD are mentioned almost anecdotally, since the sample of deteriorated cases is small. These parameters were observed in an attempt to identify a possibly associated diathesis which in some way is etiologically linked to, or at least predictive of, the tendency to deteriorate. Many additional observations will be necessary to make any such determination.

It is a common perception that hypermetropia in childhood strabismus increases prominently, leading to the recommendation that patients with accommodative esodeviation be refracted at frequent intervals and especially when their state of control is precarious. Moreover, this concept undoubtedly is at least in part responsible for the traditional preference for atropine in cycloplegic refraction, even among those ophthalmologists who would rely on an alternate drug in routine examinations.

The most widely quoted surveys of refractive errors in children are those of Brown (9) and Slataper. (10) A three- to four-day atropine regimen was employed by Brown in all examinations. He found that over the first seven years of life, hypermetropia underwent an average yearly increase, greatest over the first three years and then decreasing progressively, of between +0.41 and +0.02 D (average increase +0.18 D per year). Thereafter a trend toward decreasing hypermetropia was apparent, averaging -0.23 D per year between ages eight and 13 years, and -0.14 D per year between ages 14 and 20 years.

Slataper's study, in which the characteristics of his patients are not stated, combined his findings over the first ten years of life with those of Brown, with closely similar results. Neither of these comprehensive series indicate clearly their composition with respect to strabismus.

The prominent warnings with respect to possibly undetected hypermetropia predisposing to deterioration and requiring the intense vigilance of frequently repeated cycloplegic examinations are not well supported by the fractional increases that were revealed in the present series. Although a larger number of observations would have been preferred, cases that evolved to a deteriorated state showed increases in hypermetropia comparable to those of an age-matched population not selected for strabismus. For clinical purposes such changes in hypermetropia as were found would not appear to be of sufficient degree to influence either the prognosis or the method of management of accommodative esodeviation. It is of course true that clinically meaningful individual departures from these overall figures occur; in this group of patients, the largest average annual increase was +1.03 D. However, the results are not consistent with the suggestion that an accelerated rate of increase in hypermetropia is characteristic of most cases of deteriorated accommodative esodeviation.

SUMMARY AND CONCLUSIONS

This paper reports a retrospective analysis of the etiologic factors in accommodative esodeviation and their influence on deterioration. The records of 193 patients presenting initially with pure accommodative esodeviation and followed longitudinally were available for study. Tabulation was made of AC/A and presence or absence of deterioration and the initial refractive error and annual rate of change in deteriorated cases.

Review of these findings led to the following conclusions:

1. Contrary to traditional views, there was no significant diffference in the incidence of deterioration between cases with and without a high AC/A, although sample size was relatively small.

2. The rate of increase of hypermetropia in cases showing deterioration was small in clinical terms and similar to that found by other authors in large age-matched populations containing both normal and unclassified strabismic individuals.

3. Deterioration in accommodative esodeviation cannot be attributed solely to a high AC/A nor to large increases in hypermetropia. Other possible influences on deterioration were not investigated.

Modified portion of candidate's thesis for the American Ophthalmological Society, May 1982.

REFERENCES

1. Burian HM: Accommodative esotropia. Classification and treatment. In Ferrer OM (ed): Ocular Motility. Int Ophthalmol Clin Vol. 11 No. 4, 1971, Boston, Little Brown and Co., pp 23-26.

2. Von Noorden GK: Burian - von Noorden's Binocular Vision and Ocular Motility, 2nd ed, St. Louis, CV Mosby Co., 1980. pp 287-313.

3. Costenbader FD: Clinical course and management of esotropia. In Allen JH (ed): Strabismus Ophthalmic Symposium II. St. Louis, CV Mosby Co., 1958, pp 325-353.

4. Parks MM: Abnormal accommodative convergence in squint. Arch Ophthalmol 59:364-380, 1958.

5. Parks MM: Ocular Motility and Strabismus. Hagerstown, Harper and Row, 1975, pp 99-111.

6. Manley RR, Parks MM: Unpublished data.

7. Baker JD, Parks MM: Early-onset accommodative esotropia. Am J Ophthalmol 90:11-18, 1980.

8. Folk ER: Intermittent congenital esotropia. Ophthalmology 86:2107-2111, 1979.

9. Brown EVL: Net average yearly change in refraction of atropinized eyes from birth to beyond middle life. Arch Ophthalmol 19:719-734, 1938.

10. Slataper FJ: Age norms of refraction and vision. Arch Ophthalmol 43:446-481, 1950.

DISCUSSION BY T. K. LYLE

Accommodative esotropia is a useful retrospective study which explores the hypothesis that the longer a child's eyes are properly aligned the better the prognosis. Thus the age of the child at the onset of the deviation and the inverse of the interval between this and the commencement of proper treatment might correlate with the development of good stereopsis. Likewise, the longer the deviation is present, the more ingrained a suppression scotoma might become.

The 76 patients in the study were at least 5 years old and all sensory tests were done with the patients wearing full optical correction and they were divided into two groups: low and high AC/A ratio.

In both groups the visual acuity results, even in the worse eye, were excellent with therapy. Thirty-seven of 38 of the patients, whether in the high or low AC/A groups, had achieved a visual acuity of 20/40 or better, but stereo-acuity varied considerably. Seventeen of the total 76 patients never achieved stereopsis, although some degree of fusion was present on the synoptophore test. In this group it appeared that there was no correlation between the age of onset of the esotropia and the length of time that it had been in existence. Although the AC/A ratio groups differed in measurements of refraction and deviation, the final results in binocular function did not differ significantly.

THE ELECTRORETINOGRAM IN HIGH HYPERMETROPIA

E. Meyer and I. Perlman

ABSTRACT

The electrical response of the eye (ERG) is generally accepted to be subnormal in highly myopic eyes. This is probably due to the thinning and to the degenerative changes of the retina casued by the enlarged globe.

Hypermetropia may be associated with a globe which is smaller than usual. The ERG responses in the light and dark-adapted states were measured in 23 patients with high hypermetropia. Whereas in the light-adapted state all subjects exhibited normal responses, three patterns of responses in the dark-adapted state could be identified: Group I exhibited subnormal b-wave amplitudes with normal a-waves; Group II presented with normal responses; and Group III showed super normal b-wave amplitudes with normal a-waves.

INTRODUCTION

The electrical response of the eye (ERG) to a flash of light is commonly used for clinical evaluation of retinal function.[1] The electroretinogram is composed of two principle waves. The a-wave is the leading edge of the late receptor potential and it reflects light absorption by the photoreceptors and their integrity.[2-4] The b-wave is generated in the proximal retina[4] and, therefore, its amplitude depends on the size of the a-wave and on the integrity of signal transmission from the photoreceptors to the proximal retina. Thus the relationship between the b-wave amplitude and that of the a-wave reflects retinal function and solely depends on retinal parameters. Any ocular parameter that may attenuate the light reaching the retina such as cataract, corneal opacity and vitreous hemorrhage may affect the size of the ERG but not its pattern. Namely, the relationship between the b-wave and the a-wave will be normal. In a large number of patients with high myopia subnormal ERG responses are recorded in the light and dark-adapted states.[5-6] High myopia is usually associated with an eye globe significantly larger than the normal emmetropic eye. The gradual growth of the myopic globe results in stretching and thinning of the retina causing degenerative changes in retinal cells and deterioration of their function.[6]

STRABISMUS II
ISBN 0-8089-1424-3

High hypermetropia is sometimes associated with a smaller than normal eye globe. It has been previously shown that the size of the b-wave was inversely proportional to the axial length of the eye.[6] The present study was designed to investigate in detail the functional integrity of the retina in high hypermetropia. The hypermetropic patients could be divided into three groups according to the relationship between the b-wave amplitude and the a-wave amplitude. One group exhibited normal relationship while patients belonging to the other two groups were characterized by either subnormal or abnormally strong dependency of the b-wave on the a-wave.

METHODS

Twenty-three patients with high hypermetropia (larger than +5D) served in this study. Most of the patients were children aged 7-20 years. None of them complained of poor night vision. Twenty-six volunteers with normal or normally corrected vision served as controls. Dark adaptation curve was measured psychophysically for each of the control subjects and was found normal.

The ERG responses were recorded as previously described.[7] Briefly, an electronic camera flash was used as a photostimulator. The intensity of the stimuli was controlled by "neutral" density filters. The subjects' eyes were maximally dilated by 1/2% cyclopentolate hydrochloride and 2 1/2% phenylephrine hydrochloride. The ERG responses were recorded between a contact lens electrode placed on the cornea and an indifferent electrode placed on the forehead. The ground electrode was attached to the ear lobe.

The ERG responses were recorded in the light-adapted state with background illumination of eleven foot lambert. Then the subject was allowed to dark adapt for 20 minutes and the ERG responses evoked by stimuli of different intensities were recorded.

Data analysis was done as follows: The a-wave amplitude was measured from the base line to the trough of the negative wave. The b-wave amplitude was measured from the trough of the a-wave to the peak of the b-wave. The b-wave amplitude was then plotted as a function of the a-wave amplitude.

RESULTS

Representative ERG responses from a normal subject and three hypermetropic patients are illustrated in Figure 1. The

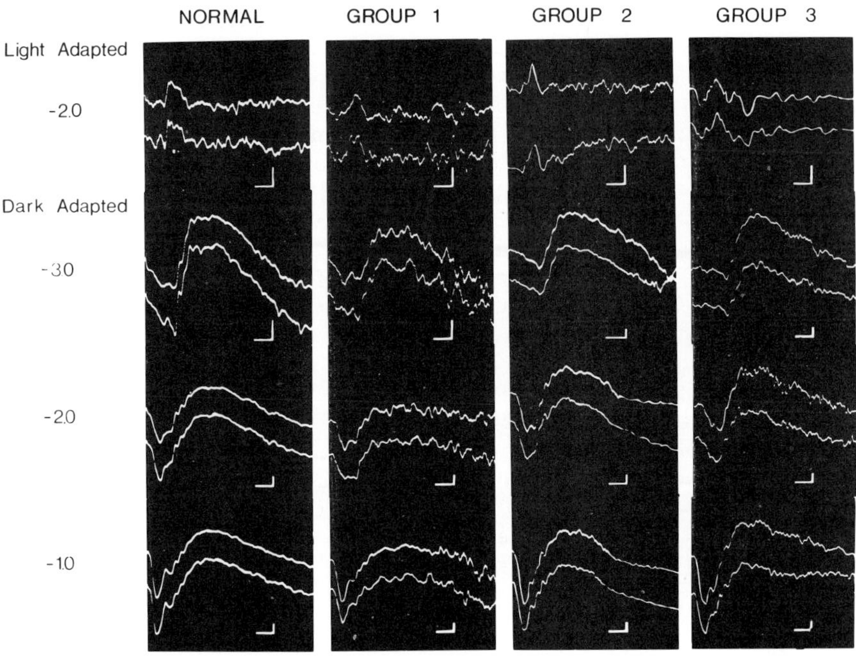

Figure 1

responses were recorded from both eyes (OS upper trace, OD lower one) in the light (1st row) and dark-adapted states. All the hypermetropic subjects exhibited light-adapted responses with normal amplitude and temporal characteristics. In the dark-adapted state the patients could be divided into three groups according to their ERG pattern. The dark-adapted ERG responses of patients belonging to Group I (Figure 2 2nd column) were characterized by relatively large a-wave and subnormal b-wave. Group II (Figure 1 3rd column) consisted of patients with normal ERG responses. While patients in Group III (Figure 1 4th column) had relatively small a-wave and abnormally large b-wave.

The ERG data of all the hypermetropic subjects are illustrated in Figure 2. Different symbols represent different patients. Each data point describes the relationship between the amplitude of the b-wave and that of the a-wave measured from a single ERG response. The two continuous lines represent the normal range given from mean -2 S.D. to mean +2 S.D. Group I patients (N = 8) are characterized by subnormal b-wave compared to the a-wave (Figure 2A). Thus, for a given a-wave amplitude, the b-wave

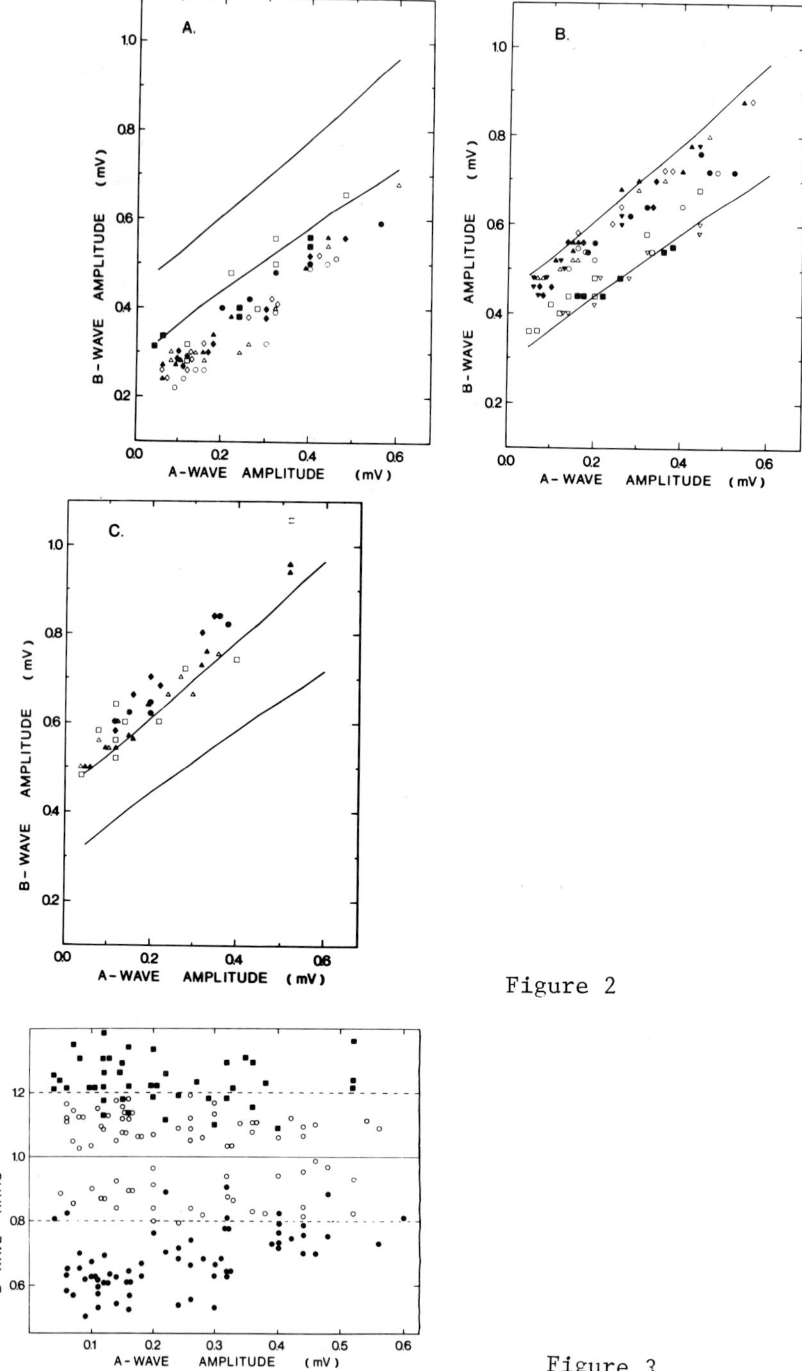

Figure 2

Figure 3

was significantly smaller in these patients than in the normal subjects. Ten patients were classified in Group II (Figure 2B). They all exhibited ERG responses of normal amplitude and pattern. Group III included five patients having abnormally large b-wave compared to their a-wave (Figure 2C).

A different way to emphasize the difference between the three groups of patients is illustrated in Figure 3. In this Figure the ratio between the measured b-wave and the expected value is plotted as a function of the a-wave amplitude. The expected b-wave amplitude was obtained from the mean normal b-wave to a-wave relationship. It is assumed here that the a-wave, the independent variable, desribes the output of the photoreceptor´s layer and, therefore, the b-wave ratio describes the integrity of signal transmission from the photoreceptors to the proximal retina. Any normal retina gives a ratio of 1.0 ± 0.2 (mean ± 2 S.D.). The data points describing Group I patients (Figure 3 solid circles) fall consistently below the normal range while data obtained from Group III patients (Figure 3 solid squares) are found above the normal range. The patients belonging to Group II (Figure 3 open circles) are characterized by normal b-wave ratios.

DISCUSSION

The data presented here demonstrate that in a large proportion of patients with high hypermetropia the ERG is significantly abnormal. It was previously reported[6] that the amplitude of the b-wave was directly proportional to the refractive power of eye. Namely, hypermetropia was characterized by a supernormal b-wave. However, recordings of the ERG responses evoked by stimuli of different intensitites in the dark-adapted state revealed here that hypermetropic patients could be divided into three distinct groups.

Twenty-three patients were examined. Only ten exhibited ERG responses with normal pattern and amplitude (Figure 2B). Eight patients were classified in Group I which was characterized by a subnormal b-wave for a given a-wave (Figure 2A). Such a relationship indicated subnormal signal transmission from the photoreceptors to the proximal retina. Such ERG pattern is reiminiscent of the one found in the Schubert-Bornschein type of nyctalopia[8-9] where abnormal signal transmission was also implicated as the cause for the defect.[10-11] However, none of the patients belonging to Group I complained of difficulties in the night. This was further supported by the normal amplitude of the ERG responses evoked by dim blue stimuli. In five patients ERG responses of supernormal amplitudes were recorded. In these patients the b-wave amplitude was significantly larger than expected from the a-wave (Figure 2C). Thus indicating stronger than normal amplification of retinal signals transmitted from the photoreceptors and the proximal retina. It should be noted that in all 23 patients, the ERG responses evoked in the light-adapted state had normal amplitude and normal b-wave implicit time. This finding excluded any progressive degenerative processes in the retina of these patients.[12]

The physiological basis of the above findings is not yet known. However, it should be mentioned that unlike a previous report,[6] no correlation was found between the b-wave amplitude or the b-wave ratio and the refractive power of the eyes.

This work was supported by Technion V.P.R. fund--M. & D. Starr Research Fund for Ophthalmology.

REFERENCES

1. Armington, JC: The Electroretinogram, Academic Press, 1974.

2. Brown, KT & Watanabe, K: Isolation and identification of a receptor potential from the pure cone fovea of the monkey retina. Nature, 193, 958, 1962.

3. Berson, EL: Electrical phenomena in the retina. Adler's physiology of the eye. Ed. Moses R.A., the C.V. Mosby Co., St. Louis, 1981, pp. 466-520.

4. Brown, KT & Wiesel, TN: Analysis of the intraretinal electroretinogram in the intact cat eye. J. Physiol., 158, 257, 1961.

5. Prijot, E, Colman I & Marechal-Courtois, C: Electroretinography and myopia. 5th ISCERG Symposium, p. 440, 1966.

6. Pallin, E: The influence of the axial size of the eye on the size of the recorded b-potential in the clinical single flash electroretinogram. Acta Ophthal. Suppl., 101, 1, 1969.

7. Perlman, I &Haim, T: Visual function of a new type of night blindness. Invest. Ophthal. Vis. Sci., in press.

8. Schubert, G & Bornschein, H: Beitrag Zur analyse de menchlichen elektroretinograms. Ophthalmologia, 123, 396, 1952.

9. Auerbach, E, Godel, V, & Rowe, H: An electrophysiological and psychophysical study of two forms of congenital nyctalopia. Invest. Ophthal., 8, 332, 1969.

10. Carr, RE, Ripps, H, Siegel, IM & Weale, RA: Rhodopsin and the electrical activity of the retina in congenital night blindness. Invest. Ophthal., 5, 497, 1966.

11. Carr, RE, Ripps, H, Siegel, IM & Weale, RA: Visual function in congenital night blindness. Invest. Ophthal., 5, 508, 1966.

12. Hill, DA, Arbel, KF & Berson, EL: Cone electroretinogram in congenital myctalopia with myopia. Am. J. Ophthal., 18, 127, 1974.

THE SURGICAL MANAGEMENT OF INTERMITTENT EXOTROPIA IN ADULTS

A. Schlossman, R. S. Muchnick, and K. S. Stern

ABSTRACT

Most studies of intermittent exotropia deal primarily with children. However, the manifestations of this disorder in adults differ considerably from those in children.

The case records of 44 adults (ages 15-70) who underwent surgery for intermittent exotropia were analyzed. Patients experienced a variety of preoperative symptoms including diplopia, headache, difficulty with reading, and ocular fatigue or pain. Cosmesis was a rare presenting complaint.

We recommend that surgery in adults be conservative, aiming at slight undercorrection. Surgical management was successful in 41 of 44 patients. All patients with post-operative exodeviations under 15 prism diopters had complete resolution of symptoms. Most patients with larger residual exodeviations did not improve symptomatically; patients with postoperative esodeviations tended to experience persistent diplopia.

INTRODUCTION

Over the past few decades, there has been a growing realization that most patients with exotropia have intermittent deviations. While this condition is common in all age groups, the presenting complaints in teenagers and adults are different from those in children. The latter are brought in by their parents chiefly because one eye appears to turn out or because they have a habit of closing one eye in bright sunlight; rarely are visual problems articulated. In sharp contrast, adults seek relief of symptoms which hinder their studies or professions; cosmetic improvement is only a secondary consideration.

Schlossman (1) noted in 1954 that divergence anomalies differ from convergence anomalies in at least one important respect: patients with exodeviations have a greater tendency to maintain fusion (i.e. deviations tend to be intermittent)

STRABISMUS II
ISBN 0-8089-1424-3

than those with esodeviations. In 1955, Schlossman and Boruchoff (2), studying a series of 200 patients, drew attention to the prevalence of intermittent extropia among patients with exodeviations and outlined the clinical characteristics of this disorder. Jampolsky (3) in 1954 described similar diagnostic features of this condition from a more theoretical viewpoint. In 1966, Burian (4) classified intermittent exodeviations into basic, simulated divergence excess, and true divergence excess types.

The natural history of intermittent exotropia is controversial Costenbader (5) stated that the exodeviation tends to remain intermittent and of constant magnitude throughout life. In contrast, Jampolsky (3) observed that although exophoria and intermittent exotropia have a common basis and usually arise during infancy, the latter may be progressive throughout life, both in degree and frequency of deviation. Knapp (6) agreed that the fundamental exodeviation is present at birth but argued that the observed deviation increases as dynamic factors change; he stressed the role of accommodative convergence in maintaining fusion at near. Burian and Spivey (7) also emphasized the role of exuberant convergence in childhood, which can mask an exodeviation; with age, convergence weakens, producing an increasingly divergent position of the eyes. Hiles et al (8) followed 48 patients with intermittent exotropia who did not undergo surgery and found that although there was general trend toward a small (5) reduction in the strabismic angle, most patients maintained deviations of approximately the same magnitude over many years.

The surgical correction of intermittent exotropia has received a great deal of attention in the literature. Burian and Spivey (7) evaluated the surgical results of 98 patients with intermittent exotropia and concluded that a good functional result is obtained provided that the deviation is reduced to within 12 prism diopters of exophoria.

Almost all other authorities advocate overcorrection. Jampolsky (9) limited overcorrections to patients over age six because of the danger of inducing sensory adaptation to esotropia in younger children; Raab and Parks, (10, 11) Cooper, (12) Knapp, (13) and Hardesty et al (14) advised overcorrection regardless of age. Scott et al (15) demonstrated that the reason for better long-term alignment in the initially over-corrected group is a general tendency toward "exophoric drift", particularly in the first six postoperative weeks.

Distinctions between children and adults with intermittent exotropia have not been emphasized, although a variable percentage of adults have been included in some studies. In Hardesty's (14) series of 100 cases of intermittent exotropia, only four are 12 years of age or older. However, in Burian and Spivey's (7) series of 98 cases, 22 are fifteen years or older. In Scott's (15) series of 65 cases, 13 are 15 years or older.

None of the previously cited papers emphasized the differences in symptomatology or management of intermittent exotropia at different ages. The present study describes the symptoms of this condition in adults and suggests guidelines for its surgical treatment.

METHODS

The records of 44 adult patients who underwent surgery for intermittent exotropia at Manhattan Eye, Ear, and Throat Hospital between 1968 and 1982 were examined. Patients were between the ages of 15 and 70, had intermittent exotropia for distance and/or near, had good (20/40 or better) vision in both eyes, had no significant hyperdeviation (6 prism diopters or less), and had no history of previous surgery. Patients with convergence insufficiency were excluded from consideration because treatment in these cases is primarily orthoptic and rarely surgical.

RESULTS

TABLE 1

AGE AT TIME OF SURGERY

Age	Number of Cases
15 - 31	30
35 - 42	7
47 - 70	7

Almost all of the patients sought help shortly before surgery. Age at time of surgery is shown in Table 1. Thirty of our patients underwent surgery between the ages of 15 and 31; another seven were between the ages of 35 and 42. Eleven patients were hyperopic (+4.00D or less), seven were emmetropic, and 26 were myopic (-8.00D or less, with the vast majority between -0.50 and -3.00D). There were 26 females and 18 males.

Table 2

PREOPERATIVE SYMPTOMS

Symptom	Number of Complaints*	% of Total Cases*
Diplopia	13	29
Headaches	9	20
Difficulty reading/focusing at near	9	20
Eye pain	6	13
Fatigue/eye strain	5	14
Cosmetic	3	7
Tearing	2	5
Excessive blinking/ closing one eye in light	2	5

*(Some patients complained of more than one symptom)

Table 3

PREOPERATIVE MEASUREMENTS

DISTANCE		NEAR	
Deviation Prism Diopters	Number of Cases	Deviation Prism Diopters	Number of Cases
10 - 30	30	10 - 30	25
31 - 60	9	31 - 60	15
61 - 80	5	61 - 80	4

Preoperative deviations, surgery, and postoperative deviations are shown in Table 4. Surgical procedures were similar for most patients. Lateral rectus recession combined with medial rectus resection was performed on 39 patients. One additional patient underwent this procedure on both eyes in a two-stage repair of a large deviation. One patient had a unilateral lateral rectus recession and another had bilateral lateral rectus recessions. A combined lateral rectus recession with bimedial resections was performed on one patient. Combined bilateral lateral rectus recessions with medial rectus resection was performed on another patient.

TABLE 4

SURGICAL MANAGEMENT

Age	Preop Deviation (diopters)	Surgery (millimeters)	Postop Deviation (diopters)
15	X(T) = 27 X' = 35 +3.00= X(T)' = 45	Recess RLR = 5.0 Resect RMR = 4.0	X = 10 E'= 6
16	XT = 20 X(T)'= 30 +3.00= X(T)' = 20	Recess RLR = 4.0 Resect RMR = 4.0	Ortho X'= 5
16	X(T) = 25 X(T)'= 15 +3.00= X(T)' = 35	Recess RLR = 4.0 Resect RMR = 4.5	Ortho Small X'
16	RX(T)= 35 RX(T)'=40	Recess RLR = 7.0 Resect RMR = 5.0	X = 5 X'= 25
16	LXT = 30 LX(T)'=30 +3.00=LX(T)' = 40	Recess LLR = 6.0 Resect LMR = 5.0	Small E Small X'
17	X(T) = 35 X' = 20 +3.00= X(T)' = 30	Recess LLR = 7.0 Resect LMR = 7.0	Ortho Ortho'
17	X(T) = 30 X(T)'= 30	Recess LR OU = 6.0	Small X Small E'
18	XT = 30 X(T)'= 30	Recess LLR = 6.0 Resect MR = 6.0	X(T) = 2 X(T)'= 5
18	X(T) = 25 X(T)'= 14	Recess LLR = 4.5 Resect LMR = 3.0	X(T) = 8 X(T)'= 4
19	X(T) = 10 X(T)'= 25	Recess RLR = 5.5 Resect RMR = 4.0	X(T) =10 X' = 6
21	X(T) = 15 X(T)'= 25 +3.00= X(T)' = 30	Recess LLR = 5.0 Resect LMR = 4.0	Ortho Ortho'
23	X(T) = 14 X(T)'= 20	Recess LLR = 4.0 Resect LMR = 3.0	X = 4 X'= 4
23	X(T) = 40-70 X(T)'= 40-70	Recess LLR = 7.0 Resect LMR = 7.0	Ortho Ortho'

TABLE 4
(continued)

Age	Preop Deviation (diopters)	Surgery (millimeters)	Postop Deviation (diopters)
24	LXT = 30 LX(T)' = 35-40	Recess LLR = 5.0 Resect LMR = 5.0	E = 6 E' = 6
24	X(T) = 25 X(T)' = 30	Recess LLR = 6.0 Resect LMR = 5.0	X(T) = 12 X(T)' = 14
25	XT = 30 X(T)' = 12 +3.00 = XT' = 35	Recess LLR = 5.0 Resect LMR = 5.0	X = 10
25	RXT = 30 RX(T) = 45 +3.00 = RX(T)' = 45	Recess RLR = 6.0 Resect RMR = 3.0	Small X Small X'
25	XT = 50 X(T)' = 48	Recess RLR = 7.0 Resect RMR = 8.0	X = 6 X' = 6
26	LXT = 60 X(T)' = 35 +3.00 = X(T)' = 65	Recess LLR = 7.5 Resect LMR = 10.0	X = 18 X' = 12
26	RX(T) = 30 RX(T)' = 25 +3.00 = XT' = 35	Recess RLR = 6.0 Resect RMR = 6.0	Ortho Ortho'
26	X(T) = 30 X(T)' = 20 +3.00 = X(T)' = 35	Recess LLR = 5.5 Resect LMR = 3.5	X = 10 X' = 8
27	X(T) = 25 X(T)' = 35	Recess RLR = 4.5 Resect RMR = 5.0	Ortho X' = 8
27	X(T) = 50 X(T)' = 40 +3.00 = X(T)' = 50	Recess LLR = 7.5 Resect LMR = 9.0	Ortho Ortho'
28	XT = 65 X(T)' = 65	Recess RLR = 7.5 Resect MR OU = 7.0	Ortho X' = 5
28	XT = 40-65 X(T)' = 45 +3.00 = X(T)' = 45	Recess RLR = 7.5 Resect RMR = 8.0	Ortho Ortho'
29	X(T)' = 25	Recess RLR = 5.0 Resect RMR = 3.5	Small X Small X'
30	RXT = 20 RX(T)' = 14	Recess RLR = 5.0 Resect RMR = 3.5	X = 7 X' = 6
30	X(T) = 30 X(T)' = 30	Recess LLR = 6.0 Resect LMR = 4.5	X(T) = 8 X(T)' = 8

TABLE 4
(continued)

Age	Preop Deviation (diopters)	Surgery (millimeters)	Postop Deviation (diopters)
30	X(T) = 18-20 X(T)' = 18-25	Recess RLR = 4.0 Resect RMR = 3.5	Small X X' = 2
31	X(T) = 45 X(T)' = 30 +3.00 = X(T)' = 40	Recess LLR = 7.0 Resect LMR = 5.5	Ortho Ortho'
35	LX(T) = 80 LX(T)'= 80	Recess LLR = 8.0 Resect LMR = 8.0 (#1)	X(T) = 45 X(T)'= 14
		Recess RLR = 7.5 Resect RMR = 7.5 (#2)	Ortho Ortho'
36	XT = 30 X(T)' = 40	Recess LLR = 7.0 Resect LMR = 7.0	X(T) = 9 X(T)'= 20
36	X(T) = 17 X(T)' = 24 +3.00 = X(T)' = 25	Recess LLR = 3.5 Resect LMR = 4.0	Ortho X' = 12-14
37	RXT = 25 X(T)' = 35 +3.00 = X(T)' = 50	Recess RLR = 6.5 Resect RMR = 5.0	Small X X' = 8
37	X(T) = 35 X' = 8 +3.00 = X(T)' = 25	Recess LLR = 7.0 Resect LMR = 7.0	ET = 15 ET' = 15
39	X(T) = 30 X(T)' = 35	Recess LLR = 6.0 Resect LMR = 6.0	Ortho Flick X(T)'
42	X(T) = 65 X(T)' = 65	Recess LR OU=7.0 Resect LMR = 6.0	X(T) = 18 X(T)'= 25
47	X(T) = 25 X(T)' = 25	Recess LLR = 5.5 Resect LMR = 5.5	X(T) = 4 X(T)'= 8
48	X(T) = 25 X' = 25 +3.00 = X(T)' = 30	Recess LLR = 4.0 Resect LMR = 3.5	X = 10 X' = 12
53	X(T) = 25 X(T)' = 20	Recess RLR = 5.0 Resect RMR = 4.0	X(T) = 14 X' = 10
64	RX(T) = 25 RX(T)'= 40	Recess RLR = 5.0 Resect RMR = 5.0	X = 4 X(T)'= 14
65	X(T) = 40 X(T)' = 40	Recess RLR = 6.0 Resect RMR = 6.0	X(T) = 14 Small X'
67	X(T) = 35 X(T)' = 40	Recess LLR = 8.0	X = 10 X' = 10
70	X(T) = 25 X(T)' = 30	Recess RLR = 5.5 Resect RMR = 4.5	Ortho Small X'

Table 5

POSTOPERATIVE RESULTS

Deviation at Distance Prism Diopters	Number of Cases	Symptoms
Esodeviation:		
E = 6 or less	2	None
ET = 15	1	Persistent diplopia
Orthophoria:	15	None
Exodeviation:		
X or X(T) less than 15	24	None
X = 18	1	None
X(T) = 18	1	Headaches

Deviation at Near Prism Diopters	Number of Cases	Symptoms Symptoms
Esodeviation:		
E' = 6 or less	3	None
ET' = 15	1	Persistent diplopia
Orthophoria:	8	None
Exodeviation:		
X or X(T)' less than 15	29	None
X' = 25	1	None
X(T)' = 20 - 25	2	Headaches blurred vision at near

Postoperative results are shown in Table 5. Symptoms were alleviated in all but three cases. One patient who was overcorrected by 15 prism diopters had persistent diplopia. Two patients who were markedly undercorrected (with more than 15 prism diopters of residual exotropia) had no improvement in their preoperative symptoms.

We have seen several additional patients who have been operated on elsewhere and overcorrected. They have had persistent esotropia and diplopia which required either additional surgery or prisms.

DISCUSSION

In the present study, 68% of our patients underwent surgery between the ages of 15 and 31, and another 16% were between the ages of 35 and 42. What are the reasons for the concentration of visual symptoms in these age groups? Burian and Spivey (7) have pointed out that the degree of exodeviation at near appears larger as the patient grows older because the convergence mechanism becomes relatively less active; therefore, exophoria at near is more difficult to control with age. Knapp (6) has suggested that the two ages when the fusion mechanism is stressed most are the late teens and twenties (when the amount of close work increases) and the early forties (when accommodation is no longer adequate for close work). In our study, the overwhelming majority of patients were in the younger age group, suggesting that educational and occupational demands can produce intolerable visual symptoms at that period.

We have shown that many adults with intermittent exotropia have visual complaints. On the other hand, there are many adults with what appear to be similar degrees of exodeviation who do not even complain of symptoms, much less seek surgery. Jampolsky (3) may have been partially correct when he stated that patients with intermittent exotropia are relatively asymptomatic. Although difficult to prove, it is our impression that only a minority of individuals with intermittent exotropia have sufficient symptoms to warrant surgical treatment. Certain individuals seem to be more susceptible to functional problems than others, perhaps due to their occupational demands or to their threshold for experiencing diplopia.

Among patients who do seek surgical correction are typically those who have unusually heavy demands for near work. One patient with a 20 prism diopters intermittent exotropia was holding a job during the day and also attending law school at night. The extra burden of reading placed an intolerable strain on her fusional control. After surgery, she was able to attend her courses comfortably. This patient's sister had a similar exodeviation; she was a housewife who read relatively little and had minimal symptoms. She would never have come to the attention of an ophthalmologist had she not accompanied her sister to the office one day.

Most patients with intermittent exotropia see themselves in the mirror with straight eyes. Therefore, the cosmetic problem is minimal, in contrast to what is usually reported in the literature. (7) Only 7% of our patients sought surgery for cosmetic reasons, even though most of them stated that they had been aware that their eyes turned out for many years.

We tend to minimize the occurrence of diplopia in comitant strabismus because we use this symptom as a chief differentiating characteristic in the diagnosis of a paralytic deviation. Nevertheless, among our patients, diplopia was the most frequent preoperative symptom. It appears that when fusion breaks, adults with intermittent exotropia may experience double vision. This finding conflicts with Jampolsky's (3) theory that hemiretinal suppression in intermittent exotropes prevents the awareness of diplopia.

As previously mentioned, most authorities advocate overcorrecting intermittent exotropes by 10 to 20 prism diopters. This may be the best option in children. However, overcorrection in adults may produce intolerable diplopia. In the present study, we were fortunate to have only one symptomatic overcorrection; this patient, predictably, experienced persistent diplopia with a 15 prism diopters esotropia. It is of interest that another patient with a 6 prism diopters esophoria was asymptomatic, suggesting that some patients may have enough fusional divergence to overcome small overcorrections.

Our success in surgical management was due to a deliberate attempt to undercorrect by a small margin. In a previous unpublished series of 22 patients (none of whom are included in this study) who underwent surgery for intermittent exotropia, one of us (A.S.) had three patients in whom 10 prism diopters or more of esotropia persisted postoperatively. All three suffered from intolerable diplopia; all were treated with prisms for a minimum of six months. Two patients were reoperated by advancement of the previously recessed lateral recti and recession of the previously resected medial recti. These procedures yielded satisfactory results. The third patient did not return for corrective surgery.

Posner and Schlossman (16) have discussed the phenomenon of postoperative diplopia. It is our experience that children under 10 years of age do not suffer from permanent diplopia even when overcorrected to postoperative esotropia. They adapt readily to the new position of the eye; areas which previously did not suppress seem to quickly make the adjustment. Adults do not have as labile a neurosensory mechanism, so they maintain postoperative diplopia indefinitely unless further surgery is performed. Even if a second operation improves the position of the eyes and the patients are well satisfied with the results, they may still experience occasional diplopia, especially in extremes of gaze.

While a small consecutive esodeviation may produce intolerable diplopia, a small residual exodeviation is compatible with complete relief of symptoms. In the present study, two patients with residual exophorias ranging from 18-25 prism diopters were asymptomatic after surgery. This suggests that in some patients, convergence may be adequate to compensate for an undercorrection if the deviation is sufficiently reduced by surgery to allow the patients to fuse with comfort.

Not all patients are able to control a large exodeviation postoperatively. In the present study, two patients with residual intermittent exotropias of 15 to 25 prism diopters for both distance and near had persistent headaches and blurred vision after surgery. In the previously cited unpublished study, surgery was inadequate to alleviate preoperative symptoms in three additional patients. However, undercorrections in adults do not appear to be as serious a problem as they are in children. (12)

Few of our patients have returned for more than two years of follow-up so we are unable to determine the stability of the postoperative results over time. However, among those patients who have been followed for more than twelve months, in only one case has the exodeviation been noted to increase by more than 5 prism diopters after the sixth postoperative week. None of the patients whose symptoms were alleviated by surgery have reported a recurrence of visual problems.

REFERENCES

1. Schlossman A: Discussion of intermittent exotropia: evaluation and therapy. Arch Ophthalmol 51:411, 1954.

2. Schlossman A, Boruchoff SA: Correlation between physiologic and clinical aspects of exotropia. Am J Ophthalmol 40:53-64, 1955.

3. Jampolsky A: Differential diagnostic characteristics of intermittent exotropia and true exophoria. Am Orthopt J 4:48-55, 1954.

4. Burian HM: Exodeviations: their classification, diagnosis, and treatment. Am J Ophthamol 62:1161-1166, 1966.

5. Costenbader FD: Symposium on intermittent exotropia. Am Orthopt J 13:33-36, 1963.

6. Knapp P: Intermittent exotropia: evaluation and therapy. Am Orthopt J 3:27-33, 1953.

7. Burian HM, Spivey BE: The surgical management of exodeviations. Am J Ophthalmol 59:603-620, 1965.

8. Hiles DE, Davies GT, Costenbader FD: Long-term observations on unoperated intermittent exotropia. Arch Ophthalmol 80:436-442, 1968.

9. Jampolsky A: Management of exodeviations. In symposium on Strabismus, Transactions of the New Orleans Academy of Ophthalmology. St. Louis: C.V. Mosby, 140-156, 1962.

10. Raab EL, Parks MM: Recession of the lateral recti. Arch Ophthalmol 82:203-208, 1969.

11. Raab EL, Parks MM: Preoperative and postoperative sensory findings and distance/near relationship, in Moore S, Mein J, Stockbridge (eds): Orothoptics: Past, Present, Future. New York, Stratton Intercontinental Medical Book Co., 1976, pp 507-513.

12. Cooper EL: Purposeful Overcorrection in Exotropia. In International Strabismus Symposium, Giessen. New York: S. Karger, 1966: 311-318.

13. Knapp P: Management of Exotropia. In Symposium on Strabismus, Transactions of the New Orleans Academy of Ophthalmology. St. Louis: C.V. Mosby, 1971: 233-241.

14. Hardesty HH, Boynton JR, Keenan JP: Treatment of intermittent exotropia. Arch Ophthalmol 96:268-274, 1978.

15. Scott WE, Keech R, Mash JL: The postoperative results and stability of exodeviations. Arch Ophthalmol 99:1814-1818, 1981.

16. Posner A, Schlossman A: Relation of diplopia to binocular vision in concomitant strabismus. Arch Ophthalmol 45:615-622, 1951.

DISCUSSION BY D. DUNLOP

Dr. Schlossman's views on undercorrection of intermittent exotropia may seem to differ markedly from presently accepted practice; but he has limited his remarks to long standing problems in adults. These patients are not used to maintaining full binocular functions constantly and are not appreciative of forcing them to give up their restful periods of suppression. The wise clinician will warn them that further treatment and perhaps surgery may be required. When using adjustable sutures, one may give the patient the option of a fairly long period of post-operative discomfort with long term stability or alternatively a short period of discomfort with the prospect of further surgery at some time in the future.

SINGLE LATERAL RECTUS MUSCLE RECESSION FOR SMALL ANGLE EXOTROPIA

J. D. Reynolds and D. A. Hiles

ABSTRACT

A single lateral rectus muscle recession for exodeviations is an infrequently utilized procedure. A retrospective consecutive series of 36 patients with small angle exodeviations were treated with a single lateral rectus recession. Nineteen patients (53%) had primary exodeviations, 15 patients (41%) had consecutive exodeviations, and two patients (6%) had recurrent exodeviations.

The mean age of surgery of patients with primary exodeviations was 9.0 years. The mean pre-operative exodeviation was 24 P.D. The mean lateral rectus recession was 6.0 mm. A minimum follow-up time was two months. A mean improvement of 11 P.D. was obtained. Of the 12 intermittent and 7 constant exotropes, 85% were converted to orthophoria or small exophorias.

The average age of surgery of the 15 consecutive exodeviators was 9.2 years. The mean pre-operative exodeviation was 16 P.D. The mean lateral rectus recession was 5.5 mm. An average improvement of 14 P.D. was obtained initially and remained throughout the study. Four patients had intermittent and eleven patients had constant exotropia and 87% were converted to orthophoria or small exophorias.

The two patients with recurrent exotropia reduced their angles by 15 P.D. and both were converted to small angle exophorias.

95% of the primary exodeviators, 93% of the consecutive exodeviators and one of the recurrent exodeviators retained or improved their stereoacuity post-operatively.

We concluded that a single lateral rectus muscle recession for exodeviations less than 18 P.D. is an effective treatment in the elimination of the tropic component, the reduction of the strabismic angle, and improvement or maintenance of stereoacuity. Despite some deterioration in angle size with time, the improvement in angle character and stereopsis appears permanent.

STRABISMUS II
ISBN 0-8089-1424-3

INTRODUCTION

The management of small angle exotropias or intermittent exotropia remains controversial. Occlusion and orthoptics is more frequently utilized than survery because of the risks of surgical overcorrection and the subsequent induction of a constant small angle esotropia and amblyopia.

The indications for surgical correction of intermittent or constant exotropia are usually considered to be angles of 20 P.D. or more, those with a significant torpic component, or those exhibiting sensory decompensation. A small subset of exotropic patients exist who exhibit angles less than 20 P.D., have angle characters which are tropic or intermittently tropic at distance and/or near and may exhibit reduced sensory functions. It is the purpose of this paper to study these patients in an attempt to answer the questions of the benefit of surgery and, more specifically, the response to a single lateral rectus muscle recession.

SUBJECTS AND METHODS

We retrospectively analyzed a consecutive 15 year series of 36 patients treated with a single lateral rectus muscle recession for angles of exodeviations between 10-20 P.D. Nineteen patients had primary exodeviations, 15 patients had consecutive exodeviations and two patients had recurrent exodeviations.

The indication for surgical intervention was the presence of a tropic phase: all patients had either a constant exotropia or an intermittent exotropia that was judged to be manifest by history at least 50% of the time.

The mean age of surgery of the 19 primary exodeviators was 9.0 years. If one 32 year old patient was excluded, the mean age was 7.3 years. Five patients were 4.0 years of age or younger. All patients received a single lateral rectus muscle recession of 5.0--6.5 mm. with a mean of 6.0 mm. The follow-up period was divided into an initial period of two to five months and a final period of 12 to 96 months. The mean follow-up time was 45 months. The one week post-operative findings were also analyzed for overcorrection.

The mean age of surgery of the 15 consecutive exodeviation patients was 9.2 years. Excluding the two adults, the mean age became 7.2 years. Only two patients were less than 4.0 years of age at surgery. All patients received a single lateral rectus muscle recession of 4.0 to 6.5 mm. with a mean of 5.5 mm. The follo-up period was again divided into an initial period of two to four months and a final period of 9 to 96 months. The mean follow-up time was 40 months. Again, the one week post-operative findings were evaluated for overcorrection

Of the two recurrent exodeviation patients, the ages at surgery were 3.4 years and 8.4 years and each patient received a single lateral rectus muscle recession of 4.0 mm. and 5.0 mm. respectively. The follow-up period was three months and seven months.

All patients had their pre-operative and post-operative angle size, angle character, and stereoacuity using the Titmus stereotest recorded. Peripheral stereoacuity was presumed to be present if the patient had 60-3000 seconds of arc while central stereoacuity was defined as 40 seconds of arc or better.

RESULTS

The 19 primary exodeviators had a pre-operative deviation range of 10-16 P.D. with a mean of 14 P.D. Twelve patients had intermittent exotropia and seven patients had constant exotropia.

After surgery, the mean improvement in angle size during the first post-operative months as 11 P.D. Of the 12 patients followed longer than one year, the mean improvement was reduced to 8 P.D. Three patients retained a stable angle size, three patients improved their angle size from 2-15 P.D., and 6 patients deteriorated between 4-12 P.D. One week post-operatively only four patients exhibited an eso angle varying from 4 to 10 P.D.

The angle character during the initial post-operative period was as follows: exophoria occurred in 16 patients, intermittent exotropia in three patients and no patient exhibited a constant tropia. In the final period of 12 to 96 months, the angle character was exophoric in ten patients, intermittent exotropia in one patient, and a constant exotropia in one patient.

Pre-operative stereoacuity was central in six patients, peripheral in 10 and absent in 3 patients. Of the 6 patients with central pre-operative stereoacuity, all retained this status post-operatively. Of the ten patients with pre-operative peripheral stereoacuity, seven remained with peripheral and three were converted to central stereopsis. Of the three patients with absent pre-operative stereoacuity, all were converted to peripheral stereoacuity. None of these patients lost stereoacuity, and there were no persistent surgical overcorrections.

The 15 consecutive exodeviators had a pre-operative angle size from 12 to 20 P.D., except one patient with a 25 P.D. angle. There was a mean of 16 P.D. After surgery the initial improvement was 14 P.D. Six patients were in the final group of 9 to 96 months follow-up and their mean improvement was 14 P.D. When the final measurement was compared with the initial measurement in these 6 patients, 4 of the patients had remained stable, 1 had improved 14 P.D. and 1 had deteriorated 4 P.D. At one week post-operatively, four patients exhibited an esodeviation. Three patients had an esodeviation of 6 to 8 P.D. while one had an esodeviation of 20 P.D.

The pre-operative angle character was an intermittent exotropia in four patients and a constant exotropia in 11 patients. In the initial post-operative period, an exophoria was noted in 13 patinets, an esophoria in one patient, and a constant esotropia resulted in one patient. In the final peirod, six patinets were followed 9 to 96 months and all remained orthophoric or exophoric.

The pre-operative stereoacuity of these patients was peripheral in four patients and absent in 11 patients. Post-operatively, three of the four remained with peripheral stereoacuity and one patinet lost peripheral stereopsis. Of the 11 with absent pre-operative stereoacuity, two patients gained peripheral stereoacuity and nine remained without.

There was one overcorrection to a constant esotropia, one patient had post-operative esophoria, and four patients had small angle esodeviations at near.

The two recurrent exotropic patients had pre-operative angle sizes of 14 and 16 P.D. Both patients were converted to phorias. Both patients had absent stereoacuity pre-operatively while post-operatively one gained peripheral stereoacuity and the other remained without stereopsis. Neither were converted to an esodeviation.

DISCUSSION

Small angle exodeviations frequently are not surgically corrected because of the small size of the deviaion and the fear of converting an exodeviation with fusional potential to a constant small angle esotropia with the possibility of the development of amblyopia in susceptible children.(1,2) The recommended treatment has, therefore, been conservative.

Many small angle exodeviators require no treatment if the patients´ fusional amplitudes maintain the deviation in a phoric state. It has also been shown that small angle intermittent exotropes do not deteriorate and some even improve.(3) The patient with a small angle exodeviation who is tropic a significant percentage of time and is cosmetically unacceptable becomes a candidate for therapy. Orthoptics may be useful for intermittent exotropias(4-7) but htis has been disputed by other authors.(8-9) Orthoptics improve the fusional amplitudes, but do not reduce the angle size. Spoor and Hiles(10) have demonstrated the efficiency of daily parttime occlusion of the dominant eye in exotropic children three years of age and younger with angles of 20P.D. or less.

The patient who possesses a small angle exotropia, either intermittent or constant, presents both a cosmetic defect and a significant barrier to single binocular vision and stereopsis. It is this subset of patients in whom a single lateral rectus muscle recession becomes a useful and successful procedure.

Recurrent residual exodeviations following exotropia surgery do not always revert to their original angle size but remain as small angle deviations. Some patients remain stable, some improve and some decompensate to larger angles and constant tropias.(11) These patients also are candidates for single alteral rectus muscle recessions. Consecutive exodeviations constitute a surgical problem(12) for there is little else to offer these patients. undoubtedly many small angle consecutive exodeviations are not treated fearing re-establishment of the original esodeviation.

The success of the procedure may be based upon the reduction of the angle size with its attendant improvement in the cosmetic appearance of the patient. Although our patients had a significant improvement in their angle size it is the conversion of an intermittent or constant exotropia to a phoric state and the retention or improvement of the pre-operative stereoacuity that are the important parameters for functional cure.

From our data it is apparent that surgery is beneficial as judged by improvement in angle size, angle character, and stereoacuity along with the absence of complications and overcorrections. Despite the fact that, of those patients who were followed long enough to be included in our final status group, 50% of the primary exodeviators and 17% of the consecutive exodeviators deteriorated slightly in angle size, there was no significant deterioration in angle character or stereoacuity.

It is important to be aware of the possibility of converting an intermittently exotropic patient to a small angle esotropia with the risk of amblyopia. This possibility occurred in none of our intermittent exotropic patients, including those operated upon at age 4.0 years or younger. This is not a concern with consecutive exotropes who basically do not have central stereoacuity.

It is also noted that there is no need for an overcorrection to be apparent one week post-operatively. If present and of small angle size, it will resolve in the primary exodeviation group. Any overcorrection in the consecutive exodeviation patient at one week post-operatively should be viewed with caution, although this, too, may resolve with time.

CONCLUSION

In conclusion, the authors felt that in the appropriate patient with a small angle exodeviation, a single lateral rectus muscle recession produced significant improvement in angle size, angle character, and stereoacuity with minimal risks. The improvement in angle character and stereoacuity appeared to be permanent.

ACKNOWLEDGEMENTS

This study was supported in part by grants to the Fight for Sight Children′s Eye Clinic of the Eye and Ear Hospital, Pittsburgh, PA, by Fight for Sight, Inc., New York, NY.

REFERENCES

1. Jampolsky A: Management of exodeviations in early childhood, in Bellows JG Contemporary Ophthalmology Honoring Sir Stewart Duke-Elder (Ed): Baltimore, Williams & Wilkins

Co., p. 429-433, 1972.

2. Pratt-Johnson JA, Barlow JM, Tillson G: Early surgery in intermittent exotropia. Am J Ophthalmol 84: 689-694, 1977.

3. Hiles DA, Davies GT, Costenbader FD: Long term observations on unoperated intermittent exotropia. Arch Ophthalmol 80: 436-442, 1968.

4. Sanfilippo S, Clahane A: The immediate and long term results of orthoptics in exodeviations. In the First International Congress of Orthoptists. St. louis, C.V. Mosby Co., p 300-312, 1968.

5. Gagnon R, Gohier L: Le Traitment orthoptique des strabismus divergents intermittents. Un Med Canada 99:1490-1492, 1970.

6. Chryssanthou G: Orthoptic management of intermittent exotropia. Am Orthopt J 24:69-72, 1974.

7. Cooper EL, Leyman I: The mangement of intermittent exotropia: A comparison of the results of surgical and nonsurgical treatment. Am Orthopt J 27:61-67, 1977.

8. Moore S: Orthoptic treatment for intermittent exotropia. Am Orthopt J 13:14-20, 1963.

9. Limon de Brown E: Treatment of intermittent exotropia. Int Ophthalmol Clinics 11(4):306-307, 1971.

10. Spoor DK, Hiles DA: Occlusion therapy for exodeviations occurring in infants and young children. Ophthalmology 86:2152-2157, 1979.

11. Weinstein GS, Biglan AW, Hiles DA: Postoperative residual small angle exodeviations. Ophthalmic Surg 13:478-482, 1982.

12. von Noorden G: Burian-von Noorden´s Binocular Vision and Ocular Motility. Theory and Management of Strabismus. St. Louis, C.V. Mosby Co., p. 326, 1980.

MASTER EYE IN EXOPHORIA

M. Kubo and O. Tamura

ABSTRACT

In the present study, it is suggested that there might exist the master-slave relationship in exophoria as in exotropia. In children, the EMG examination and forced duction on the eye are next to impossible to perform. Therefore, the EOG during the cover-uncover test is considered as a useful method to estimate the master-slave relationship.

INTRODUCTION

In constant exotropia, the "master-slave relationship" seems established. (1,2) The master eye is defined as the eye from which the magician's forceps phenomenon (MF phenomenon) discovered by Mitsui can be elicited. (1,2) When the master eye is surgically treated, excellent therapeutic results can be obtained. (3) Even when the surgical results prove inadequate, substantial improvements from constant tropia to phoria-tropia or to phoria can be observed. (3) Although there exist individual stages such as exophoria, phoria-tropia and constant tropia, it is still unknown when the master-slave relationship is established. We can not be as positive that the master-slave relationship does exist in exophoria as it does in exotropia.

The present study describes a method to determine the establishment of the master-slave relationship in exophoria.

MATERIALS AND METHODS

Eye movements in exophoria were recorded by electro-oculograms (EOG's) during the cover-uncover test using a DC preampli (Nihon Koden, RDU-5), a power amplifier (Nihon Koden, RPC-45) and a photorecorder (Yokogawa Electric Works LTD, RB-5). The EOG was recorded by a cross-talk method throughout present study, because the one eye suffered a distortion from the cross-talk of the fellow eye. (2,4) Non-polarizable silver-silverchloride disc electrodes, 10cm

STRABISMUS II
ISBN 0-8089-1424-3

in diameter, were fixed on the skin at the lateral canthi and the nasal canthi on either side. The groundlead was placed on the ear.

Subjects lay on a bed in a shielded room with head fixed. The room was illuminated to give a background adaptation with an intensity of about 200 Lux on the surface of cornea. A fixation target (5mm in diameter) was placed in median plane in front of eyes about 30cm away. The cover-uncover test was done when the eyes were actively fixed on the target. In order to know the time to cover and uncover, photocells were attached on both cheeks. The reaction of photocells did not influence the EOG.

The subjects consisted of two groups: in Group I were 5 cases of residual exophoria after master eye surgery for exotropia (Table 1) and in Group II were 5 cases of essential exophoria without a surgical history (Table 2).

Table 1. List of the residual exophoria after master eye surgery of exotropia.

Case No.	Age Sex	Vision	Fly Test	Convergence (Near Point)	Master Eye	Version by Uncover
1	49 M	R:1.5 L:1.5	+	+(10cm)	L	+(Left)
2	10 F	R:1.2 L:1.2	+	+(20cm)	R	+(Right)
3	10 F	R:1.5 L:1.5	+	+(5cm)	R	+(Bilateral)
4	39 M	R:1.0 L:1.2	+	+(20cm)	R	+(Right)
5	8 M	R:1.5 L:1.5	+	+(5cm)	R	+(Right)

Table 2. List of the essential exophoria without a surgical history.

Case No.	Age Sex	Vision	Fly Test	Convergence (Near Point)	Version by Uncover
1	18 F	R:1.2 L:1.2	+	+(5cm)	+(Left)
2	8 M	R:1.5 L:1.5	+	+(5cm)	-
3	9 M	R:1.2 L:1.2	+	+(5cm)	+(Bilateral)
4	26 F	R:1.2 L:1.2	+	+(12cm)	+(Right)
5	6 M	R:1.5 L:1.5	+	+(5cm)	-

RESULTS

1. EOG in residual exophoria after major eye surgery: Figure 1 shows the typical EOG in a case of residual exophoria after surgery of exophoria (case 1 in Table 1). In this case, the left eye was the master eye, since before surgery the left eye was the straight eye and the magician's forceps phenomenon arose from this eye only.

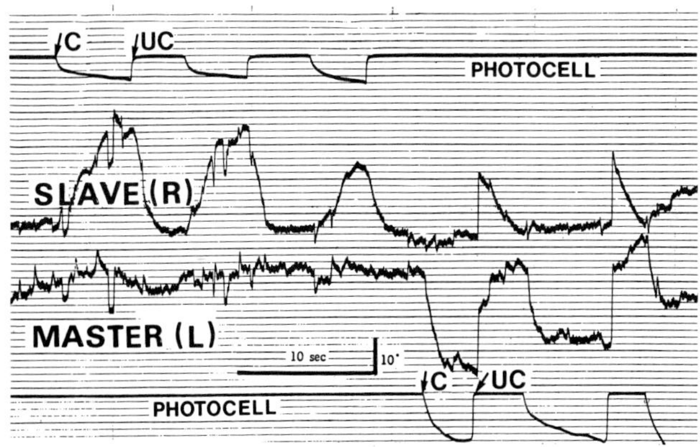

Figure 1: EOG of a case of residual exophoria and the reaction of the photocells. In this case, the left eye was the master eye.

The top line in Figure 1 shows the reaction of the photocell on the right cheek. The arrows C and UC indicate the times when the right eye was covered and uncovered three times. When the right eye was covered, this eye exodeviated gradually, and when uncovered the eye returned slowly to a straight position. However, the left eye maintained a straight position throughout. Next, the left eye, namely the master eye, was covered and uncovered three times. The left eye exodeviated, upon being covered. However, when the left eye was uncovered, both eyes showed a rapid version in the direction of the slave eye until the left eye assumed a straight position. After which, the exodeviated slave eye returned gradually to a straight position.

Figure 2 shows the EOG of the same case displayed at a high paper speed showing the portion of the version upon the uncovering of the master eye. This version occurred about 200 milliseconds after the uncovering and the eyes moved at a speed of 10 degrees in 50 milliseconds; which was equivalent to a velocity of 200 degrees per second. The results in the 5 cases examined were all similar.

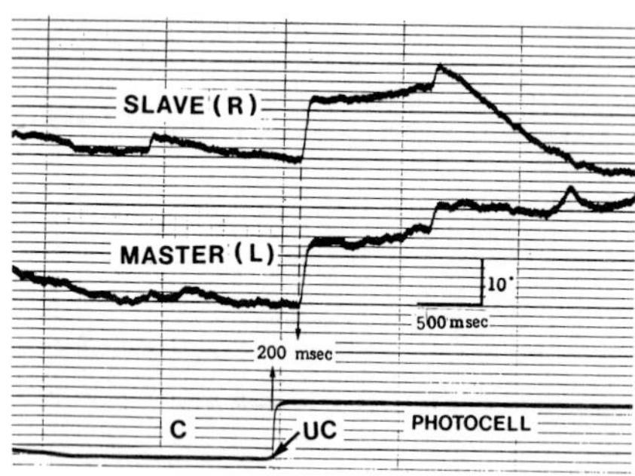

Figure 2: EOG in the same case as Fig 1 displayed at a high paper speed showing the portion of the version upon the uncovering of the master eye.

2. EOG in essential exophoria without a surgical history: Figure 3 shows the EOG obtained in a case of essential exophoria. Results of the cover-uncover test on the right eye are shown (Case 1 in Table 2). The right eye exodeviated upon being covered and returned to a straight position when uncovered, while the left eye maintained a straight position throughout. This pattern did not change even when the test was repeated. Figure 4 shows the EOG of the same case when the cover-uncover test was applied to the left eye. The eye exodeviated when it was covered. When it was uncovered, however, a rapid version occurred toward the right until the left eye assumed a straight position. After this version, the exodeviated right eye returned to a straight position. From these results, the left eye in this case was considered to be the master eye. This kind of difference in the eye movement of both eyes was seen in 2 out of 5 cases examined. Version by uncover appeared bilaterally in case 3.

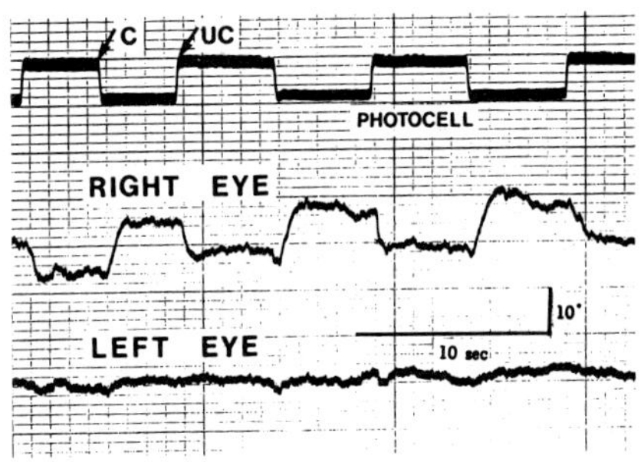

Figure 3: EOG of a case of essential exophoria during the cover-uncover test on the right eye. The left eye maintained the straight position throughout.

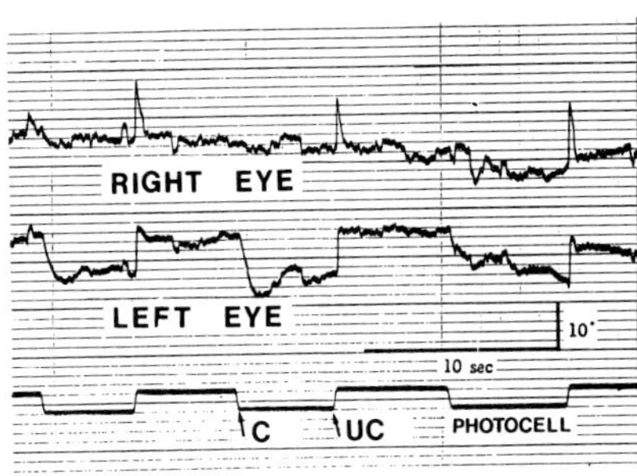

Figure 4: EOG of the same case as Fig 3 during the cover-uncover test on the left eye. When the left eye was uncovered, a rapid version occurred before orthophorization.

DISCUSSION

A series of studies by Mitsui and associates[2,3] suggested that in most cases of exotropia the "master-slave relationship" is established and that the so-called magician's forceps phenomenon (MF phenomenon) by Mitsui[1] is elicited from the master eye only. Tamura et al[4] suggested by an EMG that in most cases of alternative exotropia the master-slave relationship was not alternative, because the MF phenomenon by the change in the EMG occurred from one eye only.

The present study in exophoria showed that the eye movement by uncover of one of the eyes shows version before orthophorization, while by uncover of another eye shows immediate orthophorization. Jampolsky suggested that this may be due to the dominance of the first eye. However, this may also be a sign of the development of master-slave relationship in exophoria.

REFERENCES

1. Mitsui Y: Etiology and treatment of strabismus. Ophtalmic Plactic (Japan) 49:1151-1166, 1978.

2. Mitsui Y, Hirai K, Akazawa K, Masuda K: The sensorimotor reflex and strabismus. Jpn J Ophthalmol 23:227-256, 1979.

3. Mitsui Y, Tamura O, Hirai K, Akazawa K, Ohga M, Masuda K: Effect of master eye surgery in exodeviations. Jpn J Ophthalmol 24:221-231, 1980.

4. Kubo M, Hirai K, Mitsui Y: Method of measurement and elimination of the contralateral effect (cross-talk) in the EOG. Folia Ophthalmol Jap 30:701-704, 1979.

5. Tamura O, Mitsui Y.: Determination of the master eye in exotropia using the EMG. Rinsho Ganka (in press).

6. Jampolsky A: What can electromyography do for the ophthalmologist? Invest Ophthalmol 9:570-599, 1970.

DISCUSSION BY D. DUNLOP

Drs. Kubo's and Tamura's excellent presentation examined the question of ocular dominance, and in so doing they have presented us with an elegantly simple way of documenting and quantifying the rate of recovery of fixation after cover testing, one of the most fundamental tests in strabismology. Their method should also be valued in teaching.

SURGICAL TREATMENT OF EXOTROPIA WITH POOR VISION

G. Velez

ABSTRACT

The results of surgical treatment of exotropia with poor vision with uniocular surgery in the amblyopic eye are presented. In 29 cases a recession of the lateral rectus between 7 to 8 mm with bare sclera closure of the conjunctiva and a resection of the medial rectus between 6 to 8 mm were done. In moderate deviations of exotropia up to 45 prism diopters the final results at least one year after surgery were acceptable in most cases. An undercorrection over 15 prism diopters occurred in 17.64%. In deviations of 50 prism diopters or more the final results were poor, as 58.33% of the patients ended with an undercorrection over 15 prism diopters. In 16 cases with deviations of 50 prism diopters or more weakening of the superior and inferior oblique in the amblyopic eye was added to the horizontal rectus surgery. The final results were acceptable in a high percentage of cases. Only 18.74% of the cases ended with an undercorrection of more than 15 prism diopters.

INTRODUCTION

The surgical results of long-standing exotropia with poor vision in one eye have been contradictory. Several surgical techniques have been used regularly for such cases, including large recessions of the lateral rectus (1-2), and recession of conjunctiva of the recessed muscle (3). Jampolsky advocated surgery only in the horizontal rectus of the amblyopic eye with exotropia (4-5) and demonstrated the contracture of the obliques (5-6). Recently Raab presented a surgical approach involving in the horizontal rectus and the obliques in a large angle exotropia with poor vision in one eye (7). The purpose of this study is to show the surgical results in exotropia of moderate and large angle with surgery only on the amblyopic eye.

STRABISMUS II
ISBN 0-8089-1424-3

In 16 patients a weakening of the superior and inferior oblique of the amblyopic eye was added to the horizontal rectus surgery. An infraplacement of the horizontal rectus was done to control the hypertropia induced by weakening the two obliques in the same eye. The preoperative angle ranged in this group between 50 to 100 prism diopters.

The ages of the patients were between 10 to 59 years old. All the cases were followed for at least one year after surgery. Only those cases are reported in which the postoperative controls were followed.

The results were classified as good, acceptable and failures. Good when the final results were ortho, an overcorrection up to 5 prism diopters, or an undercorrection up to 10 prism diopters. Acceptable when the cosmetic appearance was accepted by the patient and parents and the final deviation was an overcorrection between 5 to 10 prism diopters or an undercorrection between 10 to 15 prism diopters. Those classed as failures included an overcorrection greater than 10 prism diopters or an undercorrection greater than 15 prism diopters.

The patients in which only horizontal surgery was done were divided in two groups: group one had a preoperative deviation between 30 to 45 prism diopters and group two had a deviation of 50 prism diopters or greater. The results were quite acceptable in deviations up to 45 prism diopters, failures in this group were 17.64% (Fig. 1), but in deviations of 50 prism diopters or more surgery only on the horizontal rectus with amounts of recession and resection described gave failures of 58.33% (Fig. 2).

Fig I

Nº of patients	Good	Acceptable	Failure
17	8 47.05 %	6 35.29 %	3 17.64 %

Results of lateral rectus recession, bare sclera closure of the conjuntiva and resection of the medial rectus in exotropias with poor vision between 30 and 45 prism diopters.

Fig 2

Nº of patients	Good	Acceptable	Failure
12	2 16.66%	3 25.00 %	7 58.33 %

Results of lateral rectus recession, bare sclera closure of the conjuntiva and resection of the medial rectus in exotropias with poor vision in deviations between 50 and 90 prism diopters

In the group of patients with exotropia of 50 prism diiopters or more in which a weakening of both obliques of the amblyopic eye was added to the horizontal rectus surgery the results were quite good in most cases; only 18.75% were failures (Fig. 3).

Fig 3

Nº of patients	Good	Acceptable	Failure
16	7 43.75%	6 37.50%	3 18.75 %

Results of lateral rectus recession bare sclera closure of the conjuntiva, resection of the medial rectus and weakening of the superior and inferior oblique in exotropias with poor vision between 50 and 100 prism diopters of deviation

None of the patients had an overcorrection of greater than 10 prism diopters. All failures in both groups were undercorrections. This study is in agreement with Jampolsky (4-5) who showed that there is no neccessity to do horizontal surgery on the fixing eye for exotropias with amblyopia of long standing. In cases of large angle exotropias greater than 50 prism diopters with deep amblyopia, a definitive improvement in the final results was obtained by weakening of both obliques in the amblyopic eye as an addition to the horizontal rectus muscle surgery using the Raab technique (7). The contracture of both obliques in the amblyopic exotropic eye, are logically weakened inse cases. Weakening all the abduction forces in large angle exotropias on the eye with poor vision of long standing allows acceptable final results in a high percentage of cases. I prefer this procedure over doing extra large recessions of 10 mm or more in the lateral rectus, that results in most of the cases with some limitation of abduction with a restrictive component.

The infraplacement of the horizontal rectus to control the hypertropia induced by weakening the two obliques in the same eye is important, because the weakening of both obliques in the same eye, has a net effect of creating a hypertropia. An underaction of the inferior rectus of the amblyopic eye was observed in all of the cases of large angle exotropia of long standing. The weakening of the superior oblique agravates this downward limitation and the superior rectus pulls the eye up. Using this infraplacement of the horizontal recti the hypertropia was controlled in all cases.

CONCLUSION

By working in the amblyopic eye in cases of exotropia of long-standing, the surgical results were quite acceptable using a reccession of the lateral rectus between 7 to 8 mm, a bare sclera closure of the conjuntiva and a resection of the medial rectus between 6 to 8 mm in deviations of moderate amount up to 45 prism diopters. In large angle exotropias of

REFERENCES

1. Urist MJ: Right angle exotropia. Am J Ophthalmol 58:987-1004, 1964.

2. Schwarts RL, Calhoun JH: Surgery of large angle exotropia. J Pediatr Ophthalmol Strabismus 17:359-363, 1980.

3. Cole JG, Cole HG: Recession of the conjunctiva in complicated eye muscle operations. Am J Ophthalmol 53:618-622, 1962.

4. Jamplosky A: Surgical management of exotropias. Am J Ophthalmol 46:646-648, 1958.

5. Rayner JW, Jampolsky A: Management of adult patients with large angle amblyopic exotropia. Ann Ophthalmol 5:95-99, 1973.

6. Jampolsky A: Surgical leashes and reverse leashes in strabismus surgical management. In Symposium of Strabismus. Transactions of New Orleans Academy of Ophthalmol. St Louis, CV Mosby, pp 244-268, 1978.

7. Raab LE: Unilateral four muscle surgery for large angle exotropia. Ophthalmology 86:1441-1446, 1979.

DISCUSSION BY D. DUNLOP

Inherent in Dr. Schlossman's paper and that of Dr. Velez is the concept of differentiating dominant and non-dominant eyes (a theme introduced by Dr. P. Knapp to the 1966 ISA meeting but not now regarded as of paramount importance in divergent surgery). Dr. Velez's surgical weakening of the superior and inferior obliques (Raab technique) carries the application of functional anatomy to its logical limits. It is innovative surgery and we will look forward to his long term results. Perhaps he may consider using Alan Scott's technique of Botulus injection to weaken the obliques.

MANAGEMENT OF INTERMITTENT EXOTROPIA

H. Hardesty

ABSTRACT

To study the long range results of surgically treated intermittent exotropia, 100 consecutive patients have been followed for an average of 6.7 years. In all cases, the initial procedure was bilateral recession of the lateral rectus muscles. The overall functional cure rate was 79%. However, to accomplish this result, 27 patients were operated a second time, 21 for undercorrection and six for overcorrection.

Patients who were either overcorrected or undercorrected were placed in prisms to allow constant fusion in daily life for a period of a minimum of six months before a second operation was performed. I believe that using prisms as a fusing priming device during the interval of overcorrection or undercorrection was the important factor in the high cure rate.

METHODS

One hundred surgically treated patients with intermittent exotropia have been followed for an average of 6.7 years. In all cases, the initial procedure was bilateral recssion of the lateral rectus muscles. The overall functional cure rate was 79 percent. To accomplish this result, 27 patients were operated on a second time, 21 for undercorrection and six for overcorrection.

A number of patients cooperated poorly or were lost to followup while still under treatment. Had these patients been eliminated from the series, the cure rate would have been greater than 90 percent.

To be considered a functional cure, it was necessary for the patient to meet the following criteria: (1) no tropia, constant or intermittent, at either distance or near (two patients who had small stabilized monofixational esophorias were considered cures); (2) all supplementary therapy such

STRABISMUS II
ISBN 0-8089-1424-3

as prisms, orthoptics, and cholinesterase inhibitors discontinued; (3) the patient and the parents unaware of any manifest deviation, even with extreme fatigue; and (4) the patient demonstrating some degree of stereopsis on the Titmus Stereotest.

DISCUSSION

Why have the results with this group of patients been significantly better than in previously reported series? The following line of reasoning explains the high success rate. Patients with intermittent exotropia are usually not surgically treated until the exotropia has been present for many months or years. This has permitted the establishment of deep suppression of the temporal retina with resulting poor fusional vergence amplitudes. Even through surgery results in alignment of the eyes, the low fusional amplitudes permit the eyes to diverge at times of fatigue. The patients, who still have deep suppression of the temporal retina, are not aware of diplopia.

Also, with passage of time, eyes without a fusion lock usually will slowly assume a more divergent position. Thus, the intermittent exotropia becomes more frequently manifest and increases in degree, often returning to its old angle of deviation. Understandably, parents are distressed to see a recurrence of the problem after having experienced the anxiety of having their child undergo surgery. They are reluctant to consent to a second operation, especially when we cannot promise that a second procedure will be any more effective than the first. Consequently, many months or even years pass before a second operation is performed. The continuing periods of exotropia cause the undesirable sensory factors to worsen. Under these circumstances, it is not surprising that a second operation also frequently fails to establish a permanent cure.

The goal of treatment outlined is to prevent this damaging sequence of events from occurring. Patients with undercorrections or recurrences are placed in base-in prisms to permit constant fusion in daily life. Except in rare instances, this is easy to accomplish. If the distance and near measurements are different, an amount of prism equal to the average of these two measurements usually causes the patient to fuse constantly.

Causing the patient to fuse constantly in daily life not only prevents the sensory defect from becoming worse, but also improves the quality of fusion. Stress is placed on the importance of wearing the prisms the entire waking day.

Overcorrections were managed in a similar manner. If overcorrection persisted longer than two weeks, a short trial of a cholinesterase inhibitor was given and any significantly hyperopia corrected. If despite these measures the patient remained constantly esotropic, patching was instituted. If the esotropia did not reduce with patching in one month, the patient was placed in base-out prisms to allow constant fusion. Since patients with overcorrections have little if any divergent fusional amplitudes, an amount of prism that equals or slightly exceeds the esotropia is required to accomplish this goal. With patients who remained 15 diopters or less esotropic after one month of patching, it was nearly always possible to reduce gradually and eventually eliminate the prisms. Patients with larger amounts of esotropia were required to wear prisms for a minimum of six months before further surgery was performed.

It is difficult to establish an ideal length of time for the wearing of prisms if further surgery becomes necessary. Six months has arbitrarily been selected as a minimal length of time. However, patients who have extremely poor fusion, especially if there is a vertical component, should wear their prisms for at least a year. There is no maximal time for wearing prisms as long as they are worn constantly. Parents are told this, and some choose to wait two years or longer before consenting to a second operation.

The parents were told prior to surgery that the wearing of prisms might be an essential part of the treatment of the exotropia. The patient and parential cooperation has been excellent. Many children wear their glasses by choice once constant fusion is established. Here, a word of advice is extremely important. Whenever it becomes evident that prisms should be worn for a number of months, it is advisable to have them ground into regular spectacle lenses. Fresnel press-on prisms are difficult to keep clean and become cloudy with the passage of time. Without exception, patients with prisms less than 10 prism diopters (each lens) were pleased when shifted from Fresnel press-on prisms to prisms incorporated into regular spectacles. When prism glasses are prescribed, the parents should be advised to select a small frame, and the optician instructed to grind the prisms as thin as possible.

It is believed that an overcorrection as large as 20

prism diopters frequently results in persistent overcorrection requiring further surgery. This is especially true when reestablishment of fusion is left to chance. As mentioned previously, esotropia was not allowed to remain untreated for longer than four weeks. It is particularly important to institute patching promptly if the esotropia is increasing in amount as these patients frequently develop a blind spot syndrome. A blind spot syndrome measures 25-30 diopters.

With the treatment outlined, no patient in the series of 100 cases was allowed to develop a blind spot syndrome. There were only two monofixational syndromes. It seems reasonable to assume that it was our early treatment of overcorrections with patching and prisms that caused our incidence of monofixtational patterns to be low.

CONCLUSIONS

A regimen for treating intermittent exotropia is described. Included are methods for treating both under- and overcorrection. Following these methods resulted in better than a 90 percent cure rate with fully cooperative patients. The key to obtaining this success rate was causing the patient to fuse constantly with prisms during the interval of under- or overcorrection.

REFERENCES

1. Costenbader FD: The physiology and management of divergent strabismus, in Allen GH (ed): Strabismus Ophthalmic Symposium. St. Louis, CV Mosby Co., 1950, pp. 349-366.

2. Parks MM: Comitant esodeviations in children, in Haik GM (ed): Strabismus Symposium of the New Orleans Academy of Ophthalmology. St. Louis, CV Mosby Co., 1962, pp. 31-55.

3. Knapp P: Treatment of divergent deviations in Allen GH (ed): Strabismus Ophthalmic Symposium II. St. Louis, CV Mosby Co., 1958, pp. 364-376.

4. Burian HM, Spivey BE: The surgical management of exodeviations, AM J Ophthalmol 59: 603-620, 1965.

5. von Noorden GK: Divergence excess and simulated divergence excess: diagnosis and surgical management. Doc Ophthalmol 26: 719-728, 1969.

6. Windsor CE: Surgery, fusion and accommodative convergence in exotropia. J. Pediatr Ophthalmol 8: 166-170, 1972.

7. Dunlap EA, Gaffney RB: Surgical management of intermittent exotropia. Am Orthopt J 13: 20-33, 1963.

8. Folk ER: Surgical results in intermittent exotropia. Arch Ophthalmol 55: 484-487, 1956.

9. Cooper EL: Muscle surgery and orthoptics. Am Orthoptic J 5: 5-15, 1955.

10. Hardesty HH: Treatment of overcorrected intermittent exotropia. Am J Ophthalmol 66: 80-86, 1968.

11. Hardesty HH: Treatment of under and overcorrected intermittent exotropia with prism glasses. Am Orthopt J 19: 110-119, 1969.

12. Hardesty HH: Prisms in the management of intermittent exotropia. Am Orthopt J 22: 22-30, 1972.

13. Knapp P: Use of membrane prisms. Trans Am Acad Ophthalmol Otolargyn 79: 718-721, 1975.

14. Moore S, Stockbridge L: An evaluation of the use of Fresnel press-on prisms in childhood strabismus. Am Orthoptic J 25: 62-66, 1975.

15. Jampolsky A: Management of exodeviations, in Haik GM (ed): Strabismus Symposium of the New Orleans Academy of Ophthalmology. St. Louis, CV Mosby Co., 1962, pp. 140-156.

16. Raab EL, Parks MM: Recession of the lateral recti: Early and late postoperative alignments. Arch Ophthalmol 82: 203-208, 1969.

DISCUSSION BY D. DUNLOP

We must all admire Dr. Hardesty's great industry in documenting his long term follow-up of 100 operation cases and we must compliment him on his outstanding results. His paper is a reminder that some surgeons do not follow up their cases as closely and energetically as they should. Our own experience in Australia suggests that the early post-operative period is critical to long term success. The patient should be warned pre-operatively that surgery is only one part of overall treatment and that it may have to be repeated, especially if post-op cooperation is poor.

PATTERNS OF BINOCULARITY AFTER SURGERY FOR EXOTROPIA

S. M. Wolff

ABSTRACT

Surgical overcorrection of exotropia is recommended by most authorities as a means of preventing recurrence of the exodeviation. The sensory adaptations to post-operative esotropia include the resumption of an exo-deviation, the development of a small angle esodeviation with monofixation, a larger esodeviation with significant amblyopia, or, rarely, the blind spot syndrome. The age of the patient at the time of surgery is an important determinant in the ultimate fixation pattern.

STRABISMUS II
ISBN 0-8089-1424-3

DISCUSSION BY D. DUNLOP

Dr. Wolff neatly summarizes the possible results of surgery and warns us of the dire consequences of post-operative neglect and procrastination. Again, he emphasizes the differing results with different ages of onset. Our own experience suggests that adult divergence is a different condition to early onset divergence. Our figures comparing the incidence of eso and exo deviations over a 25 year period from 1955 to 1980 show a relative decrease in incidence of divergence. This may reflect the changing habits of children in Australia who generally had no television in the 1950's and now spend several hours a day indoors that used to be spent outdoors in the sunshine. These changes may also influence the rate of recurrence of divergence post-operatively.

CONGENITAL, HEREDITARY DOWNBEAT NYSTAGMUS

W.W. Bixenman

ABSTRACT

An 8-year-old male child with congenital, hereditary downbeat nystagmus is reported. He initially presented with chin down head posturing since birth and a reading disability since starting school. He is the youngest reported case of downbeat nystagmus to date and is the first reported with a congenital, familial form of downbeat nystagmus. Interestingly, homologous base up prisms incorporated into his spectacles eliminated his torticollis, improved his vision in primary position and "cured" his reading disability.

Downbeat nystagmus has become the subject of considerable interest1-23 since Dr. Cogan's initial reports2-4 of a vertical jerk nystagmus with the fast phase directed downward that was associated with cerebellar or lower brainstem pathology at the cervicomedullary junction. As a clinical rule, one-third of patients with downbeat nystagmus have a surgical lesion, while two-thirds have nonsurgical etiologies.24

INTRODUCTION

The following case is the youngest reported to date and is presented to emphasize that a heredofamilial form of downbeat nystagmus may be one of the commonest etiologies seen in clinical practice.15

MATERIALS

Patient 1

An 8-year-old male student was first seen in consultation on 8/17/81. He was the product of a full term, uneventful gestation with a normal birth and postpartum period. Since birth, his mother had been aware that his eyes would "roll up." By the time that he was able to sit, she

STRABISMUS II
ISBN 0-8089-1424-3

noted that he would tend to keep his chin down and "look up" at people. This was repeatedly mentioned to his pediatrician who could ascertain no reason for this unusual behavior.

Although his milestones were modestly delayed in that he did not walk until 16 months of age, he developed normally thereafter. His first portrait was taken in 1974 at age 1-1/2 years (Fig 1) and demonstrates this preferred chin down head posturing.

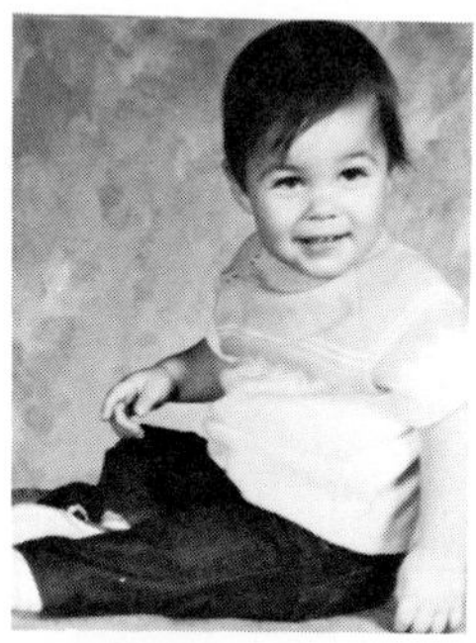

Figure 1. Patient R.B. at age 1-1/2 years demonstrating his preference to "look up."

He was first taken to an ophthalmologist at age 3 years. No cyclovertical strabismus problem could be identified which would account for this head posturing. A portrait taken shortly after that examination again demonstrates his chin down head posturing (Fig 2).

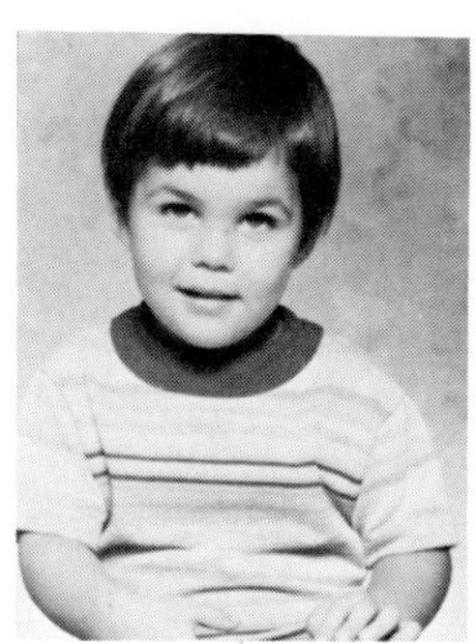

Figure 2. Patient R.B. at age 3 years with persistent chin down head posture.

Since beginning school, reading has been a major problem. He has been diagnosed as having a "learning disability" but has stayed in regular classes with tutoring. He has been quite successful in athletic competition. In the spring of 1981, he was taken for another ophthalmic evaluation. "Eye twitching" was noted and he was referred for a neurological consultation. Except for his nystagmus, his neurological examination was quite normal with no evidence of cerebellar dysfunction or ataxia. A neuro-ophthalmic opinion was requested.

The child himself was totally asymptomatic, with no suggestion that he was experiencing diplopia or oscillopsia. Family history was negative for any known ocular or neurological disorder. His parents are divorced and his father is unavailable for examination.

On examination (8/17/81), his chin down head posturing without an associated tilt was quite obvious (Fig 3). His visual acuity with his head in this position (i.e., eyes in upgaze) was 20/25-2 in either eye. His binocular vision was the same. In primary position and downgaze, his vision was 20/50-2 in either eye. He could read Jaeger 1 print with some hesitancy in upgaze, with considerable difficulty in primary position, and not at all in downgaze. His fixation was central and steady O.U. and he was fusing at both fixation distances. He was orthophoric with no A or V pattern. His ductions and versions were full. Pupillary reflexes were brisk (++++) to light and near with no anisocoria. Visual fields were full to confrontation and tangent screen examination. His stereoacuity was slightly reduced (TNO = 120 sec. arc) but equal in upgaze and downgaze. There was no apparent ocular dysmetria or flutter. His saccadic and pursuit movements were clinically normal except in the vertical plane where the nystagmus pattern was superimposed.

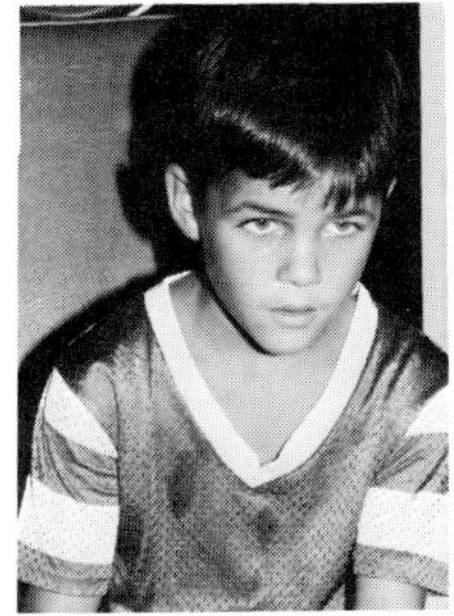

Figure 3. Patient R.B. at age 8 years.

Most remarkable was his nystagmus (Fig 4). In primary position, he manifested a constant, symmetric, low frequency downbeat nystagmus. The nystagmus was unaffected by fixation effort but was dampened by convergence. There was no latent component. His downbeat nystagmus became coarse in lateral gaze, in straight downgaze, but especially so in the oblique downgaze positions. In upgaze, his eyes were quiet with only infrequent downbeats seen.

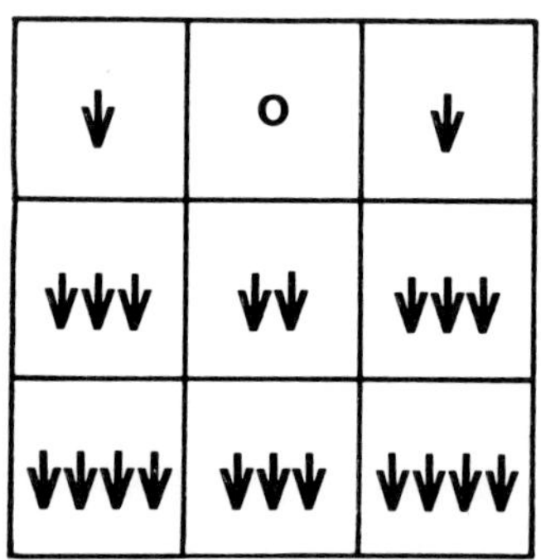

Figure 4. Pattern of downbeat nystagmus in patient R.B. Note the increased intensity in lateral gaze but especially in the oblique downgaze positions.

The pattern of his downbeat nystagmus was more evident with electronystagmography (Fig 5). The nystagmus had a frequency of 3-4 per second and demonstrated a linear slow wave configuration (Fig 6). Saccadic velocity measurements were considered to be within normal limits, both horizontally (mean = 454o/sec) and vertically (mean: up = 345o/sec, down = 333o/sec).

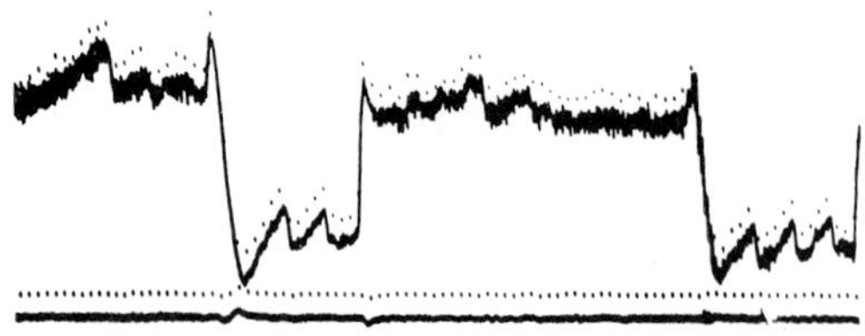

Figure 5. Electronystagmography of patient R.B. Note the 3-4/second downbeat nystagmus in downgaze and lack of nystagmus in upgaze.

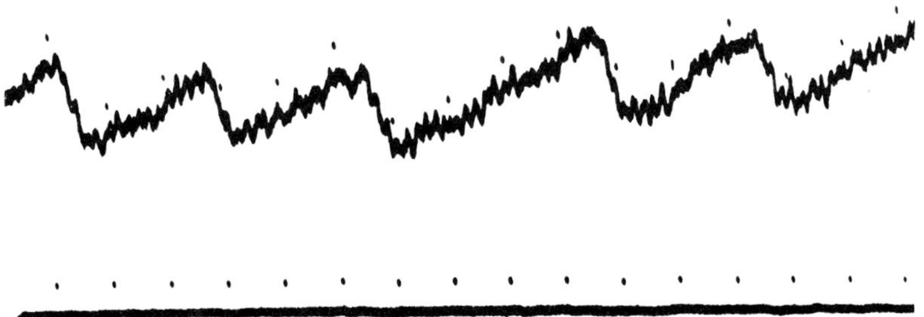

Figure 6. Electronystagmography of patient R.B. Note the linear slow wave configuration.

His fundoscopic examination was normal except for the ocular excursions which were quite dramatic with the direct ophthalmoscope.

Using a trial lens frame, various prism strengths were tried. Interestingly, base down prism of any strength had no effect on his chin down head posturing and actually worsened his vision in primary position. Base up prism improved his head posture and it appeared that 5 prism diopters base up in both eyes would permit him to assume a normal head posture and read comfortably. His refractive error was not significant (O.D.: +1.00 +0.50 X 55, O.S.: +1.25 +0.50 X 70). Glasses were prescribed with incorporated 5 base up in both lenses.

Skull X-rays and CT scans, with particular attention directed to the posterior fossa and skull base, demonstrated no abnormality.

He returned for follow-up on 10/19/81. On casual viewing, his head was straight while wearing the glasses (Fig 7) although when intent, he would occasionally assume a slight chin down head posture. Interestingly, when he took off his glasses, he now had oscillopsia in extreme downgaze. With his glasses his vision was 20/20-2 in primary position and upgaze, 20/25-2 in downgaze. Further experimentation with base up prisms indicated that 8 prism diopters would permit normal head posturing while reading. New spectacle lenses with this amount of prism were prescribed.

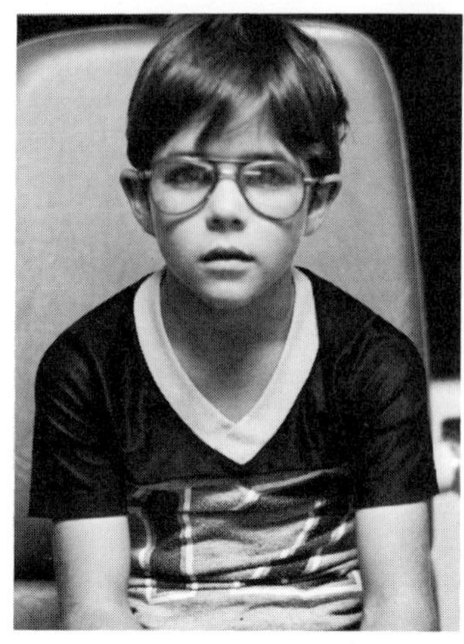

Figure 7. Patient R.B. with normal head posturing with spectacles incorporating bilateral base up prisms.

His last followup was on 8/17/82. He continues to wear his glasses constantly. He no longer has a reading problem. His athletic performance has improved tremendously. On examination, his vision remains 20/20-1 in primary position with glasses, 20/50-2 without glasses. His head posture is normal with glasses.

COMMENT

From the history provided, this child would appear to have a "congenital" form of nystagmus. On eye movement recordings, however, the slow wave configuration of his nystagmus is linear and not the increasing exponential slow wave pattern considered classical for true congenital nystagmus.25 This may be a factor as to why he responded to the base up prisms (see below).

As in other cases of asymmetric gaze nystagmus of congenital origin, this child had a "neutral zone" or "nullpoint" where the nystagmus was least pronounced. In this case, the nullpoint was in upgaze and accordingly a compensatory but anomalous chin down head posture was assumed, placing his eyes in upgaze where his vision was optimal. Indeed his vision was at its best in upgaze (20/25-2) and at its worst in downgaze (20/50-2). It is of no surprise that he had had difficulty at school with reading, for whenever he would look down to read, his vision was at its worst. Once treated with prisms, his school performance progressively improved and he is now reading at grade level. This would suggest that his nystagmus was the sole reason for his "reading disability."

Therapeutically if the nullpoint can be moved into primary position, this would eliminate the cosmetically unattractive head posturing but more importantly would maximize the vision in primary position. The first consideration when confronted with such a patient are the various prismatic and nonsurgical alternatives.26 There is some confusion however as to which is the appropriate direction to place such homologous base prisms.

At first glance, using homologous base down prisms would appear to be correct and indeed this would be the direction advised by some authors.26,27 In this patient, however, base down prisms had no effect on his chin down head posturing and actually reduced his vision in primary position.

Homologous base up prisms incorporated into spectacles eliminated the torticollis, improved his vision in primary position and over the period of a year have "cured" his reading disability. Using the technique described by von Noorden,28 homologous base down prisms would be the recommended manner in treating such a patient with a chin down head posture and null point in sursumversion. The paradoxical prism success in our patient is noteworthy.

Should such nonsurgical options prove unsuccessful or inappropriate, then surgical options may be considered which are effective in shifting nystagmus nulls toward primary position, broadening the range of the null zone and improving visual acuity.29 This child's mother has remained reluctant to consider such surgery since he continues to do well with his glasses alone.

Patient 2

Ths 5-year-old and only sibling of patient 1 was also examined on 8/17/81. His uncorrected vision was 20/30 in both eyes with linear E's. His oculomotility examination was normal with no nystagmus present and his neurological examination was normal with no ataxia or cerebellar dysfunction. There was no change present at the 8/17/82 follow-up visit.

Patient 3

The 28-year-old mother of patient 1 was also examined on 8/17/81. Her uncorrected vision was 20/20-2 O.U. and she too had normal head posturing with a normal oculomotility examination. When taken into the oblique downgaze positions, however, she developed a coarse, sustained nystagmus of a combined rotary and downbeat nature (Figure 8). In dextrodeorsumverion, she developed a combined right rotary and downbeat nystagmus, while in levodeorsumversion, a combined left rotary and downbeat nystagmus was present. In straight downgaze, no nystagmus was present. She did not report oscillopsia in these oblique downgaze positions and had been unaware that any problem existed.

On neurological assessment, there was no ataxia or evidence of cerebellar dysfunction. At her 8/17/82 follow-up, there was no change in her presentation.

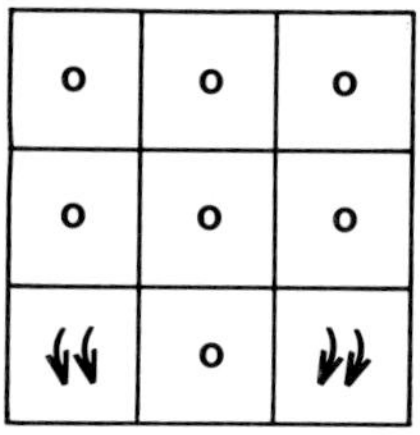

Figure 8. Pattern of nystagmus in patient P.B. Note the combined rotary-downbeat nystagmus in the oblique downgaze positions.

DISCUSSION

Vertical congenital nystagmus is unique and there are few reports available in the literature. Certainly no mention is made of a congenital downbeat nystagmus.

In 1902, William Posey described a child with nonfamilial, ideopathic vertical nystagmus, esotropia and torticollis.30 Bender and Gorman indicated that "spontaneous vertical nystagmus in direct forward gaze is (seen) almost solely in cases of congenital nystagmus"31 but mentioned no cases to substantiate this claim, nor did they differentiate between upbeat and downbeat nystagmus. In 1955, Forsythe reorted on congenital, hereditary vertical nystagmus involving five members of an Italian family over three generations.32 Clinically these cases had a pendular form of vertical nystagmus. Hoyt reported a familial form of intermittent upbeat nystagmus in a 82-year-old father and his 27-month-old son.[33] Walsh and Hoyt mention two cases of congenital vertical nystagmus[34] and cite a 1964 study by Dichgans and Kornhuber of 15 family members with a vertical congenital nystagmus of dominant inheritance.[34]

Acuired downbeat nystagmus has been clinically associated with lesions of the craniocervical junction, with platybasia or an Arnold-Chiari malformation given first diagnostic consideration. Of the approximately 130 reported cases of downbeat nystagmus in the literature to date,[1-23] 33% have been due to either platybasia or an Arnold-Chiari malformation.[2-7,11,15,17,19,20,22]

Shaw and Smith have stated that a heredofamilial form of downbeat nystagmus is the most common etiology seen in their clinical practice and is related to a familial form of spino-cerebellar degeneration.[15] Of the 38 cases of downbeat nystagmus that they reviewed, 15 (38%) were due to this etiology. Their series was skewed, however, in that half of these familial cases were from two families. It is the experience in the literature that 22% of all reported cases of acquired downbeat nystagmus have a heredofamilial form of cerebellar degeneration[12,13,15,19] which is the second most common etiology overall.

The third most common cause is an "ideopathic" variety of downbeat nystagmus,[4,7,14,15,19] constituting 17 of cases. Twenty- six percent of Shaw and Smith's more recent patient series had no apparent cause for their downbeat nystagmus.[15] When one reviews many of these patient histories,[4,7] approximately one-third have associated ataxia and/or cerebellar signs which certainly lends credence to Shaw and Smith's original contention.[15]

The remaining cases of downbeat nystagmus have been due to a large number of causes that have in common lower brainstem and/or cerebellar involvement.[1,4,10,15,16,18,19,21,22] These have been reviewed elsewhere.[18]

The case outlined in this report is the youngest in the literature to date.[1-23] In Shaw and Smith's series,[15] the youngest patient was 11 years of age but the etiology was not mentioned. In Cogan's series,[4] case #22 was a 16-year-old girl with an Arnold-Chiari malformation who had originally complained of oscillopsia at age 10. Dr. Cogan was impressed that "no children with predominantly downbeat nsytagmus were in the group" of patients that he reported.

The importance of closely checking family members in downgaze for a subclinical downbeat nystagmus has been previously stressed15 with specific reference to downbeat nystagmus due to a heredofamilial form of spinocerebellar degeneration. Affected family members may only manifest a subclinical downbeat nystagmus and not have ataxia or cerebellar dysfunction.

The mother of the reported child exemplifies this situation. She had been asymptomatic and quite unaware that any problem existed, yet manifested a constant combined rotary-downbeat nystagmus in the oblique downgaze positions. With no family history and neither the child nor the mother demonstrating any evidence of cerebellar dysfunction or ataxia, this family would appear to have an isolated form of hereditary downbeat nystagmus.

REFERENCES

1. O'Brien FH, Bender MB: Localizing value of vertical nystagmus. Arch Neuro Psych 54:378-380, 1945.

2. Cogan DG, Barrows LJ: Platybasia and the Arnold-Chiari malformation. Arch Ophthalmol 52:13-29, 1954.

3. Spillane JD, Pallis C, Jones AM: Developmental abnormalities in the region of the foramen magnum. Brain 80:11-48, 1957.

4. Cogan DG: Down-beat nystagmus. Arch ophthalmol 80:757-768, 1968.

5. Hart JCD, Sanders MD: Down beat nystagmus. Trans Ophthalmol Soc UK 90:483-490, 1970.

6. Schatz NJ: Vestibular aspects of nystagmus. Audio Dig Ophthalmol 11:1, 1973.

7. Zee DS, Friendlich AR, Robinson DA, Eng D: The mechanism of downbeat nystagmus. Arch Neurol 30:227-237, 1974.

8. Keane JR: Periodic alternating nystagmus with downward beating nystagmus. Arch Neurol 30:399-402, 1974.

9. Senelick RC, Ajax ET, van Dyk HJL: Ocular flutter and

downbeat nystagmus: A case of supratentorial origin? Neurology 24:1109-1111, 1974.

10. Shimizu N, Weinberger J, Yahr MD: Downbeat nystagmus as a sign of brainstem involvement in acute meningoencephalitis. Neurology 25:267-270, 1975.

11. Schatz NJ, Savino PJ: New Orleans Academy of Ophthalmology Symposium on neuro-ophthalmology. St. Louis: CV Mosby, 1976, pp. 87-88.

12. Zee DS, Yee RD, Cogan DG, Robinson DA, Engel WK: Ocular motor abnormalities in hereditary cerebellar ataxia. Brain 99:207-234, 1976.

13. Levin DB, Boynton JR, Smith JL: Downbeating nystagmus and hereditary cerebellar degeneration. In Smith JL (ed): Neuro-ophthalmology Update. New York: Masson, 1977, pp 337-338.

14. Doft BH, Smith JL, Ugarte TR: Inverse latent macro square wave jerks and downbeat nystagmus. In Smith LJ (ed): Neuro-ophthalmology Update. New York: Masson, 1977, pp 339-343.

15. Shaw HE, Smith JL: Downbeat nystagmus - a clinical update. In Smith JL (ed): Neuro-ophthalmology Focus 1980. New York: Masson, 1977, pp 433-436.

16. Alpert JN: Downbeat nystagmus due to anticonvulsant toxicity. Ann Neurol 4:471-473, 1978.

17. Pedersen RA, Troost BT, Abel LA, Zorub D: Intermittent downbeat nystagmus and oscillopsia reversed by suboccipital craniectomy. Neurology 30: 1239-1242, 1980.

18. Wertenbaker C, Henkind P, Keltner JL, Miller NR, Burde RM: Downbeat nystagmus. Surv Ophthalmol 25:263-269, 1981.

19. Baloh RW, Spooner JW: Downbeat nystagmus: A type of central vestibular nystagmus. Neurology 31:304-310, 1981.

20. Quencer RM: Vertical oscillopsia and blurred vision. Clin Neurol Ophthalmol 1:161-167, 1981.

21. Cox TA, Corbett JJ, Thompson HS: Upbeat nystagmus changing to downbeat nystagmus with convergence. Neurology 31:891-892, 1981.

22. Biller J, Pagano RJ: Downbeat nystagmus and pathology at cervicomedullary junction. Neurology 31:781, 1981.

23. Phadke JG, Hern JEC, Blaiklock CT: Downbeat nystagmus - a false localizing sign due to communicating hydrocephalus. J Neurol Neurosurg Psychiatry 44(5):459, 1981.

24. Smith JL: Fifty neuro-ophthalmological pearls. In Smith JL (ed): Neuro-ophthalmology Focus 1980. New York: Masson, 1979, pp 1-11.

25. Dell'Osso LF, Schmidt D, Daroff RB: Latent, manifest latent and congenital nystagmus. Arch Ophthalmol 97:1877-1885, 1979.

26. Bagolini B: Orthoptic and prismatic treatment of congenital nystagmus. In Reinecke RD (ed): Strabismus - Proceedings of the Third Meeting of the International Strabismological Association, May 10-12, 1978, Kyoto, Japan. New York: Grune & Stratton, 1978, pp 191-201.

27. Tongue AC: Childhood nystagmus. Am Orthop J 30:68-72, 1980.

28. von Noorden GK: Burian-von Noorden's Binocular Vision and Ocular Motility, 2nd ed. St. Louis: CV Mosby, 1980, pp. 416-417.

29. Dell'Osso LF, Flynn JT: Congenital nystagmus surgery A quantitative evaluation of the effects. Arch Ophthalmol 97:462-469, 1979.

30. Posey WC: Associated movements of head and eyes. JAMA 39:1365-1367, 1902.

31. Bender MB, Gorman WF: Vertical nystagmus on direct forward gaze with vertical oscillopsia. Am J Ophthalmol 32:967-972, 1949.

32. Forsythe WI: Congenital hereditary vertical nystagmus. J Neurol Neurosurg Psychiatry 18:196-198, 1955.

33. Sogg RL, Hoyt WF: Intermittent vertical nystagmus in a father and son. Arch Ophthalmol 68:515-517, 1962.

34. Walsh FB, Hoyt WF: Clinical Neuro-ophthalmology, 3rd ed. Baltimore: Williams & Wilkins, 1969, pp 279-280.

DISCUSSION BY D. GODDE-JOLLY

Dr. Bixenman has presented two cases (a mother and her 8 year old son) of apparently congenital downbeat nystagmus. Neither of them presented any sign or symptom of the more common etiologies of this condition. Four years ago, at the last Congress of the ISA, Dr. Reinecke reviewed 59 cases of downbeat nystagmus and it is noteworthy that "there were three patients who were found to have downbeat nystagmus which was alleged to have been present since infancy. Two of them (a mother and her child) were thought to have syingobulbia, but the third one was found to have the downbeat nystagmus during a routine examination and no deterioration was noted and no etiology established". Such may be the present cases.

Dr. Reinecke stressed the fact that he obtained good results in surgery in the patient who did not have an associated strabismus. So it may be asked if the best solution in such a long duration nystagmus would not be to operate in spite of the reluctance of the mother. I ask this question especially because eight glass prisms incorporated in both lenses are rather heavy; and in addition it is surprising, as the authors stressed, that base up prisms are working well in that case where the null point is in upgaze.

LATE ONSET ESOTROPIA WITH ABDUCTING NYSTAGMUS

C. Hoyt

ABSTRACT

It is now well recognized that a significant number of infants who present with a large angle esotropia demonstrate nystagmus when each eye is forced into abduction. In this paper I present 6 patients who developed a large angle esotropia with abducting nystagmus in early adulthood. These patients experienced diplopia and oscillopsia. Objective eye movement recordings in these patients do not support the use of the term "nystagmus blockage syndrome". A discussion of the possible neural mechanisms responsible for this syndrome was presented.

STRABISMUS II
ISBN 0-8089-1424-3

DISCUSSION BY D. GODDE-JOLLY

Dr. Hoyt raises an interesting question about strabismus appearing in young adults who presented previously with an abducting nystagmus. There are not many types of esotropias which may appear in adulthood. It is likely that a patho-physiological relationship exists between esotropia and nystagmus in such patients. It may well be the result of an anotomical abnormality of the opto-motor system according to Dr. Hoyt´s interesting hypothesis.

LATENT NYSTAGMUS, A DEVELOPMENTAL OCULO-MOTOR DISORDER

E. Schulz

ABSTRACT

Latent nystagmus, recorded with a high resolution technique, shows two different forms indicating a complex oculomotor disorder. This can be extended to dimensions of normal micromovements but can be distinguished from them by the characteristic temporal - nasal slow phase (drift) of the fixating eye. Latent nystagmus occurs in congenital or early childhood strabismus and non-strabismic (anisometropic) amblyopia. Binocular functions are usually absent.

Nasal-temporal optokinetic deficency in latent nystagmus is also known in cats, who were monocularly or binocularly deprived or strabismic by surgery during their sensitive period. A developmental oculomotor disorder may be considered as etiology as well.

INTRODUCTION

Latent nystagmus is a common phenomenon seen in early childhood strabismus which has been observed since the beginning of this century. The development of opinions on latent nystagmus can be summarized as follows: In 1921 Kestenbaum's observations(1) doubled the number of patients which had been described up to that time mainly by French and Dutch authors. He defined latent nystagmus as a jerk nystagmus arising on occlusion of one eye with the fast component in the direction of the uncovered (fixating) eye. He also observed a certain diminution of nystagmus in adduction, and claimed that a sharp foveal image keeps nystagmus latent and discussed a perinatal developmental anomaly as a possible cause.

In the following decades the clinical entity of latent nystagmus was denied by Sorsby in 1931(2) and propagated by Anderson in 1954.(3) The association with alternating hyperphoria was mentioned by Anderson in 1954.(3) Verhage, 1942(4) and Lang in 1967(5) and associated early childhood strabismus was stressed by Lang in 1967.(5) Adelstein and Cuppers in 1965,(6) discussed it in a rather ideological

STRABISMUS II
ISBN 0-8089-1424-3

fashion. Brain stem origin was suggested by Kornhuber in 1961(7) and van Vlieth in 1973,(8) the latter suggesting additional cortical influence. Naso-temporal defects in optokinetic nystagmus (OKN) in latent nystagmus were described by Kornhuber in 1961,(7) Doden in 1960 and Kommerell and Mehdorn in 1981,(9) through there seems to be no quantitative correlation given by Mehdorn and Kommerel in 1982(10) to nystagmus intensity. A decelerating slow phase was considered characteristic of latent nystagmus by Dell'Osso and Daroff in 1975.(11) In most cases manifest latent nystagmus was claimed to be found by high resolution techniques under binocular viewing conditions by Dell'Osso et al in 1979.(12)

However, an explanation is still lacking concerning the origin of latent nystagmus. Initially we thought there might be a key to further understanding by studying latent nystagmus using a high resolution technique and comparing it with the normal micromovement during fixation. We used a contact-lens optical lever method, which permits the identification of movements up to a few seconds or arc.

MATERIALS

We studied micromovement under varying visual conditions in 8 normal persons and found no micromovement which would fit into the criteria of latent nystagmus. If there was a certain directional preponderance of microsaccades they were always in a direction away from the leading eye. This remained constant regardless of binocular or right or left monocular viewing and regardless of direction of gaze and did not respond to binocular or monocular blue (Fig 1A, 1B). We therefore feel sure that latent nystagmus (in its definition of the fast component towards the side of the fixating eye) is different from any other form of normal micromovements under any condition.

Studying fixation movements in strabismic patients and in amblyopes we found 21 patients with latent nystagmus. Three of our findings are stressed.

1. There is latent nystagmus in the dimensions of normal micromovement which cannot be seen by any other method including funduscopy. These small movements were recorded in a 21 year old woman who had alternating convergent strabismus present since the age of 2 years, which had remained untreated until the time of examination. A slight amblyopia

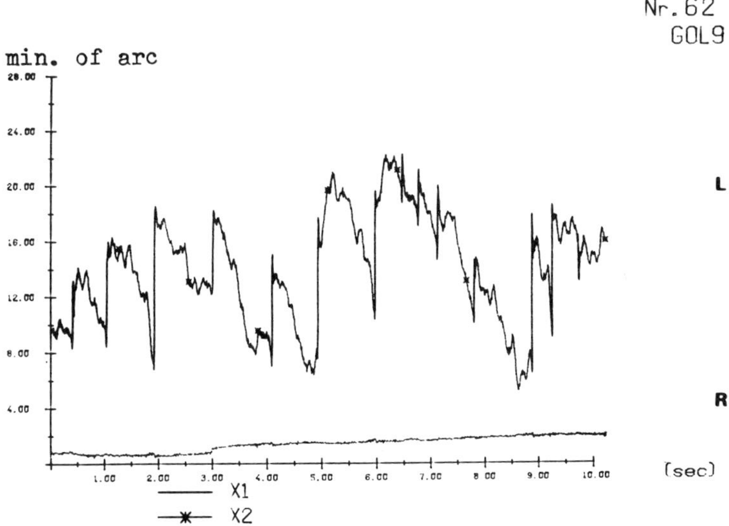

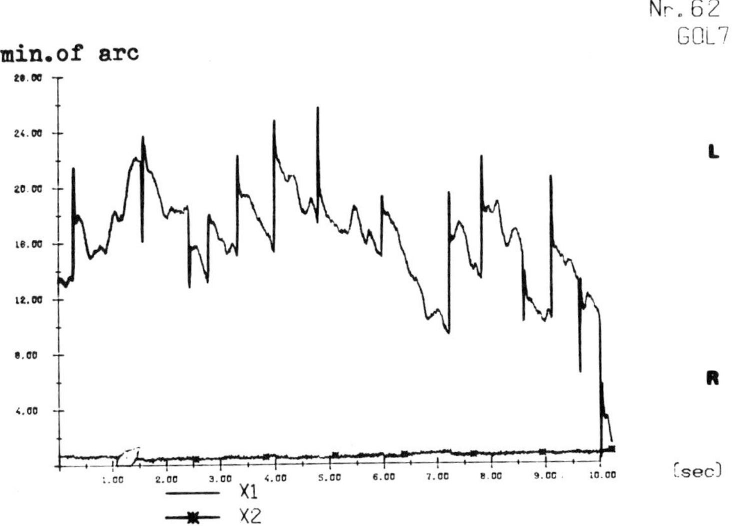

Figure 1A and 1B: Normal monocular micromovement during fixation. Right eye above, left eye below. There is a preponderance or leftward microsaccades, but no change in microsaccade direction on right or left fixation.

was present in the left eye (0.9). Monocular and binocular recordings of her eye movement during fixation showed a manifest latent nystagmus with the typical change in direction of the fast component, on alternating right or left fixation. The amplitde did not exceed 16 to 20 minutes of arc (Fig 2). It is remarkable that when her eyes were parallel postoperatively the preoperative manifest latent nystagmus became real latent nystagmus.

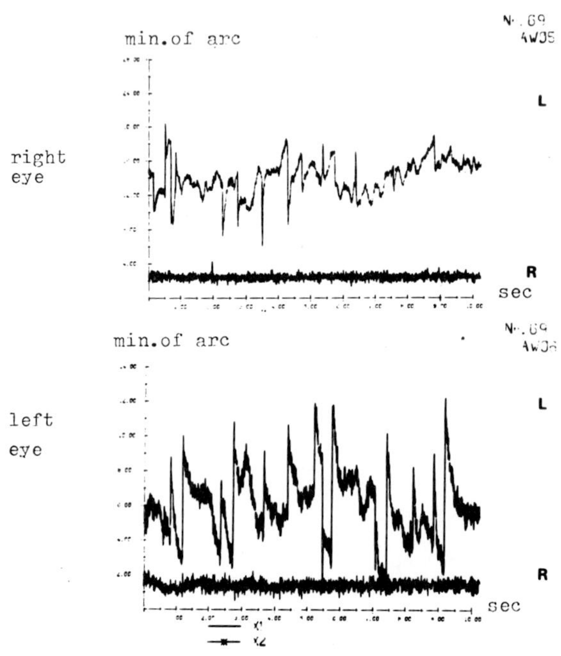

Figure 2. Latent nystagmus, slow phase wave form, which shows declerating (dec) and accelerating (ac) or both forms in one recording.

2. A 9-year-old boy who had untreated anisometropic amblyopia (0.) of the right eye (presumably from early childhood), but no strabismus, manifested latent nystagmus in his eye movement recording during fixation. This, is to our knowledge, the first case where latent nystagmus has been recorded in the absence of any strabismic deviation.

We are convinced therefore, that there is latent nystagmus in the dimensions of normal micromovement and beyond the visibility of common observation and recordings. Also that latent nystagmus can occur in the absence of strabismus and in the presence of amblyopia.

3. The third item concerns the distribution of characteristics and clinical findings: Out of our 21 patients, 6 showed real latent nystagmus, 15 manifest latent nystagmus, 9 were amblyopic, 12 were non-amblyopes. The latter group including 3 untreated patients with alternating esotropia. (In addition to our 9 amblyopes we saw 6 others in which we could not record latent nystagmus.)

In all 21 patients we found a variation of deceleration (Fig 3) and acceleration in the slow phase with increasing intensity on abduction or adduction. In 4 out of the 9 amblyopes with manifest latent nystagmus on binocular fixation there was no nystagmus but rather irregular large movements on monocular fixation with the amblyopic eye.

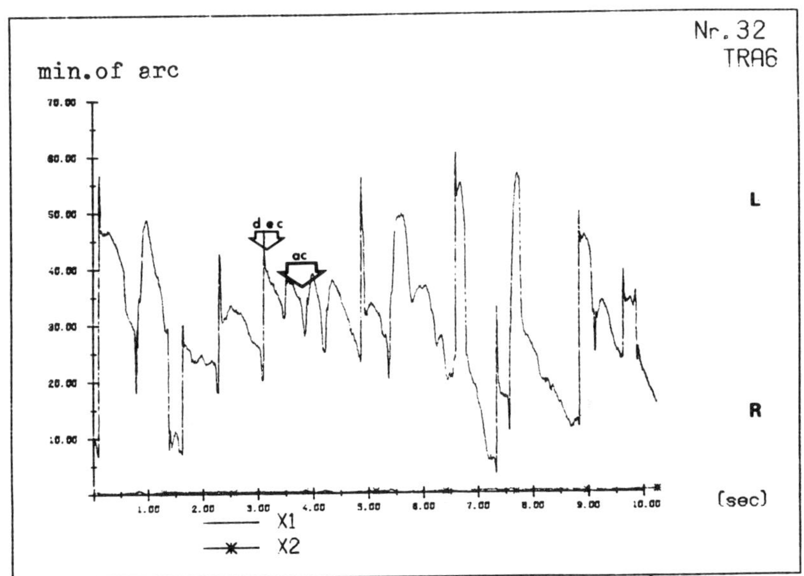

Figure 3. Latent nystagmus, slow phase wave form, which shows decelerating (dec) and accelerating (ac) or both forms in one recording.

These new findings lead to more confusion than clarification. The question is what the different forms of manifest latent nystagmus and real latent nystagmus in strabismic and nonstrabismic amblyopes and in amblyopic and non-amblyopic strabismic patients have in common. When one studies the medical history of these patients, 14 out of 21 had strabismus present at birth or within the first year of life and in 7 the strabismus lasted at least to the age of 3. In all of them an extreme deficiency of binocular vision predominates. Only 4 had a positive Bagolini test and 3 showed minimal peripheral fusion in one or more test.

From this we infer that neither amblyopia nor strabismus is the denominator for latent nystagmus but rather the deprivation of binocularity in early childhood, which to our present knowledge results in loss of binocular stimulated cells within the visual cortex. It is probably this loss of binocular cells which in experimental amblyopia leads to nasotemporal OKN defects.(13,14) These OKN deficits which also have been found in adults with cortical infarction(10) occur in latent nystagmus according to different authors.(7,9,15) Quantitative correlation to latent nystagmus intensity does not seem to exist.(10) It is remarkable that, as Nicolai in 1959(16) could show, not all amblyopic paitnets have OKN asymmetry and that our cases show the similar percentage of amblyopic patients who do not show latent nystagmus. We suggest therefore that these groups are identical and probably there is a later onset of amblyopia or a higher degree of binocularity.

SUMMARY

We believe that there is a cortical OKN related component which correlates to a deficit in early childhood binocular experience. It is highly speculative but consistent with our findings, that amblyopia or strabismus of later onset will probably not lead to an oculo-motor anomlay like latent nystagmus because of the different duration of the sensitive periods for sensory and motor disorders. There possibly is a non OKN-related component which influences the other characteristics of latent nystagmus, such as wave form, intensity and variation by innervation.

REFERENCES

1. Kestenbaum A: Latent nystagmus and fixation. Zeit f. Augenh 45:97-104, 1921.

2. Sorsby A: Latent nystagmus. Br J Ophthalmol 15:1-18, 1931.

3. Anderson JR: Latent nystagmus and alternating hyperhoria. Br J Ophthalmol 38:217-231, 1954.

4. Verhage JWC: Eine klinische Studie uber den latenten Nystagmus. Ophthalmologica 103:209-224, 1942.

5. Lang J: Der kongenitale oder fruhkindliche Strabismus. Ophthalmologica 154:201-208, 1967.

6. Adelstein F, Cuppers C: Zum Problem der echten und der scheinbaren Abducenslahmung (Das soggenannte "Blockierungssyndrom"). Buech Augenazart, 46:271-278, 1966.

7. Kornhuber HH: Uber Begleitschielen und latenten Nystagmus aus neurologischer Sicht. In Sitzungsber, Tagung Verein Rheinische-Westfalischer Augenarzte, 1960. 1961.

8. van Vliet AGM: On the central mechanism of latent nystagmus. Acta Ophthalmol 51:772-781, 1973.

9. Kommerel G, Mehdorn E: Is an optokinetic defect the cause of congenital and latent nystagmus. Vortrag Stockholm 1981.

10. Mehdorn E, Kommerell G: Uber den Zusammenhang zwischen latentem Nystagmus und symmetrischen optokinetischen Nystagmus. 80. DOG-Tagung, Munchen 19. - 22.9 (1982).

11. Dell'Osso LF, Daroff RB: Congenital nystagmus waveforms and foveation strategy. Doc Ophthalmol 39:155-182, 1975.

12. Dell'Osso LF, Schmidt D, Daroff RB: Latent, manifest latent, and congenital nystagmus. Arch Ophthalmol 97:1877-1885, 1979.

13. Hoffmann KP: Optokinetic nystagmus and single-cells responses in the nucleus tractus/opticus after early monocular deprivation in the cat. In: RD Freeman (ed) "Developmental Neurobiology of Vision", Plenum Press New York-London, 1979, pp 63-72.

14. Cynader M, Harris L: Eye movements in strabismis cats. Nature 286:64-65, 1980.

15. Doden W: Latenter Nystagmus bei Strabismus concomitans alternans. Ber Dtsch Ophthalmol 63:486-490, 1961.

16. Nicolai H: Differenzen zwischen optokinetischem Rechtsund Linksnystagmus bei einseitiger (Schiel-Amblyopie.) Klin Mbl Augenheilk 134:245-250, 1959.

DISCUSSION BY D. GODDE-JOLLY

Latent nystagmus is a puzzling condition and we must be grateful to Dr. Schulz for some new information about its pathogenesis which are founded on accurate recordings and clinical observations.

Since Keiner´s and Roelofs´ works, latent nystagmus is usually considered as the consequence of an abnormal development of the opto-motor reflexes. Dr. Schulz´s studies are leading in the same direction and support the theory Dr. Flynn developed this morning.

TORSIONAL KESTENBAUM PROCEDURE
EVOLUTION OF A SURGICAL CONCEPT

H.G. Conrad and W. de Decker

ABSTRACT

A head tilt may be or may not be the position of rest of a present nystagmus, or both tilt and nystagmus may be symptoms of a congenital strabismus syndrome. A symptomatic surgical therapy selectively cyclotorts the eyes towards the shoulder to which the head is tilted. We combine recess/resect procedures at the anterior portions of the oblique muscles with transpositions of their insertions towards the posterior/anterior pole, i.e. occipitalization/frontalization.

INTRODUCTION

The classical goal of a Kestenbaum operation is to shift the neutral zone of a nystagmus into the primary position of the eyes and consequently to make the head straight. This is clinical routine in the horizontal plane and has been done successfully also in cases with vertical head-gaze-postures. The Kestenbaum principle can also be applied to the correction of a head tilt (third or torsional plane; references see in de Decker and Conrad).1 We have already mentioned that the afflicted patients cannot be described in terms of "nystagmus and compensation" only:

a) We have seen 6 patients (9%) without strabismus who clearly tilted their heads to compensate for a congenital nystagmus beating in the horizontal or vertical or torsional plane--alone or in combination (Fig 1).

b) The majority (56) of our patients (66) showed a congenital strabismus syndrome (CIANCIA2 which ordinarily contains a head tilt to the shoulder, mainly of the dominant eye (LANG3) Table 1). This symptom is not rare but cosmetically important only in 3-5% of the patients. Within the congenital strabismus syndrome, any combination of the incomplete symptoms can be observed (Fig 2) which also means that only one-third of the sample presented with a "logical"

STRABISMUS II
ISBN 0-8089-1424-3

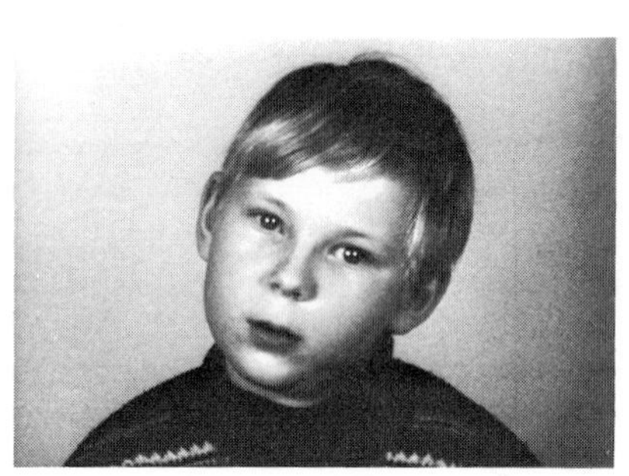

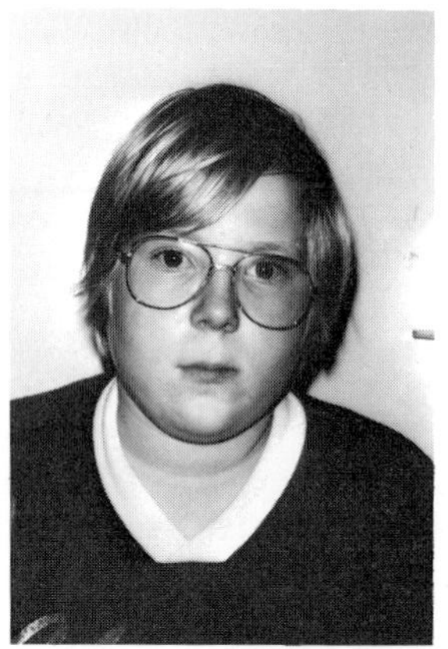

Figure 1. Left: 8-year-old boy with horizontal congenital nystagmus compensated by head tilt to the left shoulder. Right: the same patient 4 years after "torsional Kestenbaum", with small residual head tilt, and still with normal binocular vision in 9 directions of gaze.

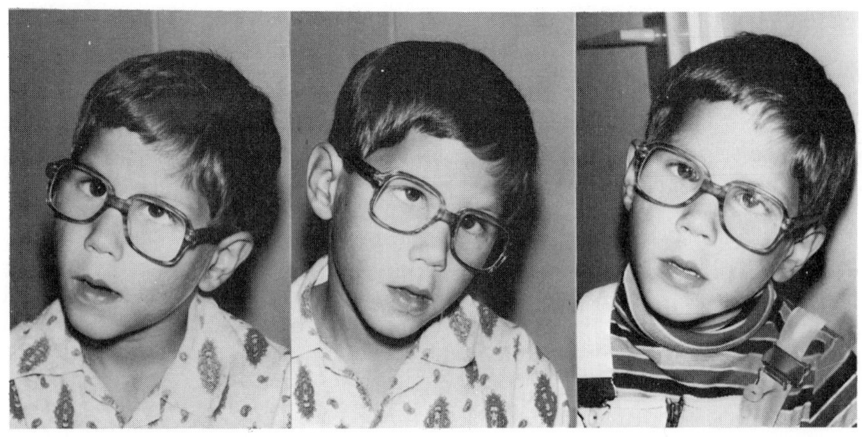

Figure 2. Left: 8-year-old boy with congenital esotropia, DVD, A-pattern, alternating face turn and head tilt but only slight "latent-type" nystagmus. Middle: same patient fixating with the other eye, while the head tilt persists. Right: persistent tilt following horizontal eye muscle surgery (bimedial Faden).

relation between the nystagmus, its beating plane, and the head tilt. One-third did not show a relevant nystagmus in any plane, 10% (6) not even a slightest degree of nystagmus (Table 2). For this reason we have used the Kestenbaum-like torsional procedure disregarding the underlying etiology and symptomatology. The idea has been simply to rotate the globes towards the side of the tilt position by shortening and lengthening the anterior parts of the oblique muscles.

Total	51	(head tilt)
	47	Strabismus
	44	Nystagmus
	26	A-V phenom.
	10	Dissoz. hypertrop.

Table 1. Evaluation of the common symptoms of the "congenital strabismus syndrome" after Ciancia and Lang. The distribution of the part symptoms herein is related to the first 51 patients.

Strabismus/Nystagmus (66 Pat.)				
Strab. conv.	56	No nystagmus	6	
		Nyst. latens	17	
		Nyst. manif.	33	
		horizontal	4	jerky
		vertical	2	jerky
		horiz. + vertical	2	jerky
		horiz. + rotat.	5	jerky
		horiz. + rotat.	10	pendular
		only rotatory	10	
		- jerky	4	
		- pendular	6	
Strab. diverg.	4	No nystagmus	1	
		Nyst. latens	3	
No strabismus	6	Nyst. latens	3	
		Nyst. manif.	3	
		partly rotatory	1	

Table 2. Distribution of different types of nystagmus in 66 patients who underwent "torsional Kestenbaum" procedures. Less than half the number showed rotatory elements of their nystagmus (26).

Surgical Concept

Our first approach had followed the principles of Harada and Ito4 and of Cuppers.5 In 1975 and 1976 we recommended an 8 mm recession and tucking of 2 or 4 oblique muscles by the anterior cyclorotating parts (today we do not operate one muscle per eye, but concentrate on the two obliques of the strictly dominant eye in patients with severe amblyopia).6-8 At that time we claimed a selective torsional efficacy without vertical side effects. Up to 19781 we could achieve better torsional results by increasing the surgical amounts to 12 and even 15 mm but had to admit vertical deviation which we compensated by recesing one superior rectus muscle. 1979 Schlossman and Muchnick9 doubted whether sufficient torsional results would be achieved by operating on the anterior fibers selectively. This argument is correct, as we had to accept an influence on the posterior fibers because we needed large amounts of surgery.

A solution of the vertical problem was found by adding a sagittal displacement as a second principle. A transposition of the whole insertion toward the anterior pole ("frontalization") or towards the posterior pole ("occipitalization") alone (Fig 3) would not give sufficient torisonal shift. But in combination with strengthening/weakening of the anterior portions we recently have obtained sufficient torsional effects without vertical side effects. Frontalization, for instance, will increase the torsional torque of the muscle but will decrease the vertical vector. This reinforces the torsional efficacy of the strengthening procedure on the anterior portion but counteracts its vertical side effect (Fig 4). Initially we missed the vertical equilibrium when adding an unnecessary advancement of the posterior fibers.

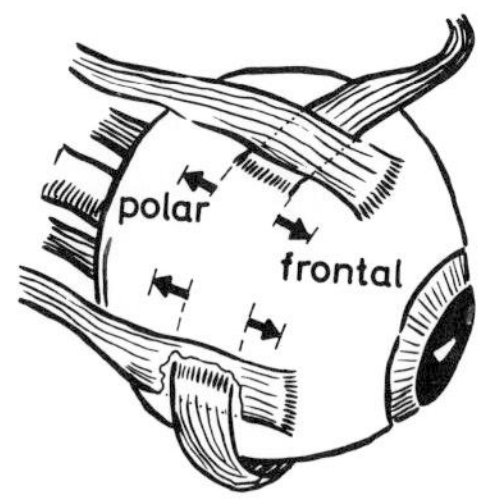

Figure 3. Principle of sagittalization, which means setting the oblique muscles more towards the posterior pole (polarization), or closer to the limbus (frontalization).

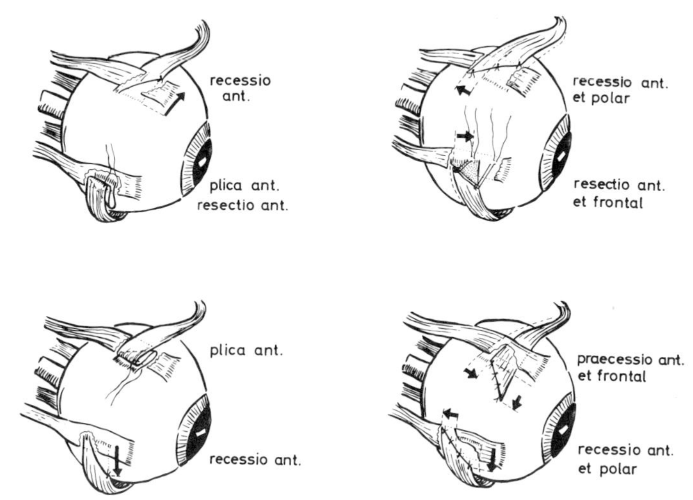

Figure 4. Extorting procedures (top) and intorting procedures (ground), without sagittal displacements (left), and with such a "sagittalization" as in Fig 3 combined with surgery on the anterior edges of the 4 obliques.

Actual Surgical Approach

Today we combine a 10-12 mm strengthening or weakening procedure on the anterior fibers with a 4 mm sagittal transposition. A full so-called torsional Kestenbaum procedure increases the torsional torque of all 4 oblique muscles. This means that in a patient who tilts his head to the right shoulder, we have to rotate the globes also towards the right (Fig 5). The two single operations on the involved superior obliques are shown in more detail (Fig 6,7). An effective variation is the split elongation at the insertion, where the anterior half is desinserted. The anterior edge of the left inferior oblique is recessed by 12 mm but "occipitalized" 6 mm instead of 4 mm. This is recommended as the posterior edge is usually too far behind for further occipitalization. The anterior fibers of the right inferior oblique are advanced rather than resected. This is less traumatic and can be done by a conjunctival approach along the upper edge of the lateral rectus. Tightening of the anterior sutures at the time of advancement normally moves the posterior parts of the muscle close to the intended place. We, therefore, only have to measure the 4 mm of "frontalization" and to attach the posterior fibers there gently. With this modification we have operated on 17 patients (Fig 8).

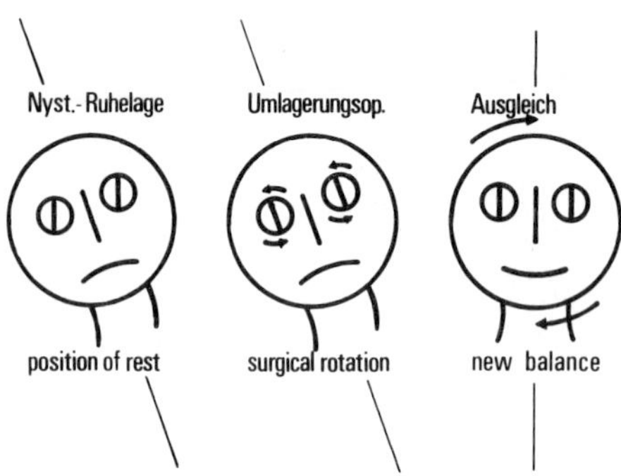

Figure 5. Eyes have to undergo a surgical torsional shift into the direction of the head tilt.

RESULTS

1) Objective torsional shift of the eyes

The average cyclotorsional effect achieved by rotating the globes has been 10-15o in primary position. A more definite evaluation does not give more clinically useful information as changes in time normally range about 5o. In addition, we must state that frequently a difference between both eyes could be observed preoperatively. A third and prevailing instability rises from gaze directions. The differences of torsional effects between adducted and abducted positions cannot yet be clearly related to the established mechanical rules which have been describing the motility since Krewson's vector-analysis.10 We have studied the distribution of the torsional components of the obliques in patients with IV nerve palsies before and after surgery. These studies (Conrad et all1) indicate that even under such basic conditions an average maximum of the torisonal effect in abduction does not exist. Further variations of the torsional measurements can be expected when we change more than one vector in patients who, suffering from a congenital strabismus syndrome, do not even completely follow Hering's Law. All these arguments, scientifically of high interest and partly unsolved, add up to the variation of about 5o. Clinically we never saw torsional diplopia induced by cyclovergence, which is important as 6 patients had normal

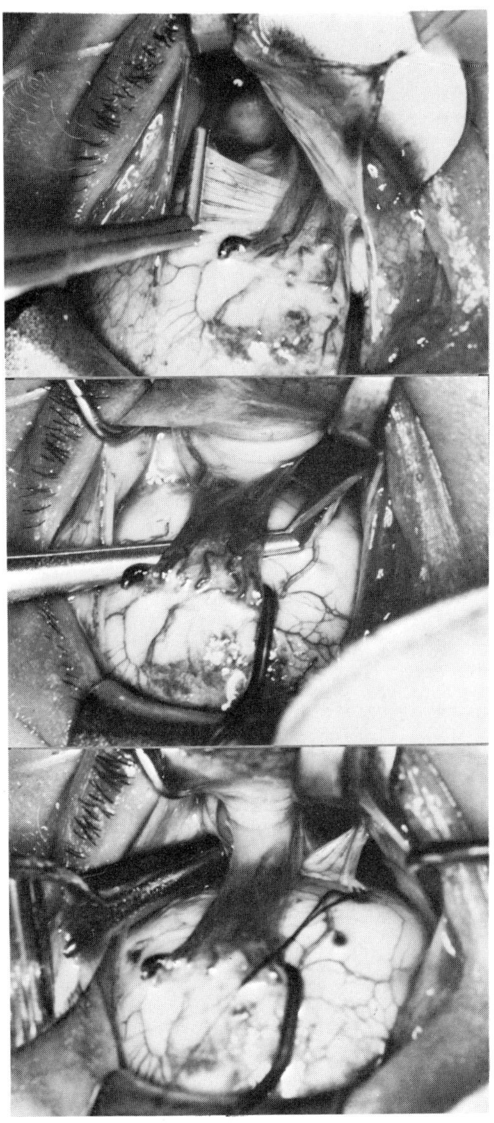

Figure 6. The right superior oblique, after hooking the superior rectus, is exposed temporally (top). The superior oblique's terminal tendon is disconnected and moved to the nasal side (middle). The anterior edge is recessed by 12 mm and "occipitalized" by 4 mm (ground). The posterior edge, guided by a forceps, becomes reattached 4 mm posteriorly, i.e., beyond the vortex vein.

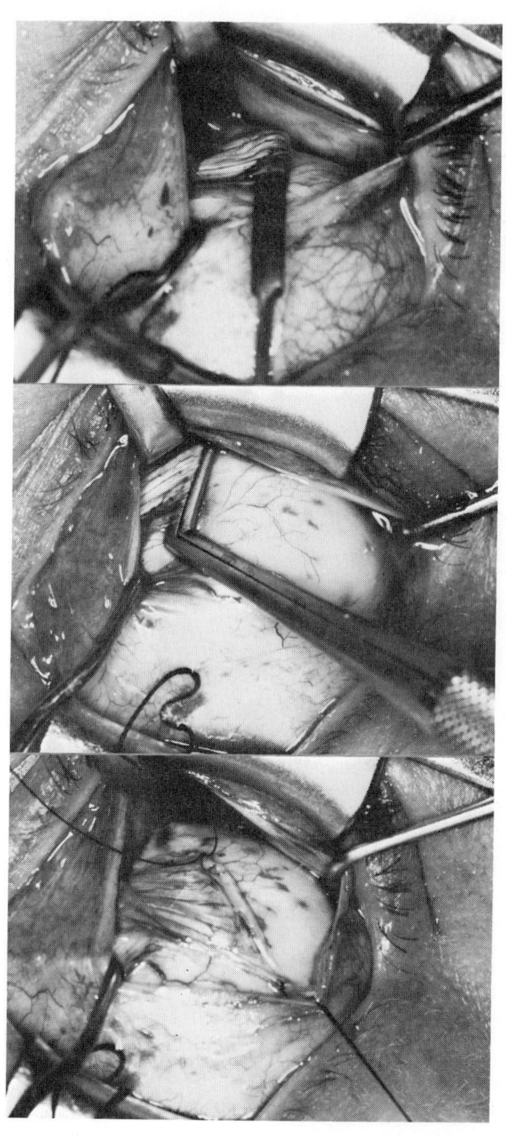

Figure 7. The tendon of the left superior oblique is found by a spatula (top) and grasped by a small clamp (Klein, Heidelberg) (middle). After disinsertion the anterior edge is advanced by 12 mm and frontalized by 4 mm, while the posterior edge is only frontalized (ground).

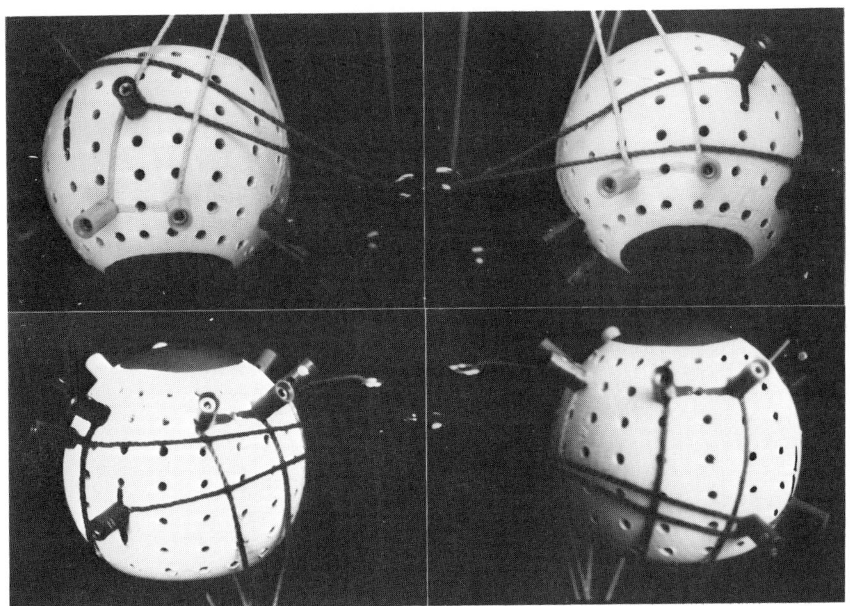

Figure 8. "Torsional Kestenbaum", shifting the globes towards the right shoulder (Ophthalmotrope). Top: Procedures on the superior obliques as in Figs 6 and 7, seen from "12 h". Ground: Procedures on the inferior obliques, seen from "6 h" (see text).

binocular vision. It is also noteworthy to say that the obtained torsional positions, with all their variations, have been stable for years.

2) Correction of the head tilt

Our patients react to the surgically induced cycloversion with quite different degrees of straightening of their heads (Fig 9). 36 (54%) show a "cure" with a residual head tilt of 0 to 5 degrees, with a tendency to tilt slightly under severe visual stress. 16 (25%) reach fair improvements with an average residual tilt of 10o. The rest (14) failed more or less, while the relatives not infrequently see some improvement under home conditions but we can confirm the unchanged tilt under examination. None was overcorrected. Fig 9 also shows that the recent technique does not give better corrections than the former one did, but the incidence of vertical side effects decreased to zero. The individual result of the operation with regard to the head tilt is not closely related to the induced cyclotorsion. Nor can we say

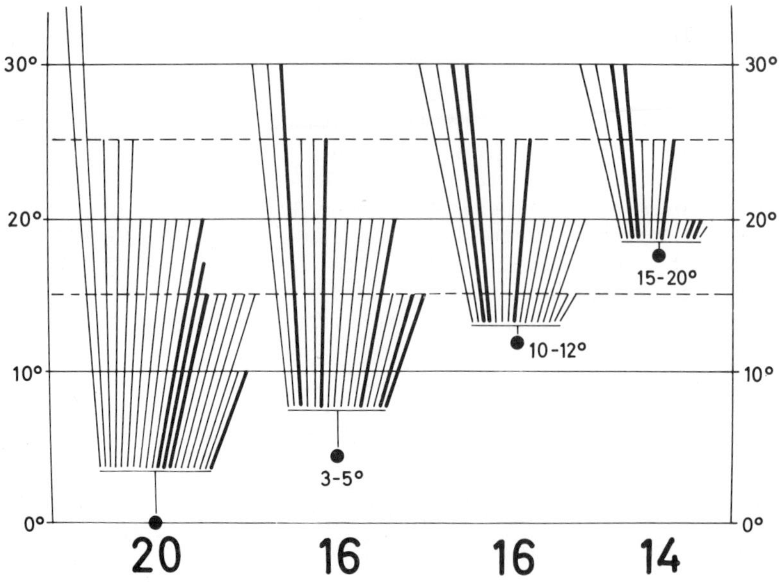

Figure 9. Results of 66 torsional Kestenbaum operations. Each vane connects the pre- and postsurgical degree of head tilt, the patients being associated to 4 success groups. Thick vanes stand for the recent, thin vanes for the former technique (see text). Please note that many cases with unsatisfactory results show still significant reductions of the tilt.

that minor degrees of original head tilt go along with better results. Surprisingly, a postsurgical sensation of inclined environment lasted--when experienced at all--only for seconds to a few hours. This is valid for cures as well as for failures, investigated with head held in any position. We have to conclude that the induced cyclotorsional shift can be compensated by two mechanisms:

a) by changing the postural balance, i.e., straightening the head b) by sensorial adaptation to inclined images.

DISCUSSION

From the natural history and the treatment of IV nerve palsies, we have learned that a sensorial adaptation to cyclo- vergence problems is not easy to reach. Much easier monocular or conjugate cyclodeviations can be overcome within weeks.12 In fact, our patients reported tilted environments only for short periods, i.e. seconds to hours. Cyclovergence problems were not reported. In this light it appears surprising that three out of four patients at least partially straightened their heads. Up to now there is no verified rule indicating which amount of aquired cyclotorsion may lead to which degree of compensatory head tilt. Even if the major part of the induced cyclodeviation should be compensated or cancelled by sensorial mechanisms, we do not have proof against the assumption that a minor resting part of the objective torsion will cause a straightening motor response.

It has been argued that the compensation of nystagmus could be triggered directly by the influence of gravity upon the statolithic mechanisms.13 If this would be valid, one should expect that the head posture would be the primary event, just followed by compensatory eye or gaze positions. We have to state that our patients with an acceptable correlation between nystagmus and head posture (those without strabismus) did not fail. The clinical evaluation shows that the neutral zone of the nystagmus comes postsurgically closer to the zero position of the head and eyes without reaching the ideal "straight" position. In those few cases the the visual acuity, too, became positively influenced by shifting the neutral zone.

Adelstein and Cuppers described horizontal and vertical gaze innervations as triggering the nystagmus.14 By the same way, they tried to understand patients who clearly reduce their nystagmus when tilting their heads. But some of our patients15 did not show the counterrotational gaze innervation of their cyclovertical muscles,16 which is dependent on gravity, i.e. statolith's inclination. In these cases we noted the lack of this "trigger" preoperatively. Nevertheless we cannot entirely rule out a postsurgical cyclotorsional gaze innervation counteracting the retinal tilt and triggering the nystagmus in the patients who have counterrotational innervation preoperatively. The complexity of the nystagmus generating system is stressed by an interesting observation: The rest of nystagmus, seemingly triggered by gravity, may be triggered by head tilt not only in the upright but also in the lying down patient--the latter behavior may even be intermittent! After all, the head tilt did reduce the nystagmus intensity only in a minority of our cases.

Thus these arguments do not concern the majority of the strabismic patients who definitely do not show a convincing connection between their head tilt and their nystagmus.

We must conclude that any attempt to bring the clinical observations--cure or failure--into a logical order in terms of "nystagmus and compensation" has failed. It does not mean a solution of the problem is impossible but gives some prospective ideas to say that there is probably a wider syndrome which includes more than strabismus, nystagmus, and head tilt. Up to now we cannot bring the facts into a convincing "hierachic" order. Our therapeutic approach is merely pragmatic.

Following the line of our surgical experience we shall try to increase the induced cyclotorsion rather by ressecting than by advancing the antagonists, i.e. the muscles to be strengthened. This would reduce the herein unwanted elasticity of the anterior, selectively rotatory fibers. On the other hand, one side effect, which we have seen in three patients, would be increased: We would have to accept restricted depressions due to Lockwood tension and, less stringent, "Brown-like-restrictions." As there is no clear interdependence between the head tilt and the other ocular symptoms, and being confronted with the limitation of the correction by the mentioned principle, we should not hesitate to try a direct approach to correct the head tilt by operating on the neck muscles. This has been done successfully in two of our patients who failed when operated on the oblique eye muscles first.

REFERENCES

1. de Decker W, Conrad HG: Rotating surgery in cases of severe head tilt. In Reinecke RD (ed): Strabismus. Proceedings of the Third Meeting of the International Strabismological Association 1978, p. 331-336.

2. Ciancia AO: La esotropia con limitation bilateral de la abduccion en el lactante. Arch Oftal B Aires 37:207-211, 1962.

3. Lang J: Der kongenitale oder fruhkindliche Strabismus. Ophthalmologica 154:201-208, 1967.

4. Harada M, Ito Y: Surgical correction of cyclotropia. Japan J Ophthalmol 8:88-96, 1964.

5. Cuppers C: Probleme der operativen Therapie des okularen Nystagmus. Klin Mbl Augenheilk 159:145-157, 1971.

6. Conrad HG: Umlagerungsoperation bei asthenopischen Beschwerden durch einseitigen Nystagmus. 131 Vers (1976) Rhein-Westf Augenarzte, p. 29.

7. de Decker W: Technische Prinzipien unserer Obliquus-Chirurgie. Proc. of the annual meeting (1976) BVA, Wiesbaden, Arbeitskreis Schielebehund lung, Weisbaden, Nov. 1976, 9,1:166, 1977.

8. Conrad HG: Umlagerungschirurgie an den Obliqui bei Komplizierten Zwangshaltungen. Proc of the annual meeting (1976) BVA, Wiesbaden, Arbeitskreis Schielbehand lung, Weisbaden, Nov. 1976, 9,1:175, 1977.

9. Schlossman A, Muchnick RS: Nystagmus blockage: classification and surgical management, in Reinecke RD (ed): Strabismus. Proceedings of the Third Meeting of the International Strabismological Association, 1978, p. 227.

10. Krewson WE: The action of the extraocular muscles. A method of vector-analysis with computations. Trans Am Ophthalmol Soc 48:443-486, 1950.

11. Conrad HG, Baranowski B, Franke C: Torsionale, vertikale, horizontale Wirkungsprofile von Obliquus-Operationen. Proc of the annual meeting (1982) BVA, Wiesbaden, Arbeitskreis Schielen. In print.

12. Guyton DL, von Noorden GK: Sensory adaptations to cyclodeviations. In Reinecke RD (ed): Strabismus. Proceedings of the Third Meeting of the International Strabismological Association, 1978, p. 399.

13. Parks MM: Surgery for nystagmus. In Hepler RS, Schatz NJ, Smith G, Lawton J, Parks MM: Nystagmus. A tape record in 1972.

14. Adelstein F, Cuppers C: Zum Problem des okular bedingten Torticollis. Bucherei des Augenarztes 46:296, 1966, Enke, Stuttgart 1977, 2nd ed.

15. Conrad HG: Rotatorische Kestenbaum-Operation. Befunde und Hypothesen. Proc of the annual meeting (1979) BVA, Wiesbaden, Arbeitskreis Schielen (reprints from the authors) 12:38, 1980.

16. Scott AB: Extraocular muscles and head tilting. Electromyografic measurement of activity of individual muscles. Arch Ophthalmol 78:397-399, 1967.

DISCUSSION BY D. GODDE-JOLLY

During the past few years the authors have improved the surgical treatment of the severe headtilt which can be associated with nystagmus. Since the headtilt often offers paradoxical peculiarities, they decided to direct their surgery directly toward the symptom of headtilt, applying the Kestenbaum operation principle to the torsional plane.

The rotation of the eyes in their previous technique was obtained by tucking the anterior fibers of one oblique muscle and recessing the anterior fibers of the antagonist oblique muscle.

If the headtilt was present with either eye fixing, the four oblique muscles had to be operated on. The results were good but a vertical side effect was sometimes observed. That is why, today, the authors brought forward an improvement which is to associate these procedures with a 4 mm transposition of the whole muscle either toward the anterior pole or toward the posterior pole, thus reducing or increasing its vertical action.

When one is familiar with the oblique muscles surgery, it is not difficult to perform a transposition of the insection toward the anterior pole but it must be difficult to do a transposition toward the posterior pole, especially in the case of the inferior oblique.

On the other hand, it may be asked if muscle surgery can lead to a perfect recovery of those severe and paradoxical headtilts which seem to be the result of a problem with the central nervous system.

ACQUIRED NYSTAGMUS IN INFANCY
A BENIGN OR THREATENING SIGN?

J. F. O'Neill, F. C. Chu, D. G. Cogan and M. K. Hammock

ABSTRACT

Acquired nystagmus and poor feeding pattern with progressive weight loss were the only presenting signs in two infants with hypothalamic astrocytomas. Tumor growth and optic nerve infiltration were significant although no other neurologic or ophthalmologic signs were present. Early CT scan may be necessary in infants with acquired nystagmus to diagnose this highly radiosensitive tumor.

INTRODUCTION

Ophthalmologists who examine great numbers of infants and young children recognize nystagmus to be an uncommon but not rare oculomotor disorder, generally benign in character. Several types of acquired infantile nystagmus are encountered with sufficient frequency and followed over long enough periods of time to be common to our experience and lull our sense of concern.

Two cases are presented of acquired nystagmus in infancy accompanied by poor feeding patterns, progressive weight loss and CT scan diagnosis of hypothalamic tumors. Nystagmus was the initial sign in each case and each presented some characteristics of spasmus nutans (head nodding, and torticollis). Both tumor masses involved the chiasm and optic nerves, consisted of low-grade astrocytoma cell type and, following biopsy and subtotal resection, were highly sensitive to radiation therapy. Optic atrophy and visual impairment occurred as part of the post-tumor/post-radiation course of each infant, although they have experienced general well-being.

Although the vast majority of cases of acquired nystagmus in the first year of life are benign, on rare occasions this oculomotor disorder, in conjunction with generalized inanition, may present as the two earliest signs of intracranial tumor. Lesions of this cell type are highly radio sensitive so that prompt diagnosis and treatment may have a good prognosis for cure.

STRABISMUS II
ISBN 0-8089-1424-3

MATERIALS

Case #1, a healthy female infant, was noted by the parents to have fine horizontal oscillations of her left eye at age six months with a similar pattern of movement beginning in the right eye one week later. The infant was the product of a full-term uncomplicated gestation, normal vaginal delivery, with a birth weight of 8 lbs. 11 oz. There are two healthy older siblings. Pediatric ophthalmologic examination confirmed the presence of an asymmetrical bilateral nystagmus described as "slow, irregular, horizontal, pendular nystagmus". Intermittent irregular head nodding movements that were not sustained were noted. No deviation of the eyes or torticollis was present. The child had good fixation and following movements of each eye, pupil responses were normal and the optic nerve heads showed no evidence of atrophy or papilledema. All growth and developmental milestones were age appropriate. A working diagnosis was acquired nystagmus, most probably spasmus nutans. Reexamination two weeks later confirmed the presence of an asymmetric slow horizontal nystagmus in this healthy seven month old infant with the additional observations of a small amplitude vertical component to the nystagmus and occasional rotary movements. Sporadic head nodding movements had been reported by the parents and were observed on only several occasions. No torticollis was observed or reported. Neuro-ophthalmologic consultation was requested.

At age eight months the infant was examined by two neuro-ophthalmologists at the National Eye Institute, noting that although the child's eyes were at times steady, a horizontal conjugate pendular nystagmus was present with a speed of 1-2 Hz and a maximum amplitude up to 5 degrees. Interspersed were episodes of smaller vertical pendular oscillations which were intermittently conjugate, disconjugate similar to "see-saw" nystagmus or monocular in such a way that one eye moved vertically while the other moved horizontally. Occasional oblique or circular oscillations were noted. Head bobbing movements were infrequent and did not appear to be correlated with the eye movements. Their opinion was that this child's nystagmus did not represent spasmus nutans because of the "relatively low frequency of the oscillations and high degree of conjugacy." They also distinguished this pattern from congenital nystagmus by its low frequency and irregular pattern. Additional history at this time was that the child had been noted to be progressively more irritable and that there was a poor eating pattern with ambivalence to nursing and formula intake, along with weight stabilization. Recommendation was made for a CT scan to be performed and for more extensive neurologic evaluation.

Several weeks elapsed during which the parents changed pediatricians to have the diet altered. At age 9 1/2 months neurologic consultation was performed at the Children's Hospital National Medical Center. This was found to be completely normal with the exception of the presence of nystagmus and a slight hypotonicity and hyperreflexia of the lower extremities. The weight stabilization by this time had become an actual weight loss, and the parents' resistance to having a CT scan accomplished was overcome at age 10 months when the scan demonstrated a large intrinsic partially cystic intracranial mass in the hypothalamic area (Fig 1).

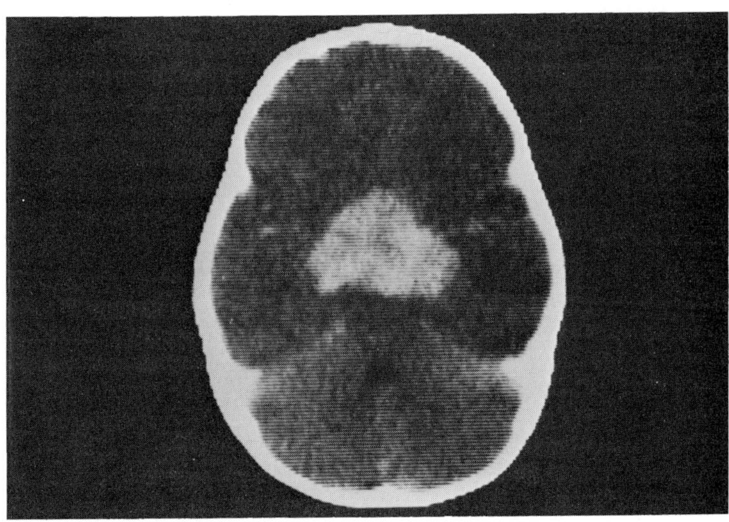

Figure 1. Case No. 1, age 10 months. Preoperative. Contrast enhanced CT scan demonstrates large midline suprasellar mass.

The following day, under general anesthesia, the neurosurgeon performed a cerebral angiogram which confirmed a suprasellar mass with elevation of both anterior cerebral arteries and stretching of both anterior choroidal arteries.

A right frontal craniotomy was performed with biopsy and subtotal resection of a hypothalamic gliomatous lesion. This consisted of a 2 cm soft encapsulated suprachiasmatic mass with infiltration into the right optic nerve. Histopathologic diagnosis was that of a low-grade astrocytoma. Radiation was started two weeks post-operatively with a total of 4500 rad administered in the related fields over a four week period.

Subsequent course over the past ten months has included one of good general health and well-being, with increased appetite, and progressive weight gain (Fig 2).

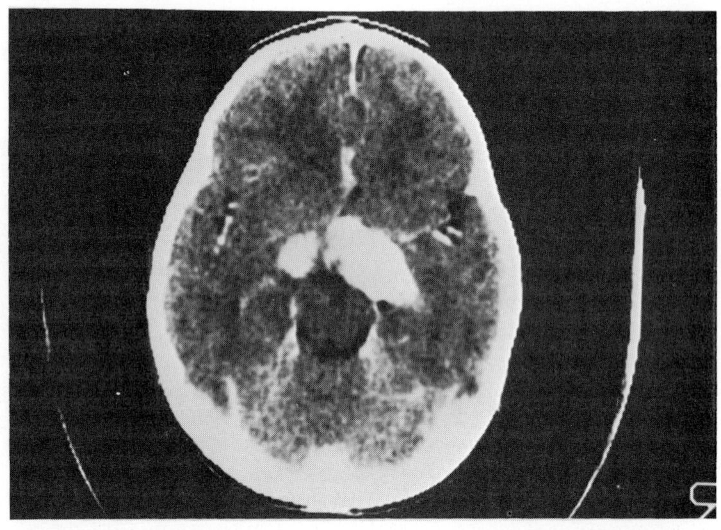

Figure 2. Case No. 1, age 20 months. Contrast enhanced CT scan. Ten months following craniotomy and radiation therapy shows shrinkage of nypothalmic glioma.

The ocular signs have been those of decreased nystagmus but a progressive course of bilateral optic atrophy, greater on the right, and increased esotropia with poor abduction of both eyes.

Case #2, a full-term black male infant with normal gestational history and vaginal delivery, had a birth weight of 7 lbs. 13 oz. The child was reported to have growth and development that were uneventful until age five months when an episode of "head turn to the right with jerky eye movements" was noted over a two week period and then subsided completely. Approximately two months later a pattern of side-to-side oscillations of both eyes was noted which persisted. At age ten months the baby was noted to not gain weight and in spite of good food intake underwent a progressive weight loss. An episode of gastroenteritis occurred and the child "began to lose ground rapidly." Concurrent examination by a pediatric neurologist was performed and a brain scan revealed a sharply demarcated uptake in the region of the third ventricle somewhat to the right of the mid-line. CT scan confirmed the tumor mass situated above the sella (Fig 3). No hydrocephalus was seen. An EEG revealed mild disorganization in the right central parietal and mid-temporal areas. The patient was admitted to the hospital with a diagnosis of gastroenteritis and diencephalic inanition syndrome of infancy.

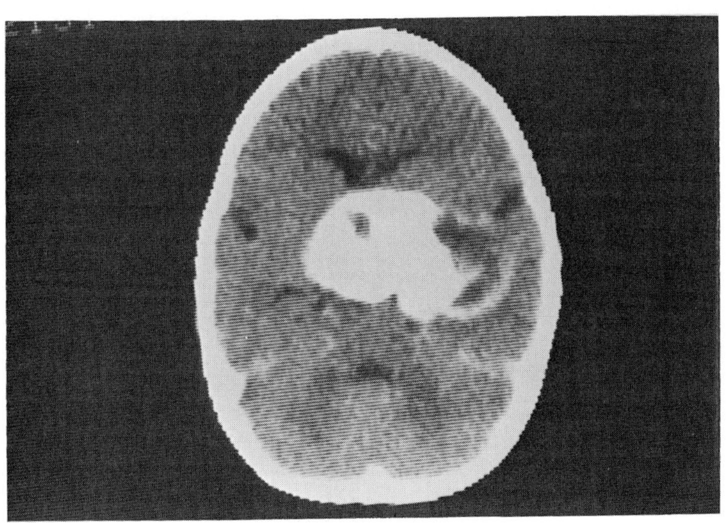

Figure 3. Case no. 2. Age 10 months. Preoperative. Contrast enchanced CT scan shows large, partially cystic suprasellar mass.

Ophthalmologic consultation noted nystagmus present only of the right eye with a slow pendular horizontal pattern of moderate amplitude. Normal fixation and following movements and equally responsive pupils were present. The fundi and optic discs were normal. An intermittent exotropia was noted with an abducted position of the right eye. Optokinetic nystagmus was equivocal. Neurosurgical examination with arteriogram was accomplished as well as a biopsy of the hypothalamic glioma with drainage of the tumor cyst. The tumor mass was noted to extend medial to the right optic nerve and to blend into both the right optic nerve posteriorly and the optic chiasm. Histopathologic diagnosis was that of a low-grade astrocytoma.

In a 3 1/2 year follow-up of this child, complete resolution of the tumor mass was noted by annual CT scan (Figs 4 & 5).

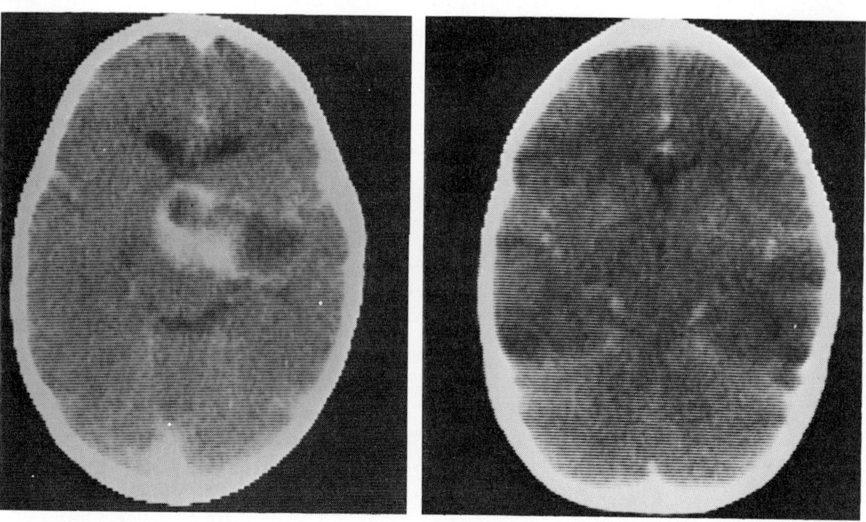

Figure 4. (left) Case No. 2. Age 1 year. Two months postoperative and one month post radiation. Contrast enhanced CT scan shows decreased size of partially cystic hypothalamic glioma.

Figure 5. (right) Case No. 2. Age 4 years. Three years postoperative and postradiation. Contrast enhanced CT scan shows reolution of tumor mass in hypothalmic area.

There has been a delayed growth pattern with chronologic age of 4 years 6 months and bone age of 3 years 6 months. Optic atrophy of the right eye has been total, with no light perception recorded, and a recession and resection of the right eye was accomplished at age two for a large angle exodeviation.

DISCUSSION

Although clinical experience in pediatric ophthalmology has strongly suggested that nystagmus beginning in the first year of life is a benign condition, several reports in recent years have cited cases in which acquired nystagmus was the earliest presenting sign of hypothalamic astrocytoma.[1-4]

In their less severe form these tumors may infiltrate the optic nerve and chiasm causing damage to the nerve fibers, optic atrophy and irrecoverable visual impairment.[5] When enlargement and extension of the hypothalamic tumor mass occurs, the diencephalic or "wasting" syndrome may result including progressive inanition, neuroendocrine disorders, hydrocephalus and death.[1,3,4,6]

Even though definitive histopathologic diagnosis was made and radiation therapy initiated by age 10 months in our two reported cases, severe optic atrophy developed in three of the four eyes. Because the predominant cell type, low-grade pilocytic astrocytoma, is highly radiosensitive, it is essential that accurate diagnosis be made and radiation therapy initiated on a timely basis to minimize damage to the anterior visual pathway and infiltration of the adjacent hypothalamic structures.

When infantile nystagmus has been observed in the past, the primary diagnostic consideration has been to differentiate one of the forms of congenital nystagmus, a constant lifetime affliction, from spasmus nutans, a transient form of asymmetric nystagmus known to have a benign, self limited course. Indeed, that distinction was the initial consideration in our first case. Following the first examination it was suggested to the parents that this form of acquired nystagmus starting at age six months, first in one eye and then the other with occasional head bobbing, might gradually diminish and disappear over the next years time. An awareness of these recent reports however, would demand that observations of acquired nystagmus in infancy include intracranial tumor as a major consideration in the process of differential diagnosis.

Many authors have addressed early onset nystagmus[7-11] with particular emphasis on the distinguishing characteristics. Spasmus nutans is generally considered to be an acquired neurophysiologic disorder of infancy, which in its complete form includes nystagmus, head bobbing and torticollis. Onset may occur any time during the first year with gradual disappearance, usually before the third year. Specific etiology has never been established but it is accepted to be a benign, self-limited condition. Norton and Cogan in their review and follow up of 20 cases of spasmus nutans cited diagnostic criteria which are most important when applied to our first case. They state that "The nystagmus is not identical in all patients and may vary in the same patient, but in general it tends (1) to be asymmetric in the two eyes, (2) to vary for different directions of gaze, and (3) to have extraordinarily fine and rapid excursions, often simulating a quiver".9 It is this last characteristic that Cogan and Chu singled out as the primary source of concern in our first patient where the nystagmus was slow (1-2 Hz) and had a broader amplitude (up to 5 degrees). That observation coupled with the relative conjugacy of the nystagmus prompted their recommendation for CT scan and more extensive neurologic evaluation.

In each of the two reported cases there are characteristics of spasmus nutans. The first case one exhibited the onset of monocular nystagmus at age 6 months followed one week later in the second eye. Although not sustained there were periods of head nodding and definite asymmetry of the oscillations between the two eyes. The second case had the initial episode start at age 5 months with a two week period of "jerky eye movements" and head turn to the right. After an interval of two months with normal eye movements the nystagmus began again and persisted until the ophthalmologic examination at the time of hospitalization when only monocular nystagmus in the right eye was noted. Surgical exploration revealed the large tumor mass to "blend imperceptibly" into the right optic nerve posteriorly. Subsequent examinations have revealed total atrophy of the right optic nerve head and no light perception in that eye.

Jayalakshmi et al reviewed 52 children with nystagmus in infancy but did not find the "character of the eye movements" to be a reliable predictor between spasmus nutans and other types of nystagmus that would have a prolonged course. Although several of their cases had other serious neurologic disorders (cerebral palsy, microcephaly, cerebral atrophy, Downs syndrome), there were no cases of intracranial tumor.12

An important factor in the diagnosis of diencephalic syndrome and the second "sign" in chronology of both of our cases is the pattern of poor feeding, and weight stabilization followed by gradual weight loss. In each case this pattern followed one to two months after the onset of sustained nystagmus. This additional history was a compelling factor to Cogan and Chu in our first case, while in case number two the child was losing weight in spite of good food intake and "began to lose ground rapidly" when a course of gastroenteritis intervened.

An important clinical question is raised by these two reported cases and the several similar cases cited with diencepthalic syndrome. Does every infant presenting with nystagmus and/or elements of spasmus nutans require a cranial CT scan and extensive neurologic evaluation?

In neither of these cases were there other localizing neurologic signs to aid in the diagnosis. Neither is careful ophthalmologic examination helpful except to note the specific characteristics of the nystagmus. Slow pendular nystagmus with medium or large amplitude is not compatible with spasmus nutans. In each of our cases preoperative fundus examination by a pediatric ophthalmologist did not identify any abnormality in the appearance of the optic nerve heads although surgical exploration revealed tumor infiltration into the posterior optic nerve and chiasm in each case. There was also a subsequent development of optic atrophy in each child.

A recent radiologic review states that cranial CT scan has become the single most effective method of evaluating gliomas of the anterior optic pathways in children whether they are confined to the intraorbital segment of the optic nerve, extend intracranially, or originate in the intracranial anterior optic pathways themselves.[13] Contrast enhanced CT scan is also an excellent method of demonstrating lesions of the hypothalamic and chiasmatic area.

Both of these cases illustrate the fact that tumor growth and invasion of the anterior optic pathways may be extensive before the development of diagnostic nerologic or ophthalmologic signs. Cranial computed tomography may be required before parents can be assured that the infant with acquired nystagmus has a benign process that may not be life threatening.

REFERENCES

1. White PT, Ross AT: Inanition syndrome in infants with anterior hypothalamic neoplasms. Neurology 13:974-981, 1963.

2. Kelly TW: Optic glioma presenting as spasmus nutans. Pediatrics 45:295-296, 1970.

3. Antony JH, Ouvrier RA, Wise G: Spasmus nutans: A mistaken identity. Arch Neurol 37:373-375, 1980.

4. Koenig SB, Naidich TP, Zaparackas Z: Optic glioma maquerading as spasmus nutans. J Pediatr Ophthalmol Strabismus 19:20-24, 1982.

5. Udvarhelyi GB, Khodadoust AA, Walsh FB: Gliomas of the optic nerve and chiasm in children: An unusual series of cases. Clin Neurosurg 13:204-237, 1965.

6. Russell A: A diencephalic syndrome of emaciation in infancy and childhood. Arch Dis Child 26:274, 1951.

7. Cox RA: Congenital head nodding and nystagmus. Report of a case. Arch Ophthalmol 15:1032-1036, 1936.

8. Osterberg G: On spasmas nutans. Acta Ophthalmol 15, part 4:451-467, 1937.

9. Norton WD, Cogan DG: Spasmus nutans: A clinical study of twenty cases followed two years or more since onset. Arch Ophthalmol 52:442-446, 1954.

10. Cogan DG: Neurology of the visual system. Springfield, Ill, Chas. C. Thomas. 1966, pp 191-194.

11. Walsh FB, Hoyt WF: Clinical Neuro-ophthalmology. Vol. 1, 3rd ed. Baltimore, Williams and Wilkins Co, 1969, pp 274-277.

12. Jayalakshmi P, Scott TF, Tucker SH: Infantile nystagmus: A prospective study of spasmus nutans, congentital nystagmus, and unclassfied nystagmus of infancy. J. Pediatr 77:177-187, 1970.

13. Savoiardo M, Harwood-Nash DC, Tadmor R, Scotti G, Musgrave MA: Gliomas of the intracranial anterior optic pathways in children. Radiology 138:601-610, 1981.

DISCUSSION BY D. GODDE-JOLLY

Dr. O'Neill's paper is of the utmost importance since one must not miss a Russel syndrome which is secondary to a hypothalamic astrocytoma. An acquired jerking nystagmus in infancy may be a problem, especially after the age of 5 or 6 months, when the etiology cannot be established. Even if there is no sign of intracrannial lesion, one has to keep in mind that it may well be the first sign of such a lesion.

The diagnosis of spasmus nutans is often unsatisfying. In the classical triad no sign is really specific. The best is certainly the high frequency nystagmus but the only assurance is the perfect recovery. It is rather a later diagnosis and the authors have well stressed the importance of the neuro-ophthlamological examination including a CT scan, which in one of their cases revealed the hypothalamic astrocytoma.

Other serious diseases may be found. The diagnosis of stasmus mutans was made in two of our cases which later turned out to be two cases of Pelizaeus Merzbacher syndrome. In neither case the nystagmus had the distinctive appearance of the "rolling eyes" and there was an abnormal head position in one of them. The optic atrophy appeared more than two years later and the pyramidal and cerebellar symptoms appeared still later.

So we can conclude that an acquired nystagmus in infancy without an established etiology must not be considered a benign condition until a complete examination has been performed and a long follow up remains negative.

COMBINATION OF ARTIFICIAL DIVERGENCE WITH KESTENBAUM OPERATION IN CASES OF TORTICOLLIS CAUSED BY NYSTAGMUS

P. Roggenkamper

ABSTRACT

For patients with anomalous head position caused by nystagmus and associated with strabismus there are two main principles of surgical treatment: the Kestenbaum/Anderson-procedure and the "artificial divergence" of Cuppers. The latter is advantageous in cases with good binocular functions, because less surgery is needed and an further improvement of visual acuity is often possible. In those cases, which are not appropriate to the surgical treatment using artificial divergence (especially because of insufficient range of fusion) we combine both principles to maintain the advantage of the artificial divergence procedure. Patients operated in this way showed good results.

INTRODUCTION

There are two different methods of treating patients with torticollis, which is not caused by a paretic squint or an orthopedic disease, but is caused by nystagmus having a null point at the anomalous head posture: One is the operation after the Kestenbaum-principle and the other uses the principle of the artificial divergence.

The Kestenbaum-principle is well-known (fig. 1a, 1b): in 1953 Kestenbaum proposed a four-muscle-surgery in case of torticollis caused by nystagmus of the sort that, postoperatively in primary position achieves the same innervational situation as preoperatively with anomalous head-posture.(1) A comparable operation was developed by Anderson, and also was published in 1953.(2)

STRABISMUS II
ISBN 0-8089-1424-3

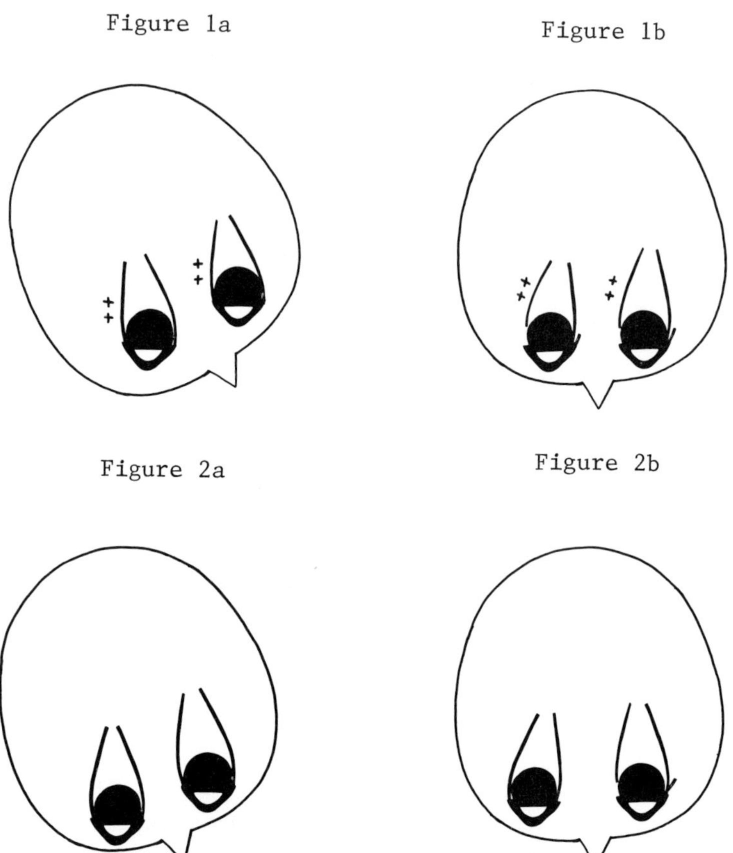
Figure 1a Figure 1b

Figure 2a Figure 2b

The principle of the artificial divergence (Fig. 2a, 2b), published by Cuppers in 1971 is based on the fact that in many nystagmus-patients with binocular functions there is less nystagmus in convergence and therefore the near visual acuity is relatively better than the distance visual acuity. Also, while fixating a near target less or no torticollis is present.(3) Such observations had been made in 1914 by laFont. The latter is based on dampening the nystagmus by increasing the innervation of the internal recti. If the fusion range is sufficient - which can be easily examined by the use of prisms base-out (if necessary for a longer time) -

one eye can be placed surgically into divergence. This should result in a greater expenditure of innervation in the convergent direction. Cuppers emphasized that his operation was indicated when the eye is in adduction when the patient demonstrates his habitual torticollis. Surgery which follows the Kestenbaum-principle would result in this eye being shifted in the same direction. For this reason also the term of "half Kestenbaum" is occassionally used, however this is confusing because Kestenbaum's principle is not used but the principle of artificial divergence which is basically different. If no anomalous head-posture is present and only improved visual acuity is sought this can be achieved by a recession of both internal recti (of course a sufficient fusional range is required) (Fig. 3).

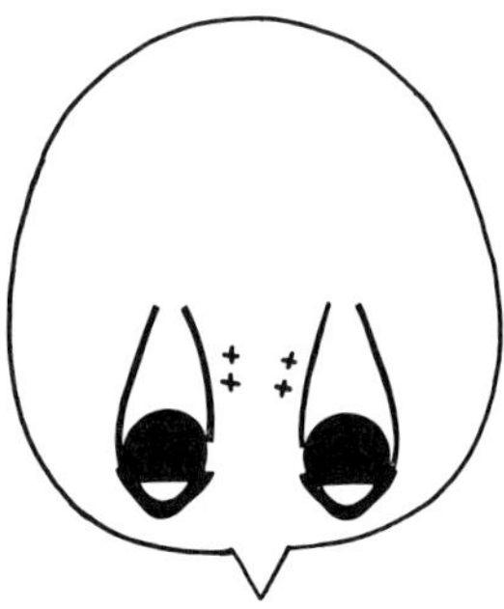

Figure 3

Strained fusion usually doe not cause asthenopic complaints in patients with congenital nystagmus who have binocular function. When the nystagmus is dampened with better visual acuity or less torticollis, our patients are more comfortable.

Over the last ten years we have applied both surgical concepts successfully. In all cases the surgery was preceded by the use of prisms to simulate the postoperative situation up to a certain amount. Before a operation Kestenbaum parallel shifting prisms base-right or base-left side are used. In the Cupper's operation, prisms in one or both sides base-out are tried. The amount of surgery accoding to Kestenbaum does not follow the amount of prisms used but the amount of the torticollis. Large prisms are not practical. We share the opinion of Kaufmann that priority should be given to the artificial divergence, because there is less surgery required, and there as opposed to the Kestenbaum's is further chance for improvement of visual acuity.(4)

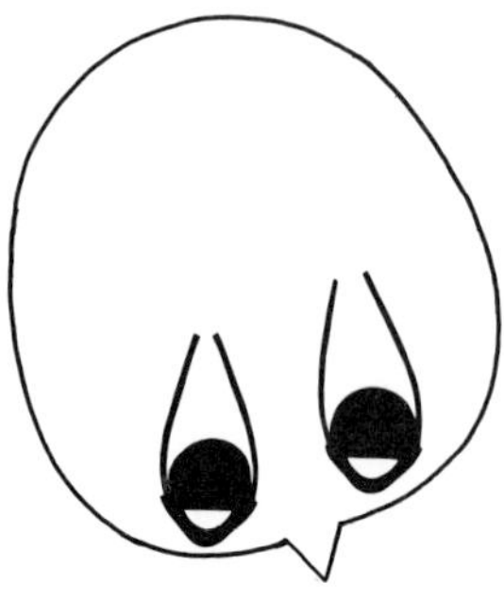

Figure 4a

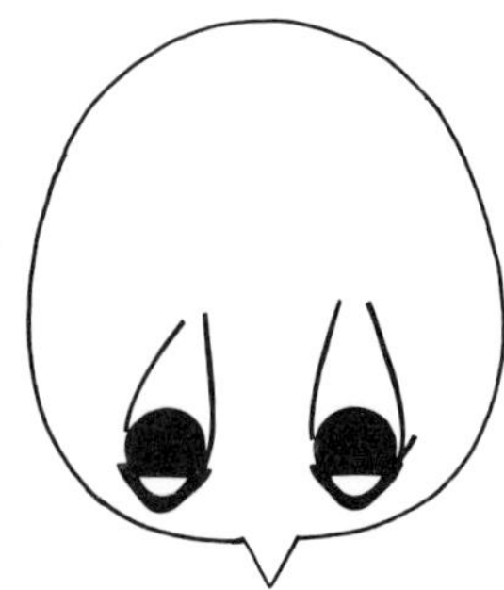

Figure 4b

Three years ago we combined the principle of Kestenbaum with that of the artificial divergence (that is in those cases in which the artificial divergence would not release the torticollis completely because of an insufficient range of fusion). Preoperatively we used prisms: both in the sense of parallel shifting, and in order to know the maximal possible artificial divergence we could create. For example, to treat an anomalous head-posture of twenty degree left head turn: The left eye would have the medial rectus recessed 4 mm, and the resection of lateral rectus 8mm, the right eye would have only recession of the lateral rectus of 4 mm (fig. 4a, 4b). Because the medial rectus of the right eye was not resected there was convergence required, which provided an additional contribution to dampening the nystagmus. That has nothing to do with the so called three-muscle-surgery which Cuppers applied in former times and Sevrin more recently in order to have left one muscle, which could be operated if needed in more exact dosage in a second procedure.(3, 5) The latter was not in order to combine the artificial divergence with the Kestenbaum's principle and Cuppers renounced this in connection the recession of the adducted medial rectus in anomalous head-posture, which would be equivalent to an artificial convergence.(6, 7)

We have operated on five patients in which the principle of artificial divergence was used where usually only the Kestenbaum procedure would have been applied. The following advantage was seen: less surgery than in the Kestenbaum's procedure was required. Thus, instead of four muscle only three were needed. In contrast to the Kestenbaum results a better visual acuity at least of far vision is to be expected (that means not only the same visual acuity in primary position postoperatively as preoperatively in abnormal head-posture, but better acuity) and because of the addition of two principles the anomalous head-posture should be influenced in a safer way over a longer time.

Postoperative follow-up of our five cases is relatively short, however all patients are without complaint, the anomalous head-posture has mostly disappeared. In one patient the postoperative visual acuity is unchanged 1.2. In case of the other four patients the visual acuity improved from one to three lines.

Editors Note: No further specific data are given.

REFERENCES

1. Kestenbaum, A.: Nouvelle Operation du nystagmus. Bull Soc Ophthalmol Fr. 6:599-602, 1953.

2. Anderson, J.R.: Causes and treatment of congenital eccentric nystagmus. Br J Ophthalmol 37:267-281, 1953.

3. Cuppers, C.: Probleme der oiperativen Therapie des ocularen Nystagmus. Klin. Monatsbl Augenheilkd 159:145-157, 1971. 145-157.

4. Kaufmann, H., Kolling, G.: Operative Therapie bei Nystagmuspatienten mit Binokularfunktionen mit und ohne Kopfzwangshaltung. Ber. Dtsch. Ophthalmol. Ges. 78:815-819, 1981.

5. Sevrin, G. and Corte, H. de: L'usage des prismes dans le nystagmus. Ann. Ocul. 203:437-443, 1970.

6. Kommerell, G.: Nystagmusoperationen zur Korrektur verschidener Kopfzwangshaltungen. Klin. Monatsbl Augenheilkd 164:172-191, 1974.

7. Muhlendyck, H.: Therapeutische Moglichkeiten bei Nystagmuspatienten mit guter Binokularfunktion und Abnahme der Nystagmusintensitat in der Nahe. Arbeitskreis Schielbehandlung, (hrsg. M. Freigang) Nurnberg, Bd. 11:133-144, 1979.

DISCUSSION BY D. GODDE-JOLLY

Dr. Roggenkamper suggests that we add the benefit of the Kestenbaum procedure with "artificial divergence" in the treatment of the horizontal head turn secondary to nystagmus. The Kestenbaum procedure will be shifting the image to the front position, while "artifical divergence" stimulates convergence. This seems reasonable. The question is to make sure that, although the binocular vision exists in 50% of nystagmus patients, the fusion range is large enough to make a void divergent strabismus after surgery.

PROGRESSIVE, EXAGGERATED A-PATTERN STRABISMUS WITH PRESUMED FIBROSIS OF EXTRAOCULAR MUSCLES

P. Fells, E. Waddell, and M. Alvares

ABSTRACT

Eight children are described who were born with unilateral or bilateral ptoses and strabismus. Two patients, personally observed from early life have had a progressive loss of vertical movements of both eyes although the condition presented unilaterally. All patients now ehibit an A-pattern of their ocular movements which was not apparent before two years of age in any patient and appeared in most cases between three and five years of age. This development of A-pattern movements implies progressive involvement of the extraocular muscles in all cases even though unequivocal worsening of vertical ocular rotations was seen in only two patients. Positive traction tests demonstrated grossly limited or absent elevation in seven cases and surgery confirmed the causative tight inferior recti.

Do these cases represent yet another sub-group of "congenital fibrosis of the extraocular muscles" which already includes at least five groups? Do they represent another form of "perverted ocular movements"? Detailed consideration of each child shows that despite certain common features with both these groups the progressive A-pattern strabismus appears to be new. Furthermore, the intriguing question arises as to how tight inferior recti can produce an A-pattern unless abnormal supranuclear innervation is invoked.

The various types of "congenital fibrosis of the extraocular muscles" are reviewed briefly and the features of this new group discussed.

INTRODUCTION

Progressive ptosis with ophthalmoplegia has been described over the past century and until 1951 was regarded as secondary to neuronal degeneration as suggested by Mobius. In 1951 Kiloh and Nevin concluded that the ocular changes were due to myopathy because of histological signs in limb and ocular muscle biopsies.1 Two separate reports in 1968 by

STRABISMUS II
ISBN 0-8089-1424-3

Rosenberg, and by Drachman presented evidence of neural disease in these patients with 'ocular myopathy' with the implication that the ophthalmoplegia could also be neurogenic in origin.[2,3] Progressive external ophthalmoplegia currently is used descriptively by many neurologists with the acknowledgement that several disease processes may have the same end result.

General fibrosis of the extraocular muscles was described in 1950 by Brown as a rare, congenital anomaly.[4] Since 1950 several ophthalmolotists have included a number of ocular conditions under the same generic heading e.g. strabismus fixus, congenital fibrosis of inferior rectus with ptosis, vertical retraction syndrome, Duane's syndrome, Mobius' syndrome, to name but a few.

We shall describe eight patients, all children, who were born with unilateral or bilateral ptoses and strabismus. All showed an A-pattern of their ocular movements after two years of age, usually appearing between age three to five years. Two patients personally observed by one of us (P.F.) from early life with unilateral ptosis showed progressive worsening of ocular rotations in both eyes.

CASE REPORTS

Case 1, a six month old girl, was seen for the left ptosis and left hypotropia and occasional left esotropia. She had been a full-term baby after a normal pregnancy and had had a left ptosis which was first attributed to birth trauma. The left eye elevated poorly. The right eye moved normally. By eleven months no elevation of the right eye could be elicited and depression was poor. The pupil reacted normally to light and near stimuli. Attempted elevation caused convergence of the eyes. Neurological examination at twenty-one months was normal apart from the eyes. Surgery was done at two and a half years for left ptosis. The traction test was positive bilaterally on attempted upward rotation of eyes. The left levator muscle was resected 15 mm.

At three years a second operation was tried to improve the left hypotropia. Traction tests for elevation were still positive. A tight left inferior rectus was biopsied and recessed 5 mm. Post-operatively the left hypotropia persisted but now a shallow A-pattern was seen. No retraction nystagmus was elicited with O.K.N. At age three the second general and neurological evaluation was normal including skull X-rays, encephalogram, Tensilon test, creatine phosphokinase, pyruvate, lactate, T4 and T.S.H. levels. The inferior rectus biopsy showed normal histochemistry and normal electromicrography compared with matched controls. By age six the best corrected acuities were right 6/9, left 6/18. The patient continues to use the left eye for reading and the right eye for distance. Neither eye elevates but both move horizontally with a marked wide-angled A-pattern.

Case 2, an eleven month boy, was seen for slight left ptosis and limited elevation of left eye which had been seen a few months after birth. He was the result of a normal pregnancy. When seen at Moorfields he was found to have left ptosis, left hypotropia and left esotropia.

Surgery at age 14 months showed limited elevation of left eye in traction test with tight inferior rectus. The inferior rectus was recessed 4 mm and the left medial rectus recessed 5 mm. Right eye traction test showed minimal limitation of ele- vation. At age 20 months, because left eye was still hypotropic, a left superior rectus resection of 4mm was performed. By age 26 months, increasing chin elevation as a compensatory posture for limited right eye elevation was seen. Full pediatric evaluation showed normal neurological examination apart from eyes.

Other data included: normal skull EMI scan, blood lactate, pyruvate and creative phosphokinase levels all normal, and negative Tensilon test.

By age five a definite A-pattern esotropia on upgaze and exotropia on downgaze could be demonstrated.

At age six a wider A-pattern with slight elevation of each eye in adduction was found but no elevation found in the abducted position. Vision OD and OS were 6/5 and 6/9.

Case 3, a 2 year old girl, was said to have had esotropia, right ptosis and limited elevation of each eye of age two months. E.U.A. at another hospital revealed resolving disc edema but she had normal E.R.G. and V.E.R. The history included a normal full term gestation. She was found to have a large compensatory posture of chin elevation and turn to right to allow right fixation. Limited elevation of right and left eyes, horizontal nystagmus of right eye, vertical and rotatory nystagmus of left eye were noted. Occlusion therapy was not tolerated.

At age 3 an operation of left medial rectus muscle

recession 5 mm and left lateral rectus muscle resection 8mm was done and the A-pattern was first seen.

She continued to use the hypotropic right eye for fixation at age 4. And by age 5 she had a chin elevation which was large. No right levator action and no Bell's phenomenon could be demonstrated.

At age 6 at operation, a strongly postitive traction tests with grossly limited elevation on the right and left, as well as some restriction to depression were found. Horizontal rotations were normal. The right inferior rectus muscle was recessed 5 mm and the right ptotic lid was moderately elevated by a silastic band, but not fully, to avoid corneal exposure.

At age 7 the right vision was only 6/36 and left vision 2/60. No reason for low right vision has been found. Fundi are normal. The child is hyperactive and will not co-operate with electrodiagnostic tests when awake. A large A-pattern with limited elevation, limited depression and slight restriction of abduction bilaterally are seen.

Case 4, a 2 year old boy, was said to have had full gestation and forceps delivery. Right ptosis and left esotropia were noted at birth. When seen at Moorfields Eye Hospital a 30o esotropia, and right ptosis were found. Right and left vision was 6/12 with glasses for myopic astigmatism. No right Bell's phenomenon could be demonstrated. Rotatory nystagmus was present.

At age 3 operation showed a positive right traction test with restricted elevation which improved a little on pressing the eyeball into the orbit. The right medial rectus was recessed 5 mm, the right inferior rectus was tight and an abnormally wide insertion was recessed 4 mm.

By age 4 an A-pattern esotropia was seen when admitted for a second operation. Strongly positive right traction test was found and exploration of already recessed right inferior rectus revealed an abnormal second head of inferior rectus 10 mm from the limbus. Its further medial than normal location had caused it to have been missed at the first operation. Both parts of the inferior rectus were recessed to 14 mm from the limbus. At age 4 1/2 improved elevation of right eye and a good Bell's phenomenon were seen.

At age 5 an operation consisting of right levator muscle

resection of 12 mm by the anterior route was done.

At age 7 the right vision was 6/9 and left vision was 6/7.5 while wearing glasses. The cosmetic appearance was satisfactory with 4 prism diopters of esotropia and right hypotropia with retraction of right eye on maximal elevation.

Case 5, a six year old girl, was said to have been born with a right ptosis. When seen at Moorfields Eye Hospital she had a right ptosis, right esotropia, and amblyopia of 2/60. Left vision was 6/9. Bilateral vertical retraction syndromes were seen with the left more than the right. There was no response to left occlusion. No right Bell's phenomenon could be elicated.

At operation age 6, a right levator resection of 16 mm was done and a positive right traction test with limited elevation was found. Postoperatively a poor response to surgery was seen. Some bilateral orbicularis oculi weakness was noted as well as an absent reight Bell's phenomenon. The left eye tended to go up and in on forced lid closure and an A-pattern was seen with a right hypotropia. No change was seen at age 7.

Case 6, a 4 year old girl, had a history of being born after induction of labour at forty-two weeks. Pregnancy had been complicated by mild pre-eclamptic toxemia but there were no neonatal problems. A right ptosis was present at birth with right esotropia and no elevation of the right eye.

Right levator resection had been done at age 3. When seen at Moorfields Eye Hospital, right esotropia, hypotropia with right ptosis, and no elevation of the right eye were seen. Attempted elevation produced right convergence. There was a slight decrease in left elevation and poor left depression. The chin was elevated. Poor abduction was noted.

At age 4 the right medial rectus was recessed and the right lateral rectus was resected.

At age 7 a right fascia lata sling for right ptosis was placed followed 6 months later by a right inferior rectus recession after a positive traction test.

At age 9 she was seen at Moorfields Eye Hospital with shallow A-Pattern going from esotropia on upgaze to exotropia on looking down. Manifest horizontal nystagmus was noted.

Absent right elevation persisted. Now only limited left elevation and left abduction were found. No right Bell's phenomenon was present. Adduction of each eye was decreased and the left eye depressed poorly.

Case 7, a 3 year girl, was seen at St. Thomas' Hospital with bilateral ptoses and internuclear palsies with exotropia. No elevation of either eye and no Bell's phenomenon could be elecited. She was the result of a normal, full-term pregnancy. At age 4 she had right and left lateral recti recessions. And subsequently had right and left ptoses operations.

At age 8 she was seen at Moorfields Eye Hospital where bilateral ptoses, no elevation right or left, marked chin elevation, and depression of the abducting eye with slight elevation of the lids on the abducting side were documented. Convergence was good with associated nystagmus. And vision was 6/6 OD and 6/18 OS. Right fixation was preferred with face turn to left. A wide A-pattern was noted.

At age 13 right and left traction tests were positive except for some slight right elevation in abduction. The right lateral rectus was tenotomized centrally as it was already fully recessed and the right medial rectus was resected 5 mm. Little change post-operatively was seen.

By age 17, marked face turn and tilt to left with chin elevation, a wide A-pattern, and slowness in reading were found.

Case 8, a one year old girl was seen at Moorfield Eye hospital with exotropia, manifest nystagmus, and ptoses. She was born of Turkish parents at full term. Divergent eyes had been seen at birth with bilateral slight ptoses. Talipes calcaneo valgus was also present at birth. Pediatric assessment had showed that she was slow to walk and generally hypotonic with normal reflexes.

Some left corneal exposure at night was suspected. She moved her head to use the left eye most of the time with an elevated chin. No upward movement could be elicited by following or doll's head movements. A wide A-pattern was noted.

At age 3, convergence with retraction was seen. Traction tests were quite normal in all directions with no restriction to elevation right or left and normal fundi were seen at examination under anesthesia.

Figure 1. Patient B. J. showing the 9 gaze positions

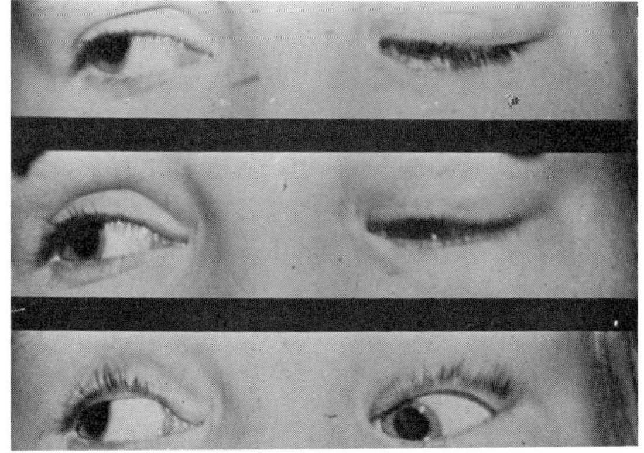

Figure 1a.
Right gaze

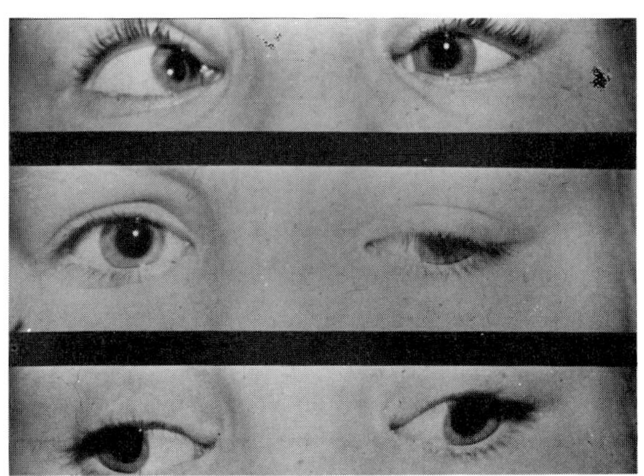

Figure 1b.
Straight ahead

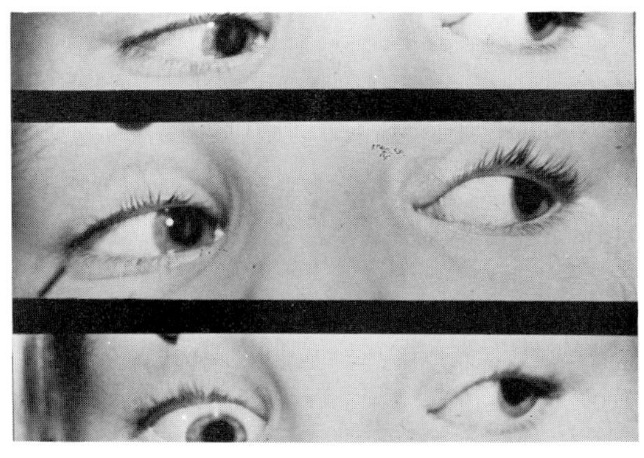

Figure 1c.
Left gaze

Note the limited total vertical excursion of the eyes

Figure 2. Patient D. C. showing the 9 gaze positions

Straight ahead

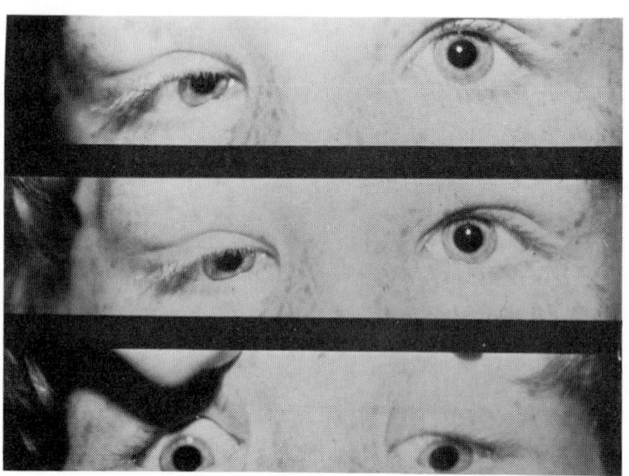

Note the limited total vertical excursion of the eyes

DISCUSSION

All eight patients were born with uni- or bi-lateral ptoses and had no elevation on the side with the ptosis and absent Bell's phenomenon. There was no family history of ptosis in any of the cases, and all patients had normal pupils and normal fundi without evidence of pigmentary retinopathy. None showed signs of associated neural disease except for the slight developmental retardation in the youngest one, Case 8, who surprisingly had normal traction tests. Cases 1 to 7 had limited elevation on the traction test and some showed limited depression on the traction tests where voluntary depression was also reduced. Five patients had manifest nystagmus and three of these showed retraction on attempted convergence. Only Case 4 had an anatomical anomaly of double insertion of the inferior rectus with a second, deeper and more posterior attachment.

These patients do not fit the classical description of progressive external ophthalmoplegia, 50% of which is familial, nor can they all be regarded as general ocular muscle fibrosis since tight inferior recti should produce V- and not A-patterns. Normal pupils and positive traction tests eliminate third nerve palsies. The associated nystagmus and convergence retraction are suggestive of midbrain involvement.5 The wide A-pattern movements, highly exaggerated in going from exotropia to esotropia over a small vertical range, must also be evidence of abnormal innervation, presumably supranuclear. The two year old Case 8, with the A-pattern but normal traction tests, may develop secondary inferior rectus contractures later.

CONCLUSION

These cases support Rowland's contention that more than one disease process may result in the syndrome of progressive external ophthalmoplegia.6 The neurogenic/myopathic controversy continues. The wide A-patterns developing two to five years after the ptoses must be due to a combination of abnormal innervation and ocular muscle fibrosis which may be primary or secondary.

REFERENCES

1. Kiloh LG, Nevin S: Progressive dystrophy of the external ocular muscles (ocular myopathy). Brain 74:115-143, 1951.

2. Drachman, DA: Ophthalmoplegia plus. The neurodegenerative disorders associated with progressive external ophthalmoplegia. Arch Neurol 18:654-674, 1968.

3. Rosenberg, RN, Schotland DL, Lovelace RE, Rowland LP: Progressive Ophthalmoplegia. Arch Neurol 19:362-376, 1968.

4. Brown, H.W. (1950). Congenital Structural Muscle Anomalies In Strabismus Ophthalmic Symposium (I) Allen J (ed): St. Louis, CV Mosby, 1950 pp 205-236.

5. Ferrer JA: General Fibrosis Syndrome in Fells P (ed): 2nd Congress of the International Strabismological Association Marseille, Diffusion Generale de Librairie, 1976.

6. Rowland, LP: Progressive External Ophthalmoplegia in Vinken, P. J. and Bryn, B. W., (eds): Handbook of Clinical Neurology, vol. 22: System disorders and atrophies, part II, chapter 8, Amsterdam, North Holland Publishing Company, 1977.

DISCUSSION BY T. MARUO

The authors observed many cases of fibrosis of extraocular muscles in detail, and frequently found A-patterns.

My only question is: Does the A-pattern result from the imperfect ocular movements in the fibrotic condition of these extraocular muscles? I believe one cause of this A-pattern is perverted convergence movements of slight degree on attempted upward gaze, which are often seen in the condition of fibrosis of extraocular muscles.

DUANE'S RETRACTION SYNDROME
CONSIDERATION ON PATHOPHYSIOLOGY AND ETIOLOGY

A. Huber

ABSTRACT

Duane's syndrome in recent years has been most frequently interpreted as the consequence of a paradoxic abnormal innervation of the affected external rectus muscle which according to electromyographic findings behaves like a muscle double innervated by a weak abducens nerve and a stronger oculomotor nerve branch or like a muscle only innervated by a oculomotor nerve branch. Histological proof of this electrophysiological concept was only given recently by the interesting observation of a case of Duane's syndrome by Neil Miller who was able to demonstrate the absence of the abducens nerve nucleus in the brainstem and at the same time the innervation of the affected external rectus by an oculomotor nerve branch.

We present the case of a young patient with unilateral Duane's syndrome and a acoustic nerve tumor on the same side. On exploration of the cerebellopontine angle, no abducens nerve (or only a thin fibrous string) could be found on the pathologic side. This important observation supports again the concept of Duane's syndrome being due to congenital aplasia of the abducens nucleus and/or nerve. It seems that always a branch of the inferior division of the oculomotor nerve steps in for this defect.

INTRODUCTION

The congenital retraction syndrome, as first described by Stilling1 (1887), Turk (1896)2 and Duane (1905)3, is characterized in its typical and most frequently observed form by abduction deficiency, globe retraction and palpebral fissure narrowing on attempted adduction, widening of the palpebral fissure on attempted abduction and normal or only slightly defective adduction. It is, however, commonly accepted that many cases of congenital retraction syndromes in one way or other do not fit into this pattern, and that there exists a whole spectrum of various types, especially

STRABISMUS II
ISBN 0-8089-1424-3

with regard to the nature of the defective horizontal movements. They all present the constant and pathognomonic features of retraction of the globe and palpebral fissure narrowing on attempted adduction. Thus following the suggestions of Lyle4 and Malbran5 we have classified the syndrome into three types.

Types of Duane's Retraction Syndrome

Duane I, By far the most frequent form, is the classical one as mentioned above: Apart from the defective abduction, the retraction of the globe and the palpebral fissure narrowing on adduction, there may sometimes be additional abnormalities like A or V phenomena, updrift or downdrift of the affected eye on adduction or attempted abduction.

Duane II: Instead of an impairment of the abduction there is a limitation or complete palsy of adduction with exotropia of the paretic eye; abduction appears to be normal or only slightly limited. There is, as in Duane I, distinct narrowing of the palpebral fissure and retraction of the globe on attempted adduction.

Duane III: This rare form of retraction syndrome is characterized by a combination of limitation or absence of both abduction and adduction of the affected eye; here abduction and adduction may be defective in the same degree (affected eye in parallel position), or adduction more defective than abduction (affected eye in divergent position). Also in Duane III there is characteristic globe retraction and palpebral fissure narrowing on attempted adduction. There is no doubt that between these three retraction syndromes patterns exist numerous transient forms of atypical symptomatology (as for instance Malbran's type of vertical retraction syndrome with limitation of elevation and depression of one eye). Most patients with Duane's syndrome demonstrate a peculiar sensory adaptation with excellent binocular function in directions of gaze where visual axes are aligned, and usually suppression without diplopia in the field of the paretic muscles; in about a third of the cases compensatory head positions are necessary for obtaining binocular single vision. Unilateral retraction syndromes are the rule; the left eye is distinctly (60%) more often involved than the right eye (20%). Bilateral involvement occurs only in about 20%. Slight female preponderance (3:2) is a fact without explanation.

PATHOPHYSIOLOGY, PATHOGENESIS

Early histopathologic studies and surgical observations led to the conclusion that Duane's syndrome was a local, purely myogenic phenomenon. Thus a generally accepted concept was that the cause of the abduction deficiency was fibrosis of the external rectus muscle and that the limitation of adduction was caused by a false posterior insertion of the internal rectus muscle[8,12,13,14,11], or by adhesions between the medial rectus muscle and the orbital wall[15].

However, electromyographic studies of recent years have shown that the explanation given by the majority of earlier authors was based on rather mechanical facts and is not a satisfactory solution to the pathogenetic problem. These investigations[15,16,17,18,19,17A,17B] first of all demonstrated, in the case of a retraction syndrome with a congenital muscle palsy, that a muscle was indeed present and it usually had a functioning, although abnormal nerve supply. Simultaneous electromyographic recording of both the internal and external recti of the affected eye revealed a paradoxical innervation of the external rectus to be the pathogenetic principle of all forms of Duane's retraction syndrome.

In Duane I the intention of abduction leads to normal reciprocal inhibition of the internal rectus, but to a quite insufficeint activity of motor units in the external rectus. Adduction of the affected eye produces normal activity of the internal rectus, whereas the external rectus shows a paradoxic activity contradicting Sherrington's Law of Reciprocal Innervation. In other words, the external rectus has its maximum of innervation on adduction, whereas there is a defective activity on abduction. The clinically observed abducens palsy explains itself by the insufficient innervation of the external rectus on attempted abduction. The co-contraction of the two normally antagonistic recti on adduction produces the retraction of the globe.

In Duane II in spite of the impaired or absent adduction the internal rectus of the affected eye manifests a normal innervation pattern in all directions (full action on attempted adduction, inhibition on abduction). But its contraction cannot become effective because it is counterbalanced by an equally strong innervation and contraction of the external rectus on adduction. Abduction

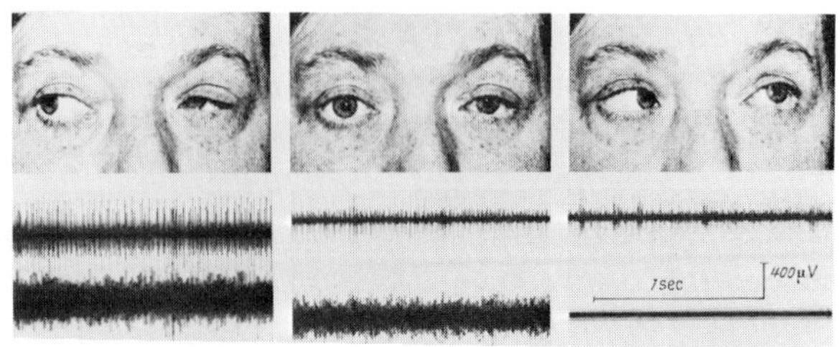

Figure 1. - Duane Syndrome I. - Limitation of abduction of the left eye, normal adduction, narrowing of the palpebral fissure and retraction of the globe on adduction. Electromyogram: Simultaneous recording of external rectus (Upper curve) and internal rectus (Lower curve) of left eye: Paradoxical innervation of the external rectus which manifests a maximum of innervation on adduction and defective innervation on attempting abduction. Normal electric behaviour of internal rectus: Maximum of innervation on adduction, complete inhibition on abduction.

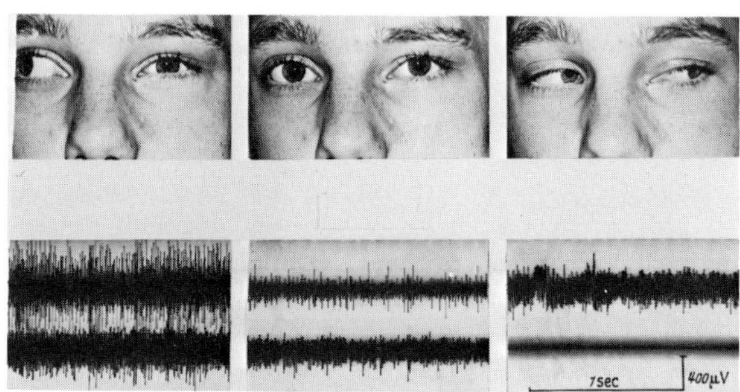

Figure 2. - Duane Syndrome II. - Complete absence of adduction, normal abduction. Narrowing of the palpebral fissure and retraction of the globe on attempting adduction. Electro- myogram: Simultaneous recording of external rectus (upper curve) and internal rectus (lower curve) of left eye: the external rectus manifests a physiological maximum of innervation on abduction and a second paradoxical maximum of innervation on attempting adduction. Normal electric behaviour of internal rectus with maximum of innervation on attempting adduction and complete inhibition on abduction.

in Duane II is possible, because the external rectus has not only a maximum of innervation on attempted adduction, but another maximum on abduction. In other terms, the external rectus muscle behaves in two ways: In a physiological way on aduction and in a paradoxic way on adduction.

In Duane III the internal rectus again manifests normal innervation on adduction and inhibition on abduction, but its contraction in adduction is again counterbalanced by an equally strong activity of the external rectus on adduction. Therefore no adduction is possible. So far Duane III repeats Duane II, but in contrast to the latter there is no abduction or at least limited abduction. The EMG gives the obvious explanation: on attempting abduction there is apart from some nystagmoid bursts, no innervation of the external rectus. Not only these few synchronous discharges on attempted abduction, but also the whole discharge pattern and discharge level of the external and internal rectus in primary position and in adduction are so similar that one is tempted to assume that the recording actually is taken from two separate eye muscles but actually takes place from two close sites of one and the same muscle (Innervated by one and the same nerve).

There are still other forms of paradoxical innervation of the external rectus to be observed20, namely: pathological co-activity of the external rectus with the superior rectus (Divergence on looking upwards); or the inferior rectus (Divergence on looking downwards); all syndromes with distinct abduction paralysis; but less pronounced retraction of the globe and palpebral fissure narrowing on adduction.

In conclusion, the Duane syndromes are characterized by a considerable variability of symptoms, however always based on the phenomenon of a anomalous innervation of the external rectus leading to a paradoxical synergistic innervation of eye muscles which are innervated by different nerves. In the beginning of our observations we ascribed the paradoxical coinnervation of the eye muscles in Duane's Syndrome to a supranuclear oculomotor defect among the connections of the medial longitudinal fasciculus. In spite of numerous associated developmental anomalies (Klippel- Feil Syndrome, ptosis, heterochromia, Horner Syndrome, nystagmus etc.) there were never any accompanying signs of a brain stem lesion in authentic cases; the supranuclear theory therefore had to be abandoned. We also discussed the possibility of a peripheral innervational anomaly in the sense of a misdirection of nerve branches during embryogenesis.

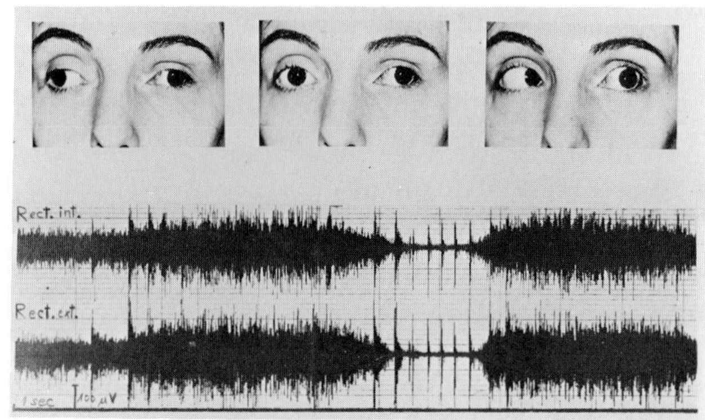

Figure 3. - Duane Syndrome III. - Complete absence of adduction and distinct limitation of abduction of left eye; exophoria of affected eye in primary position. Narrowing of palpebral fissure and retraction of globe on attempting adduction. Electromyogram: Simultaneous recording of external and internal recti of the left eye: In the primary position of right fixating eye rather intensive innervation of both recti with slight preference of external rectus (left outer part of both upper curves)- on attempting adduction (gaze to the right) intensive activation of both recti with striking similarity of discharge pattern. On abduction (gaze to the left) complete inhibition of asynchronous discharges and appearance of completely synchronous discharge (3-4 per sec.) of 30-60 m./sec. duration in both muscles. These synchronous discharges are so similar that one could assume that the recording takes place from the same muscle by two electrodes placed one not far from the other one (see details especially in both lower curves).

The extrinsic eye muscles are developed by a condensation of the mesoderm around the eye. At first (when the embryo is 7 mm long), they form one mass which is supplied by the third nerve only. Later (at embryo length of 8-12 mm) when the fourth and sixth nerve arrive, this mass divides into separate muscles.

It is conceivable that, due to an absence or aplasia of the abducens nerve, a branch of the oculomotor nerve, as a substitute, goes into that part of the muscle mass which is to become the external rectus. When first considering this pathogenetic possibility, we were not aware that such a sixth nerve anomaly had already been observed. Hoyt and Nachtigaller21,22 succeeded to find in anatomy literature about half a dozen observations of branches of the oculomotor nerve innervating the external rectus muscle, not only in cases with intact abducens nerve (in other words double innervation of the external rectus), but also in cases of aplastic or absent abducens nerve.[23,24,25,26,27]

In some other anatomic reports there are observations on anastomoses between the oculomotor and abducens nerve within the cavernous sinus or the orbit[28,29,24]. However, these were just casual observations in the anatomy theatre and unfortunately not at all related to a clinical observation of a Duane's Syndrome.

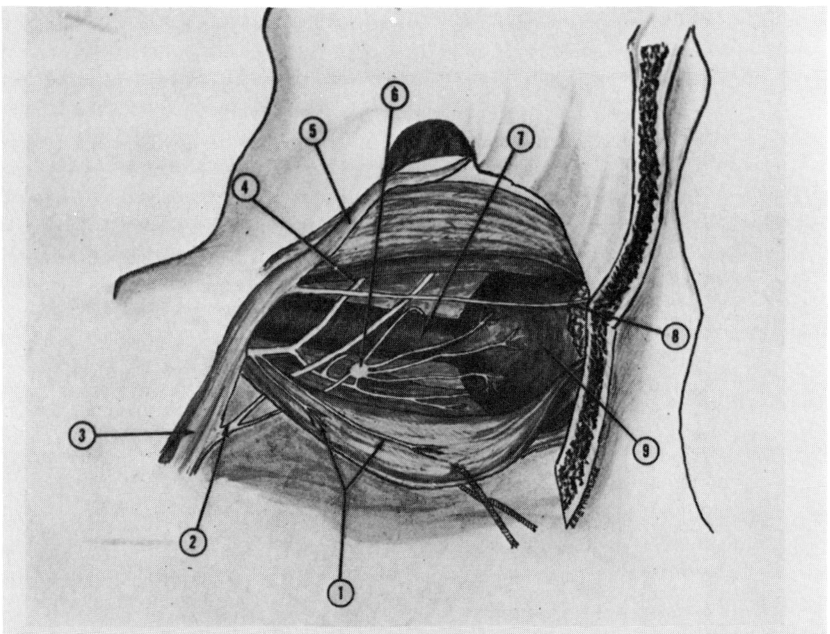

Figure 4. - Anatomical observation from literature (after Tillack,26:) Absence of right abducens nerve and substitute innervation of lateral rectus by branches of oculomotor nerve.

HISTOPATHOLOGY (Autopsy Findings)

Until recently the only reported necropsy of a patient with well documented unilateral Duane's Syndrome was that of Matteucci[30]: There was no sixth nerve on the involved side, and histopatho- logically the abducens nucleus was hypoplastic, the lateral rectus muscle was fibrotic and the medial rectus hypertrophic. Unfortunately the terminal branches of the oculomotor nerve were not examined. It is to the great merit of N. R. Miller and co-workers[31] from John Hopkins University to have found two clinically well documented cases of Duane's Syndrome, where after death complete intracranial and orbital pathological examination was possible[31, 32]. The first case was a bilateral Duane of Type III with limitation of both abduction and adduction and with retraction and palpebral fissure narrowing on attempted adduction. Postmortem examination of the brainstem and the posterior parts of the orbits revealed bilateral absence of the abducens nuclei and the abducens nerves. No large motor neurons were identified at levels normally occupied by the abducens nuclei. No intra-axial fibers referable to the sixth cranial nerve could be identified with the brainstem. Both oculomotor nuclei and nerves were normal. At the level of the ciliary ganglion, the inferior division of the oculomotor nerve bifurcated and than divided into several branches penetrating the inferior medial aspect of the lateral rectus muscle.

Just recently we were able to observe the intracranial pathology of a unilateral Duane's Syndrome during intracranial surgery. The patient with a well known congenital left abducens nerve paralysis was admitted to the neurosurgical unit of the University Hospital Zurich (Prof. G. Yasargil) with signs and symptoms of a left sided acoustic neurinoma (loss of hearing, slightly horizontal jerking gaze nystagmus, facial and trigeminal nerve intact, positive CT findings of a space occupying lesion within the cerebello-pontine angle). Clinically there was a typical Duane's Syndrome Type I on the left side with total abduction deficiency, widening of the palpebral fissure on attempted abduction and retraction as well as palpebral fissure narrowing on adduction, which was only slightly reduced in intensity. The patient had binocular single vision with a head turn of 16o to the left. After surgical exploration of the left cerebello-pontine angle (Prof. G. Yasargil) a big solid acoustic neurinoma was removed. After the extirpation of the tumor the nerve groups IX, X, XI and VII, VIII could easily be identified; however the left abducens nerves, which

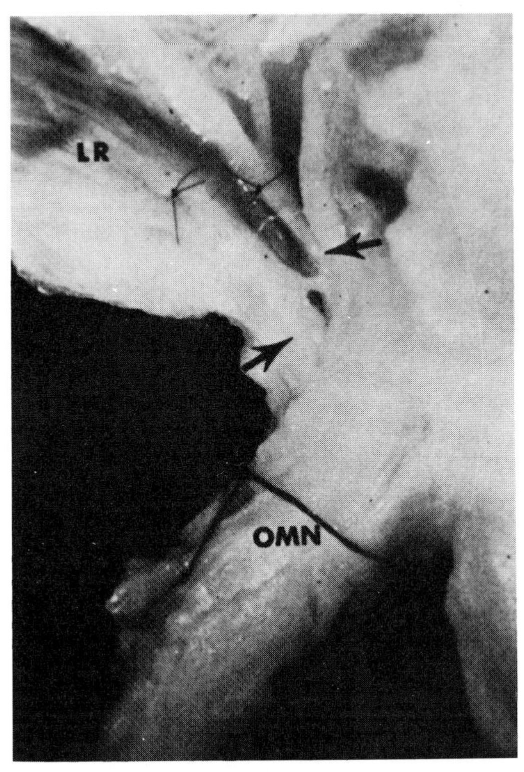

Figure 5. - Case of bilateral Duane's Syndrome (courtesy of Drs. N. Miller and Hotchkiss, John Hopkins Medical Institutions, Baltimore): Oculomotor nerve (OMN) sends several branches (marked by arrows and dark sutures) to lateral rectus muscle (LR). The region of the external rectus muscle innervated by fibers from the third nerve demonstrated healthy, well formed muscle bundles, whereas the poorly innervated muscle mass revealed distinct fibrosis. The internal rectus muscles were normal in size and structure on both sides. The second case was a clinically documented case of unilateral Duane's Syndrome with abduction deficiency, globe retraction and palpebral fissure narrowing on attempted adduction on the left side. Here the left abducens nucleus contained no cell bodies to form motor neurons, but in its rostral portion were found several small cell bodies felt to be compatible with intranuclear neurons. The left abducens nerve was absent.

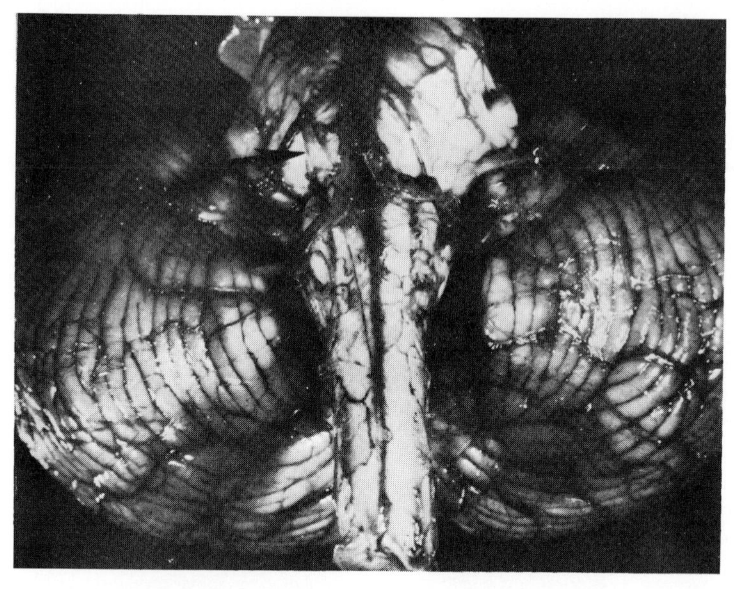

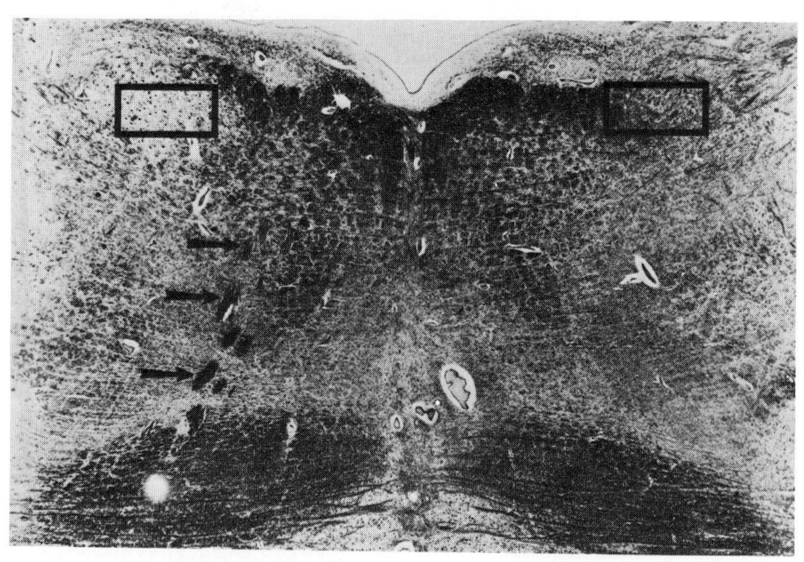

was not under a presure effect of the tumor, was difficult to find, as it consisted only of two thin atrophic fibers of 0.1 mm diameter which had separate exits (1 cm distance between them) from the dura. The further course of these atrophic abducens nerve portions towards the orbit, of course, could not be examined during surgery: The question is open, whether they actually reached, as aplastic nerves, the external rectus muscle on the left side or not.

COMMENT

From the above mentioned electromyographic data and the clinical-pathological correlations obtained from post mortem examinations and in vivo observations of clinically documented cases of Duane's Syndrome it is evident that a cranial nerve anomaly is responsible for the clinical picture of paradoxical innervation. The congenital anomaly consists of absence or aplasia of the abducens nerve and a substitute innervation of the external rectus muscle by extra branches of the oculomotor nerve (inferior division). The clinical spectrum of the different types of Duane's Syndrome results from the variability of the three innervational portions of the external rectus, namely the normal abducens innervated portion, the abnormal oculomotor innervated portion and the non-innervated fibrotic portion.

In Duane II the external rectus has a dual character: On adduction it behaves like an internal rectus innervated by the oculomotor nerve, on abduction like an external rectus innervated by the abducens nerve. Here one could assume a sort of double innervation of the external rectus in the sense that the single muscle fibers have two end-plates, one innervated via an end twig of the third nerve, the other via

Figure 6. - Case of unilateral left sided Duane's Syndrome (courtesy Dr. N. Miller et al., Wilmer Ophthalmological Institute, John Hopkins Hospital, Baltimore): Above: Ventral brainstem showing intact right abducens nerve (Dark arrow), but absence of left abducens nerve. Below: Section through pons at level of abducens nuclei: Right abducens nucleus and portions of abducens nerve fascicle are present; absence of left abducens nucleus, no portions of left abducens fascicle visible. The left external rectus muscle was partially innervated by branches from the inferior division of the oculomotor nerve. Again the poorly innervated protions of the external rectus muscle on the left side turned out to be distinctly fibrotic.

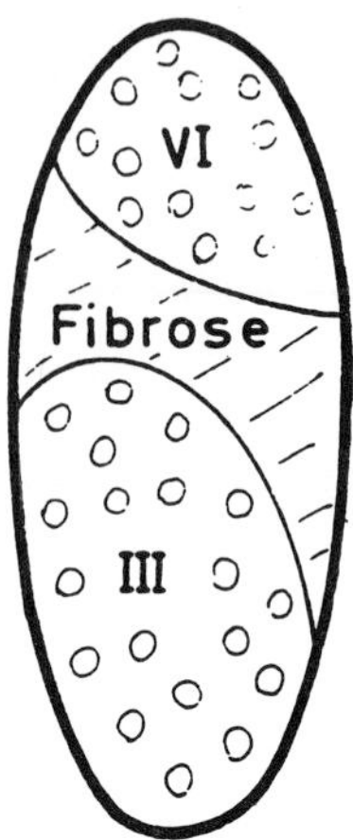

Figure 7. - Schematic cross section through lateral rectus muscle in Duane's Syndrome: The clinical spectrum of the different types of Duane's Syndrome results from the variability of the three innervational portions of the external rectus, namely the normal abducens (VI) innervated portion, the abnormal oculomotor (III) innervated portion and the non-innervated fibrotic portion. On the basis of such knowledge the clinical and electromyographic symptomatology of Duane III is the easiest to explain. The astonishing similarity of the discharge pattern of the external and internal recti can be explained perfectly by the assumption the a branch of the oculomotor nerve exclusively supplies the external rectus which does not receive any innervation from the abducens nerve because its complete absence.

an end twig of the sixth nerve. For this model of double innervation the old anatomical findings of an additional oculomotor branch of the external rectus with preservation of the sixth cranial nerve give satisfactory explanation.

Duane I finally has to be interpreted on the hypothesis of a partial double innervation of the external rectus with pronounced efficiency of fibers of the third nerve. Hereby the quantitative relation between the two type of fibers (third and sixth nerve) can vary from case to case thus explaining not only the varying degree of the abducens paresis, but also the occasional occurrence of an adduction paresis.

Paradoxical innervation of the external rectus during upward or downward gaze in Duane's syndromes with minimal retraction and palpebral fissure narrowing is a variation where the additional nerve to the external rectus is derived from the superior or inferior divisions of the oculomotor nerve, respectively.

The hypothesis that a disturbance in normal embryological development is the cause of Duane's Syndrome is further sub- stantiated by the frequent (approximately 30-50% of the patients) association with other ocular anomalies (Persistent pupillary membrane, microphthalmus, heterochromia iridis, congenital cataract, coloboma) as well as with congenital abnormalities of facial, skeletal or nerual development (Goldenhar's Syndrome, facial asymmetry, abnormal ears, Klippel-Feil anomaly, cervical spina bifida, limb anomalies, cleft palate, facial palsy, deafness, spinal miningocele and syringomyelia).33,34 The differentiation of these frequently affected structures occurs between the fourth and the eight week of gestation, coincidentally with the development of the third, fourth and sixth cranial nerve, and their contact with their respective muscles. It seems evident that a teratogenic event during the second month of gestation could cause the majority of ocular and extraocular abnormalities found in combination with Duane's syndrome. One of the consequences of such a disturbance of embryogenesis is the abnormal development of the abducens nerve and its nucleus: Therefore presumably during the second fetal month the external rectus muscle fibers await in vain innervation by abducens nerve elements and finally for their full differentiation attract branches of the oculomotor nerve although these are predisposed for other muscles. Variations in pathogenecity and timing of noxious stimuli, whether genetic or environmental, may account for the spectrum of malformations and abnormalities in ocular motility observed in the different types of Duane's Syndrome.

Unsolved remains the problem which circumstances lead to the distrubance of embryogenesis during the second month of gestation resulting in Duane's Syndrome. No significant history of maternal illness or drug ingestion during pregnancy could be obtained, at least in our own cases. However Pabst16 among 55 cases of Thalidomid embryopathy found 19 children with severe disorders of ocular motility: seven with Moebius-syndrome, five with norizontal gaze palsy, three with bilateral abducens paresis and four with typical Duane's syndrome. It could be demonstrated that ocular motility disorders including retraction syndromes occur after

Thalidomid poisoning of the embryo between the 35th and the 39th day post menstruation. There is no doubt that more detailed and more numerous gestational histories might provide additional insight into the causes of disturbed embryogenesis and thus into the etiology of Duane's retraction syndromes.

REFERENCES

1. Stilling J: Untersuchungen uber die Entstehung der Kurzsichtigkeit Wiesbaden (Germany), JF Bergmann, 1887, p. 13.

2. Turk S: Bemerkungen zu einem Falle von Retractions bewegung des Auges Zentralbl Prakt Augenheilkd. 23:14-18, 1899.

3. Duane A: Congenital deficiency of abduction, associated with impairment of adduction, retraction movements, contraction of the palpebral fissure and oblique movements of the eye. Arch Ophthalmol 34:133-159, 1905.

4. Lyle KT, Bridgeman MC: Worth and Chavasse's Squint The Binocular Reflexes and the Treatment of Strabismus. 9th ed. London, Bailliere, Tindall & Cox, 1959.

5. Malbran J: Strabismes et paralysies. Heraly, Charleroi, 1963.

6. Wolff J: The occurence of retraction movements of the eye ball together with congenital defects in the external ocular muscles. Arch Ophthalmol 29:297-309, 1900.

7. Wolff J: Ueber Retraktionsbewegungen des Augapfels bei angeborenen Defekten der aussern Augenmuskeln. Arch Augenheilkd 44:79-84, 1902.

8. Gifford H: Congenital defects of abduction and other ocular movements and their relation to birth injuries. Am J Ophthalmol 9:3-22, 1926.

9. Mayou MS: Presidential address and discussion on squint. Trans Ophthalmol Soc UK 54:3-75, 1934.

10. Spaeth EB.: Surgical aspects of defective abduction Arch Ophthalmol 49:49-62, 1953.

11. Axenfeld TH, Schurenber E: Beitrag zur Kenntnis der

angeborenen Beweglichkeitsdefekte der Augen. III. Angeborene Retractionsbewegungen. Klin. Monatsol Augenheilkd 39:851-859, 1901.

12. Apple C: Congenital abducens paralysis Am J Ophthalmol 22:169-173, 1939.

13. Bahr K: Vorstellung eines Falles von eigenartigen Muskelanomalien eines Auges Ber. dtsch. ophthal. Ges. 25:334, 1896.

14. Heuck G: Ueber angeborenen verebten Beweglichkeits-defekt der augen. Klin Monatbsl Augenheilkd 27:253-278, 1879.

15. Breinin GM: Elektromyography - A tool in ocular and neurologic diagnosis: II. Muscle palsy. Arch Ophthalmol 57:165-175, 1957.

16. Papst W: Thalidomid und knogenitale Anomalien der Augen, Ber. Dtsch Ophthalmol Ges 65:209-215, 1963.

17. Huber A, Esslen E, Kloti R, Martenet AC: Zum Problem des Duane Syndrome Albrecht von Graefes Arch Ophthalmol Arch Augenheilkd 167:169-191, 1964.

17A. Huber A: Electrophysiology of the retraction syndromes Br J Ophthalmol 58:293-300, 1974.

17B. Huber A: Duane's Retraction Syndrome. Doc Ophthalmol 26:619-628, 1969.

18. Blodi FC, Van Allen MW, Yarbrough JC: Duane's syndrome: A brain stem lesion. Arch Ophthalmol 72:171-177, 1964.

19. Scott AB, Wong GY: Duane's syndrome: An electromyographic study. Arch Ophthalmol 87:140-147, 1972.

20. Papst W, Esslen E: Zur Aetiologie der angeborenen Abduzens-lahmungen. Klin Monatsbl Augenheilkd 137:306-327, 1960.

21. Hoyt WF, Nachtigaller H: Anomalies of ocular motor nerves. Neuroanatomic correlates of paradoxical innervation in Duane's syndrome 2nd related congenital ocular motor disorders. Am J Ophthalmol 60:443-448, 1965.

22. Hoyt WF, Nachtigaller H: Zur Frage peripherer

Fehlkontakte der Augenmuskelnerven am Musculus rectus lateralis im Duane-Syndrom Klin Monatsbl Augenheilkd 146:625-628, 1965.

23. Fasebeck GF: Einige anatomische beobachtungen. Muller's Archiv Anat, Fisal Wissenschaften Med 473-476, 1842.

24. Henle J: Handbuch der Nervenlehre des Menscher in: Handbuch der Systematischen Anatomie des Menschen Braunschweig, F. Viehweg and Son, 1879, p. 384-501.

25. Generali G: Considerazioni anatomiche, fisiiologiche e patologiche intorno il nervo gran simpatico; del progessore. Annali Universali di Medicina gia compilati dal dottore Annibale Omedei, 104: Fasc. 310, 60-90, 1842.

26. Tillack TW, Winer JA: Anomaly of the abducens nerve. Yale J Biol and Med 34:620-624, 1962.

27. Bremer JL: Recurrent branches of the abducens nerve in human embryos. Amer J of Anatomy, 28:371-390, 1921.

28. Schobinger: Dissertatio de telae cellulosae dignitae Gottingae 1748, cit. by E. Svitzer.

29. Svitzer, E.: Bericht von einigen nicht haufig vorkommenden und einigen noch nicht beobachteten Variationen der Verzweigungen der Augennerven und ihrer Verbindungen miteinander. Kopenhagen, 1945.

30. Matteuci, P.: I difetti congenti di abduzione con particolare riguardo alla patogenesi Rassegna Ital Ottalmol 15:345-380, 1946.

31. Miller NR, Kiel SM, Green WR, Clark AW: Unilateral Duane's retraction syndrome (Type 1) Arch Ophthalmol 100:1468-1472, 1982.

32. Hotchkiss MD, Miller NR, Clark AW, Green WR: Bilateral Duane's retraction syndrome Arch Ophthalmol 98:870-874, 1980.

33. Paffenbach DD, Cross HE, Kearns TP: Congenital anomalies in Duane's retraction syndrome Arch Ophthalmol 88:635-639, 1972.

34. Cross HE, Paffenbach DD: Duane's retraction syndrome and associated congenital malformations. Am J Ophthalmol 73:442-450, 1972.

DISCUSSION BY T. MARUO

I thank the author heartily for explaining the pathophysiology of Duane's syndrome.

I also observed 361 cases of this disease over a 19-year period from May 1963 through April 1982, and performed EMG examinations in 143 cases of the 361.

Clinical types are not always consistent with electrical findings. This can be explained by the varying number of branches of the oculomotor nerve that go to the lateral rectus muscle. In these cases the medial rectus muscle is often seen to be taut and firmly attached to the sclera at surgery and is lacking in extensibility.

ORBITAL AND FACIAL ANTHROPOMETRY IN A AND V PATTERN STRABISMUS

M. Ruttum and G. K. von Noorden

ABSTRACT

Fifty-one patients with A or V strabismus and 109 non-strabismic age and sex-matched subjsects were anthropometrically analyzed with respect to 10 standard orbital and upper facial measurements in an attempt to evaluate the contribution of structural factors in this form of strabismus. We conclude from the data that certain orbital features may be important in the pathogenesis of A and V pattern strabismus and deserve further investigation by other means, but we do not feel that the categorization of all facial types into broad and arbitrary clases is either clinically useful or instructive regarding the etiology of this form of strabismus.

INTRODUCTION

A and V patterns occur in approximately 1/4 to 1/3 of cases of horizontal strabismus. Explanations of these phenomena of vertical incomitance have included dysfunction or anomalous insertion of extraocular muscles;(1-5) primary central nervous system abnormalities(6) (e.g., A pattern in hydrocephalus with myelomeningocele); and orbitofacial structural variations(7) (e.g. V patterns with craniofacial anomalies such as Crouzon's and Apert's syndromes).

Urrets-Zavalia(8) offered another structural hypothesis for A and V patterns in strabismic but otherwise normal children. He studied a population of Bolivian Indian children who manifested an upward, mongoloid appearing slant of the palpebral fissure due to malar hyperplasia and found 62 cases of strabismus; esotropia was associated with A pattern and inferior oblique underaction, whereas exotropia was associated with V patttern and inferior oblique overaction. Conversely, in Caucasian children in whom malar hypoplasia led to a downward slanting and antimongoloid appearance of the palpebral fissure, esotropia was seen with V pattern and exotropia with A pattern. He added, however, that not every patient with A or V pattern will display characteristic facial traits.

STRABISMUS II
ISBN 0-8089-1424-3

Von Noorden(9) found 20% of cases to go "against the rule," that is antimongoloid facies with A-esotropia and V-exotropia and mongoloid facies with V-esotropia and A-exotropia. He suggested the need for further clarification of this matter.

Helveston(10) defined mongoloid palpebral fissures as having outer canthi higher than inner canthi and vice versa for antimongoloid. He noted that both Caucasians and Orientals tend to have an upward slanting palpebral fissure, but that in Orientals this slant is deceptively high due to differences in skin folds of the upper lids. In his experience with esotropic patients, A pattern was associated with mongoloid palpebral fissures and V pattern with antimongoloid, but no such correlation was found with exotropes.

Because of curiosity about these relationships in a heterogeneous population and uncertainty about whether such external facial features can be a reflection of oblique muscle function, as suggested by Urrets-Zavalia, we undertook a prospective study of this matter.

SUBJECT AND METHODS

We examined a total of 51 A and V pattern patients without hydrocephalus, craniofacial abnormalities, or previous ocular surgery who were old enough to allow an accurate orthoptic and anthropometric evaluation. The standard criteria of at least 15 prism diopters of vertical incomitance between upgaze and downgaze of 25 degrees for V patterns and 10 prism diopters for A patterns were adhered to in this study.

The well-standardized measurements listed in the Table were selected as being representative of malar (zygomatic anatomically) and external orbital development. Palpebral fissure obliquity was measured from photographs. The rest were measured directly from the patients with standard anthropometric calipers. One hundred and nine nonstrabismic children of similar age distribution were measured to provide further comparative data.

RESULTS

We found a statistically significant difference at $p < 0.05$ between the mean palpebral fissure obliquity of A and V estropes (Table), the A esotropes having greater or more

TABLE. RESULTS OF OPHTHALMOLOGIC AND ANTHROPOMETRIC MEASUREMENTS

Pattern	Number	Mean Age (Years)	Vertical Incomitance (Prism Diopters) (±S.D.)	Palpebral Fissure Obliquity (Degrees) (±S.D.)	Inter-pupillary* Distance	Intercanthal* Distance		Width* of Face	Depth of Face*		Exophthal-mometry (millimeters)
						Lateral	Medial		Upper	Middle	
V-Esotropia	24	5.9	24(10)	4.8(3.4)	0.96	1.0	0.99	0.98	0.98	0.99	12.9
A-Esotropia	12	6.9	33(13)	7.3(2.6)	1.0	1.0	1.02	0.98	0.96	0.97	14.0
V-Exotropia	5	11.2	31(17)	4.2(3.0)	1.02	1.01	1.06	0.98	0.98	0.96	14.0
A-Exotropia	10	13.1	22(5.4)	7.2(2.4)	1.02	1.02	1.08	1.0	0.98	0.99	15.9
Normals†	109	5.8	-	7.4(2.4)	1.0	1.0	1.0	1.0	1.0	1.0	-

*Ratio of patient measurement to normal measurement for age; corrected for head circumference
†Normal data for measurements other than palpebral fissures obliquity supplemented by published standardized measurements (References 11, 12).

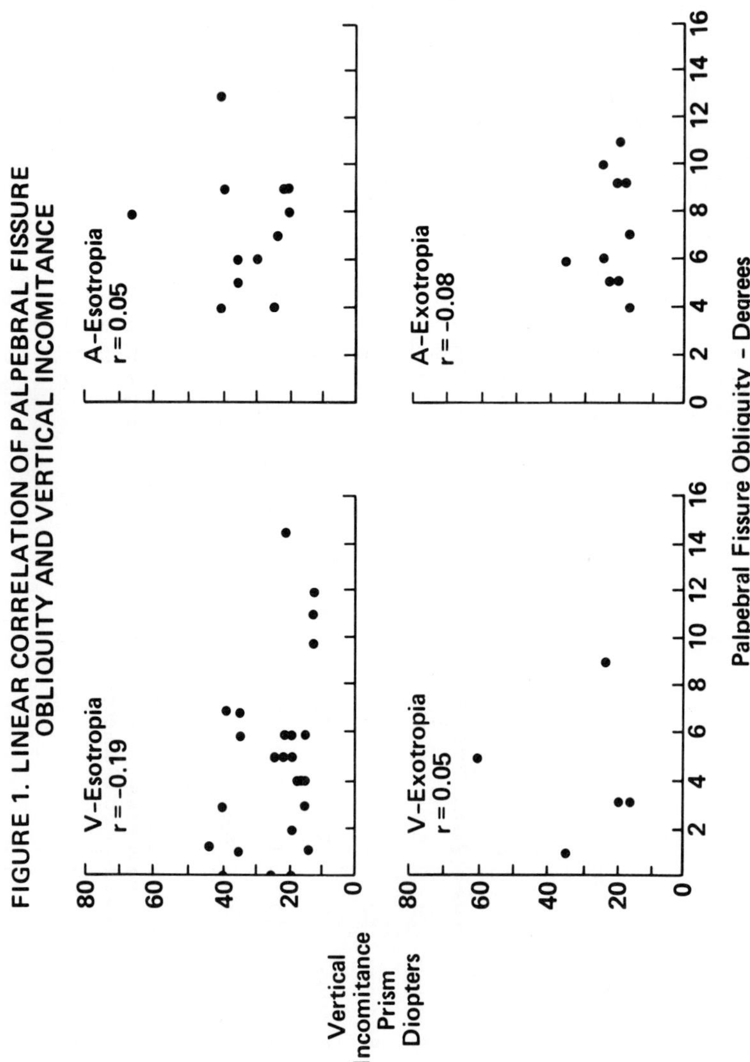

FIGURE 1. LINEAR CORRELATION OF PALPEBRAL FISSURE OBLIQUITY AND VERTICAL INCOMITANCE

"mongoloid" obliquity. For A and V exotropes the difference was not significant and indeed, showed a tendency toward the opposite of the hypothesized relationship.

Correlation coeffiecients relating the amount of vertical incomitance with the degree of palpebral fissure obliquity in each group (Figure 1) showed virtually no linear trend between the two measurement within any group.

The A and V esotropes were subdivided into those with abnormal and normal oblique muscle function (Figure 2), as defined practically by our decision to perform either oblique muscle surgery or vertical transpositions of the horizontal recti to correct the vertical incomitance. The V estropes with abnormal oblique muscle function had significantly more vertical incomitance than those with normally acting obliques, but they had the same amount of palpebral fissure obliquity. The opposite was seen among the A esotropes in whom the patients with abnormal oblique function had significantly more palpebral fissure obliquity but no difference in amount of vertical incomitance.

FIGURE 2. RELATIONSHIP OF OBLIQUE MUSCLE FUNCTION TO PALPEBRAL FISSURE OBLIQUITY AND VERTICAL INCOMITANCE IN "A" AND "V" ESOTROPES

Pattern	Oblique Muscle Function	Number of Patients	Palpebral Fissure Obliquity (Degrees)	Vertical Incomitance (Prism Diopters)
"V"	Normal	13	5.0	20*
"V"	Abnormal	11	4.5	29*
"A"	Normal	9	6.3†	32
"A"	Abnormal	3	10.3†	33

*$p < 0.05$
†$p < 0.05$

None of the other anthropmetric or ophthalmologic measurements differed significantly among the various groups.

DISCUSSION

We have demonstrated in a nonhomogeneous, largely Caucasian population that there is a small but statistically significant difference between palpebral fissure obliquity in A and V esotropes but no such relation with exotropes, thus agreeing with Helveston.(10) We did not find a linear correlation between palpebral fissure obliquity and amount of vertical incomitance or a consistent relationship between these measures and oblique muscle function. Finally, we were also unable to find anthropometric differences related to external orbital and facial development between groups.

The 2.5 degree difference in palpebral fissure obliquity between A and V esotropes is probably clinically undetectable. Furthermore, since several studies, including Helveston's and ours, have shown that nearly all eyes tend to have palpebral fissure obliquity of well above horizontal, the dividing line between facial types cannot be zero degrees, and thus it is not clear where antimongoloid obliquity ends and mongoloid begins. To then attempt to relate these facial types to particular esotropic patterns seems to be arbitrary. It would be folly to speculate on how such a small difference in one measurement could be related to mucular and orbital factors responsible for each pattern.

The frequent association of V pattern in cases of facial and orbital dysgenesis, however, leads one to the conclusion that orbitofacial structural factors do function interdependently with ocular alignment, though many other factors are undoubtedly involved as well.

REFERENCES

1. Urist MJ: Horizontal squint with secondary vertical deviations. Arch Ophthalmol 46:245-267, 1951.

2. Brown HW: Vertical Deviations. In symposium, Strabismus, Trans Am Acad Ophthalmol Otolaryngol 57:157-162, 1953.

3. Jampolsky A: Oblique muscle surgery of the A-V patterns. J Pediatr Ophthalmol 2:31-36, 1965.

4. Postic G: Contribution a l' etude de O'etiopathogenie des syndromes A et V. Bull Mem Soc Fr Ophthalmol 78:240-252, 1965.

5. Gobin MH: Sagittalization of the oblique muscles as a possible cause for the "A," "V," and "X" phenomena. Br J Ophthalmol 52:13-18, 1968.

6. France TD: In Moore S, Meins J, Stockbridge L (eds), Orthoptics: Past, Present, Future. New York, Stratton International Medical Book Corp, 1975, p 287.

7. Miller M, Folk E: Strabismus associated with craniofacial anomalies. Am Orthoptic J 25:27-37, 1975.

8. Urrets-Zavalia Jr A, Solares-Zamora J, Olmos HR: Anthropological studies on the nature of cyclovertical squint. Br J Ophthalmol 45:578-596, 1961.

9. von Noorden GK: Burian-von Noorden's Binocular Vision and Ocular Motility: Theory and Management of Strabismus. 2nd ed, St. Louis, CV Mosby, 1980, p. 341.

10. Helveston E: Atlas of Strabismus Surgery. St. Louis, CV Mosby, 1977, p. 4.

11. Farkas LG: Anthropmetry of the Head and Face in Medicine. New York, Elsevier North Holland Inc., 1981, p. 190.

12. Smith DW: Recognizable Patterns of Human Malformation. Philadelphia, WB Saunders Company, 1970.

DISCUSSION BY T. MARUO

A-V pattern strabismus is often associated with craniofacial dysostosis, hydrocephalus, and others. This is a problem of structural factors and a specific case. A-V pattern strabismus, however, is observed even in the cases without these abnormalities and there may be racial difference of race explaining these pattern strabismies.

PRESENT STATUS OF STRABISMUS IN CRANIOFACIAL ANOMALIES

E. L. deBrown and F. O. Monasterio

ABSTRACT

The strabismus in the craniofacial dysostosis was analyzed in relation to the anatomical alterations of the orbital bones. These anomalies produce displacements around the two principle planes of the skull: the fronto-parallel plane and the sagital plane, and also around the three orbital axes: the horizontal, the vertical, and the anteroposterior axes.

Examples are given with patients showing the different craniofacial anomalies related with the misalignment disturbances of the mentioned planes and axes of the orbit and the related specific strabismologic pictures.

I. Strabismus in Holoprocencephaly

Eleven cases of holoprocencephaly were presented which show varying degrees of cerebral facial deterioration. In the six stillborn cases, the autopsy showed the partially artophied central nervous system. In the five cases which survived, the occurence of a neurological strabismus was discovered.

The pathological study of the extraocular muscles proved the correlation between the atrophy of the central nervous system and the absence of the nervous fibers in the extraocular muscles.

II. Strabismus in Treacher Collins Disease

Three patients suffering from this orbital fissure anomaly were shown in connection with the "V" Syndrome. The outward and downward displacements of the orbit, the eyeball and the soft tissues (antimongoloid inclination of the palpebral fissure) are pointed out as the pathogenesis of "V" Syndrome. The craniofacial surgery, which consisted in the closure of the orbital fissures with bone implants and the realignment of the external canthus, proved to control the "V" Syndrome.

STRABISMUS II
ISBN 0-8089-1424-3

VERTICAL STRABISMUS ASSOCIATED WITH PLAGIOCEPHALY

R. M. Robb and W. P. Boger III

ABSTRACT

Thirty-three patients with plagiocephaly due to unilateral coronal synostosis have been studied because of a high incidence of vertical strabismus. Twenty-seven of the 33 patients were found to have an ipsilateral hypertropia. In two patients the hypertropia disappeared after early neurosurgical correction of the coronal synostosis, but in most patients the hypertropia persisted, mimicking a fourth cranial nerve palsy with overaction of the inferior oblique muscle and a head tilt to the opposite shoulder. We think the vertical muscle imbalance is due to structural abnormalities of the orbit induced by the cranial synostosis. Appropriate strabismus surgery reduced the ocular deviation in five patients.

INTRODUCTION

Unilateral coronal synostosis occurs sporadically as a limited form of cranial synostosis.[1] Although lower facial malformations do not accompany this type of isolated cranial synostosis, a distinctive asymmetrical growth of the head usually draws attention to the condition. The mis-shapen head, a form of plagiocephaly, is characterized by elevation of the brow and flattening of the forehead on the involved side. Roentgenograms of the skull reveal a harlequin deformity of the affected orbit with exagerated obliquity of the orbital roof, an updrawn lesser wing of the sphenoid bone, and absence of the ipsilateral coronal suture. Bilateral coronal synostosis is also known to occur, either in isolated form or as part of one of the more extensive craniofacial dysostoses.[2] The ocular features of the latter have been described extensively.[3-8] During the past twelve years we have come to recognize a type of vertical strabismus associated with the unilateral form of coronal synostosis. This type of vertical ocular deviation has received relatively little attention in the ophthalmic literature.[9] A recent paper, the only specific report of the condition known to us, describes four patients with plagiocephaly and varying degrees of involvement of ocular motility.[10]

STRABISMUS II
ISBN 0-8089-1424-3

MATERIALS AND METHODS

Between 1969 and 1981 thirty-seven patients with plagiocephaly due to unilateral coronal synostosis were seen for ophthalmological evaluation at the Children's Hospital Medical Center. Most of the patients were referred from the neurosurgical service, but not all patients admitted to that service with the diagnosis of plagiocephaly were seen by us. At least ten patients who had surgery for unilateral coronal synostosis during this same period of time did not have ophthalmological consultations. Therefore, our estimate of the frequency of the ocular complications of plagiocephaly must remain aproximate. Visual acuity and ocular motility measurements were made in a manner consistent with patient age, which ranged from one month to seventeen years. Cycloplegic refractions and fundus examinations by indirect ophthalmoscopy were performed on all patients. Seven patients had only one examination; the others were seen on multiple occasions for diagnosis and management of their ocular problems. Four patients were excluded from this study, three because of imcomplete clinical data and one because strabismus surgery had been performed elsewhere before we examined the patient. This study is, therefore, based on data from 33 patients.

OBSERVATIONS

Twenty-seven of the 33 patients were found to have hypertropia of the eye on the side of the coronal synostosis. The hypertropia ranged from 10 to 30 prism diopters in those patients on whom measurements could be made. In one patient the vertical deviation was apparent only when the head was tilted to the side of the hypertropic eye. Of the six patients without a vertical deviation three had no apparent strabismus, two had esotropia, and one had Duane Syndrome in the eye contralateral to the coronal synostosis.

The hypertropia was accompanied by a head tilt to the opposite side in 15 patents and to the same side in one patient. The head tilt did not allow all patients to achieve binocular vision and it was oftwen present intermittently. In only four patients was the hypertropia clearly increased by forced head tilt to the ipsilateral side (positive Bielschowsky test[11]).

Ten patients were noted to have overaction of the inferior oblique muscle on the side of the hypertropia with or without underaction of the antagonist superior oblique, and an additional four patients had bilateral inferior oblique overaction. One patient had bilateral underaction of the inferior oblique muscles. When there was inferior oblique overaction on the side of the hypertropia some patients tended to turn the head away from that side, thereby reducing the vertical deviation. On the other hand two patients without oblique overaction had an habitual head turn toward the side of the coronal synostosis and in this position appeared to have a smaller hypertropia.

Five of our patients have had strabismus surgery, either weakening of one or both inferior oblique muscles or recession of the ipsilateral superior rectus. Surgery improved the vertical deviation and head position in most cases, but it did not render any patient orthophoric in all positions of gaze.

Twenty-eight of the 33 patients had neurosurgical correction of the coronal synostosis in infancy, mostly during the first year of life. Five patients had late remodelling of cranial defects and three had no corrective surgery. Early opening of the closed coronal suture and advancement of the supraorbital margin is generally felt to offer the best opportunity for symmetrical growth of the head.[1,2] Two of our patients who were noted to have a definite vertical deviation prior to cranial surgery had no apparent vertical strabismus postoperatively. In these two patients cranial surgery was performed at one month and eight months of age, respectively, and the vertical deviation was found to have disappeared six weeks to three months postoperatively. On the other hand a vertical deviation persisted in 20 patients who underwent early surgical correction of their coronal synostosis, and in these cases it was not possible to recognize any change in ocular alignment coincident with the cranial surgery.

A number of other anomalies were present in the patients we studied. In individual patients each of the following was found: the Pierre Robin anomaly, an ipsilateral lymphangioma of the forehead, and bilateral congenital absence of the radial bones. Another patient had multiple anomalies including the tetralogy of Fallot, thoracic and lumbar hemivertebrae, and congenital dislocation of the hips. Four patients had unilateral or bilateral blepharoptosis. Three patients had unilateral congenital obstruction of the nasolacrimal duct, and one had bilateral obstruction. The latter patient required dacryocystorhinostomies when simple probing failed because of bony abnormalities beyond the lacrimal sac. Refractive errors were often present in our patients, but the ametropia was not more frequent on the side of the synostosis.

DISCUSSION

The ipsilateral hypertropia seen in a large percentage of patients with unilateral coronal synostosis simulates a fourth cranial nerve palsy. We feel that the hypertropia is not due to an actual nerve palsy because of the infrequency of a positive Bielschowsky test. More likely the vertical deviation is caused by underaction of the superior oblique muscle due to distortion of the orbital anatomy. The roof of the orbit is foreshortened, and, as suggested by Bagolini, Campos, and Chiesi[9], the trochlea is probably displaced posteriorly, weakening the depressive action of the reflected superior oblique tendon. The inferior oblique muscle would not be similarly weakened since the orbital floor is much less affected by the cranial anomaly than is the orbital roof. Our efforts to document an altered course of the superior oblique tendon by computerized orbital tomography have not yet been conclusive, but such studies dramatically illustrate the asymmetry of orbital development. A number of forms of strabismus, both horizontal and vertical, have been attributed to altered orbtal configuration.[13-14] Although early neurosurgical correction of unilateral coronal synostosis undoubtedly allows the skull to assume a more symmetrical contour,[1] some orbital asymmetry usually remains. Our experience suggests that a large proportion of patients with unilateral coronal synostosis, with or without early neurosurgical intervention, can be expected to have vertical ocular deviations.

ACKNOWLEGEMENTS

Elizabeth D. Hampton and Dorothy W. Rodier assisted in retrieving data for this paper. John F.Bowers, M.D., Richard J. Blocker, M.D., Robert L. Bahr, M.D., and Robert A. Peterson, M.D. provided ophthalmological information on individual patients.

Supported in part by The Children's Eye Fund and by the Massachusets Lions Eye Research Fund, Inc.

REFERENCES

1. Shillito, J. Jr., and Matson, D.D.: Craniosynostosis: a review of 519 surgical patients. Pediatrics 41: 829-853, 1968.

2. Tessier, P.: Relationship of craniostenoses to craniofacial dysostoses and to faciostenoses. Plastic and Reconstructive Surgery 48: 224-237, 1971.

3. Howell, S.C.: The craniostenoses. Am J. Ophthalmol. 37: 359-379, 1954.

4. Laitinen, L., Miettinen, P. and Sulamaa, M.: Ophthalmological observations in craniosynostosis. Acta Ophthalmologica 34: 121-132, 1956.

5. Archer, D.B., Gordon, D.S., Maguire, C.J.F., et al: Ophthalmic aspects of craniosynostosis. Trans. Ophthalmol. Soc. U.K. 94: 172-196, 1974.

6. Walker, J. and Wybar, K.: Ocular motility problems in craniofacial dysostosis. S. Moore, J. Mein, and L. Stockbridge (Ed.) In _Orthoptics: Past, Present, Future_. Stratton, NY, 1976. p. 299-310.

7. Miller, M. and Folk, E.: Strabismus associated with craniofacial anomalies. Am. Orthopt. J. 25: 27-37, 1975.

8. Nelson, R.B., Ingoglia, S., and Breinin, G.M.: Sensorimotor disturbances in craniostenosis. J. Pediatr, Ophthal. Strabis. 18: 32-41, 1981.

9. Koziak, P.H.: Craniostenosis. Report of 22 cases, Am. J. Ophthalmol. 37: 380-390, 1954.

10. Bagolini, B., Campos, E.C., and Chiesi, C.: Plagiocephaly causing superior oblique deficiency and ocular torticollis. Arch. Ophthalmol. 100: 1093-1096, 1982.

11. Bielschowsky, A.: Disturbances of the vertical motor muscles of the eyes. Arch. Ophthalmol.: 20: 175-200, 1938.

12. Hoffman, H.J., Mohr, G.: Lateral canthal advancement of the supraorbital margin. A new corrective technique in the treatment of coronal synostosis. J. Neurosurg. 45: 376-381, 1976.

13. Zaki, H.A.A., and Keeney, A.H.: The bony orbital walls in horizontal strabismus. Arch. Ophthalmol. 57: 418-424, 1957.

14. Urrets-Zavalia, A., Solares-Zamora, S., and Olmos, h.R.: Anthropological studies on the nature of cyclovertical squint. Br. j. Ophthalmol. 45: 578-596, 1961.

ELECTROMYOGROPHY IN CONGENITAL FAMILIAL OPHTHALMOPLEGIA

G. W. Cibis, R. Kies, T. Lawwill, and G. Varghese

ABSTRACT

The etiology of congenital familial opthalmoplegia including the levator muscle is unclear. Fibrous tissue replacing muscle in such cases lead to the term congenital familial fibrosis. As the intrinsic muscles of the eye, two of which are derived from epithelium, are usually spared it is thought that the condition is a primary abiotrophy of mesodermally derived extraocular muscles. A nuclear or supranuclear etiology however is possible. We report on two non-related families that provide evidence of a nuclear or supranuclear etiology.

INTRODUCTION

The etiology of congenital familial ophthalmoplegia including the levator muscle is unclear leading to an appellation of names for what may or may not be the same condition. The basic clinical entity is a congenital ophthalmoplegia including the lid. Internal ophthalmoplegia is separated from external ophthalmoplegia with total ophthalmoplegia meaning paralysis of all extra- and intraocular muscles. If one or more external muscles including the lid is spared it is a partial or incomplete ophthalmoplegia. This classification implies a neurogenic etiology.

A second etiologic possibility is primary abiotrophy of the mesodermally derived extraocular muscles resulting in clinical fibrosis. Even with this presumtive etiologic classification system however confusion exists as to the inclusion of total, internal versus external, vertical but not horizontal, and familial versus non-familial (sporatic) cases in the congenital familial, fibrosis group. Harley et al (9) included "various forms" of extraocular muscle fibrosis such as; (1) general fibrosis syndrome (3) (2) congenital fibrosis of the inferior rectus muscle with blepharoptosis, (3) strabismus fixus, (4) vertical retraction syndrome, (13) (5) congenital unilateral fibrosis, enophthalmos and

STRABISMUS II
ISBN 0-8089-1424-3

blepharoptosis, (16) as a clinical spectrum of the "fibrosis group." Parks, in discussing this paper questioned the validity of including groups 2-5, which are usually sporatic within the general fibrosis syndrome. The general fibrosis syndrome is usually dominant in inheritance and within a family does not show a great deal of variability of expression.(18)

We report two unrelated families with dominantly inherited congenital familial fibrosis. Each family has distinctive clinical findings which we feel so differentiate these two fammilies from each other as to constitute separate diseases. Because of their apparent neurogenic etiology they are also not part of the fibrosis group but more truely congenital ophthalmoplegias with secondary fibrosis akin to Duane's syndrome.

CASE REPORTS

Family M (Fig 1): A mother and her three children all had total internal and external ophthalmoplegia (Fig 2). All have the typical chin up, eyes down and slight exotropic position with ptosis. No noticeable horizontal or vertical movement of the eyes were seen in the mother and two daughters and only slight, less than five degrees, movement

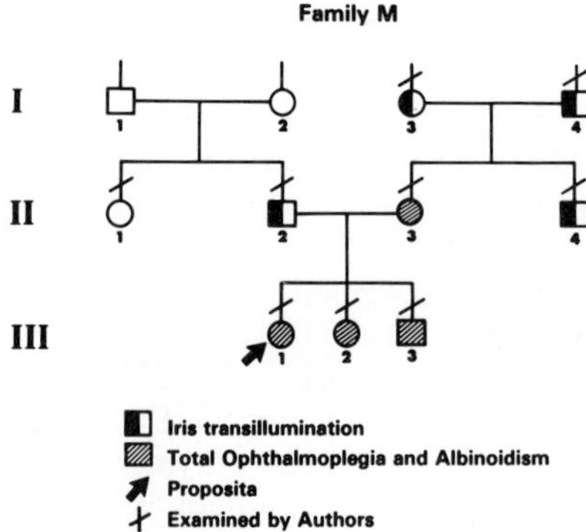

Figure 1. Family tree of Family M showing a dominant hereditary pattern of ophthalmoplegia.

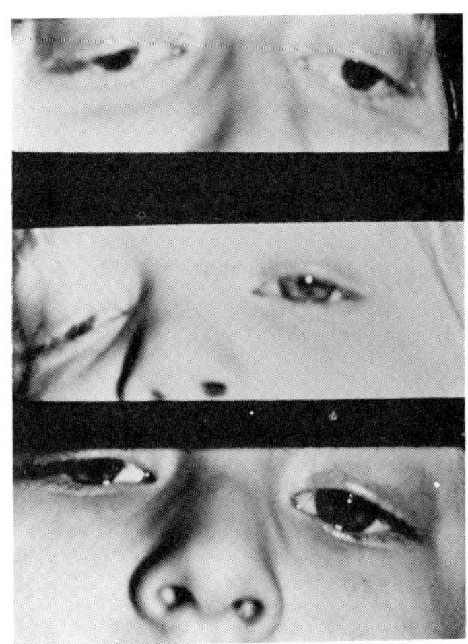

Figure 2. Mother (top) and daughters Family M with total internal and external ophthalmoplegia. Note ptosis and exotropia.

was seen in the infant son. All patients had rotary nystagmus. None of the patients had amblyopia. Best corrected visions in the mother and daughters was 20/30 with appropriate myopic astigmatic corrections. The pupils of these patients are fixed, slightly dilated and fail to respond to light or attempted accommodation. The patients all need bifocal corrections for near vision because of the lack of accommodation. The pupils responded to mydriatics but never reached full dilation. The pupils constricted with 1/8% pilocarpine indicating denervation sensitivity of the parasympathetic system. The two daughters were operated for ptosis and exotropia. Both had markedly positive forced ductions with white fibrotic tight abnormal appearing extraocular muscles. Electromyography of the lateral rectus of the mother showed marked reduction in the available motor units with normal amplitudes and durations of potentials (Fig 3). No fibrillation or sharp positive waves were noted at rest. Increased amplitudes and polyphasicity of the available motor units as occurs with lower motor neuron type lesions were not seen, indicating the lesions as either primary fibrotic muscle or supranuclear. Activity did not change with attempted eye movement.

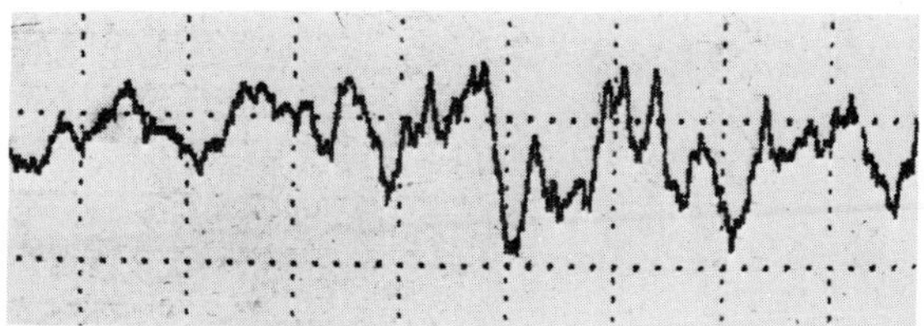

Figure 3. Electromyogram of the right lateral rectus of patient 11-3 Family M. There is a reduction in the number of motor units. Amplitude and duration of such action potentials as exist are normal. Vertical scale 100 microvolts/Div, horizontal 10ms/Div.

Family S (Fig 4): A second unrelated family had larger horizontal movements (20 degrees), but on attempted upgaze had spastic convergence-like movements (Fig 5-8). The affected father and two daughters were all slightly exotropic in the chin tilt up, eyes down position (Figs. 5-7). Electromyography on the left lateral rectus of the father showed a marked decrease in motor unit activity both during clonic and voluntary activity. The amplitude and duration of the motor units were within normal limits (Fig 9). The left inferior rectus showed normal decreased motor unit activity on downgaze (Fig 10). However, on attempted upgaze recruitment was increased in the inferior rectus (Fig 11), clinically reflected as spastic convergence-like movements indicating recruitment of the medial rectus as well with visible retraction.

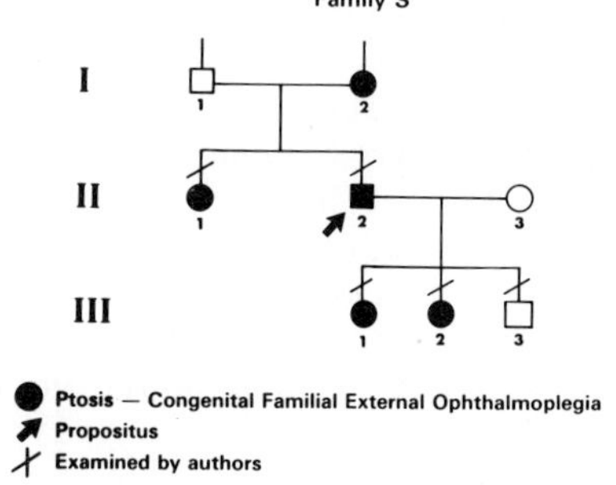

Figure 4. Family tree of Family S showing dominant heredity of the ophthalmoplegia.

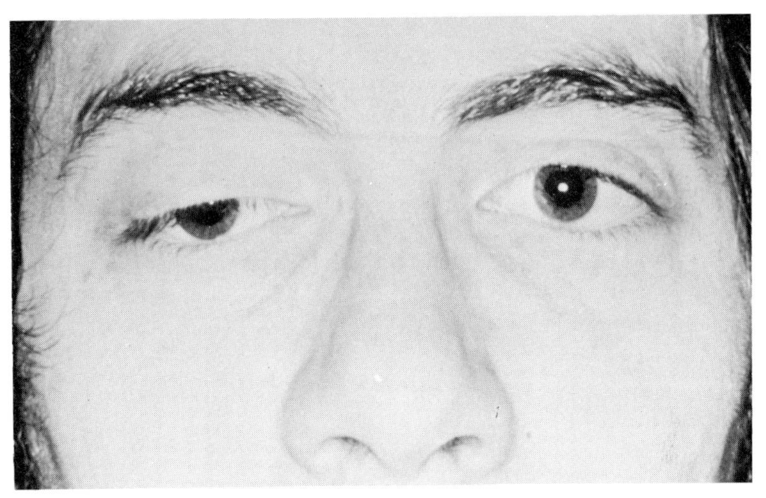

Figure 5. Propositus of Family S (II-2) in straight ahead gaze. Note assymetric ptosis and chin tilt up position.

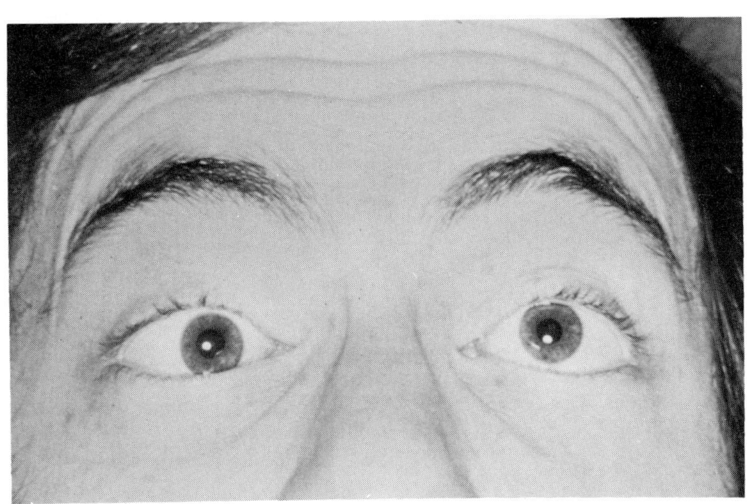

Figure 6. Same patient as in Fig 5 on attempted upgaze (no wrinkling of forehead). There is spastic convergence with retraction.

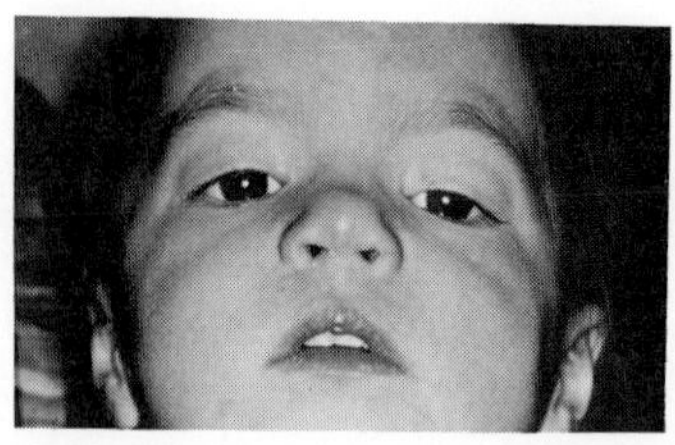

Figure 7. Patient III-2 Family S. Note exotropia with chin tilt up eyes down position and ptosis.

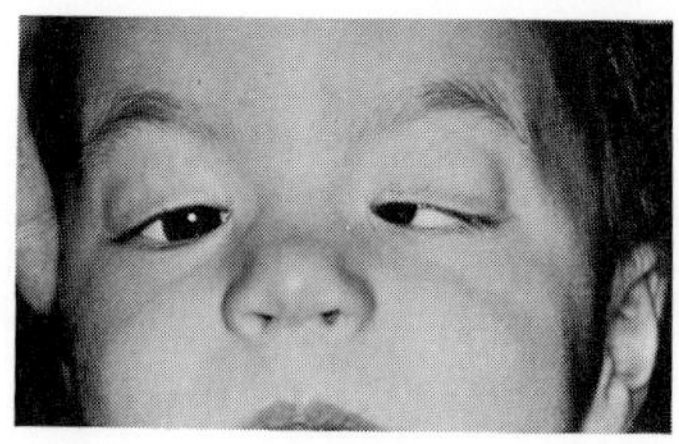

Figure 8. Patient III-2 Family S on attempted upgaze has spastic convergence movements with retraction. Note narrowing of lid tissue left eye.

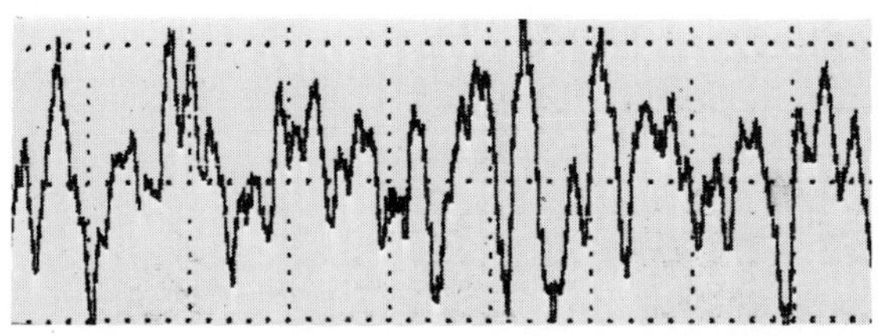

Figure 9. Electromyogram of the left lateral rectus in its field of action. (Patient II-2 Family S). There is a marked decrease in motor unit activity with normal amplitude and duration indicating fibrosis. Vertical scale 100 microvolts/Div, horizontal 10 ms/Div.

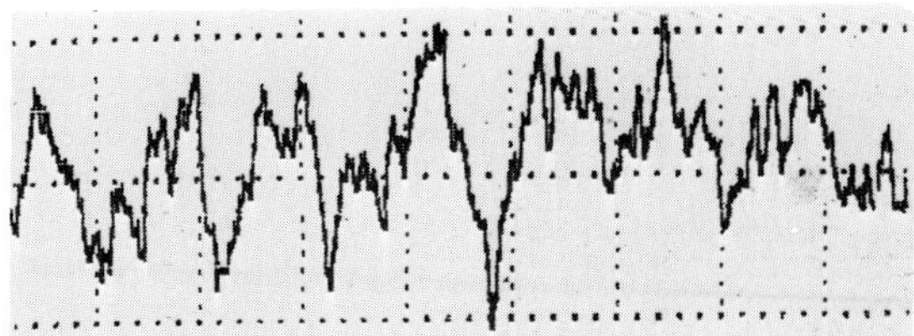

Figure 10. EMG left inferior rectus of patient II-2 Family S shows decreased motor unit activity on down gaze. Vertical scale 100 microvolts/Div, horizontal 10ms/Div.

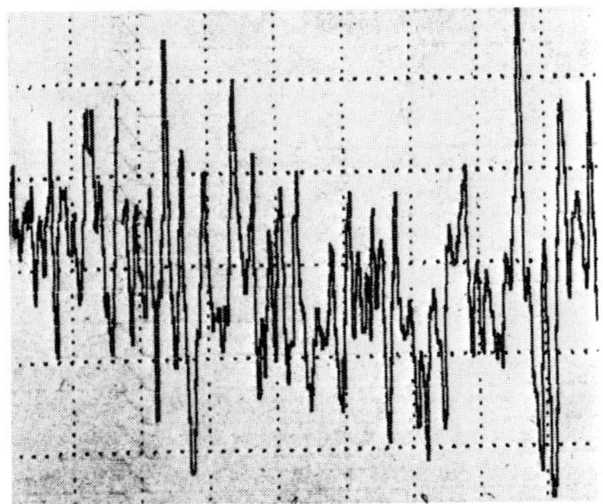

Figure 11. EMG same muscle as Fig 10 shows increased recruitment of motor unit firing in the left inferior rectus of patient II-2 on attempted upgaze. Clinically this was reflected as retraction with convergence spasm. horizontal 10 ms/Div, vertical 100 microvolts/Div.

The findings in the lateral rectus most likely indicate either a fibrosis or an upper motor neuron lesion. If this is a lower motor neuron lesion we would expect increased amplitude and duration of the motor unit potential. The increase in motor unit activity in the inferior rectus on upgaze suggests an anomolous innervation of the inferior rectus muscle akin to Duane's syndrome.

Recession of the inferior rectus muscle and ptosis surgery was performed on all three patients. Prior to surgery the father had had a forced duction test which was markedly positive when told to look up but less so when asked to look down. We interpret this clinically as a sign of the co-contraction as first pointed out by Dr. Andrea Tongue in Duane's patients.

At the time of surgery the father and one daughter had fair forced duction movement. The second daughter's eye, however, was bound down tight with an abnormal double headed posteriorly inserted fibrotic appearing inferior rectus muscles bilaterally.

DISCUSSION

The term general fibrosis syndrome was introduced by Brown in 19503 in describing four congenital nonfamilial instances of fibrosis of all extraocular muscles leading to a mechanical restriction of movement. The term subsequently persisted in the literature even though ophthalmoplegia had historically been applied to cases of this type (see Waardenburg et al for a historical review (22)). The difference in terminology related to a difference in opinion as to the etiology of this condition with Brown clearly favoring a mechanical peripheral orbital cause. He classified the following syndromes based on the muscles involved: (1) typical and atypical retraction syndrome (medial and lateral rectus muscles), (2) strabismus fixus (medial and lateral rectus muscles), (3) vertical retraction syndrome (superior and inferior rectus muscles), (4) superior oblique tendon sheath syndrome (inferior and superior oblique muscles) and (5) general fibrosis syndrome (involvement of three or more of the extraocular muscles).

The advent of electromyogrophy clarified the true etiology of Duane's typical retraction syndrome as neurogenic. (2) Autopsy cases of Duane's syndrome show an absence of abducens nerve nuclei with partial innervation of the lateral rectus by branches of the oculomotor nerve. (11,12) Fibrosis of the lateral rectus muscles and secondarily of the antagonist medial rectus muscle occurred in all cases examined by electronmicroscopy4. Hotchkiss, et al, in their case found fibrosis of both lateral recti muscles to be confined to those areas with the poorest innervation. Extraocular muscle fibrosis in the typical retraction syndrome (Duane's) as Brown described it has therefore clearly been shown to be secondary to a brainstem nuclear etiology. This brings into question the etiologic significance of fibrosis into the "general fibrosis syndrome" and its "variants" and whether or not one should use fibrosis as a diagnostic criterion to differentiate Duane's from congenital familial ophthalmoplegia.

The electromyogram of the lateral rectus of both patient III-2 Family S and patient II-3 Family M showed decreased motor unit activity with normal amplitude and duration of the motor units. Histopathological islands of normal muscle interspersed with areas of fibrosis as found by Apt in cases of congenital fibrosis would account for our EMG findings as would Hotchkiss, et al's correlation of lateral rectus fibrosis to the areas with poorest innervation (anomalous) in their case of Duane's syndrome. Increased amplitude and duration of the motor unit potentials seen with lower motor neuron lesions were not present. This and the co-contraction anomolous innervation shown in Family S along with the rotary nystagmus and total ophthalmoplegia in Family M place the site of the lesion in both families at the nuclear and supranuclear level.

Clinically the two families presented fit the criterion of familial congenital fibrosis with both having evidence of extraocular muscle fibrosis at the time of surgery. EMG and other evidence in our families indicates that the muscle fibrosis in congenital familial fibrosis may be secondary to innervational abnormalities similar to Duane's syndrome. We feel that extraocular muscle fibrosis as a primary etiologic entity for familial cases such as our remains to be proven.

Ptosis which is not found in Duane's syndrome differentiates Family S from "vertical retraction syndrome" (13,16,20) most case reports of which are non-familial and unilateral. Fibrosis and positive forced ductions were found in all of our patients but were much less marked in the father and one daughter of Family S than in the other child indicating an intrafamilial variability of expression for the fibrosis. The spasmic convergence in Family S, in our opinion due to co-contraction, has been described by other authors in families with congenital familial fibrosis. (6,7,8,9)

The rotary nystagmus and total ophthalmoplegia in Family M speaks in favor of a nuclear or supranuclear etiology. Similar families with total ophthalmoplegia have been reported by LI17 and by Popoviciul (9). Most cases of congenital familial fibrosis spare the intrinsic muscles of the eye two of which are derived from epithelium rather than mesoderm. This has been used as a major argument in favor of a primary abiotrophy of medodermally derived extraocular muscles as the etiology of congenital fibrosis. Cogan (5) in discussing Holmes (10) paper felt the nystagmus present in many of the reported cases of congenital familial fibrosis, as in our Family M, to favor a supranuclear brainstem involvement. We feel that Family M with total ophthalmoplegia must be categorized separately from Family S where more typically the intrinsic muscles were spared but co-contraction could be demonstrated. We recommend using the terms Congenital Familial Total Ophthalmoplegia for Family M and Congenital Familial External Ophthalmoplegia with Co-Contraction to describe Family S. Such a classification is most similar to that of Waardenburg (22) and ignores the misleading concept of fibrosis. The terms familial and congenital are necessary to separate these cases from acquired and sporatic ones. We would restrict the term general fibrosis to sporatic cases as described by Brown in 1950, Laughlin in 1956, Apt in 1978, without rotary nystagmus, evidence of co-contraction, or internal ophthalmoplegia.

REFERENCES

1. Apt L, Axelrod RN: Genralized fibrosis of the extraocular muscles. Am J Ophthalmol 85:822-829, 1978.

2. Blodi FC, Van Allen MW, Yarbrough JC: Duane's Syndrome: A brain stem lesion. Arch Ophthalmol 72:171-177, 1964.

3. Brown HW: Congenital Structural Muscle Anomalies. In Allen JH (ed): Strabismus Ophthalmic Symposium. St. Louis, CV Mosby Co, 1950, p. 205-236.

4. Celic M, Dorn V: Clinical electromyographic and electro-oculographic examination in Stilling-Turk-Duane's retraction syndrome. In Mein J, Moore S, (eds): Transaction of the IV International Orthoptic Congress, Kimpton H, Publisher London, 1981, p. 145-150.

5. Cogan DG: Discussion remarks. Trans Am Ophthalmol Soc, 1954, 41:368.

6. Crawford JS: Congenital fibrosis syndrome. Can J Ophthalmol 5:331-336, 1970.

7. Hansen E: Congenital general fibrosis of the extraocular muscles. Acta Ophthalmol (Kbh) 46:469-476, 1968.

8. Harley RD, Rodriques MM, Crawford JS: Congenital fibrosis of the extraocular muscles. Trans Am Ophthalmol Soc 76:197-226, 1978.

9. Harley RD, Rodriques MM, Crawford JS: Congenital fibrosis of the extraocular muscles. J Pediatr Ophthalmol 15:346-358, 1978.

10. Holmes WJ: Hereditary congenital ophthalmoplegia: Trans Am Ophthalmol Soc 53:245-253, 1955.

11. Hotchkiss MG, Miller NR, Clark AW, Green WR: Bilateral Duane's syndrome. Arch Ophthalmol 98:870-874, 1980.

12. Hoyt WF, Nachtigaller H: Anomalies of ocular motor nerves. Am J Ophthalmol 60:443-448, 1965.

13. Khodadoust AA, von Noorden GK: Bilateral vertical retraction syndrome. Arch Ophthalmol 78:606-612, 1967.

14. Laughlin RC: Congenital fibrosis of the extraocular muscles. Am J Ophthalmol 41:432-438, 1956.

15. Lees F: Congenital, static familial ophthalmoplegia. J Neurol Neurosurg Psychiatry 23:46-51, 1960.

16. Leone CR, Weinstein GW: Orbital fibrosis with enophthalmos. Ophthalmic Surg 3:71-75, 1973.

17. Li TM: Congenital total bilateral ophthalmoplegia. Am J Ophthalmol 6:816-821, 1923.

18. Parks MM: Discussion remarks. Trans Am Ophthalmol Soc LXXVI, p. 222-223, 1978.

19. Popoviciu M, Popoviciu M: Familial hereditary nuclear ophthalmoplegia. Oftalmologia (Bucharest) 5:339-344, 1961.

20. Pruksacholawit K, Ishikawa S: Atypical vertical retraction syndrome: A case study. J Pediatr Ophthalmol 13:215-220, 1976.

21. von Noorden GK: Congenital hereditary ptosis with inferior rectus fibrosis. Arch Ophthalmol 83:378-380, 1970.

22. Waardenburg PJ: Genetics and Ophthalmology Vol II: p. 1091-1104, Van Gorcum Publishers, Assen, Netherlands 1963.

23. Oritz de Zarate JC: Recessive sex linked inheritance of congenital external ophthalmoplegia and myopia coincident with other dysplasias. Br J Ophthalmol 50:606-607, 1966.

DISCUSSION BY T. MARUO

As I also have observed cases of general fibrosis syndrome with paradoxical divergence during lateral gaze, I would like to add some words. Both EOG and EMG examinations revealed paradoxical divergence in my study. This result supports the authors' view that supranuclear abnormalities are involved in the general fibrosis syndrome.

Although a neurogenic etiology and a myogenic one can be discriminated in the EMG examinations, it is difficult to distinguish where the cause of neurogenic palsy is, in the upper motor neuron or in the lower. It seems reasonable to consider that the supranuclear origin also may be added to the causes of general fibrosis syndrome because paradoxical innervation of the inferior rectus is present. Some questions remain: a) What is the evidence that the electrode is inserted not into the inferior oblique but into the inferior rectus exactly? and b) Since there is either a supranuclear or nuclear etiology of internal ophthalmoplegia, can the abnormalities of the internal ocular muscle itself, e.g., fibrosis, be considered as another etiology?

ISOLATED PALSY OF THE INFERIOR DIVISION OF THE OCULOMOTOR NERVE: A CASE REPORT AND REVIEW OF THE LITERATURE

M. A. Musarella, J.R. Buncic

ABSTRACT

The clinical entity of paralysis of only the inferior division of the third cranial nerve is a rare phenomenon. Our case and the three cases reported in the literature suggest that the development of the tonic pupil is characteristic of this clinical entity, presumed to be a viral etiology.

INTRODUCTION

The oculomotor nerve divides into superior and inferior divisions as it passes through the superior orbital fissure. The superior branch supplies the superior rectus and levator palpebrae. The inferior branch supplies the medial and inferior recti, inferior oblique and parawympathetic ciliary ganglion fibers which are destined for the iris sphincter and ciliary muscles. Palsies affecting each division have been described, but are indeed rare.[1,2] Inferior branch palsies occurred spontaneously[3], with trauma[4,5] following viral illness[1,6,7] and with neoplasial. We describe herein the clinical signs and course of an isolated inferior oculomotor branch palsy in a seven year old child which occurred following a flu-like illness.

Case report.

This 7-year old girl, who had a febrile, flu-like illness 2 weeks previously, complained of "sore eyes" to her mother. The child was seen by a local physician who noted bilaterally injected conjunctiva and prescribed neosporin drops. The following day the patient was noted by her mother to have a dilated left pupil. She was referred to another physician who observed a sluggishly reactive left pupil, but preserved ocular motility. Ten days later she developed horizontal diplopia, external deviation of the left eye, and a dilated, nonreactive left pupil and was referred to the Hospital for Sick Children for consultation.

STRABISMUS II
ISBN 0-8089-1424-3

The patients visual acuity was R.E.: 20/20/ and L.E.: 20/70. Refraction of L.E.: plano +0.50X 180o improved vision to 20/40+1.

The left eye was exotropic 45 prism diopters and hypertropic 12 prism diopters. Total paralysis of the left medial and left inferior recti, and palsy of the left inferior oblique muscle was seen. The superior rectus and levator palpebrae were intact. The pupil of the left eye was dilated, measuring 7 mm. in diameter and did not constrict to any stimuli. The left IV and VI N. muscles were preserved as were the branches of the trigeminal and facial nerves. The examination of the anterior segments and fundus were unremarkable. The ocular motility and pupillary function of the right eye were intact.

Specific inquiry revealed the child to be free of headaches. Family history and past health were nocontributory. No other signs of sinus, orbital or neurological involvement could be elicted. Diagnostic studies, including hemogram, erythrocyte sedimentation rate and SMA-12 gave normal values. Lumbar puncture revealed normal cerebrospinal fluid with no cells or elevated protein level. Computed tomographic examinations of the orbits and cranium were interpreted as normal. Metrizamide cisternogram was performed to examine the interpeduncular fossa and revealed no abnormalities.

The child was observed with treatment and w months later had visual acuity of R.E.: 20/20 and L.E.: 20/40. Near point of accommodation (NPA) of R.E.: 3 cms. and L.E.: 7 cms. Ocular motility showed improvement of the left exotropia to 25 prism diopters and left hypertropia to 8 prism diopters. Biomicroscopy of the iris revealed segmental areas of contractions. Pupils measured R.E.: 4 mm. and L.E.: 7 mms. Hypersensitivity to .1% pilocarpine ws noted in the left pupil.

In the following four months the patients inferior branch oculomotor palsy had cleared completely except for the pupil, which had developed aberrant regeneration and pharmacological features of pupillary myotonia.

DISCUSSION

Isolated oculomotor nerve palsy may complicate various virus infections and has been recorded following viral meningitis[9] infectious mononucleosis[10], maxillary sinusitis[11], varicella[6,12], mumps[12,13], and coxsackie-virus[14]. Miller[7] noted that in 4 cases of acquired oculomotor nerve palsy in children, the palsy was due to an infectious process. One child (8 years of age), with a preceding viral syndrome, had involvement of the inferior division of the third nerve which resolved within 2 months. Sharf and Hyman[6] reported a case of unilateral transient internal ophthalmoplegia and medial rectus palsy, but prominent paralysis of the inferior oblique muscle in a 2 year old girl following a mild attack of varicella. Internal ophthalmoplegia following varicella has been described by several authors[15-19]. Susac and Hoyt[1], described 3 patients with inferior branch palsies of the oculomotor nerve. All 3 presented with painless diplopia. The palsy cleared within a short time in 2 patients. One child was a 5 year old girl who had a febrile, flu-like illness two weeks prior to onset of her diplopia nd unilateral mydriasis. Although ocular motility recovered in 2 patients they had residual tonic pupils suggesting a postviral illness. Tonic pupils are frequent sequelae of a viral process. Our patient may represent another of these postinfectious neuropathies of the inferior division of the third nerve. The previous mild flu-like illness suggests a possible postinfectious etiology but we cannot prove this. The hypersensitivity of the pupil to dilute pilocarpine in our case indicates a lesion in the peripheral portion of the oculomotor nerve which contains the parasympathetic root to the ciliary ganglion. The question to be asked is why is the inferior division selected by an infectious process? Possibly the ciliary ganglion may act as a reservoir for virus particles as the gasserion ganglion does for herpes simplex. Isolated inferior branch palsies not due to trauma may not be so rare and most likely may go unrecognized. In its early stages it may present only as a unilateral mydriasis which can be intermittent. The extraocular muscle palsy may not be present in the early stages. We hope this report will make pediatric ophthalmologists more aware of this condition. We suggest only observation since our case and those in the literature have adhered to the favorable course of patients with this post infectious neuropathy of the inferior branch of the oculomotor nerve.

REFERENCES

1. Susac JD, Hoyt WF: Inferior branch palsy of the oculomotor nerve. Ann Nerol 2:336-339, 1977.

2. Derakhshan I: Superior branch palsy of the oculomotor nerve with spontaneous recovery. Ann Neurol 4:478-479, 1978.

3. Walsh FB, Hoyt WF: Clinical Neuro-Ophthalmoloty, 3rd ed. Baltimore, Williams and Wilkins, 1969, Vol. 1, p. 255.

4. Cross AG: The ocular sequelae of head trauma. Ann R Coll Surg Engl 2:233-240, 1948.

5. Heinze J: Cranial nerve avulsion and other neural injuries in road accidents. Med J Aust 2:1246-1249, 1969.

6. Sharf B, Hyams S: Oculomotor palsy following varicella. J Ped Ophthalmol 9:245-247, 1972.

7. Miller NR: Solitary oculomotor nerve palsy in childhood. Am J Ophthalmol 83:106-111, 1977.

8. Duke-Elder: System of Ophthalmoloty, Vol. XII, Neuro-Ophthalmology, C.V. Mosby Company, 1971, St. Louis, pp. 730-753.

9. Walsh FW, Hoyt WF: Clinical Neuro-Ophthalmology, 3rd ed. Baltimore, Williams and Wilkins, 1969, Vol. 3, pp 2340, 2387-2389.

10. Nellhaus G: Isolated oculomotor nerve palsy in infectious mononucleosis. Neurology 16:221-223, 1966.

11. Green WR, Hackett ER, Schlezinger NS: Neuro-ophthalmologic evaluation of oculomotor nerve paralysis. Arch Ophthalmol 72:154-167, 1964.

12. Butler TH: Third nerve paralysis after mumps and chicken-pox. Br Med J 1:1095, 1930.

13. Butler TH, Wilson AJ: Ocular paralysis following mumps. Br Med J 1:752, 1937.

14. Marzetti G, Midulla M, Balducci L: Monolateral paralysis of the third cranial nerve associated with A9 coxsackie virusinfection. Minerva Pediat 20:943-947, 1968.

15. Ross JVM: Ocular varicella with an unusual complication. Am J Ophthalmol 51:1307-1308, 1961.

16. Rogers JW: Internal ophthalmoplegia following chicken pox. Arch Ophthalmol, 71:617-618, 1964.

17. Laha PN, Srivastava JR: Unilateral ophthalmoplegia Interna - a complication of chickenpox. J Indian Med Ass 22:334, 1955.

18. Monod MF: Concerning a case of tonic pupil in the course of varicella. Bull Soc Ophthal Franc 11:754-756, 1958.

19. Clavel MA: Unilateral mydriasis a result of varicella. Bull Soc Ophthal Franc 11:756-757, 1958.

DISCUSSION BY T. MARUO

Many doctors treat isolated palsy of the inferior division of the oculomotor nerve as partial or incomplete oculomotor palsy. That's why there are few case reports about it.

I have a high regard for the authors' detailed observations. It is interesting that misdirection is seen in these cases. The misdirection syndrome is often observed in the condition of complete oculomotor palsy. I believe that misdirection can be caused by complete palsy even in those cases of seeming isolated palsy of the inferior division.

OCULOMOTOR PARALYSIS IN ASSOCIATION WITH PERIORBITAL HEMANGIOMA

E. A. Palmer

ABSTRACT

Paralytic exotropia due to unilateral third cranial nerve palsy was observed in two infants with massive periorbital hemangiomas. The pupil was fixed and dilated in both cases. Computerized tomography demonstrated no intracranial abnormalities.

The involved eye was occluded by the eyelids during early infancy in both patients. Because of the presence of strabismus, anisometropia, and stimulus deprivation, treatment for amblyopia was required in both cases. These children have been observed until age 18 months and 4 years, and one or both have also experienced trichiasis, fundus changes, respiratory obstruction, and failure to thrive. The younger child has not developed good fixation with either eye and has not yet shown dramatic overall improvement in eith the hamangioma or the paralytic strabismus. The hamartomatous mass has undergone marked regression in the older patient, but the visual acuity remains poor in the paretic eye; strabismus surgery provided cosmetic benefit to this patient.

STRABISMUS II
ISBN 0-8089-1424-3

BENIGN RECURRENT SIXTH NERVE PALSIES IN CHILDHOOD: SECONDARY TO IMMUNIZATION OR VIRAL ILLNESS

D. B. Werner and P. J. Savino

ABSTRACT

Four children with benign, isolated, and recurrent sixth nerve palsies are presented. Two of the children had palsies which ccurred following immunizations; the other two patients had palsies that followed mild, febrile illnesses which were assumed to be of viral etiology. In all patients, the palsy resolved without other associate neurologic signs or symptoms. If a child presents with an atraumatic sixth nerve palsy, a tumor, hydrocephalus, and meningitis must be considered. If the neurologic exam shows no associated abnormalities, invasive testing is not indicated. The patient should be followed closely by the ophthalmologist and pediatrician for spontaneous recovery.

STRABISMUS II
ISBN 0-8089-1424-3

SIMILARITIES AND DIFFERENCES BETWEEN STRABISMUS AND AMBLYOPIA: AN EYE MOVEMENT STUDY

L. W. Stark, K. J. Ciuffreda and R. V. Kenyon

INTRODUCTION

Strabismus and amblyopia are two common ocular conditions that routinely confront the clinical eye specialist. Strabismus is an anomaly of binocular vision in which the visual axis of one eye fails to intersect the object of regard. Recognition of strabismus dates back to 3000 B.C. in Egypt and is responsible for giving rise to the term "evil eye"(1). While many early attempts to cure strabismus involved use of potions and diets, the first reasonable treatment involved use of a strabismus mask (Figure 1), developed by Paul of Egina (450 A.D.) to "straighten the eyes out". It is interesting that a similar clinical procedure, binasal occlusion(2) is presently used by some otpometrists to promote fusion in esotropes with anomalous retinal correspondence.

Amblyopia is an anomaly of monocular vision in which the reduced vision cannot be attriburted to uncorrected refractive error, structural abnormalities, or ocular or neurological disease, and was a much later discovery. deBuffron is credited with being the first to recognize that the squinting eye had poor vision(3). Furthermore, to improve vision, he recommended occlusion therapy to improve this vision, not unlike modern practice. These two ocular conditions frequently occur together, 66% of amblyopes having strabismus (M. Flom, personal communication).

In our research we sought to define and document the eye movement deficits attributable either to amblyopia or to strbismus. If one studies patients having amblyopia without strabismus, the "amblyopic" defects may be determined. In such patients, amblyopia is generally the result of uncorrected anisometropia or unequal refractive error, producing unilateral retinal-image blue during the early years of life. This may be considered akin to a mild form of stimulus deprivation amblyopia in which monocular contrast deprivation occurs. Amblyopia is characterized by a deficit in central visual acuity(4) and contrast sensitivity(5). Recent evidence also points to monocular spatial distortions(6) and "scrambling" of patterned visual

STRABISMUS II
ISBN 0-8089-1424-3

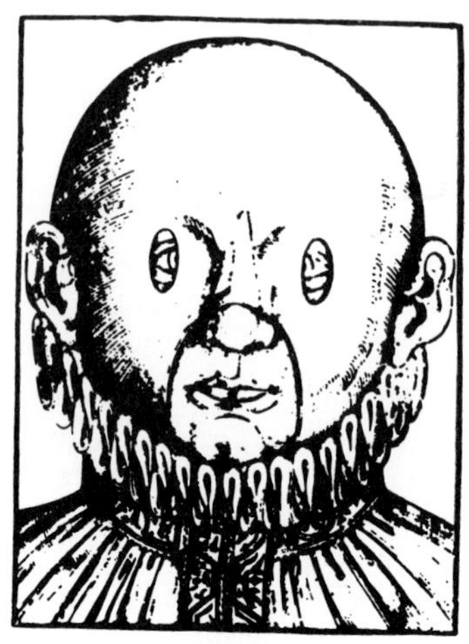

Figure 1. Strabismus Mask

stimuli(7); i.e. spatial phase deficits(8), as additional primary contribution factors leading to reduced visual acuity pattern perception in the amblyopic eye. That amblyopia primarily affects central and near peripheral vision is deduced from eye-nad reaction time experiments of Mackenson showing relatively minor latency increases for peripheral stimuli but marked latency increases for central stimuli(9). An additional central vision abnormality (present in 80% of amblyopic eyes(10)) is eccentric fixation, an anomaly of monocular vision in which the time-average position of the fovea is off the object-of-regard. Similarly, one may determine "strabismic" defects if eye movements are studied in patients having strabismus without amblyopia. This is accomplished most easily by using patients having intermittent strabismus, tyupically exotropia, in which the large neural non-Hering law bias, i.e. strabismus, is manifest only some of the time. This intermittency apparently allows for development of normal visual acuity in each eye. In the simplest cases of strabismus, the same image falls binocularly on grossly non-corresponding retinal elements producing diplopia and different parts of the image falls on corresponding retinal elements producing confusion. However, adaptive processes frequently occur to reduce the unfavorable perceptual consequences resulting from diplopia and confusion. These include suppression, the process whereby all or part of the ocular image of one eye is prevented from contributing to the binocular percept and anomalous correspondence, a type of correspondence in which a pseudo-fovea develops.

Classically, amblyopia has been divided into strabismic amblyopia and anisometropic amblyopia. However, in our attempt to determine eye movement defects attributed primarily either to amblyopia or to strabismus, we developed slightly difference "diagnostic" categories which we believe best suit such a goal. As detailed in the tables of section I, our categories included amblyopia without strabismus with very mild amblyopia and constant strabismus with amblyopia. The first two categories allowed us to determine the eye movement defects resulting either from amblyopia or from strabismus alone, while te latter two categories allowed us to determine effects resultsing from both conditions. The problem with the classical breakdown is that separation of defects related to either amblyopia besides having both conditions may also have anisometropia. A patient with anisometropia amblyopia may and generally does have strabismus. With the classical breakdown, if one studies eye movements inthe amblyopic eye of a strabismic amblyope, is the oculomotor defect a result of amblyopia or strabismus? One cannot make such a differentiation in many instances with complete confidence. Section II presents the similar effects on disparity vergence produced by the suppression of strabismus and by that of amblyopia. Section III presents the differences in versional eye movement abnormalities produced on the one hand by the monocular sensory defects of amblyopia, Section IIIa, and on the other hand by the binocular motor defects of strabismus, Section IIIb.

I. Diagnostic Categories

We agree with authorities in the field that, "An adequate classificaiton of amblyopia presents difficulties, caused in the main by our lack of knowledge of the mechanisms underlying amblyopia,"(11) and, furthermore, we are aware of at lease two classifications of amblyopia(12,13), both based on the clinical conditions responsible for producing the amblyopia. In contrast, in our classification (Table I), we group patients according to the presence or absence of either amblyopia or strabismus. This classification has worked out quite nicely for us, especially in terms of relating the versional eye movements defects in our patients to either the presence of amblyopia (increased saccadic latencies, increased drift) or strabismus (saccadic intrusions, latent nystagmus, manifest nystagmus). (See Table II-V). We feel that both classifications (See Table I), i.e., the more traditional one

TABLE 1 - Overview of clinical data and diagnostic group comparison in patients with versional and vergence eye abnormalities.

Patient	Age (yrs)	Refractive Status	Visual Acuity	Strabismic Deviation (prism diopters)
Constant strabismus amblyopia				
1	25	LE+2.00=-0.25x130	20/25	2 ET LE
		RE+2.25	20/15	
2	23	LE+3.75=-0.50x165	20/30	18 ET LE
		RE+0.50	20/15	
3	29	LE+1.25=-0.50x10=3ΔBD	20/25	27 const. alt. XT
		RE+1.00=-0.75x135=2ΔBU	20/50	and 5 HT LE
4	28	LE+2.25	20/80	55 ET LE
		RE+2.75=-1.00x180	20/40	
5	15	LE-1.50	20/122	10 ET LE and
		RE-1.75	20/20	1 HT LE
6	32	LE+4.00	20/277	4 ET LE
		RE plano	20/20	
7	33	LE+0.75=-0.50x40	20/630	6 ET LE and
		RE+0.25=-0.50x180	20/10	2 HT LE
8	26	LE-3.00=-2.25x38	20/20	6 ET RE and
		RE+0.25=-3.75x136	20/30	15 alt HPH
Amblyopia without strabismus				
9	24	LE+0.75=-2.00x90	20/38	None
		RE pl =-0.50x19	20/20	
10	25	LE-2.50=-1.25x172	20/25	None
		RE=5.00=-0.75x5	20/40	
11	19	LE+5.00	20/110	None
		RE+3.00	20/15	
Intermittent strabismus with or without mild amblyopia				
12	22	LE-0.75=-0.25x148	20/20	18 ALT XT
		RE-3.00=-0.25x100	20/20	and 12 HT LE
13	31	LE-5.00	20/20	15 XT LE
		RE-4.50=-0.75x20	20/20	
14	13	LE+0.75	20/20	20 ET RE and
		RE+0.50	20/20	6 HT RE
15	32	LE+0.75=-1.75x180	20/20	50 XT RE
		RE+1.25=-3.50x5	20/23	
16	25	LE plano	20/32	10 XT LE and
		RE-1.00	20/16	20 HT LE
Former strabismic patients				
17	24	LE-5.00	20/15	6 EPH
		RE-2.50=-0.75x165	20/25	
18	25	LE-0.75=-0.50x8	20/25	10 EPH and
		RE-2.75=-0.75x90	20/30	2 HPH
19	18	LE-1.75=-0.50x135	20/30	4 EPH and
		RE-0.75=-1.50x10	20/30	20 alt HPH

Eccentric Fixation (prism diopters)	Correspondence & Stereoacuity	Amblyopia Therapy/ Corrective Surgery	Traditional Diagnosis Categories
Constant strabismus amblyopia			
1/2 nasal LE	ARC 200"	Surgery, age 16	SA
1 nasal LE	-- 400"	Surgery, age 6	SA
manifest nystagmus	Parad. ARC --	Surgery, age 3 & 16	SA
manifest nystagmus	ARC --	Surgery, age 2	SA
2.5 nasal and 2 superior LE	ARC 300"	No	SA
16 nasal and 4 superior LE	-- --	No	AA
2.5 and 3.5 nasal and 3.4 superior LE	--	Surgery, age 6	SA
latent nystagmus	-- --	Surgery, age 1	AA
Amblyopia without strabismus			
2 nasal and 2 inferior LE	NRC 100"	No	AA
2 nasal and 2 inferior RE	NRC 60"	No	AA
2 temporal LE	NRC 400"	Amblyopia therapy before and during study	AA
Intermittent strabismus with or without mild amblyopia			
slight unsteady central LE RE	-- --	No	SwoA
central steady LE RE	ARC 40"	Surgery, age 16	SwoA
manifest nystagmus	UHARC+ --	Surgery, age 2	SwoA
1 nasal and superior RE	-- --	Therapy initiated 1 month before study	SwoA
1/2 nasal LE	-- --	No	SA
Former strabismic patients			
manifest nystagmus	NRC 140"	Surgery, age 3	AA
None	NRC --	Surgery, age 8	AA
latent nystagmus	-- --	Surgery, age 5	SA

Key: ET = esotropia XT = exotropia ARC = anomalous retinal correspondence NRC = normal retinal correspondence HT = hypertropia SA = strabismic amblyopia AA = anisometropic amblyopia SwoA = strabismus without amblyopia EPH = esophoria HPH = hyperphoria

+ Unharmonious ARC

Table II - Absence of Normal Disparity Vergence in Cross-section of Patients Tested

Patient	Absence of Normal Disparity Vergence
Constant-strabismus amblyopia	
1	Yes
2	Yes
5	Yes
7	Yes
Amblyopia without strabismus	
9	Most of the time
10	No
11	Yes
Intermittent strabismus without amblyopia	
13	Yes
14	Yes
Former strabismus patients	
17	Most of the time
18	Yes

Table III - Versional Eye Movement Abnormalities in Patients Having Intermittent strabismus With or Without Mild Amblyopia

Patient	Nystagmus	Saccadic Intrusions	Increased Saccadic Latencies	Abnormal Saccadic Substitution	Increased Drift
12	No	Yes	No	No	Very little in non-dominant eye
13	No	Yes	Each eye	No	Very little in non-dominant eye
14	No	No	Mildly Amblyopic Eye Only	Mildly Amblyopic Eye Only	Some of the time in mildly amblyopic eye
15	No	Yes	No	No	Some of the time in mildly amblyopic eye
16	Yes; Manifest Nystagmus	No	-	-	No

Table IV - Versional Eye Movement Abnormalities in Patients Having Amblyopia Without Strabismus

Patient	Nystagmus	Saccadic Intrusions	Increased Saccadic Latencies	Abnormal Saccadic Substitution	Increased Drift
9	No	No	Yes	No	Yes
10	No	No	No	No	Yes
11	No	No	Yes	Yes	Yes

Table V - Versional Eye Movement Abnormalities in Patients Having Constant Strabismic Amblyopia or Formerly Having Strabismus

Patient	Nystagmus	Saccadic Intrusions	Increased Saccadic Latencies	Abnormal Saccadic Substitution	Increased Drift
1	No	Yes	No	No	Yes
2	No	Yes	No	Yes	Yes
3	Yes; manifest nystagmus	No	No	No	No
4	Yes; manifest nystagmus	No	Yes	-	No
5	No	Yes	Yes	Yes	Yes
6	No	No	Yes	Yes	Yes
7	No	Yes	Yes	Yes	Yes
8	Yes; latent nystagmus	No	No	-	No
17*	Yes; manifest nystagmus	No	No	-	No
18*	No	-	-	-	-
19*	Yes; latent nystagmus	No	No	No	No

*Formerly Strabismic Patient

in which strabismic or anisometropic amblyopia are the two basic functional amblyopic categories, or ours which is based simply on the presence of strabismus or amblyopia, serve as a difference way of approaching the same problem.

II. Similar Effects on Disparity Vergence by the Suppression of Strabismus and by that of Ambylopia

Absence of disparity vergence

Most patients with strabismus and/or amblyopia exhibit normal disparity vergence responses(14,15). Although latencies were normal, patients made unequal vergence movements in each eye. Vergence amplitudes were always smaller in the dominant eye than in the fellow eye; the average vergence amplitude of the dominant eye was approximately 18% of that of the fellow eye. The unequal vergences were accompanied by a binocular saccade that served to place the fovea of the dominant eye close to the new target. The combination of this saccade and the small amplitude vergence functioned to place and maintain the dominant eye on the new target (Figure 2).

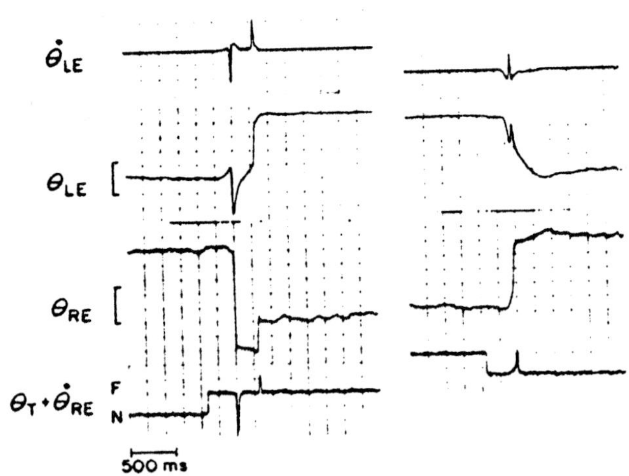

Figure 2. Abnormal vergence in amblyopia and in strabismus: absence of disparity vergence, with presence of asymmetrical accommodative vergence and monocularly driven saccades; note inequality of saccades due to muscular interaction.

When one eye was occluded, responses of control subjects to the symmetric vergence stimuli resembled responses recorded in our patients under binocular viewing conditions. Each contained unequal vergence with the smaller amplotude occurring the viewing eye of the control subjects and the dominant eye of the patients. Each used a binocular saccade, triggered by the monocular retinal error in the viewing or dominant eye to bring the fovea of that eye near the new target. In the control subject we know that accommodative vergence produces the unequal vergence amplotudes since occluding one eye "opens the loop" of the disparity vergence control system. We suspect accommodative vergence is also responsible for the unequal vergence movements in the patients, as will be shown below.

When patients were monocularly occluded so that only the dominant eye viewed the symmetrically positioned targets, responses agreed both qualitatively and quantitatively with the symmetric vergence responses from these patients under binocular viewing conditions. As with the control subjects, blocking of one eye caused accommodation to drive vergence, producing unequal vergence amplitudes(16). The monocular retinal error produced by the target change caused a binocular saccade placing the dominant eye on the new target.

Neither degree of strabismus nor grade of amblyopia in patients with constant strabismus amblyopia had any effect on the responses to the symmetric vergence stimuli. Patients with small angle strabismus and deep amblyopia produced symmetric vergence responses similar to those of patients who had mild amblyopia and small angle strbismus. Furthermore, the presence of ARC did not alter the basic response. Within our group of patients three were successfully treated for amblyopia or strabismus. One patient received orthoptics therapy for amblyopia and eccentric fixation in the left eye. After training his visual acuity increased from 20/110 to 20/20 and his eccentric fixation reduced from 2 prism diopters to zero. His vergence movements recorded shortly after termination of orthoptics treatment contained the same characteristic abnormal verence response recorded in most of our patients. Thus, even after normalization of visual acuity and centralization of fixation, normal disparity vergence responses were never recorded in this former amblyope. Interestingly, some other oculomotor findings such as saccadic latency also remained abnormal in this patient during and subsequent to successful amblyopia therapy. Patients with a history of strabismus as a child and surgical correction to reduce the strabismus were also included in our sample and again showed the typical abnormal vergence responses. Another patient who now has an exophoria was operated on at age 8 to correct a squint of his left eye. His symmetric vergence responses were similarto those of the other patients in our study having strabismus but who were not surgically corrected. However, still another patient who had an esotropia surgically corrected at age 3 and presently has esophoria, had intermittent episodes of normal convergence interspersed with more frequent abnormal responses. The striking absence of disparity vergence in our patients may be related to stimulus form. If we had used large field stimuli(17) or if we had equalized perceptual efficacy of the stimulus to each eye (for example, by using neutral density filters in front of the dominant eye) we might have observed true disparity responses. This possibility is consistent with our notion of suppression as a common factor in strabismics and in amblyopes. Further research with careful eye movement recordings will decide whether the slow, irregular and inconsistent changes clinically observed with strabismic amblyopic patients in amblyoscopes are in fact true disparity vergence reponses or perhaps reflect slow changes in tonic or proximal innervational levels. These results in our patients demonstrate the absence of disparity vergence and the presence of normal accommodative vergence that together with monocularly generated binocular saccades are able to move the dominant eye onto target. Similar results have been found by Quere(18,18a) and colleagues in the laboratory and Pickwell and Hampshire(19) in the clinic on strabismic and amblyopic subjects.

Accommodative vergence

Disparity vergence is part of the near triad: accommodation, vergence and pupil (all linked synkinetically by fixed CNS connections). Thus, a disparity stimulus driving vergence also produces a vergence accommodative response (with a gain of about 0.7 equivalent to an AC/C of 4 prism D/D); conversely, a blue stimulus driving accommodation also produces an accommodative vergence response (with a gain of about 0.6 equivalent to a CAC ratio of 0.1 D/prism D). Maddox(20) conjectures that accomodative vergence was primary and "fusion supplement" completed the triadic response; Fincham and Walton(21) measured the active vergence accommodation and speculated that it was primary. Stark, following Donders and Hering(22), felt that both accommodative vergence and vergence accommodation were always active and suggested that for a large enough disparity (a few degrees) the stimulus would lie off the fovea and the accommodation system would then be unable to appreciate target blur. This allowed vergence accommodation to play a dominant role by providing a mechanism that acts on sensory input and not by changing synkinetic gains. Accommodative vergence was first studied by Mueller(23); he observed that if one eye were covered, and the viewing eye changed fixation from a far to a near target along its line of sight, the covered eye rotated inward.

During accommodative vergence binocular vergence movements were first observed and recorded by us in all of the several hundred eye movements analyzed in five subjects. This included viewing with the dominant and non-dominant eye, predictable and non-predictable stimulus presentations, and for convergence and non-predictable stimulus presentations, and for convergence and divergence. These records clearly demonstrate the binocular nature of accommodative vergence(16).

Our patients′ recordings show the unexpected predominance of accommodative vergence. The absence of disparity vergence leave open the accommodative vergence triadic synkinesis mechanisms as a continuing and powerful vergence response controller. The arguments for the presence of accommodative vergence in our patients are that the patients′ monocular response is the same as their binocular response, that the patients′ monocular response is the same as the normal subjects′ monocular response, and the binocularity of the patients′ response is about the same amplitude of the normal subjects′ response. The amplitude of vergence in the dominant eye is about 18% of that of the non-dominant eye; in normal controls the amplitude of the viewing eye movement is about 12% of that of the covered eye.

Monocular-error-driven binocular saccades

The presence of the monocular driven binocular saccade in our patients is easily understood. Disparity may not be perceived because of the suppression of the non-dominant eye. The retinal eccentricity in the dominant eye is calculated as a horizontal position error that requires a horizontal saccade to correct it. The saccade should, of course, be binocular according to Hering′s Law.

Unequal saccades: not a violation of Hering′s Law

The occurrence of monocularly driven saccades upon a background of ongoing accommodative vergence in our patients with striking absence of disparity vergence provided the opportunity for a further exciting observation--the presence of apparently non-Hering's Law saccades during vergence(24,25,15,26) (Kenyon and Stark, in press). These unequal saccades were present in at least 85% of the vergence movements found in all diagnostic groups of patients. In each saccadic pair the smaller saccade opposes the vergency movement. Saccades that occur before and after the vergence have equal amplitudes, indicating that these unequal saccades are not an artifact of the recording system. The inequalities of these saccades are not restricted to our patients, since apparently non-Hering's Law saccades are present during vergence movements in normals. From Hering's Law of equal innervation we would expect binocular saccades to be equal. If the neurophysiological controller signals to the two eyes are different, then this would be a violation of Hering's Law. How can we identify the mechanism of production of the inequality of these saccades? One way is to simulate the interaction with linearly additive saccadic and vergence controller signals, thus obeying Hering's Law, acting on a biomechanical model of eye muscle and globe. Our studies showed (Kenyon and Stark, in press) the saccades in the simulation to show inequalities similar to those seen in our patient group and in normal subjects with ongoing accommodative vergence or ongoing asymmetrical disparity vergence (Figure 3). The same qualitative rule applies: saccades directed opposite the vergence are truncated in amplitude and velocity and the opposite occurs for saccades going in the same direction as the vergence. Since the model obeys Hering's Law of Equal Innervation and uses only linear summation of controller signals, non-linear summation of saccadic amplitudes with the ongoing vergence seen in these simulations must occur as the result of interactions within the biomechanical mechanisms of the plant model. We conclude that the inequality of saccades is due not to a violation of Hering's Law per se at the neural level but to a biomechanical interaction in the muscle globe peripheral apparatus (i.e. plant).

III. Different Effects on Versional Eye Movement Function Produced by Binocular Motor Deficits of Strabismus and by Monocular Sensory Deficits of Amblyopia

Saccadic intrusions

Saccadic intrusions are generally executed in opposite directions separted by 150-500 msec, occasionally less. The second saccade of an intrusion generally brings the eye back

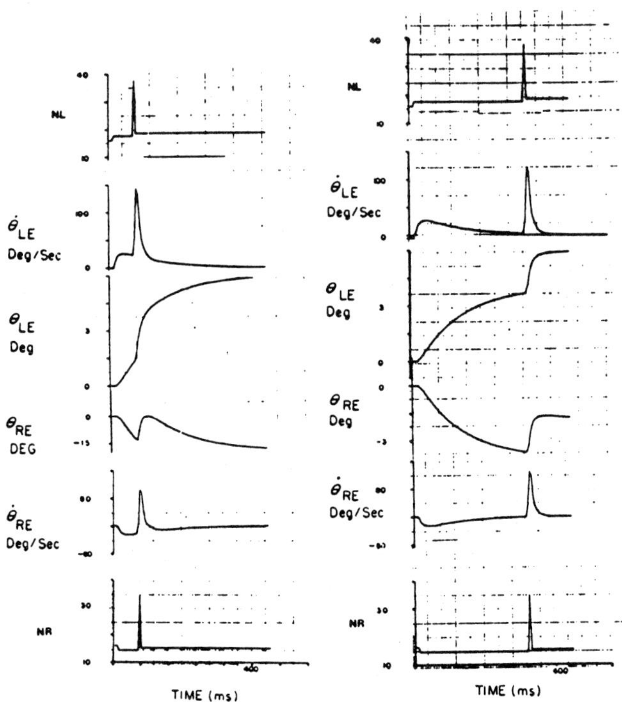

Figure 3. Simulation producing unequal saccades by muscular interaction. Note linear addition of reciprocally innervated controller signals obeying Hering's law.

towards the baseline, resulting in little net change in eye position(27,28). Average intrusion amplitude was 0.7 degrees with a frequency about 1 per second (Figure 4). In most instances, the baseline position before and immediately after completion of a saccadic intrusion was similar. Subjects were able to follow random target step displacements to the left or right as small as 0.4 degrees in amplitude. In many instances, considerable drift did not precede initiation of the intrusion. When drifts did occur, the accumulated position error was usually corrected by a single saccade. These could be as small as 5 minutes in amplitude, as measured during high-gain recordings. Therefore, it is clear that saccadic intrusions are a pair (sometimes three) of pre-programmed saccades not serving that oculomotor function of correcting for drift-induced position errors. Since saccadic intrusions were rarely found in amblyopia without strabismus, but typically found in strabismus without amblyopia, the intrusions appear to be related to the presence of strabismus and not amblyopia. However, the presence of saccadic intrusions is not unique to strabismus. They are frequently found in patients wit neurological disorders, specific dyslexia, and schizophrenia and are also observed less frequently in normal subject.

Special maneuvers with saccadic intrusions

Saccadic intrusions were found during monocular fixation with the amblyopic eye in four of five subjects with constant strabismus amblyopia. When a large amount of drift occurred with target fading, saccadic intrusions appear to be unrelated to abnormal eye position or error detection in the amblyopic eye (Figure 4). Saccadic intrusions were not at all the pattern of correction of drift eror, but rather this was carried out by one or more unidirectional corrective saccades. Significantly, saccadic intrusions then occurred after reappearance of the target. Thus this finding does not provide strong evidence to relate saccadic intrusions to a "Lawwill(29) adaptive phenomenon"--to prevent fading or to "revive" a faded retinal image.

Steinman, Cunitz, Timberlake and Herman(30) observed that microsaccades could be suppressed when experienced subjects were instructed to "hold their eye steady" rather than "fixate" in the presence of a visible target. During the "hold" command, our patients sometimes remarked that they did not pay as much attention to target detail and perhaps position errors as they did during the "fixate" command. However, during both sets of instructions, attention and motivation to perform the prescribed task successfully was high. Some stated that the amblyopic eye seemded more unsteady during the "hold" command, but that target clarity was similar for both condition. One patient noted that at

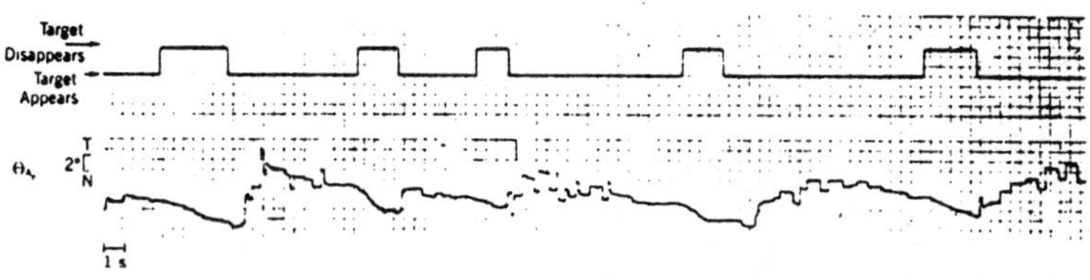

Figure 4. Saccadic intrusions are not produced when fixation target "fades" or disappears.

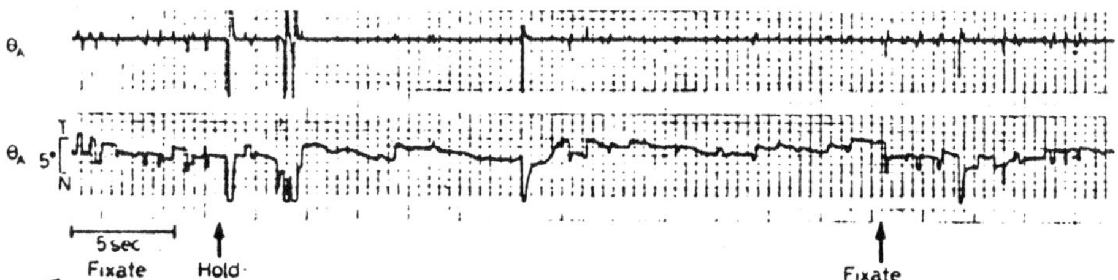

Figure 5. Saccadic intrusions are suppressed with "hold" command.

times she relaxed accommodation and maintained relatively steady, "saccade free" fixation by concentrating on the defocused image; at other times, defocusing was not essential to suppress her fixational saccades.

The observation most pertinent to our patients was that during the "hold" command, there was a marked reduction in saccadic intrusion frequency (Figure 5) especially which is easy to see in the velocity traces(28). An earlier report of our work(31) was confirmed by Schor and Hallmark(32). In contrast, during the "fixate" command saccadic intrusions occurred at usual rates and amplitudes. Thus, oculomotor intentional fixational gaze, rather than a sensory-related phenomenon such as might result from strabismus-induced "fixation degradation", is implicated in the saccadic intrusion generating mechanism in our strabismus patient. At times saccadic intrustions could be suppressed, but with occurrence of increased drift amplitude and velocity. At other times and in other patients suppression of saccadic intrusions was possible without occurrence of markedly increased drift. Again, this implicates an intentional gaze mechanism for saccadic intrusion and relates them to fixational microsaccades that have been suspected to have other than error-correcting functions. Interestingly, changes in instruction to strabismic or amblyopic subjects from "fixate carefully on the target" to "hold theeye steady" (in the presence of the target) could decrease fixational saccadic frequency by 50% to 90%, similar to that found for normal persons.

Latent nystagmus

Latent nystagmus is a disorder of the oculomotor system wherein the nystagmus is either absent or normally present during binocular viewing, but upon occlusion of an eye, a conjugate jerk then ensues. The slow phase in the "gazing" eye is nasal (Figure 6 left). The term "gazing" eye is used instead of viewing eye since it is suspected that a motor control deficit and not a sensory abnormality underlies the genesis of latent nystagmus. Evidence for this comes from van Vliet´s(33) experiment with an Ewald pseudoscope. Here the latent nystagmus occurred with the slow phase nasally in the eye through which the subject directed his gaze and which he incorrectly thought he was viewing! The association of latent nystagmus with alternating hyperphoria(34) again suggests a motor gaze deficit and not a sensory one. Burian and von Noorden(11) prefer the term dissociated vertiacal deviation to emphasize the noncomitant and nonvergence nature of the

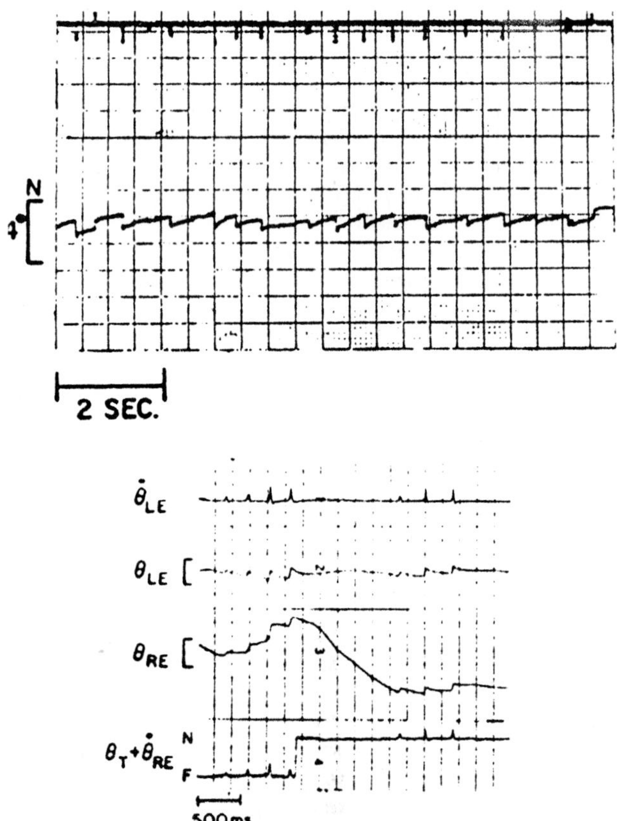

Figure 6. Latent nystagmus (left) with nasal drift of gazing and Manifest nystagmus (right) superimposed on ongoing vergence.

deficit wherein "either eye turns up when the fellow eye fixates". Pure latent nystgmus was found in two out of eighteen patients with strabismus; it was not found in any patients having amblyopia only. Latent nystagmus had a mean frequency of 1.7 Hz, a mean amplitude of 1.0 degree and a mean slow phase velocity of 2.0 deg./sec.; dominant eye fixated. With our precise recording techniques we could be quite sure that our cases of latent nystagmus did not conceal a manifest nystagmus of very low amplitude(35).

Manifest nystagmus

Manifest nystagmus is a disorder of the oculomotor system wherein jerk nystagmus is present during monocular and binocular conditions in patients with strabismus. Again, as with latent nystagmus, manifest nystagmus was found in four out of eighteen patients with strabismus; and, in agreement with Gillies(36), not in patients having only amblyopia(28a). Monocular fixtion with the amblyopic eye in a patient increased the amplitude of manifest nystagmus to 5 degrees as compared with 1.5 degrees with monocular fixation with the dominant eye ofr 2.5 degrees with binocular fixation. When one patient changed from fixation in the light to "fixation" in total darkness, mean nystagmus amplitude increased. This suggests that in the light a velocity-correcting system (probalby smooth pursuit) requiring visual feedback was operating to counteract the tru nystagmus as revealed in the dark; again, evidence pointing to a motor gaze defect rather than to a sensory deficit underlying manifest nystagmus. Nystagmus in strabismic patients could also be reduced by use of the "hold" command(37) and by eye movement auditory feedback(38).

When one of our patients with manifest nystagmus made vergence eye movements, the slow phase of the nystagmuc summated algebraically with that of a vergence. In the divergence movement (Figure 6 right) the slow phase of the nystagmus and the accommodative vergence in the viewing eye oppose each other. This interaction counteracts the slow phase of the nystagmus, keeping the viewing eye stationary on the target. With no drift of the eye off the target, the saccadic phase of this nystagmus was absent. This shows thatthe slow phase in this patient's nystagmus is primary and that the saccade is used to correct for the retinal error produced by the drift.

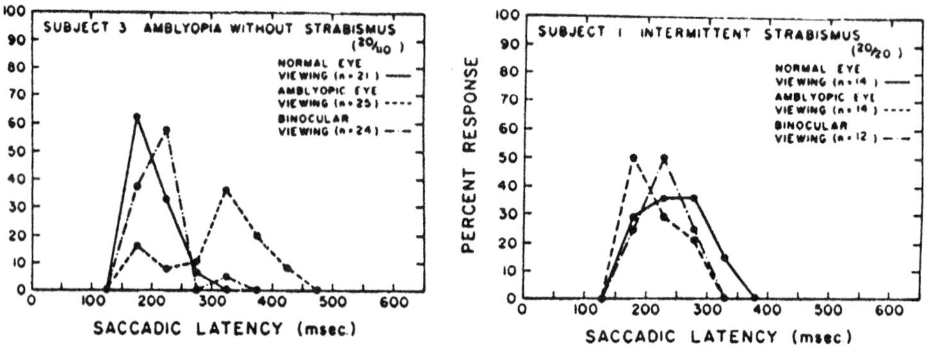

Figure 7. Increased saccadic latency in amblyopia contrasted with normal saccadic latency in strabismus.

Increased saccadic latency

An important function of the saccadic eye movement system is foveation of peripheral retinal stimuli. Saccadic latency has been extensively studied in normal human subjects, whereas few investigations of saccadic latency have been conducted in subjects having amblyopia and strabismus.

Increased saccadic latencies (horizontal movements) were observed in amblyopic eyes in 6 of 11 subjects having amblyopia with or without strabismus(39,40). Significant increases in latency or differences between dominant and nondominant eyes in our two subjects having intermittent strabismus without amblyopia were not observed (Figure 7).

We studied targets in the "near periphery" and found significant effects. Mackensen(9) used more peripheral stimuli, greater than 15 degrees, and reported no significant increase (250 vs 225 ms); he theorized that the peripheral retina was little, if at all, affected in amblyopia and turned to eye-hand reaction time measures to study the centrl retina. He now found drammatic differences in reaction time between the amblyopic and normal eye (325 vs 225 ms), and this was confirmed by von Noorden(41) and Goldstein and Greenstein(42). Recently, evidence of increased saccadic latency for vertical eye movements in amblyopic eyes have been established(43), as well as results suggesting the amblyopic delay involves visual but not auditory sensory modalities(44).

Increased fixational drift

Drift refers to slow movement of the eye during attempted steady fixation. Drift was considered abnormal if the amplitude exceeded 12 min arc and/or the velocity exceeded 20 min arc/sec; these criteria were developed in our oculomotor laboratory following resting of several hundred individuals, including experienced normal subjects, aive normal subjects and clinic patients. Increased drift was related to the presence of amblyopia since it was found in amblyuopia without strabismus but not in strabismus without amblyopia(28,45). Increased drift amplitude and velocity in the amblyopic eye was in strong contrast to steady monocular fixation with the dominant eye or with binocular fixation.

Recordings of binocular eyue movement during monocular fixation with the amblyopic eye clearly show that the large slow movement in the amblyopic eye is drift and is not due solely to accommodative vergence, as reflected by increased accommodation variability in amblyopic eyes(46), since the movement is largest in the viewing eye (Figure 8). It is not due solely to smooth pursuit, since the movements are nonconjugate. Finally, it is not due to disparity (fusional) vergence, since the movements are not symmetrical and occur with one eye occluded.

The paucity of corrective fixational saccades with amplitudes comparable to the drifts meant that errors created by abnormal drift were generally corrected by driftmovements in the opposite direction. This suggests that the microsaccadic system, one of whose normal functions is to correct for drift-induced fixation errors, may be less effective in amblyopic eyes, perhaps related to increased saccadic latencies. Drift may also be due to delayed or reduced velocity error detection in the smooth pursuit velocity-correcting system or to normal drift characteristics for fixation with a non-foveal region(47), as most patients

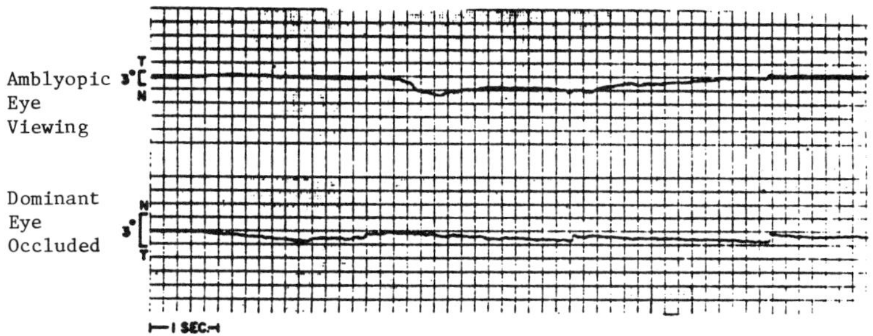

Figure 8. Increased fixational drift.

had eccentric fixation. Increased drift might degrade visual acuity not by producing retinal-image motion across the fovea, but by moving the retinal image on to more eccentric positions, while increased drift amplitudes would also contribute to increased variability in any acuity measure.

Decreased smooth pursuit gain

Pursuit gain for tracking of targets having larger amplitudes (4 and 8 deg) was also of interest. When visual acuity was decreased, low gain pursuit, followed by large saccades correcting for position errors, was observed(48,49,50,31). However, once visual acuity reached 2/25, pursuit gain was generally higher and less variable. Pursuit gain for monocular tracking with the dominant eye generally was within normal limits for our laboratory standards.

Saccadic substitution

The results of small amplitude (less than 2 degrees) ramp tracking with the amblyopic eye clearly demonstrated that patients primarily sued saccades rather than smooth pursuit movements to follow the target (Figure 9)(51). Substitution of abnormally large saccades for small amplitude smoot pursuit movements occurred during small amplitude, constant velocity tracking with the amblyopic eye in response to both nasalward and templeward target motions on the retina (Figure 9). That tracking small amplitude stimuli binocularly or monocularly with the dominant eye never resulted in abnormal saccadic substitution further points to a sensory rather than motor basis for this pursuit defect.

Although there is no clear mechanism to explain the phenomenon of abnormal saccadic substitution, there are at

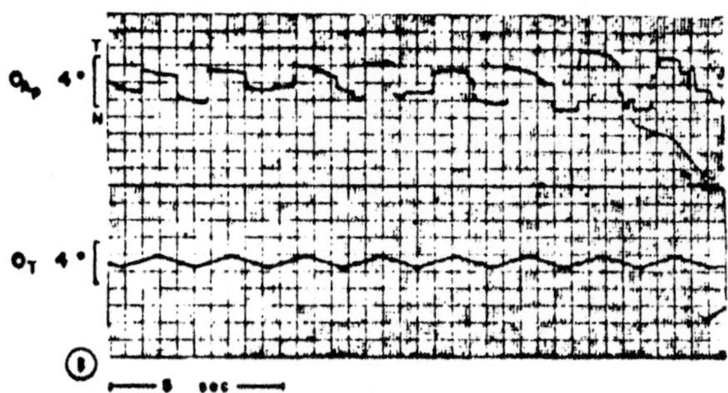

Figure 9. Abnormal saccadic substitution.

least three possibilities. The first is abnormal direction sense in amblyopic eyes. As a result of amblyopia, a depression of the directional-sensitivity gradient over the central retina may occur. This could result in impaired and/or markedvariability of direction sense, including errors or biases in estimation of angular distance of targets relative to the preferred fixation locus. In the present situation, overestimation of small angle target movements on the retina would result in the inappropriately large eye movement exhibited by our patients. It is interesting to speculate that our notion of abnormal direction sense in amblyopic eyes, based upon dynamic test results, may be related to eccentric fixation, which is based upon statis test results. Eccentric fixation is found in the majority of amblyopic eyes, and its presence suggests a shift in the zero sensorimotor directional reference point under "steady-state" monocular test conditions. A second mechanism is suppression, commonly found in amblyopic eyes under binocular test conditions. A sensorially depressed central zone would correspond to all or part of the area undergoind suppression in the amblyopic eye during binocular viewing. If this is true, a strategy of placing the target just outside this depressed region might be adopted during monocular tracking with the amblyopic eye. Direction, amplitude and velocity of target movement could be processed for a longer period of time and could provide a possible explanation for the abnormal tracking response, consistent with otherdelays in amblyopic eyes. A third explanation might simply be that abnormal saccadic substitution represents a normal phenomenon for small amplitude pursuit tracking with the peripheral retina. However, the persistence of this abnormal response in one subject whose fixation centralized during orthoptic therapy does not lend support to this idea.

Orthoptics

Quantitative eye movement analysis was carried out in an amblyope during an extended period of orthoptics treatment(52). Several aspects of eye movement control improved in the amblyopic eye during treatment: decrease in drift amplitude, decrease in drift velocity, increase in pursuit gain (Figure 10). These findings demonstrate that as amblyopia decreased and fixation became centralized, certain aspects of eye movement control, primarily under the province of the smooth-pursuit system, could be modified by the orthoptics therapy. Furthermore, the findings suggest that the "critical period" for oculomotor plasticity for these aspects of eye movement our amblyope extended into adulthood.

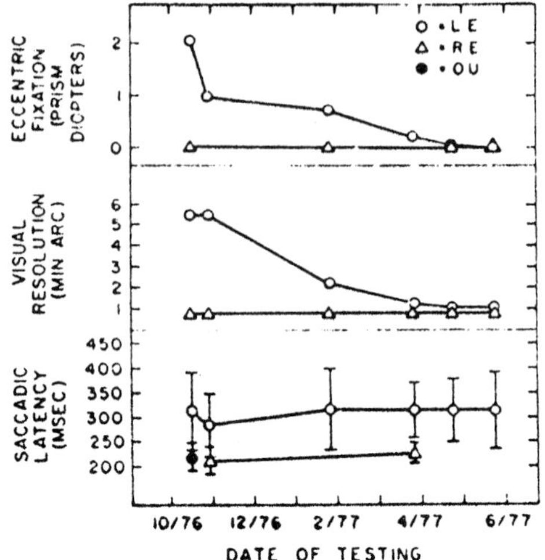

Figure 10. Orthoptics treatment of amblyope showing amelioration of visual functions without normalization of prolonged saccadic latencies.

However, other aspects of eye movement control in the amblyopic eye remained abnormal throughout treatment: increased saccadic latencies, abnormal saccadic substitution, and static overshooting. Perhaps those neural channels and neural elements used for spatial resolution and responsible for eccentric fixation can be functionally modified in the adult amblyope and require a relatively short course of therapy for recovery (the visual acuity recovery function for our adult amblyope was similar to that measured in a young amblyope). Perhaps for certain other neural channels and neural elements (probably "transient" channels) involved in saccadic initiation recovery in an adult amblyope is either very slow or no lonerpossible. The increase in saccadic latencies suggests a processing delay over the central retina in the amblyopic eye involving pathways from the amblyopic eye to centers controlling saccadic initiation, such as the superior colliculus, although involvement of parietal lobe mechanisms underlying directed visual attention remains a distinct possibility.

Although only one patient was studied, we believe that our results and their clinical implications are of interest to those involved in clinical as well as theoretical aspects of amblyopia. However, recently similare results have been obtained in older amblyopes (ages 6-28 years) following intensive orthoptic therapy(53) (Hokoda and Ciuffreda, in preparation). In addition, static aspects of accommodation and other vision functions improve during and following such therapy.

IV. Future Questions

These results provoke many interesting questions. How can our simple separation of amblyopia without strabismus from strabismus without amblyopia be reconciled with more classical classifications? Will our findings be robust to further more extensive surveys with many more patients? What clues to the underlying deficits in neurological control of binocular vision can be extracted from our studies? Is suppression in strabismus and amblyopia the common mechanism blocking disparity vergence? Where are the neuroanatomical loci of the deficits? What are the neuropathophysiological mechanisms?

ACKNOWLEDGEMENTS

We would like to thank NASA-Ames Research Center (NCC 2-86) and NIH Grant EY03541 for partial support.

REFERENCES

1. Duke-Elder S, Wybar K: System of Ophthalmology, Vol VI, London, Henry Kimpton, 1973.

2. Griffin JR: Binocular Anomalies: Procedures for Vision Therapy, Professional Press, Chicago, 1976.

3. deBuffon GL: Dissertation sur les causes du strabisme ou des yeux louches. Memoires de l'Academie Royale des Sciences, Paris, 1746.

4. Kirschen DK, Flom MC: Visual acuity at different retinal loci of eccentrically fixating functional amblyopes. Am J Opt Physiol Optics 55:144-150, 1978.

5. Levi DM, Harwerth RS: Spatio-temporal interactions in anisometropic and strabismic amblyopia. Invest Ophthalmol Vis Sci 16:90-95, 1977.

6. Bedell HE, Flom MC: Monocular spatial distrotion in strabismic amblyopia. Invest Ophthalmol Vis Sci 20:263-268, 1981.

7. Hess RF, Campbell FW, Greenhalgh T: On the nature of the neural abnormality in human amblyopia; neural aberrations and neural sensitivity loss. Pflugers Arch 377:201-207, 1978.

8. Lawden MC, Hess RF, Campbell FW: The discriminability of spatial phase relationships in amblyopia. Vision Research 22:1005-1016, 1982.

9. Mackensen G: Reaktionszeitmessungen bei amblyopie. Albrecht von Graefes. Arch Ophthalmol 159:636-642, 1958.

10. Brock FW, Givner I: Fixation anomalies in amblyopia. Arch Ophthalmol 47:775-786, 1952.

11. Burian HM, von Noorden GK: Binocular Vision and Ocular Motility, C.V. Mosby Co., St. Louis, 1974.

12. Amos JF: Refractice amblyopia: its classification, etiology and epidemiology. J Am Opt Assn 48:489-497, 1977.

13. von Noorden GK: Classification of amblyopia. Am J Ophthalmol 63:238-244, 1967.

14. Kenyon RV, Ciuffreda KJ, Stark L: Dynamic vergence eye movements in strabismus and amblyopia: symmetric vergence. Invest Ophthalmol Vis Sci 19:60-74, 1980.

15. Kenyon RV, Ciuffreda KJ, Stark L: Dynamic vergence eye movements in strabismus and amblyopia: asymmetric vergence. Br J Ophthalmol 65:167-176, 1981.

16. Kenyon RV, Ciuffreda KJ, Stark L: Binocular eye movements during accommodative vergence. Vis Res 18:546-555, 1978.

17. Hooten K, Myers E, Worrall R, Stark L: Cyclovergence: the motor response to cyclodisparity. Graefes Arch Clin Exp Ophthalmol 210:65-68, 1979.

18. Quere MA: Abnormal ocular movements in amblyopia. Trans Ophthalmol Soc UK 99:401-406, 1979.

18a. Quere MA, Pechereau A, Lavenant F: Etude electro-oculographique des mouvements de vergence. Premiere Partie: La vergence symetrique. J Fr Ophthalmol 4:25-32, 1981.

19. Pickwell LD, Hampshire R: Jump convergence test in strabismus. Ophthalmic Physiol Opt 1:123-124, 1981.

20. Maddox EE: Investigations on the relationship between

convergence and accommodation of the eyes. J Anat 20:475-505, 565-584, 1886.

21. Fincham EF, Walton J: The reciprocal actions of accomodation and convergence. J Physiol 137:488-508, 1957.

22. Hering E: The Theory of Binocular Vision, Bridgeman B and Stark L (eds.): Plenum Press, New York, NY 1977.

23. Meuller J: Elements of Physiology, trans. by Baly W (1843), Vol 2, Taylor & Walton, London, 1826.

24. Kenyon RV, Ciuffreda KJ, Stark L: Binocular eye movements during accommodative vergence. Ass Res Vis Ophthalmol, Sarasota, FL, 1976.

25. Kenyon RV, Ciuffreda KJ, Stark L: Unequal saccades during vergence. Am J Optom Physiol Opt 57:586-594, 1980.

26. Ono H, Nakamizo S, Steinback M: Nonadditivity of vergence and saccadic eye movements. Vision Res 18:735-739, 1978.

27. Ciuffreda KJ, Kenyon RV, Stark L: Saccadic intrusions in strabismus. Arch Ophthalmol 97:1673-1679, 1979.

28. Ciuffreda KJ, Kenyon RV, Stark L: Suppression of fixational saccades in strabismic and anisometropic amblyopia. Ophthalmic Res 11:31-39, 1979.

28a. Ciuffreda KJ, Kenyon RV, Stark L: Fixational eye movements in amblyopia and strabismus. J Am Optom Assoc 50:1251-1258, 1979.

29. Lawwill T: Local adaptation in functional amblyopia. Am J Ophthalmol 65:903-906, 1968.

30. Steinman RM, Cunitz RJ, Timberlake GT, Herman M: Voluntary control of microsaccades during maintained monocular fixation. Science 155:1577-1579, 1967.

31. Ciuffreda KJ: Eye movements in amblyopia and strabismus. Ph.D. Dissertation, University of California, School of Optometry, Berkeley, 1977.

32. Schor C, Hallmark W: Slow control of eye position in strabismic amblyopia. Invest Ophthalmol Vis Sci 17:577-581, 1978.

33. Van Vliet, AGM: On the central mechanism of latent nystagmus. Acta Ophthalmol 51:772-781, 1973.

34. Anderson JR: Latent nystagmus and alternating hyperphoria. Br J Ophthalmol 38:217-231, 1954.

35. Dell'Osso, LF, Schmidt D, Daroff RB: Latent, manifest latent and congenital nystagmus. Arch Ophthalmol 97:1877-1885, 1979.

36. Gillies WE: The significance of nystagmoid movement in amblyopia. Arruga A In International Strabismus Symposium, New York, Skarger(ed), 1968.

37. Ciuffreda KJ: Jerk nystagmus: some new findings. Am J Optom Physiol Optics 56:521-530, 1979.

38. Ciuffreda KJ, Goldrich SG, Neary C: Use of eye movements auditory biofeedback in the control of nystagmus. Am J Optom Physiol Optics 59:396-409, 1982.

39. Ciuffreda KJ, Kenyon RV, Stark L: Increased saccadic latencies in amblyopic eyes. Invest Ophthalmol 17:697-702, 1978a.

40. Ciuffreda KJ, Kenyon RV, Stark L: Processing delays in amblyopic eyes: evidence from saccadic latencies. Am J Opt Physiol Opt 55:187-196, 1978.

41. von Noorden GK: Reaction time in normal and amblyopic eyes. Arch Ophthalmol 66:695-703, 1961.

42. Goldstein JH, Greenstein F: Eye-hand coordination in strabismus. In P. Fells (ed): The First Congress of the International Strabismological Assocation, C. V. Mosby Co., St. Louis, 1971.

43. Mimura O, Kato H, Kani K, Shimo-oku M: Saccadic latencies in amblyopia using infrared television fundus camera with two dimensional stimuli. Jpn J Ophthlamol 25:248-257, 1981.

44. Fukushima M, Tsutsui J: Visually and auditory evoked saccadic reaction time in amblyopia. In Strabismus Vol II, Reinecke RD (ed), Grune & Stratton, New York, NY (in press).

45. Ciuffreds KJ, Kenyon RV, Stark L: Increased drift in amblyopic eyes. Br J Ophthalmol 64:7-14, 1980.

46. Ciuffreds KJ, Kenyon RV: Accommodative vergence and accommodation in normals, amblyopes, and strabismics. In Vergence Eye Movements: Basic and Clinical Aspects, Ciuffreda and Schor (eds.), Butterworth, Boston, 101-173, 1983.

47. Zeevi YY, Peli E, Stark L: Study of eccentric fixation with secondary visual feedback. J Opt Soc Am 69:669-675, 1979.

48. von Noorden GK, Mackensen G: Pursuit movements of normal and amblyopic eyes: an electro-ophthalmographic study. II. Pursuit movements in amblyopic patients. Am J Ophthalmol 53:477-487, 1962.

49. Fukai S, Tsutsui J, Nakamura Y: Abnormal pursuit movements of the fellow eye in amblyopia with strabismus, in Orthoptics: Past Present Future, Moore S, Mein J, Stockbridge L (eds.): New York, NY, Stratton Intercontinental Medical Book Corporation, 1976.

50. Schor CM: A directional impairment of eye movement control in strabismus amblyopia. Invest Ophthalmol 14:692-697, 1975.

51. Ciuffreda KJ, Kenyon RV, Stark L: Abnormal saccadic substitution during small-amplitude pursuit tracking in amblyopic eyes. Invest Ophthalmol 18:506-516, 1979.

52. Ciuffreda KJ, Kenyon RV, Stark L: Different rates of functional recovery of eye movement during orthoptics treatment in adult amblyope. Invest Ophthalmol 18:213-219, 1979.

53. Selenow A, Ciuffreda KJ: Vision function recovery during orthoptic therapy in an exotropic amblyope with high unilateral myopia. Am J Opt Physiol Optics, (in press).

DISCUSSION BY G. KOMMERELL

Dr. Stark summarized his wide experience in exact eye movement recordings applied to strabismic patients. Clearly, the essential feature of constant strabismus is the lack of normal disparity vergence. The so-called pathological fusional movements, known to the ophthalmologists as "eating up prisms", are disparity responses which take alot more time than the normal disparity vergence. Nevertheless, they may be subject to future analysis with Dr. Stark´s fine instrumentation.

OPTOMOTOR EFFECT IN ESOTROPIA UNDER GENERAL ANESTHESIA

Y. Mitsui, O. Tamura, P.V. Berard, R. Reydy

ABSTRACT

The active discharges in electromyograms from bilateral medial recti in esotropia under general anesthesia taper off in the dark after 5 to 10 minutes and re-appear after re-exposure to the light. The re-firing by high illumination is not greater than that by low illumination; however, the lag time until re-firing appears is shorter when illumination is high, ranging from 20 seconds by 10,000 lux to 130 seconds by 1 lux. This optomotor effect is ipsilateral. It is supposed that there is a subcortical optomotor effect pathway extending to the extra-ocular muscles where the visual input possibly accelerates muscle afferent transmission.

INTRODUCTION

In esotropia active discharges from the medial recti muscles are frequently recorded in electromyograms (EMGs) done under general anesthesia.[1] Considerable evidence shows that an optomotor reflex plays an important role in the manifestation of esotropia.[2,3,4] Berard and his associates[5] found that a similar optomotor reflex occurs under general anesthesia. The purpose of this paper is to describe the optomotor effect in the EMG of esotropic subjects under general anesthesia.

MATERIALS AND METHODS

Subjects: EMGs of the four horizontal recti were examined in 20 cases of constant esotropia while the patients were under general anesthesia, in 16 of which active discharges from the medial recti appeared. These 16 cases were selected as subjects. They consisted of 9 males and 7 females, ranging in age from 6 months to 15 years.

Method: EMGs of the four horizontal recti were recorded while the patients were under general anesthesia by the same method and conditions reported previously.[1] After

STRABISMUS II
ISBN 0-8089-1424-3

confirmation of the presence of active discharges from the medial recti, the operating light (about 10,000 lux) and all lights in the room were turned off except for the minimum local illumination needed by the anesthetist to observe necessary meters. Illumination to the cornea of the patient was thus essentially zero. The procedure followed after the subjects had been in the dark for 10 minutes differed by case, the 14 cases being divided into three groups:

Group I, 10 cases: After 10 minutes in darkness, the right eye was spot-lighted useing a hand-ophthalmoscope placed close to the eye (about 300 lux to the cornea). Two minutes later the operating light was turned on so that both eyes were illuminated. The EMG recording was continued throughout.

Group II, 2 cases: After 10 minutes in the dark, the room was indirectly illuminated to a brightness of 1 lux at the cornea of the patient. Three minutes later the operating light was turned on.

Group III, 2 cases: After 10 minutes in the dark, the operating light was turned on.

Group IV, 2 cases: After 10 minutes in darkness, the right eye was spot lighted by a hand-ophthalmoscope placed close to the eye. The brightness of ophthalmoscope was reduced to 1 lux by the use of a filter. The left eye was covered by a black contact lens. Three minutes later the left eye was spot-lighted similarly after removing the contact lens while the spot-lighting on the right eye was continued.

RESULTS

The influence of light and dark on the EMG of esotropic patients while under general anesthesia showed the same pattern in all of the ten cases of group I. Examples of the pattern are shown in Figure 1, 2, and 3.

The active discharges from the medial recti began to taper off after 5 minutes in the dark and reached their minimum in 5 to 10 minutes (Fig 1-a). When the right eye was then spot-lighted in the dark, the discharge from the medial rectus of this eye began to increase after 40 to 50 seconds and reached the maximum in a few seconds thereafter, while the discharge from the left medial rectus remained unchanged

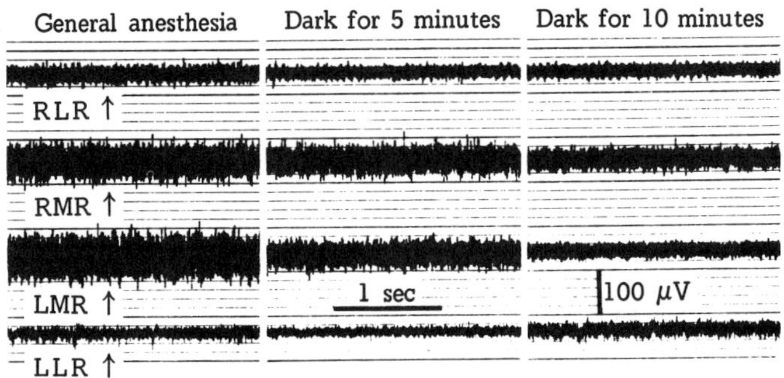

Figure 1. a: EMG of the four horizontal recti of an esotropic case under general anesthesia.

Left: under operating light. Center: after 5 minutes in the dark. Right: after 10 minutes in the dark.

Right eye spot-lighted

RLR ↓

RMR ↓

LMR ↓ 1 sec 100 μV

LLR ↓

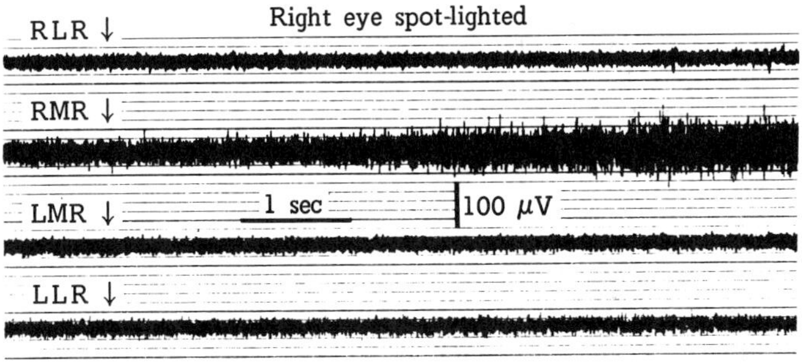

Figure 1. b: The same as above when the right eye was spot-lighted after 10 minutes in the dark.

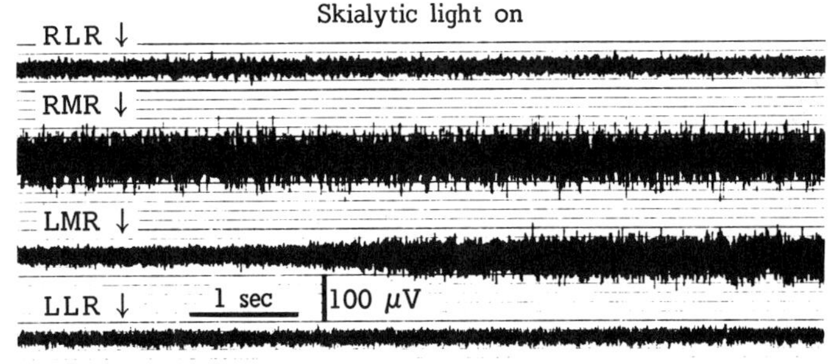

Figure 1. c: The same as above when the operating light was turned on after 2 minutes of spot-lighting on the right eye.

RLR ↓
RMR ↓
LMR ↓
LLR ↓
↓ Light turned off
60 sec
100 μV
1
6
7
Time in absolute darkness (minutes)

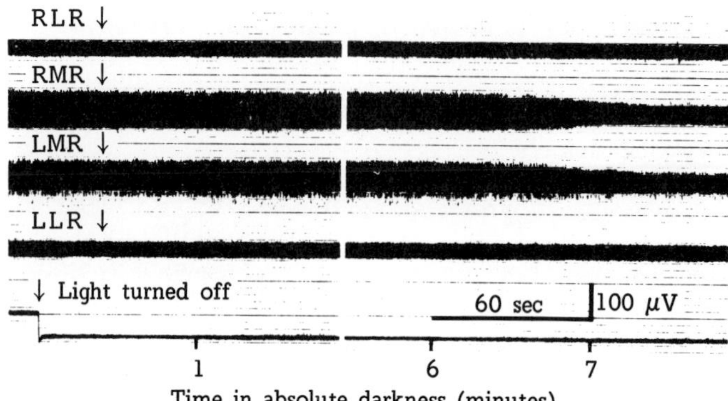

Figure 2. a: EMG of the four horizontal recti recorded at a low paper speed, showing the section of maintainance of darkness.

RLR ↓
RMR ↓
LMR ↓
LLR ↓
60 sec
100 μV
60 sec
↑
Spot-light turned on (right eye)
↑
Skialytic light turned on

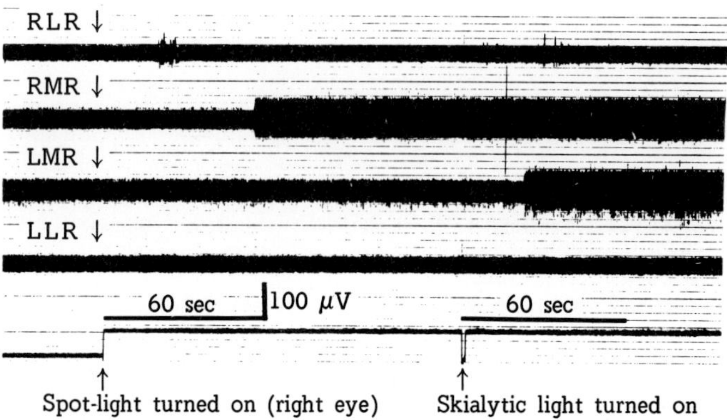

Figure 2. b: The same as above, showing the section starting from the time where the right eye was spot-lighted after darkness.

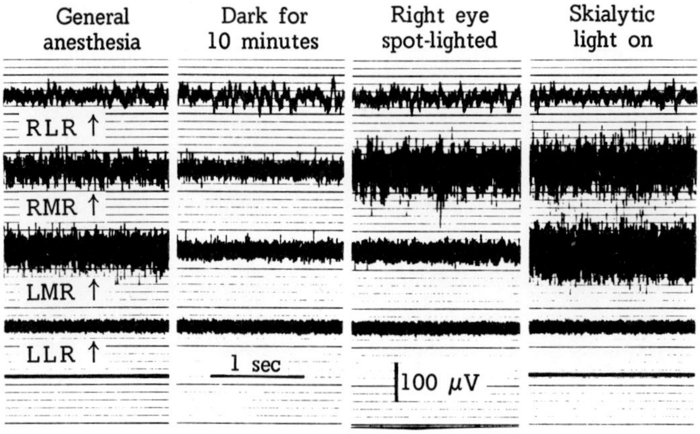

General anesthesia
Dark for 10 minutes
Right eye spot-lighted
Skialytic light on
RLR ↑
RMR ↑
LMR ↑
LLR ↑
1 sec
100 μV

(Fig 1-b). When the operating light was turned back on, an increased discharge from the left medial rectus also appeared (Fig 1-c).

The tapering off of discharges in the dark occurs insidiously and the reduction is visible only by comparing two distant sections of the usual EMG (Fig 1-a), or in one continuous section of the EMG when recorded at an extremely low paper speed (Fig 2-a). The increase of discharges by re-exposure to the light occurs rather suddenly and it is clearly visible even in one continuous section of the usual EMG (Fig 1-b and c), but is more obvious when recorded at a low paper speed (Fig 2-b).

A general tendency was to show rebound; that is, discharges from the medial recti under re-exposure to the light were apt to be greater than those recorded originally. An example is shown in Fig 3. This rebound was seen in 8 of the 10 cases examined.

No obvious changes in discharges from both lateral recti muscles were seen during the experiment.

Results in the 2 cases of group II showed that, 1) re-firing of the medial recti muscles was brought about by re-exposure to illumination as weak as 1 lux, 2) the lag time until re-firing appeared was long, lasting between 100 and 130 seconds, respectively; and 3) re-firing did not further increase when the operating room light was turned on (Fig 4).

Results in the 2 cases of group III showed that the lag time was shortened to 21 and 28 seconds, respectively, by re-exposure to 10,000 lux (Fig 5).

Results in the 2 cases of group IV were similar to those in the group I except that a decrease in the discharge from the right medial rectus appeared when the left medial rectus began to fire, suggesting the reciprocity in the firing from the both medial recti muscles (Fig 6). This decrease was not lasting, however. In one case it disappeared gradually during the period from 18 to 25 seconds (Fig 6) and in the other case it lasted for about 12 seconds, and then disappeared rather suddenly.

Figure 3. EMG of the four horizontal recti of an esotropic case. From the left to the right, 1) under general anesthesia under operating light, 2) after 10 minutes in the dark, 3) after the right eye was spot-lighted, and 4) after the operating light was turned on. A rebound is obvious.

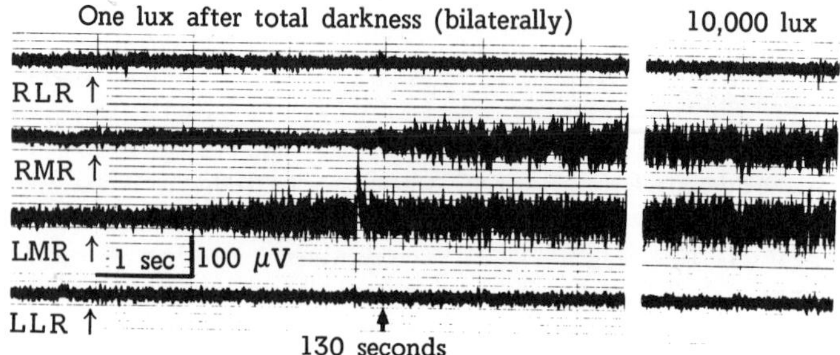

Figure 4. EMG of the four horizontal recti of an esotropic case in which the re-exposure to the light was bilateral with indirect illumination at a brightness of 1 lux at the cornea, followed by illumination with operating light of 10,000 lux. For details see the text.

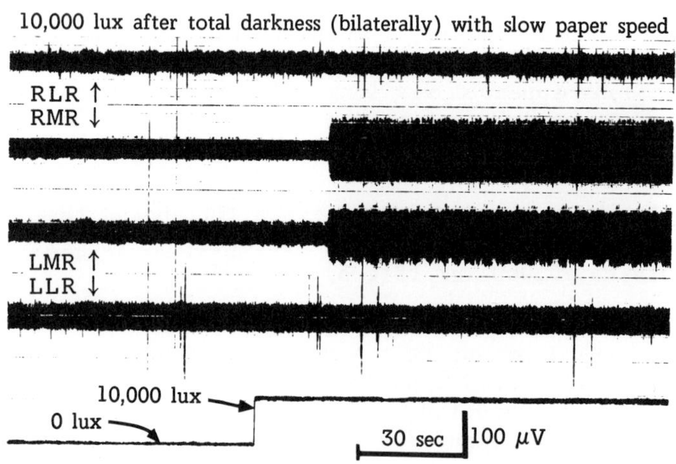

Figure 5. EMG of the four horizontal recti of an esotropic case when re-exposed to operating light (10,000 lux) after 10 minutes in the dark, recorded at a low paper speed, showing the time lag for re-firing shortened to about 20 seconds.

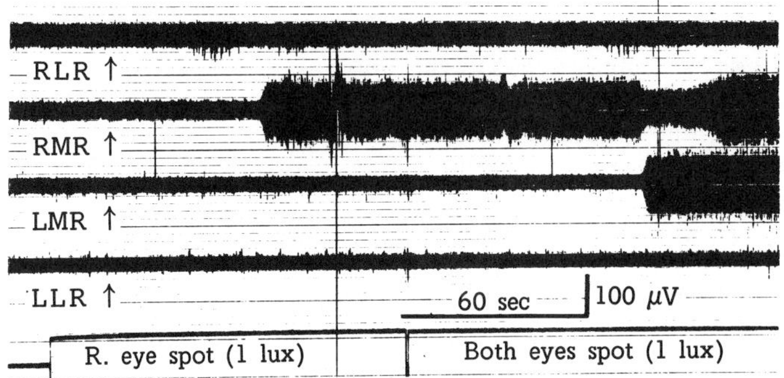

Figure 6. Reciprocity in the firing from both medial recti muscles in a case of group IV. For details see the text.

DISCUSSION

Much evidence indicates that optomotor reflexes play a role in the development of strabismus.2,3 However, nothing is known with certainty as to the pathway of these reflexes.

That pupillary reactions to light persist under general anesthesia at surgical planes is well known, though the reflexes become slightly sluggish. The sluggishness is attributed to the subcortical transmission of this reaction. It is therefore not unreasonable to tentatively conclude from the present experiment that a subcortical optomotor reflex pathway in esotropia is present in addition to a transcortical pathway. However, another experiment1 suggests that the muscle afferent is involved in signals passing through the subcortical pathway by causing firing from the medial recti muscles. The reciprocity in the firing from both medial recti muscles, which suggested the involvement of muscle afferent,1 was also demonstrated in the present study, although under a certain limited condition (Group IV). Therefore, an interaction between the muscle afferent and visual input is suspected in this pathway. The superior colliculus might be the site, or a site, where this kind of interaction takes place.6,7

Our results showed that the optomotor reactions in esotropia, which appear in a fraction of a second in the awakened state,3 are much delayed under general anesthesia, that 1 lux is enough to cause re-firing from the medial recti, and that the re-firing caused by 1 lux is not smaller than that caused by 10,000 lux, although the lag time is longer, lasting 2 minutes or more with 1 lux. By re-exposure to 10,000 lux, the lag time can be shortened to 20 seconds. All of theses characteristics may be related to the mechanism of interaction. It may be supposed that the role of visual input in this pathway is related to the synthesis of a "transmission substance" or the like at the synapse where the interaction is taking place, The muscle afferent acts when a signal is transmitted only in the presence of this substance. All phenomena observed in the present experiment can be understood, if we assume that it take 5 to 10 minutes before the stock of this substance is exhausted in darkness and that the rate of synthesis of this substance upon re-exposure to light depends on the brightness of illumination, ranging from 20 seconds at 10,000 lux to 2 minutes or over at 1 lux to

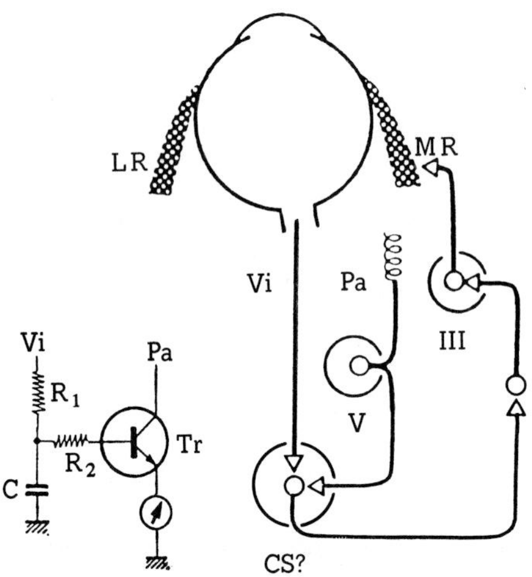

Figure 7. A hypothetical subcortical optomotor effect transmission pathway and interaction between proprioceptive afferent and visual input. Signals may come from the former (Pa), while the latter (Vi) may be involved in the synthesis of a "transmitting substance".

LR: lateral rectus
MR: medial rectus
Pa: proprioceptive afferent (discharging spontaneously)
Vi: visual input
CS: colliculus superior
V: trigeminus
III: oculomotor nerve

Inset: Electronic simulation of the possible interaction at the colliculus superior where Vi: 0 V for 0 lux, 10 V for 300 lux and 17 V for 10,000 lux. R_1 = 500 K , R_2 = 150 K , C = 1,000 uF, Tr = silicon bipolar transistor with 0.7 V threshold.

reach the threshold. The muscle afferent involved here may come from spontaneously discharging receptors8 and is not necessarily a result of the stretch reflex. Fig 7 illustrates a hypothetical subcortical optomotor reflex pathway in esotropia, superimposed on the probable proprioceptive pathway described elsewhere.1 The contralateral pathway is deleted for simplicity. An electronic simulation of the possible interaction between the proprioceptive impulse and visual input is also shown as an inset in the same illustration. In this simulation the proprioceptive afferent (Pa) continues to pass through the transitor (Tr) for about 7 minutes after the visual input (Vi) is turned off, and begins again to pass through Tr about 40 seconds (or 20 seconds) after Vi is turned back on, when Vi = 10 V (or 17 V), R_1 = 500 , R_2 = 150 K , C = 1000 uF, and Tr is a silicon bipolar transistor. Fig 8 shows the off- and on-effect of Vi on the transmision of Pa through the Tr, according to the electronic simulation.

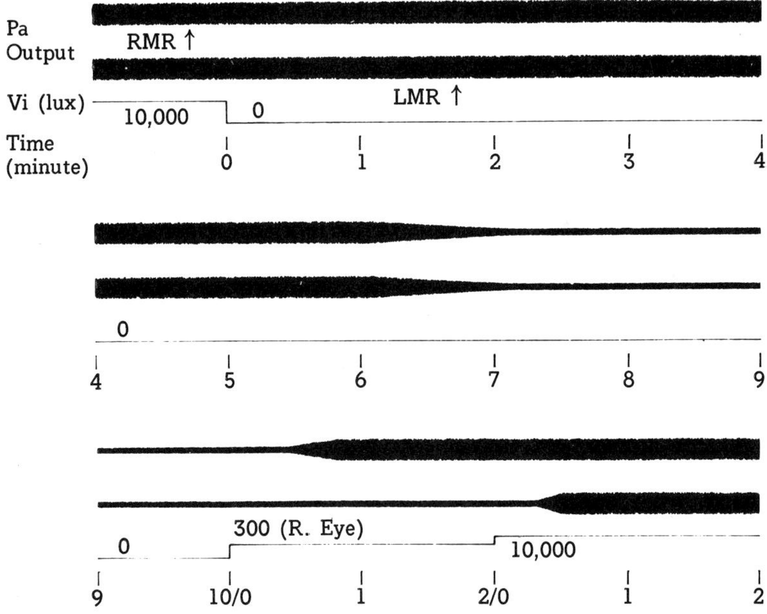

Figure 8. Relation between the transmission of proprioceptive afferent (Pa) and visual input (Vi) drawn according to the simulation shown in Fig 6. Continuously discharging randomized pulses were used as Pa-input.

CREDITS

Authors wish to thank Dr. Takao Saito, Professor of Anesthesiology, Tokushima University, who undertook the general anesthesia in absolute darkness throughout the study.

REFERENCES

1. Mitsui Y, Tamura O, Hirai K, Akazawa K, Ohga M, Masuda K: An eletromyographic study of esotropia. Br J Ophthalmol 65:161-166, 1981.

2. Keiner GBJ: New Viewpoints on the Origin of Squint. The Hague, Martinus Nijhoff, 1951.

3. Mitsui Y, Hirai K, Akazawa K, Masuda K: The sensorimotor reflex and strabismus. Jpn J Ophthalmol 23:227-256, 1979.

4. Gobin MH: Limitation of suppression to one half of the visual field in the pathogenesis of horizontal deviation of squint. Ophthalmologica 155:297-298, 1968.

5. Berard PV, Reydy R, Mouillac-Gambarelli N: Le reflexe opto-moteur (eclairment-obscuration) et le test d'elongation sous anesthesie generale dans les esotropies. Lecture given in Nice, June 27, 1981. Bull Soc Ophthalmol 82(8-9):1037-1042, 1982. France (in press).

6. Abrahams VC, Rose PK: Projections of extraocular, neck muscles, and retinal afferents to superior colliculus in the cat: Their connections to cells of origin of tectospinal tract. J Neurophysiol 38:10-18, 1975.

7. Donaldson IML, Long AC: Interactions between extraocular proprioceptive and visual signals in the superior colliculus of the cat. J Physiol (Lond) 298:85-110, 1980.

8. Bach-Y-Rita P, Ito F: Properties of stretch receptors in cat extraocular muscles. J Physiol (Lond) 186: 663-688, 1966.

DISCUSSION BY G. KOMMERELL

Dr. Mitsui´s paper raises a controversial issue of immediate clinical importance. The basic question at stake is the following: Does proprioceptive muscle afference play a role in the pathogenesis of strabismus? I have been discussing this question with Dr. Mitsui for three years in several letters, but our conclusions remain different. Dr. Mitsui´s answer to the above question is "probably yes", and mine is "probably no". In my opinion, most of Dr. Mitsui´s findings can be interpreted as the effect of retinal, rather than proprioceptive, afference.

Before explaining the problem to you, I would like to emphasize that Dr. Mitsui always responded in an extremely kind manner to my scepticism and repeatedly allowed me to share his findings and thoughts before publication.

As the paper presented by Dr. Mitsui at this meeting is only one link in a chain of articles from his laboratory, it will be necessary to refer to his previous work. There were two observations which suggested proprioceptive muscle afference to Dr. Mitsui. The first was the "magician´s forceps phenomenon" (Mitsui 1979) and the second the "reverse phase reflex movement" (Ishikawa 1978).

Dr. Mitsui (1979) demonstrated the magician´s forceps phenomenon in patients with exotropia. When the fixing right eye was slightly adducted with forceps, the strabismic left eye assumed the straight ahead position. As the movement of the strabismic eye was only obtained in the light, not in the dark, Dr. Mitsui concedes that retinal input is a necessary condition for the efficacy of muscle afference, whereas I assume that retinal input suffices to explain the whole phenomenon. The forced adduction of the right eye brings about a shift of the image on the retina and displaces the fixation point from the fovea. When the patient tries to refixate, he will not be able to do so with his restrained eye. Thus, the position error will persist, and a series of saccades will be elicited which then brings the strabismic left eye to the middle position. If the right eye is further adducted by forced traction, the left eye may take over fixation, or if the left eye is amblyopic, the patient may simply give up his efforts to refixate. The series of saccades which leads the left eye to the middle position can be seen in an EOG recording published by Dr. Mitsui (1981b, Fig. 4). In patients with intermittent exotropia, fusional attempts may also intervene.

The reverse phase reflex movement is elicited by mechanically oscillating the fixing eye. These forced oscillations result in reversed movements of the strabismic eye. As does the magician's forceps phenomenon, the reverse phase reflex movement also requires visual input and does not occur in the dark. It is clear that forced oscillations result in a corresponding slip of the retinal image, thus providing a strong visual pursuit stimulus. However, I must admit that the responses which Dr. Mitsui recorded at higher frequencies, that is at three, six and nine Hertz, cannot be explained as pursuit attempts. Looking closely at Dr. Mitsui's records written at higher paper speed, I was struck by the machine-like responses which were exactly opposite to the stimulus, without any latency, and showed constant amplitudes over many cycles. If these responses can be reproduced with a different recording technique, then this finding would indeed be a point in favor of Dr. Mitsui's hypothesis.

Important doubts about the role of proprioceptive afference in the reverse phase reflex movement were raised by Yamazaki (1980) who did strabismus surgery under superficial local anesthesia. When he oscillated only the eyeball with the horizontal muscles detached from the globe, a reverse phase movement of the other eye occurred. But pulling at the muscles without oscillating the globe failed to produce a movement of the other eye.

Dr. Mitsui, taking into account that visual input is important but objecting to the idea that the magician's forceps phenomenon and the reverse phase reflex movement are in fact visually elicited saccades, pursuit movements and/or fusional vergences, hypothesizes that light thrown on the retinal might work through a subcortical rather than cortical pathway. Thus, he became interested in the effect of light in general anesthesia, a state in which the visual cortex would be expected to function only minimally. Today, Dr. Mitsui and also Dr. Tamura in Session 8B showed to us that in general anesthesia eye muscle innervation slowly tapers off when the light is turned off and comes back after re-illumination. However, after re-illumination, one to two minutes are needed before the EMG suddenly shows increased firing. This long latency and the restriction of the effect to only one muscle (to the ipsilateral medial rectus without any reciprocal changes in the opposing lateral rectus) leads me to doubt that the effects recorded in general anesthesia are related to the magician's forceps phenomenon in the awake patient. Rather, light in general anesthesia may act as an unspecific arousal stimulus and may have nothing to do with muscle afference.

In an electromyographic study of esotropia, Dr. Mitsui (1981a) reported that under general anesthesia an additional unilateral retrobulbar anesthesia increased the firing of the contralateral medial rectus. This finding would indeed suggest afferent impulses from one orbit influencing contralateral eye muscle innervation. However, as the amount of firing in the EMG depends so much on the position of the needle electrode and a stable level of general anesthesia is difficult to maintain, confirmation of this finding should be awaited before general conclusions are drawn.

Coming to the end, I would like to express my personal admiration to Dr. Mitsui who has decided not to follow traditional paths and has instigated a whole new line of research trying to illucidate the pathogenesis of strabismus. I think Dr. Mitsui and his co-workers may finally succeed in proving a role of proprioceptive muscle afference in strabismus. However, at the present time, it appears to me that the evidence is still insufficient and partly conflicting.

Moreover, it should be mentioned that the role of proprioceptive muscle afference has remained an unsolved puzzle not only in strabismus but also in the normal ocular motor system (Keller and Robinson 1971, Manni and Bortolami 1982). Current models of this system do not require proprioceptive muscle afference (Berthoz, 1981).

REFERENCES

1. Berthoz A: Metrics and models of saccadic eye movements. Discussion summary. In: Fuchs AF, Becker W: Progress in oculomotor research. Elsevier/Northholland. New York, Amsterdam, Oxford, 1981.

2. Ishikawa S: Proprioception of the extraocular muscle, a review and recent findings. Acta Soc Ophthalmol Jpn 82:233-249, 1978.

3. Keller EL, Robinson DR: Absence of a stretch reflex in extraocular muscles of the monkey. J Neurophysiol 34:908-919, 1971.

4. Manni E, Bortaolam R: Proprioception in eye muscles. In: Lennerstrand G, Zee DS, Keller EL: Functional basis of ocular motility disorders. Oxford, New York, Toronto, Sydney, Paris,

Frankfurt, 1982.

5. Mitsui Y, Hirai KI, Akazawa K, Masuda K: The sensorimotor reflex and strabismus. Jap J Ophthalmol 23:227-256, 1979.

6. Mitsui Y, Tamura O, Hirai KI, Akazawa K, Ohga M, Masuda K: An electromyographic study of esotropia. Brit J Ophthalmol 65:161-166, 1981a.

7. Mitsui Y, Tamura O: Proprioception and exodeviations. Brit J Ophthalmol 65:578-584, 1981b.

8. Yamazaki A: The mechanism of the reverse phase reflex movement and magician's forceps phenomenon in patients with exotropia. Acta Soc Ophthalmol Jpn 84:1650-1663, 1980.

VISUALLY AND AUDITORY EVOKED SACCADIC REACTION TIME IN AMBLYOPIA

M. Fukushima, J. Tsutsui

ABSTRACT

Visually evoked saccadic reaction time (V-SRT) was compared with auditory evoked saccadic reaction time (A-SRT) in amblyopic and normal fellow eyes, and the mechanism of increase of V-SRT in the amblyopia was studied and compared with certain central nervous system diseases. Both of V-SRT and A-SRT were measured in 11 of normal subjects, 8 of strabismic amblyopes, 10 of anisometric amblyopes and 4 subjects of strabismus without amblyopia. In the subjects of normal and strabismus without amblyopia, there was no V-SRT and A-SRT difference between fellow eyes. In the strabismic and anisometropic amblyopes, V-SRT of the amblyopic eyes were significantly increased as compared with that of the normal fellow eyes, but A-SRT showed no difference. Thus, we conclude that the characteristic increase of V-SRT in the amblyopic eye depends on a visually procesing delay in the sensory pathway rather than a delay in the motor pathway, and the delay was caused by dysfunction of the occipital visual sensory area.

INTRODUCTION

Increase of saccadic reaction times (SRT) in amblyopic eyes have been reported,1-6 although the reason for the increase has not been explained. In this study, visually evoked SRT (V-SRT) was compared with auditory evoked SRT (A-SRT) in amblyopic and normal fellow eyes.

MATERIALS AND METHODS

Both of V-SRT and A-SRT were measured in 11 normal subjects, 8 of strabismic amblyopia, 10 of anisometropic amblyopia and 4 of strabismus without amblyopia. The clinical data are shown in Table 1. The range of age was 9 to 20 years old (mean:13.6) in the normal subjects, 6 to 22 years old (mean:11.1) in the amblyopic groups and 8 to 17 years old (mean:12.3) in strabismus without amblyopia. The

STRABISMUS II
ISBN 0-8089-1424-3

visual acuity of the amblyopic eye was from 0.1 to 0.6, and the mean value was 0.2 by a crowded target. The visual acuity was 0.1 or 0.2 in most cases. The visual acuity of the normal fellow eye was 1.0 to 1.5. The visual acuity of both normal subjects and strabimus without amblyopia was 1.0 or over.

Case NO.	SRT NO.	Age (Y)	Sex	Visual Acuity (R / L)	Squint Angle		Fixation
NORMAL SUBJECTS							
1	101	9	F	1.5 / 1.5	-	-	F
2	119	9	M	1.5 / 1.5	-	-	F
3	102	11	F	1.5 / 1.5	-	-	F
4	117	11	F	1.2 / 1.2	-	-	F
5	122	12	F	1.0 / 1.0	-	-	F
6	91	13	F	1.5 / 1.5	-	-	F
7	92	13	F	1.5 / 2.0	-	-	F
8	118	15	F	1.5 / 1.5	-	-	F
9	121	17	M	1.5 / 1.5	-	-	F
10	88	20	F	1.5 / 1.5	-	-	F
11	98	20	F	1.2 / 1.2	-	-	F
STRABISMIC AMBLYOPES							
1	115	6	M	1.0 / 0.3p	10ΔET'	10ΔET	M
2	104	8	F	0.1 / 1.0	25ΔET'	25ΔET	Pf
3	120	9	M	1.5 / 0.3	40ΔXT'	40ΔXT	Pf
4	79	10	M	1.2 / 0.2p	16ΔET'	14ΔET	F
5	82	10	F	1.5 / 0.1	12ΔET'	18ΔET	M
6	94	10	F	1.2 / 0.6	18ΔET'	18ΔET	F(us)
7	77	21	M	0.2p / 1.5	30ΔET'	35ΔET	Pf
8	93	22	F	1.0 / 0.1	60ΔET'	60ΔET	Pf
ANISOMETROPIC AMBLYOPES							
1	105	7	F	1.2 / 0.2	8ΔX'	18ΔXT	F
2	114	7	F	0.6 / 1.5	-	-	F
3	90	8	F	1.5p / 0.2p	-	-	F(us)
4	116	8	F	1.5 / 0.1	-	-	F
5	84	10	F	0.3 / 1.5	-	-	F
6	95	10	F	0.3p / 1.5	-	-	F
7	96	10	F	0.1 / 1.2	-	-	F(us)
8	85	13	F	1.5 / 0.3	-	-	F
9	109	13	M	0.4 / 1.2	-	-	F
10	83	17	M	0.3p / 1.5	-	-	F
STRABISMUS WITHOUT AMBLYOPIA							
1	123	8	F	1.5 / 1.5	25ΔXT'	40ΔXT	F
2	125	15	F	1.5 / 2.0	16ΔX(T)'	30ΔXT	F
3	124	9	M	1.5 / 1.5	20ΔET'	20ΔET	F
4	127	17	M	1.0 / 1.0	30ΔET'	30ΔET	F

Sex M: Male, F: Female
Fixation F: Foveal, Pf: Parafoveal, M: Macular
(us): unstable

Table 1: Clinical data of normal subjects, strabismic amblyopes, anisometropic amblyopes and strabismus without amblyopia.

The saccadic eye movements were recorded with DC-EOG and a storage oscilloscope. A subject at 1 m distance from a screen under photopic condition was examined by using small spot of light target projecting on the screen. A chin- and head-rest stabilized the head. The spot size was 34 min arc and the luminance of the spot and the background were 45.5 cd/m2 and 30.0 cd/m2 respectively. In visually evoked saccade, a subject tracked the target monocularly which moved at random interval with horizontal step displacement between a central fixation of point and points of 10 degrees to right and left. This step displacement was elicited with a visual target generator (a Hamamatsu TV Instrument, HTV-C773). In the auditory evoked saccades, the subject was commanded to look at the same fixation points immediately after a click sound of 4000 Hz, which was applied randomly by headphones. After several practice trials, 40 measurements in total of V- and A-SRT were made for each eye, measuring the normal eye first and followed by the fellow amblyopic eye. The data analysis was performed on a digitizer (Talos) and microcomputer system (NEC). A T-test (two-tailed test) was used for a statistical analysis.

RESULTS

Normals, strabismic amblyopes, anisometropic amblyopes and strabisics without amblyopia, mean V-SRT and A-SRTs, and differences of V-SRT and A-SRT between the two eyes (ΔV-SRT, A-SRT) are shown in Table 2.

	EYE	V-SRT (msec)	ΔV-SRT (msec)	A-SRT (msec)	ΔA-SRT (msec)
NORMAL SUBJECT (N=11)	RIGHT	180.8 ± 23.2	5.8 ± 4.0 ($p<0.84$)	189.2 ± 16.9	6.8 ± 5.8 ($p<0.30$)
	LEFT	181.2 ± 21.9		186.3 ± 13.6	
STRABISMIC AMBLYOPIA (N=8)	FELLOW	187.1 ± 21.3	53.1 ± 31.0 ($p<0.003$)	209.4 ± 19.4	8.0 ± 7.3 ($p<0.84$)
	AMBLY	240.2 ± 44.9		208.6 ± 24.0	
ANISOMETROPIC AMBLYOPIA (N=10)	FELLOW	185.3 ± 23.4	40.4 ± 26.5 ($p<0.002$)	210.7 ± 20.9	8.1 ± 6.1 ($p<0.10$)
	AMBLY	225.7 ± 37.1		205.2 ± 17.2	
STRABISMUS WITHOUT AMBLYOPIA (N=4)	RIGHT	175.2 ± 12.0	1.1 ± 0.6 ($p<0.26$)	196.6 ± 34.0	2.1 ± 1.3 ($p<0.61$)
	LEFT	174.3 ± 12.2		195.8 ± 32.8	

V-SRT : Visually evoked Saccadic Reaction Time
A-SRT : Auditory evoked Saccadic Reaction Time
ΔSRT : Difference of SRT between amblyopic (or right) and fellow (or left) eye

Table 2: The mean V-SRT and A-SRT in the amblyopic and normal fellow eye.

In ten normal subjects, V-SRT was ranged from 148.6 to 223.6 msec with the mean of 180.8 + 23.2 msec (Mean + S.D.) for the right eyes and 181.2 + 21.9 msec for the left eyes. The ΔV-SRT was 5.8 + 4.0 msec ($p < 0.84$). The A-SRT of normal subjects ranged from 167.4 to 222.0 msec with the mean of 189.2 + 16.9 msec for the right eyes and 186.3 + 13.4 msec for the left eyes. The ΔA-SRT was 6.8 + 5.8 msec ($p < 0.30$). The normals showed no difference between right and left eyes of V-SRT and A-SRT.

In eight strabismic amblyopes (2 foveal fixators and 6 eccentric fixators), mean V-SRT was 187.1 + 21.3 msec for the normal fellow eyes and was 240.2 + 44.9 msec for the amblyopic eyes. The ΔV-SRT between the amblyopic and normal fellow eyes was 53.1 msec. The mean A-SRT was 209.4 + 19.4 msec for the normal fellow eyes and 208.6 + 24.0 msec for the amblyopic eyes, and ΔA-SRT was 8.0 msec. The V-SRT in the strabismic amblyopes was significantly increased as compared with that of normal fellow eyes ($p < 0.003$), but A-SRT showed no difference ($p < 0.84$).

In ten anisometropic amblyopes (foveal in all), V-SRT of the amblyopic eyes was increased as compared with that of the normal fellow eyes. The mean V-SRT was 185.3 + 23.4 msec for the normal fellow eyes and 225.7 + 37.1 msec for the amblyopic eyes, and ΔV-SRT was 40.4 msec. The mean A-SRT of anisometropic amblyopes was 210.7 + 20.9 msec for the normal fellow eyes and 205.2 + 17.2 msec for the amblyopic eyes, and ΔA-SRT was 8.1 msec. In anisometropic amblyopes, V-SRT of the amblyopic eyes was significantly increased as compared with that of the normal fellow eyes ($p < 0.002$), but A-SRT showed no diference ($p < 0.10$). In four strabismics without amblyopia and all foveal fixators, mean V-SRT was 175.2 + 12.0 msec for the right eyes and 174.3 + 12.2 msec for the left eyes, and ΔV-SRT was 1.1 msec ($p < 0.26$). The mean A-SRT ws 196.6 + 34.0 msec for the right eyes and 195.8 + 32.8 msec for the left eyes, and Δ A-SRT was 2.1 msec ($p < 0.61$). No difference was found between the right and left eyes of V-SRT and A-SRT.

No V-SRT difference was detected between normal subjects and normal fellow eyes in anisometropic and strabismic amblyopes, but V-SRT of the amblyopic eyes was longer than that of the normals as well being longer than the normal fellow eyes, and ΔV-SRT of strabismic amblyopes was longer than that of anisometropic amblyopes. Both A-SRTs of the amblyopic and normal fellow eyes were always within normal range and had no relation to the type of amblyopia. In the

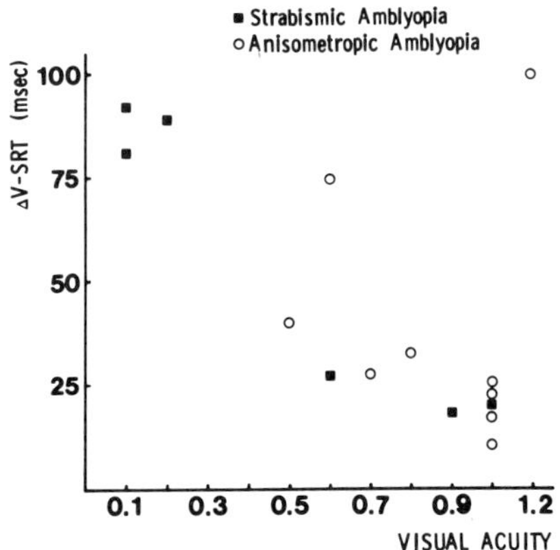

Figure 1: Relationship between ΔV-SRT before treatment and visual recovery.

subjects of strabismus without amblyopia, V-SRT and A-SRT showed no difference between each eye. It is suggested that amblyopia was a necessary condition for the increased V-SRT but not for strabismus.

The relationship between ΔV-SRT before treatment and visual recovery in 15 amblyopes who had been observed for 6 months is shown in Figure 1. When ΔV-SRT was shorter, the visual recovery had improved to 0.9 or over, but the visual recovery was poor when ΔV-SRT was longer. A tendency to longer ΔV-SRTs was seen in deeper amblyopia.

DISCUSSION

Previous studies on the binocular V-SRT and A-SRT in the various lesions of the brain revealed that the sensory pathway of the saccadic eye movements elicited by visual inputs differed from those made in response to auditory inputs, but the motor signals from oculomotor center reached the extraocular muscles through the same pathway.[7,8,9] For example, when the lesion was located in the visual cortex of the occipital lobe and parietal subcortex, V-SRT was increased but A-SRT was not. When the lesion was present in the auditory cortex of the temporal lobe, A-SRT was increased with normal V-SRT. When the lesion occupied in the parietal cortex, both of V-SRT and A-SRT were increased because sensory signals of visual and auditory inputs altered to motor signals in the cortex. Conversely, when the lesion ws located in the hemilateral motor area or the cerebral pyramidal tract, both of V-SRT and A-SRT toward the contralateral side of the lesion were delayed and those toward the ipsilateral side were normal. By analysing the relation between V-SRT and A-SRT, the lesion of the sensory and/or motor pathway could be separated and the functional site of lesion in cerebral disease could also be identified.

In this study, the V-SRT was increased whereas A-SRT was not, and differences of SRT of right- and left-ward saccades in a few amblyopes were within a normal range. Thus we conclude that the characteristic increase of V-SRT in the amblyopic eyes depends on visually processing delay in the sensory pathway rather than in the motor pathway, and is caused by dysfunction of the occipital visual sensory area.

REFERENCES

1. Mackensen, G.: Reactionszeitmesungen bei Amblyopie. Albrecht Von Graefes Arch Klin Exp Ophthlmol 159:636-642, 1958.

2. Von Noorden, G.K.: Reaction time in normal and amblyopic eyes. Arch Ophthalmol 66:695-701, 1961.

3. Schor C: A directional impairment of eye movement control in strabismus amblyopia. Invest Ophthalmol 14:692-697, 1975.

4. Ciuffreda KJ, Kenyon RV, Stark L: Increased saccadic latencies in amblyopic eyes. Invest Ophthalmol 17:697-702, 1978.

5. Mimura O., Kato H, Kani K, Shimo-oku M: Saccadic latencies in amblyopia using infrared television fundus camera with two-dimensional stimuli. Jpn J Ophthalmol 25:248-257, 1981.

6. Hamasaki DI, Flynn JT: Amblyopic eyes have longer reaction times. Invest Ophthalmol 21:846-853, 1981.

7. Fukushima M.: The studies on saccadic reaction time. I. Methodology and normal subjects. Nippon Ganka Gakkai Zasshi 86: 36-41, 1982.

8. Fukushima M: The studies on saccadic reaction time. II. Cases with mental deficiency, diffuse cerebral atrophy and parietal lobe lesion. Nippon Ganka Gakkai Zasshi 86:510-518, 1982.

9. Fukushima, M.: The studies on saccadic reaction time. III. Cases with occipital lobe lesion. Acta Soc Ophthalmol Jpn in press.

DISCUSSION BY G. KOMMERELL

Dr. Fukushima tested the saccadic reaction time to visual and auditory stimuli. His conclusion that the increased latency of amblyopic eyes is due to a sensory rather than motor processing delay appears to be well supported.

DYNAMIC CHANGES OF OCULAR MOTILITY IN THE TIGHT LATERAL RECTUS SYNDROME

P. Nemet, S. Ron and S. Gur

ABSTRACT

In the tight lateral rectus syndrome a mechanical restriction limits adduction of the involved eye. However, when both eyes are following a target within a certain range and the healthy eye is fixating, the subject performs normal saccadic movements with both eyes. The temporal changes of the ocular motility were studied before and after surgery using a conventional DC EOG monocular recording method. Fixation was binocular or monocular. Twelve days post-operatively the restriction in adduction was no longer present. In addition, when the eyes moved away from the operated lateral rectus there was, in both eyes, an overshoot of 20% of the amplitude in 20% of the saccades, followed by a correcting saccade after about 120 msec. The incidence of this overshoot increased to 50% of all saccades after 5 months. When the operated eye was fixating, an undershoot of the saccade in both eyes was in the direction of the operated lateral rectus, followed 200 msec later by a correcting saccade. The incidence of this pattern also increased with time.

Two major findings of the study were as follows:

1) The motility of the operated eye as well as of the intact eye changed in time in an effort to bring them to some degree of committence, despite the former being amblyopic and squinting.

2) A saccadic overshoot occurred when both eyes moved in the direction away from the operated eye. A saccadic undershoot was found when they moved in the direction of the operated eye. Both were compensated by corecting saccades.

These results indicate that a neural reorganization of the spatial code to a temporal movement has taken place, which affects the yoke muscles rather than the adaptation of the saccadic generator of the involved eye.

STRABISMUS II
ISBN 0-8089-1424-3

INTRODUCTION

The tight lateral rectus syndrome (TLR) is characterized by mechanical limitation of adduction of the involved eye associated with exotropia and overaction of both oblique muscles of that eye. While this syndrome can be tested by force generation tests4, an EOG examination might provide a time course for the eye movements.

In an attempt to evaluate the dynamic change of ocular motility in this particular entity we have studied eye movements in two patients with TLR syndrome prior to and following surgery. The temporal changes recorded during a period of several month following surgery indicate that the plastic adaptation of the ocular motility continues following surgery.

METHOD AND PATIENTS

Eye movements were measured using a standard electro-oculogram technique. Electrodes (Ag-AgCl) were placed at the outer and inner canthi of each eye. The signal was amplified through a DC amplifier and conveyed to a FM tape recorder. The overall bandwidth of the system was better than 100 HZ. The target was a LASER beam with a subtending angle of 5 deg increasing to 25 deg in increments of 5 deg. A total of at least 15 eye movements were recorded for each experimental condition. The target moved left or right of a central fixation point. The target was presented in a quasi-random mode to avoid prediction. With each target movement a pulse was also generated proportional to the target movement and recorded on the tape recorder. The recorded eye movements and the pulse signals were reproduced on UV paper for analysis.

The patient was seated with his head restrained and his chin resting in a holder. Eye movements were measured when the patient fixated monocularly and binocularly. In patient #1, eye movements were recorded prior to surgery, 11 days, and 5 months post-operatively; in patient #2, eye movements were measured prior to surgery, 14 days, and 2 months post-operatively.

Patient #1, a 22-year-old male, underwent recess-resect surgery at age 5 for left esotropia. At age 7 a recession of LLR ws performed for correcting secondary left exotropia. A year ago his eye examination revealed: Visual acuity of 6/6 in his RE, and 6/36 in his LE, not improvable, with only negligible refractive error. The left eye had limitation of adduction, and overaction of both oblique muscles. Left exotropia of 50 prism diopters for distance and 60 prism diopters for near was present with X pattern. The exotropia increased with gaze to right and decreased with gaze to left. Traction test on adduction of the LE was positive.

The LE was operated. The LLR ws found 16mm from the limbus and was covered with a thick fibrotic tissue which was removed. Two marginal myotomies of the LR were performed and the conjuctiva was recessed. The LMR was resected 10mm. One year post-operatively the patient has 4 prism diopters of left esotropia and mild limitation of his LLR.

Patient #2, a 21 year old male, underwent recess-resect surgery of his right eye at age 4 for right esotropia. On his recent admission visual acuity was 6/6 in each eye. A right exotropia of 50 prism diopters for near and distance was present with an X pattern and mild limitation of adduction of this eye.

The RE was operated. The lateral rectus was recessed and the medial rectus was resected and advanced to the original insertion. Following surgery there was a residual exotropia of 20 prism diopters.

RESULTS

It might be presumed that in TLR syndrome when the non-involved eye is moving right or left from central fixation, normal saccades will be performed with only minor post-operative changes. Even these changes might be expected to disappear in time. We found that eye movements of both the involved and non-involved eyes changed following surgery.

The results of both cases are similar and therefore eye movements of patient #1 only are shown. The results shown are the typical formats similar to other published studies1,2,3. In Fig 1, eye movement to right are shown in three different tests: pre-operatively, and twice post-operatively at 11 days and 5 months. Preoperatively, when both eyes or the non-involved (RE) looked to a right target and back to center, the saccadic response of the RE was normal; however, post-operatively the saccades were different. Eleven days post-operatively the saccades, when above 15o of target displacement, undershot and drifted to target. Five months post-operatively the RE either made a correct response when moving to the right or overshot the target and made a corrective saccade in the opposite direction.

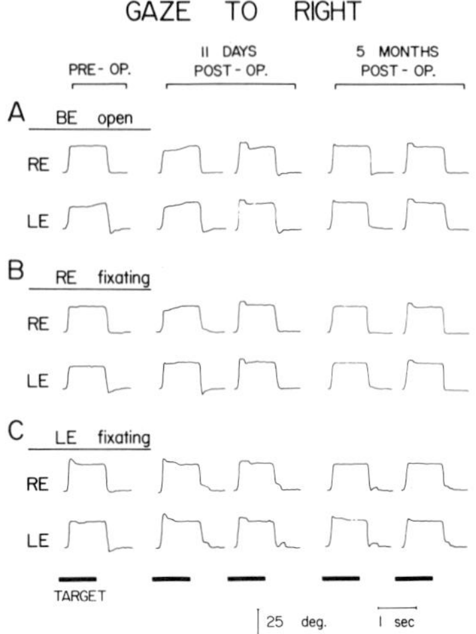

Figure 1. Eye movements to right, recorded when both eyes were opened (A), right eye fixating (B) and left eye fixating (C). The records were from patient #1 in three experiments: Pre-operatively (left panel), 11 days (middle panel) and 5 months post-operatively (right panel). The bar indicates the stimulus duration.

When the non-involved eye or both eyes were open pre-operatively the involved eye (LE) made a normal saccade to the right but overshot the target when moving back to center and corrected it with a slow drift towards the center (Fig 1, left panel). Post-operatively, on gaze to the right, the RE either undershot the target and made a correcting drift (Fig 1, midddle panel), or made a dysmetric saccade (Fig 1, middle and right panels). On movement back to the center when the RE undershot and drifted to the center, the LE always made a larger saccade and drifted to the opposite direction (Fig 1, middle panel).

When the involved eye (LE) was fixating, pre-operatively when moving to the right, RE made a hypermetric saccade with drift in the opposite direction. When returning to the center, the LE overshot the center and made a corrective drift to the center. Post-operatively both eyes performed similarly grossly overshooting the target with multiple saccades when moving back to the center. Both the overshooting and the multiple saccades decreased significantly in time (Fig 1C). It might be expected on gaze to the left from the center, when either eye or both eyes are

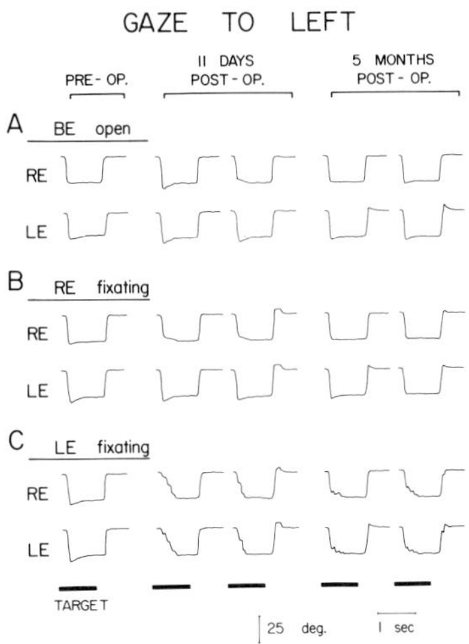

Figure 2. Same as Fig 1 but gaze to left.

fixating, the response would result in a normal saccade. However, in both pre- and post-operative eye movement responses, drift corrections were present either from overshooting or undershooting saccades (Fig 2) when moving from the center, or back to the central position. When the LE was fixating, post-operatively multiple saccades appeared with relative decreasing amounts in time (Fig 2C).

DISCUSSION

Some of the temporal changes in both the RE and LE might be explained, at least in part based on TLR, the weakness of the LLR post-operatively and the changes during the development of comitance after surgery. It has long been recognized that in the paralysis of an extrocular muscle (e.g. LLR), if a saccadic movement is made from the right to the center, the involved eye (LE) will perform a slow "floating" movement when compared to saccadic movement of the non-involved eye (RE)4. The eye will drift to a steady state determined by the pulse-step command of the saccade generator. In our study, the LLR was severed surgically (myotomized) and this undoubtedly greatly weakened the ability of the muscle to generate a response appropriate to a pulse-step command. The saccade undershot the target and was corrected with a slow movement to the primary position (Fig 1,C, central panel).

As stated in the method, the deviation of the left eye was greater on gaze to the left and the TLR led to increased limitation of the gaze to the right. When the eyes moved to the left the LLR pulled the eye against a recessed LMR following the original operation. Thus, in movement to the left, when the healthy eye (RE) was fixating, the involved eye (LE) overshot and drifted to a steady state position. This overshoot persisted even eleven days post-operatively, since apparently the spread of comitance did not yet occur (Figs. 1 and 2, A and B). However, five months post-operatively the overshoot disappeared in the majority of eye movements, indicating that the spread of comitance might take even longer.

The spread of comitance has theoretical bases when the involved eye is fixating, possible through a mechanism of adaptation to the new situation (e.g. paresis), while not violating Hering's law. The temporal changes when the healthy eye is fixating shown in this study are much more difficult to explain. For a pre-operative hypometric eye movement to occur, the healthy eye must be aware, at least in part, of the limitation that the TLR is having on the movement of the involved eye; it must adapt or contribute to the comitance through plasticity of the CNS which modifies the neural signals. The eye movement changes might be only for an intermediate period post-operatively until the neural rearrangement takes place resulting in a normal saccade (as observed, five months post-operatively, Fig 1 and 2A and B, right panel). Part of the rearrangement is probably the result of peripheral binocular vision which was found in both patients months after surgery. Thus, surgery did not only correct the mechanical restriction, but also created dynamic changes in the motility of both eyes.

REFERENCES

1. Metz, HS: III Nerve palsy: I. Saccadic velocity studies. Ann Ophthalmol 5:526-528, 1973.

2. Metz HS, Rice LS: Human eye movements following horizontal rectus muscle disinsertion. Arch Ophthalmol 90:265-267, 1973.

3. Metz HS, Scott AB, O'Meara D, Stewart HL: Ocular saccades in lateral rectus palsy. Arch Ophthalmol 84:453-460, 1970.

4. Scott AB: Force and velocity tests in strabismus. Tr Am Acad Ophthalmol Otolaryngol 79:727-732, 1975.

DISCUSSION BY G. KOMMERELL

Dr. Nemet examined goal-directed saccades in patients with constant strabismus before and after surgery on the strabismic eye. Surprisingly, the non-operated eye showed dysmetria and post-saccadic drift when used for refixations after surgery on the strabismic eye. These changes cannot be explained by the current understanding of the ocular motor system.

PURSUIT MOVEMENT DISORDERS AND THE PROGNOSIS OF STRABISMUS TREATMENT

J. Tsutsui, S. Fukai, and H. Kimura

ABSTRACT

Since eye tracking pursuit is dependant on the foveal projection and optokinetic nystagmus can be evoked by extrafoveal projection, the double anomaly means the existence of sensory-motor disorder in two visuomotor systems. Especially, the asymmetric pursuit and the asymmetric OKN were considered to be due to the asymmetric innervation from the occipital hemisphere. These intensive innervational anomalies seemed to disturb the cure status of strabismus. Fortunately, these peculiar cases are only 9% of strabismus.

The relationship between pursuit movement disorders and the therapeutic prognosis of strabismus was investigated retrospectively in 49 cases of esotropia and 54 cases of exotropia. The incidence of double anomaly was 19.4% of the total 103 cases, that is, 28.6% of esotropia and 11.1% of exotropia. Cases with poor prognosis showed the double anomaly in 54.5% of esotropia and 25.0% of exotropia. The disorders of pursuit movements indicate the existence of intensive innervational anomalies in strabismus.

INTRODUCTION

Among various eye movement disorders in strabismus, pursuit movements, including optokinetic nystagmus (OKN) and the eye tracking movement, are of great significance.(1,2,3,4,5) In this study the relationship between pursuit movement disorders and the therapeutic prognosis was investigated retrospectively. Eye tracking seems to be evoked by the foveal X cell system, and OKN by the extrafoveal Y cell system. There have been few investigations of the therapeutic effect of eye movement disorders in strabismus.(6)

CASES AND METHODS

This study includes 103 randomly selected patients treated for strabismus including 49 with esotropia and 54

STRABISMUS II
ISBN 0-8089-1424-3

with exotropia. Patients were observed for 3 to 6 years. The average age was 9.5 years, with a standard deviation of 6.4 years at the first visit. The rule of treatment was 1) preoperative orthoptics to establish a binocularity base, 2) surgery, 3) postoperative orthoptics to complete binocularity and 4) follow-up with minimum home training for 3 to 6 years. The status was classified as follows: cure 1 was complete cure, cure 2 achieved an inactive state of deviation and binocularity at the primary position, and cure 3 showed continued activity of the main strabismic problems. The therapeutic results were graded after more than 3 years of follow-up.

Ocular movements were analyzed by means of EOG, and were evoked by a horizontal eye tracking test and an optokinetic drum. The velocity of eye tracking target was 16 degrees/sec to 48 degrees/sec and that of the OKN drum was 10 degrees/sec to 180 degrees/sec. For the screening test, a simple pendulum and hand-operated OKN drum were used routinely. These procedures are convenient and useful for the repeated examination of a large number of patients.

The ocular movements were recorded by means of EOG at the pre-treated and post-treated stages and were evaluated retrospectively.

The abnormal pursuit movements were classified into three grades: grade 1 was normal, grade 2 was mildly irregular and showed partial deterioration and grade 3 showed smooth defect asymmetry, inverse OKN and marked deterioration. Grade 3, which showed both eye tracking and OKN defects, was called the "double anomaly" and it was selected as the target of disorder in this study.

RESULTS

In 49 cases of estropia, 24.4% were classed as cure 1, 53.1% for cure 2, and 22.5% for cure 3. The double anomaly of pursuit was found in 16.6% of cure 1, 23.0% of cure 2 and 54.5% of cure 3 (Fig. 1). The incidence of double anomaly was significantly high in the cure 3 group compared with cure 1 group ($P < 0.1$). The EOG showed a marked smooth defect and deterioration of OKN. These findings were not improved after the treatment (Fig. 2).

Pursuit disorder and cure status: Esotropia (49)

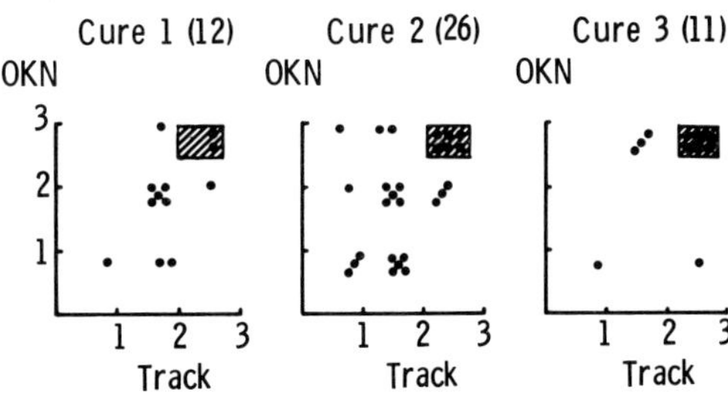

Figure 1. Pursuit disorders and cure status in esotropia. Square of oblique line indicates the double anomaly.

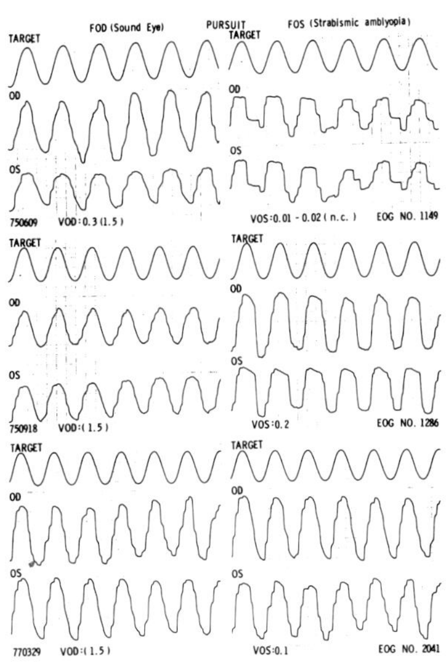

Figure 2. Eye tracking movements showing no therapeutic effect in a case of esotropia and possible decussation anomaly.

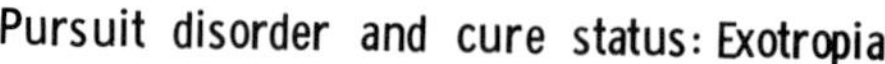

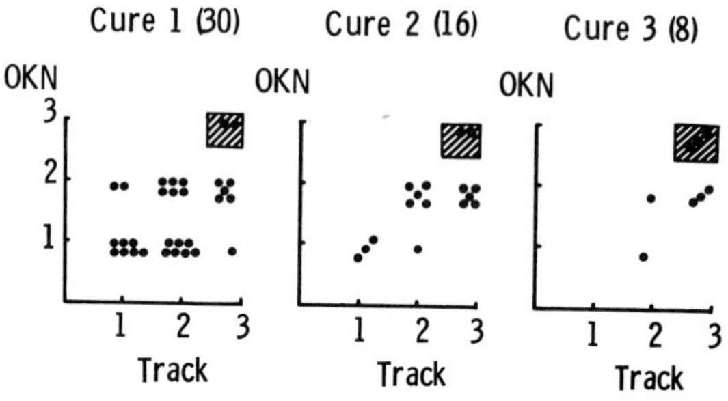

Figure 3. Pursuit disorders and cure status in exotropia. Square of oblique line indicates the double anomaly.

In 54 cases of extropia, 55.6% be classed as cure 1, 29.6% for cure 2 and 14.8% for cure 3 (Fig. 3). Compared to esotropia, the rate of complete cure was significantly higher (P < 0.05). The incidence of double anomaly was relatively low (12.9%) in exotropia and high (28.0%) in esotropia (P<0.2). The double anomaly of pursuit was present in 6.6% of the cure 1, 13.3% of cure 2 and 37.5% of cure 3 (P < 0.05 compared with cure 1).

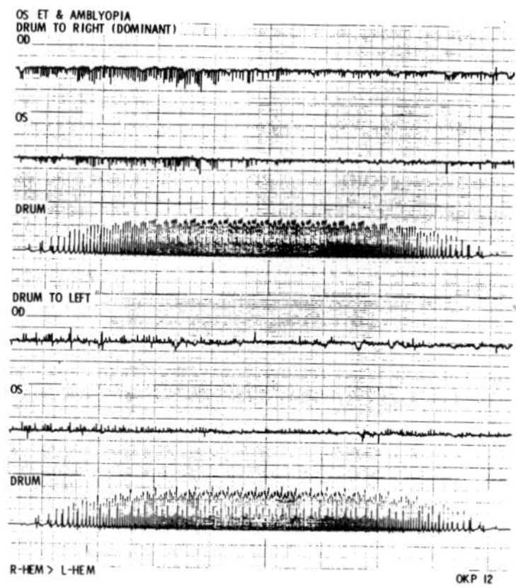

Figure 4. Asymmetric deterioration of OKN (drum to left).

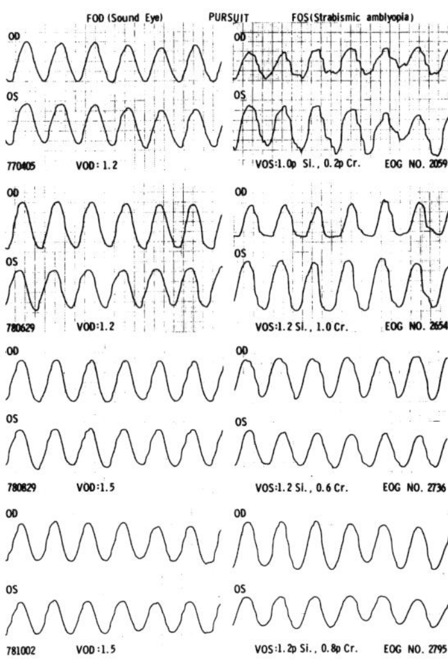

Figure 5. Eye tracking movements showing an improvement in a case of esotropia with amblyopia.

The pattern of double anomaly in cure 1, only 4 cases, depended on the unstable fixation due to the pre-existing amblyopia. On the other hand, in cure 3, definite innervational anomalies, such as asymmetric deterioration of smooth pursuit and OKN (Fig. 4), inverse OKN or ataxic eye tracking were found in all cases. The asymmetric pursuit and the asymmetric OKN suggest the existence of asymmetric innervation from the occipital hemisphere. These peculiar cases were only 9.0% of the entire series. A normalization of pursuit movements by the amblyopia treatment was recognized in cases with a visual improvement (Fig. 5). Cases with a characteristic innervational anomaly showed no improvement with treatment.

DISCUSSION

In the last congress of ISA(7), I reported "Human strabismic cases suggestive of asymmetric projection of the visual pathway." For the detection of those innervational anomalies, the routine pursuit tests are useful. In the routine examination of strabismus and amblyopia, simple routine tests such as the pendulum test and the OKN test are necessary for all cases. These tests can reveal the peculiar innervational anomaly. Among the various pursuit movement disorders, the double anomaly indicates a severe innervational anomaly both in X cell and Y cell systems. I would like to speculate that the X and Y systems may have a connection with the occipital eye movement system. The incidence of double anomaly is much higher in esotropia than in exotropia. Only 20.0% of cases with double anomaly achieved complete cure, while 80.0% of them had an incomplete cure or an intractable result. The abnormality of pursuits in the cure 1 group depended on the unstable fixation of the amblyopic eye, a technical error due to the short attention span of young children. These double anomalies were normalized after the treatment. However, the abnormality of pursuits in the cure 3 group depended on the severe innervational anomaly and treatment brought little improvement. My conclusions as to the meaning of double anomaly are as follows: An innervational anomaly, such as a possible decussation anomaly of the optic chiasm shows a specific pattern of asymmetry of pursuits and the prognosis of strabismus treatment is poor. The ddep amblyopia also shows a sensory motor dysfunction, detected through the pursuit movements and only partial improvement could be obtained. The double anomaly indicates hidden neurological evidence, a malformation of the extraocular muscle, such as fibrosis, and poor attention capacity due to cerebral dysfunctions.

REFERENCES

1. von Noorden GK, Mackensen G: Pursuit movements of normal and amblyopic eyes. An electro-ophthalmographic study I. Physiology of pursuit movements. Am J Ophthalmol 53:325-336, 1962.

2. von Noorden GK, Mackensen, G: Persuit movements of normal and amblyopic patients. Am J Ophthalmol 53:477-487, 1962.

3. Fukai S, Tsutsui J: Asymmetric version in pursuit eye movement under extrafoveal fixation. Jpn J Ophthalmol 17:30-39, 1973.

4. Schor C: A directional impairment of eyemovement control in strabismus amblyopia. Invest Ophthalmol 14:692-697, 1975.

5. Fukai S, Tsutsui J, Nakamura, Y.: Abnormal pursuit movements of the fellow eye in amblyopia with strabismus. In Moore S, Mein J, Stockbridge L (eds): Orthoptics, Past, Present, Future. NY Stratton Intercontinental Medical Book Corporation, pp. 75-91, 1975.

6. Ciuffreda KJ, Kenyon RV, Stark L: Different rates of functional recovery of eye movements during orthoptics treatment in an adult amblyope. Invest Ophthalmol Visual Sci 18:213-219, 1979.

7. Tsutsui J, Fukai S: Human strabismic cases suggestive of asymmetric projection of the visual pathway. In Reinecke RD (ed): Strabismus NY, Grune & Stratton, pp. 79-88, 1978.

DISCUSSION BY G. KOMMERELL

Dr. Tsutsui showed that disturbances of the pursuit and optokinetic systems suggest a bad prognosis for the achievement of binocular vision. Apparently, Dr. Tsutsui applied binocular stimulation. The asymmetries of the pursuit and optokinetic systems may have shown up even more clearly with monocular stimulation, as demonstrated in Dr. Flynn's paper at this symposium.

EFFICACY OF THE FADENOPERATION

H. G. Conrad, G. Kluge and H. Treumer

ABSTRACT

The typical profile of efficacy of the Fadenoperation of the medial rectus muscle shows a slight exponential increase when the eye is adducted. A 40 degrees/60 degrees adduction will be reduced by about 25 degrees after a Fadenoperation 13 mm behind the insertion. The stretch of the anterior muscle segment during the operation creates a recession of the posterior segment. Therefore, a basic effect in the primary position of the eye can be avoided or achieved. The quadrifold efficacy of the Fadenoperation is shown by examples and samples: 1. a possible "static" angle reduction; 2. marked incomitance pattern; 3. reduction of (over) convergence; 4. reduction of "dynamic" variations of ET angles. The profile of a recession-plus-Fadenoperation resembles classical recess-resect operations. The profile of the pure Fadenoperation ("unstretch" technique) is distinct from the efficacy of any other operation.

INTRODUCTION

1977/81 we derived the profile of efficacy from the surgical correction of medium angle esotropia. Average data for let´s say left medial rectus muscle Fadenoperation (12.5 mm) are: 2 degrees at 20 degrees levoversion, 4 degrees in primary position, 13 degrees at 20 degrees dextroversion. Angle reduction mainly depends on the degree of adduction of the globe i.e. on the innervation of the medial recti muscles. The incomitance pattern is described by a slight exponential curve. This paper deals with the profiles best suiting each of the clinical conditions which should allow calculations of surgical measures. If the dosage suffices, the efficacy of the Fadenoperation may be called quadrifold: 1. some static angle reduction, 2. marked incomitance pattern, 3. reduction of (over) convergence, 4. reduction of "dynamic" changes of esotropia. Any 20 degrees/30 degrees adduction will be reduced by about 13 degrees.

DEFINITION OF EFFICACY

Efficacy means pattern of angle reduction achieved by the Fadenoperation (Cuppers)(1) on medial recti muscles. It depends on the degree of adduction of the operated eyes.

STRABISMUS II
ISBN 0-8089-1424-3

Therefore, it is incomitant in different directions of gaze, and it varies with the distance of fixation as well as with variable ET angles in time.

MATERIAL AND METHODS

Our standard surgical technique is shown in Fig 1. The efficacy of the original technique of Cuppers(1) and Muhlendyck(4) is equal if we suture equally fast. Smoother techniques need more millimeters or give less reliable results.

Measurements of the angles of squint were performed before and after medial rectus Fadenoperations by alternate or simultaneous prism-and-cover test, by Synoptometer, and by photography of corneal reflections at various positions of gaze, distances, times. Examples and samples (x + s) out of numerous patients are given.

Physiological and mechanical hypotheses were based on findings of CT scans, at a simple but useful model (23 cm disc

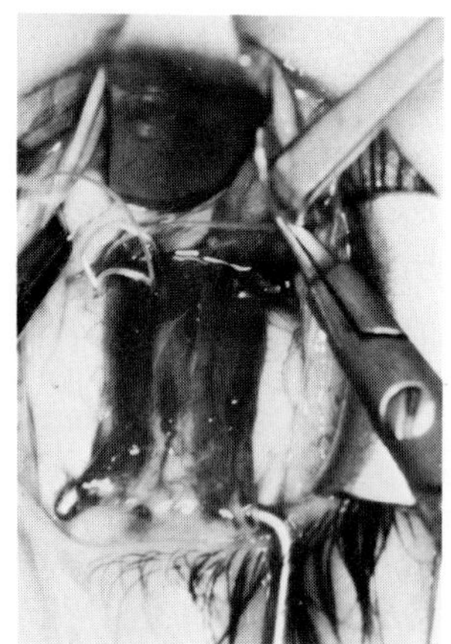

Figure 1. Technique recommended by de Decker and Conrad(2) 1975 described in detail by Conrad and de Decker(3) 1977. Unless there is an additional recession, the muscle is not desinserted. 13 mm behind the insertion on either side 1/5 to 1/4 of the muscle´s width is caught by a triple Faden loop of Suturamid 3/0. Left hand side: 3 scleral bites, 3 open loops, right: locked fixation suture.

with a rubber band), on observations during operations, on frog muscle experiments, and on extensive interdisciplinary discussions.

CLINICAL DATA

Incomitant pattern at lateral gaze

Figures 2 and 3 demonstrate the typical shape of efficacy of the Fadenoperation in two patients. The high effect at right gaze is explained by the high total adduction: 40 degrees of ET plus 40 degrees of right gaze. The larger the ET angle and the more of right gaze, the higher the effect. The resulting incomitance pattern follows a slight exponential curve. Adduction is mainly a function of "innervational factors".

If total adduction (ET + gaze + convergence) was the only factor influencing the efficacy, we would be able for instance to derive the effects in case of a 5 degree ET by shifting the curve 40 degrees downward and 40 degrees to the right side. This curve, however, would become too low and would grow exponentially too late. Mechanical characteristics must be taken in account, as for instance, the lack of restriction of overadduction on large angle ET.

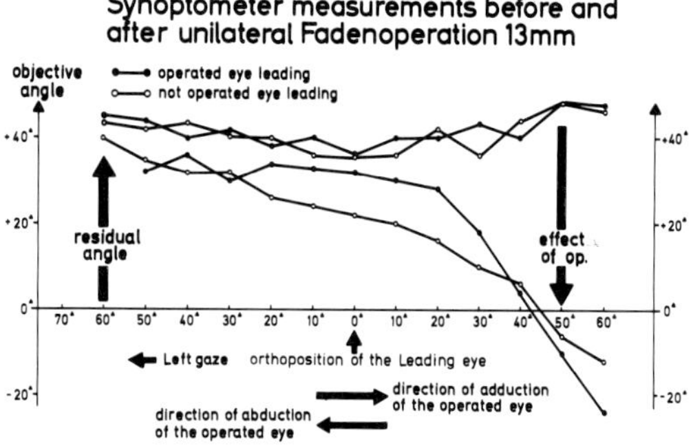

Figure 2. Our standard technique reduces any 40° - 60° total adduction by about 25° (See figures 4 and 5).

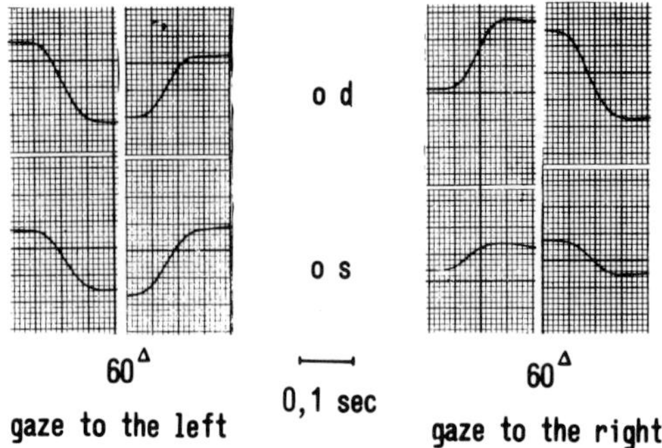

Figure 3. ENG record of smooth pursuit movements. ET + 45°, unilateral Fadenoperation at 13.5 mm: With increasing adduction of the operated left eye, the loss of torque becomes significant: Speed and excursion are reduced. This may balance the dyskinetic version, if the deviating eye hesitates to abduct (so-called Nystagmus Block Syndrome)(4).

Figures 4, 5, and 6 present comparable data, taken one month after standard Fadenoperations. In the primary position there are some basic effects (Fig 4, 6), which are doubled by a mild additional recession of the insertion (Fig 5). Consequently the exponential profiles in Figures 2 and 4 are distinct from those seen in the case of convential recess and/or resect operations. Figure 5 resembles conventional recess-resect operation with equal basic effects. Only the exponential end of the Faden profile is a bit steeper.

The effects in the primary position are lasting, the incomitance is reduced by 1/3 within two years. Since incomitant ET with excessive convergence or varying angle the incomitant profile is to be regarded as a side effect (Fig 4, 5), we prefer bilateral operations (Fig 6). Still adults may suffer from diplopia due to overcorrections at lateral gaze positions. Hence the dosage shall be careful. On the other hand, if there is a congruent profile of a paresis, we apply a Fadenoperation to the yoke muscle of the sound eye.

Convergence

The reduction of the (over) convergence is shown in Figures 7 and 8. The effect at distance may be called

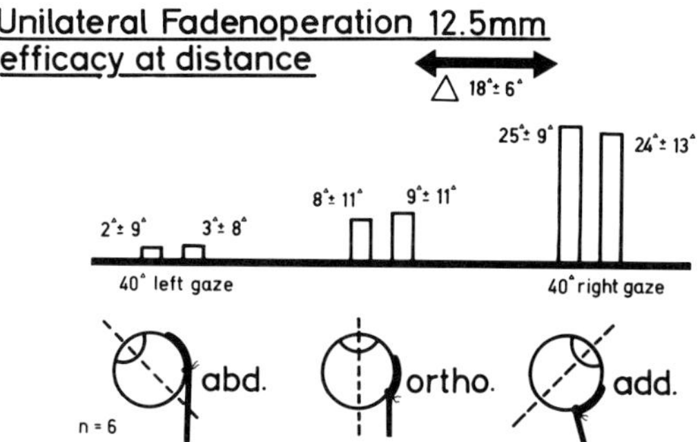

Figure 4. Effects, measured by alternating prism-and-cover test (Prism in front of the fixating eye). Left columns: left (operated) eye fixating, right columns: right eye fixating. Small-medium angle ET. Fewer millimeters or loose suture loops would lower and flatten the profile. The standard deviation indicates angle variations in time besides individual responses. But the difference between primary and adduction position is a rather constant factor.

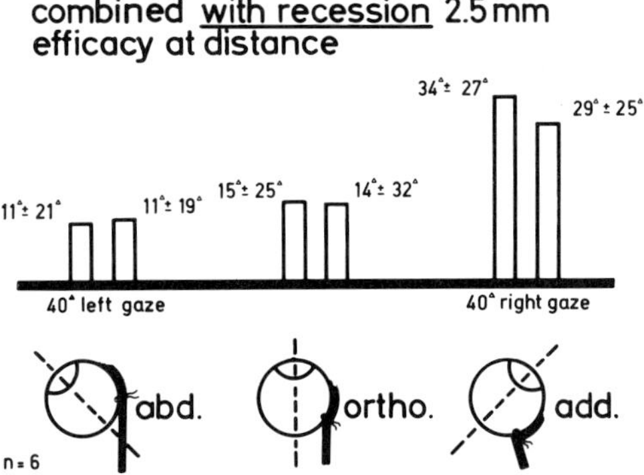

Figure 5. Medium angle ET. The additional recession was performed at the insertion. The mean values are representative, the high standard error of this sample, however, demonstrates clinical problems. One operation produced an excessive overcorrection, the mere removal of the sutures gave a satisfactory result. Another one was insufficient: at reoperation we found the sutures to have gone out of the sclera. This we had diagnosed in advance because of the persisting overadduction. We successfully renewed the Fadenfixation.

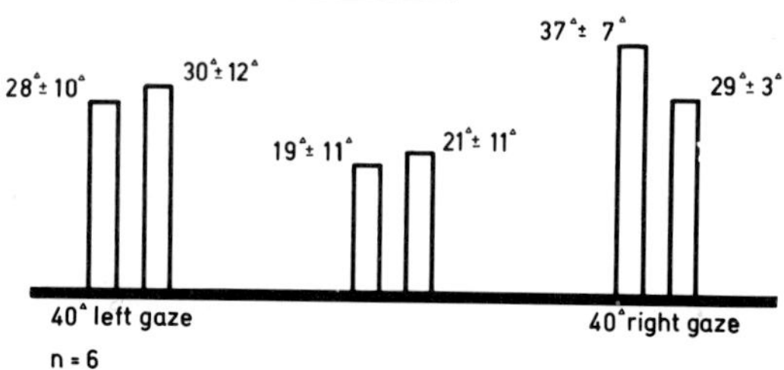

Figure 6. Standard technique. Medium angle ET. The incomitance pattern is less prominent than in unilateral procedures.

"static", the additional effect at near "dynamic". Our indication is the primary or postsurgical nonaccommodative convergence excess, since an absolute accommodative convergence excess can be perfectly cured by Varilux glasses. The majority of cases, however, do not sufficiently respond to bifocals (i.e. are only partly accommodative). The Fadenoperation does not replace the full hyperopic correction, and some patients reach their optimum reduction of squint when bifocals and bilateral Fadenoperation are combined. (Conrad)(5).

Variable angles

"Variable angles" vary at a given direction and distance of fixation. They are caused neither by fusional nor by accommodative factors, but by fixation effort, fatigue, psychic stress, and by "time itself". Similary observations were described by Seitz and Zehender(6). Cuppers(1) 1974 and Muhlendyck and Linnen(4,7) 1975 called the minimum degree of varying angles "static" and the amplitude towards the maximum "dynamic component". Von Noorden(8) calls the minimum of a "variable" angle "basic" or "constant" deviation, because he used the term "dynamic" for fusional and accommodative variations (9).

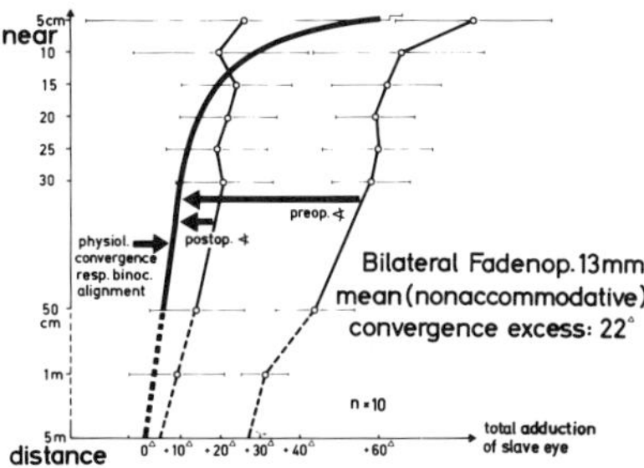

Figure 7. Measurements done by simultaneous prism-and-cover test in order not to elicit "latent components". We see the typical profile of efficacy of the standard Fadenoperation depending largely on the actual adduction of the operated eye(s). Note that the physiological convergence (total adduction) of either eye is only 10° at a fixation distance of 30 cm! Only with excessive convergence the increase of the effects is early and significant. The average maximum of the convergence excess is at a fixation distance of 25 cm. The profile, however, continues to grow exponentially. Therefore, it "comes late", giving a chance for recess-resect operations in case of a large angle at distance. If, however, there is a small angle at distance, conventional surgery would correct the angle either at distance or at near.

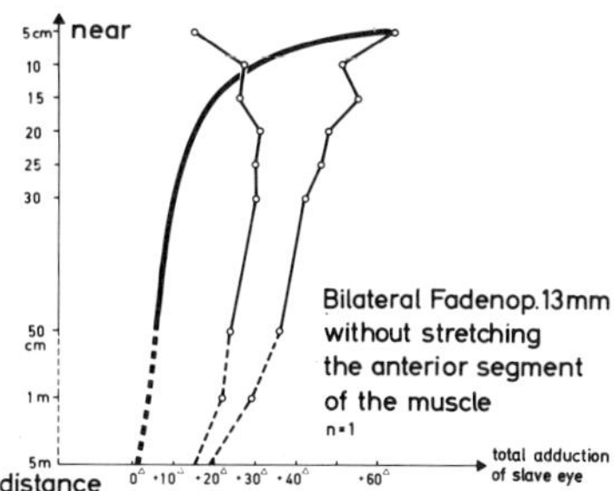

Figure 8. Illustration like Figure 7, but "unstretch" technique: The sutures passed through the exposed (Fig 11) muscle at 15.5 mm behind the insertion, the sclera at 13 mm. The loops were closed with the globe in its orthoposition by means of a push-suture instrument (prod.: Grosse). The basic effect of Figures 6 and 7 is reduced to 4°, the typical slight exponential increase of the effect is preserved. In a second step a resection of one lateral rectus muscle was performed to correct the residual basic angle.

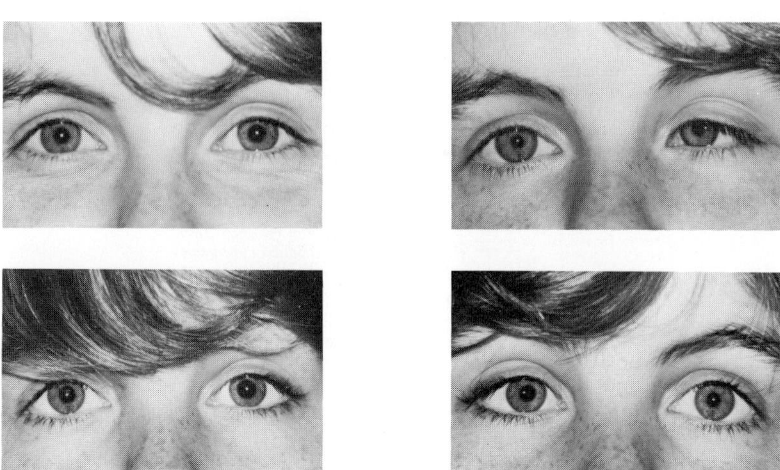

Figure 9. Upper row (preop): persistent variable angle after recess-resect procedures on both eyes. The range of variation does not depend on different distances of fixation. Emmetropia.
Lower row (postop): After additional Fadenoperation on both medial recti (12.5 mm, standard technique), the basic microtropia (left) is undisturbed. The maximum angle (right) appears reduced from 40^ to 20^. In case of instable eye positions without fusional ability or if the surgeon produced too much of the stretch effect, the minimum angle would have been turned into an XT: Compare Figure 7 with Figure 8 and 10.

Figure 9 demonstrates the lacking effect at times of the minimum angle, and the reduction of the maximum by about 50%. This varying efficacy depends on the varying amount of adduction of the globe during angle variations (Fig 10). On the other hand, if the mere Fadenoperation is 100% successful in a static angle, this is explained by the static effect of stretching the anterior segment - i.e. recessing the posterior segment (Fig 8, 11). It does not give proof to the hypothesis of de Decker(10) and Muhlendyck(11) which say that such an angle must have been entirely variable since the Fadenoperation works on "dynamic" components only. If the Faden worked only in the adducted eye, the deviating forces in the primary position would persist after the operation, requiring a superb fusional capability. This indeed would raise the question of Knapp(12): "Why did they squint at all?" The same arguments refute the application of a pure (unstretch) Fadenoperation for decompensating esophorias.

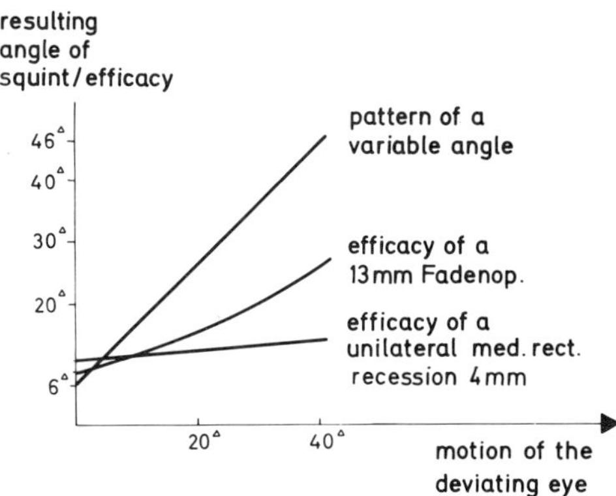

Figure 10. The abolition of dynamic components would demand absolute immobilization. Still the Fadenoperation creates marked reduction of the amplitude of angle variations. Some overcorrection of the minimum angle (beware of diplopia!) augments the reduction of the maximum angle. On the other hand, operating without any stretch of the anterior segment can even undercorrect a minimum angle (See figure 8).

"Unstretch" technique without static effects

Figure 8 demonstrates the efficacy of the pure Fadenoperation: No basic effect, but the same increasing shape at near as in Figure 7. The additional static effect in Figure 7 is due to our standard technique which stretches the anterior segment (Fig 11).

Clinical conclusions

The efficacy of the Fadenoperation of the medial rectus muscle is quadrifold: 1. typical incomitance pattern at lateral gaze; 2. reduction of (over) convergence; 3. reduction of the amplitude of variable esotropic angles; and 4. reduction of "static" angles if anterior segment is stretched.

The surgeon analyses the motility and decides: Suitable efficacy or unwanted side effects?

With firm fixation sutures the calculations are reliable. As well those of the typical "dynamic" curves, as those of the "static effect: zero (unstretch), moderate (stretch), marked (stretch of anterior segment plus recession at insertion or resection of antagonist). The "unstretch" profile is distinct from conventional recess-resect operations. There is no operation to compete with the pure Fadenoperation.

"Static" overcorrections can be compensated by recessing the antagonist, "dynamic" ones by removing the fixation sutures.

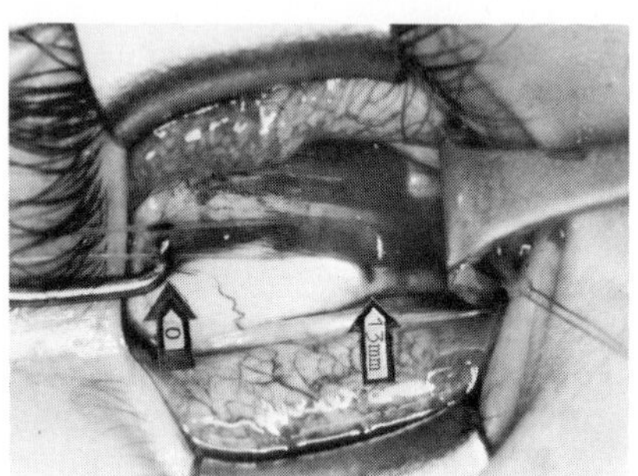

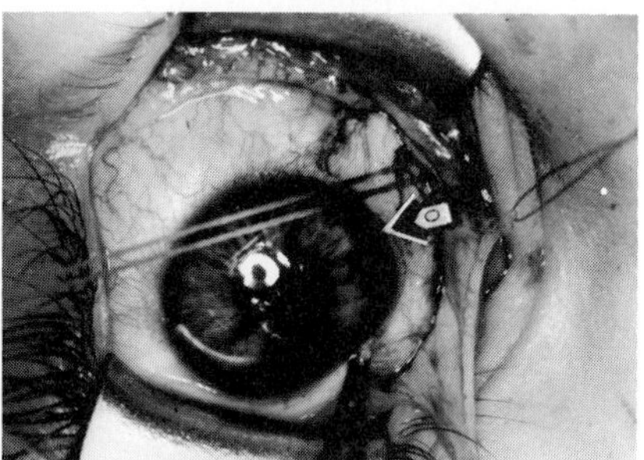

Figure 11. Left: To expose the muscle, the eye is abducted some 20 mm. The stretched(13) medial rectus muscle is marked by a thread 13 mm behind its insertion, beside the 13 mm ink point on the sclera. The ink spots on the threads mark their zero points above the insertion.
Right: When the globe is allowed to return to its primary position the muscle takes up some slack. The zero marks on the threads arrive at the limbus, indicating the shrunk length of the anterior muscle segment. Of which the borderline measures 8 mm now, instead of 13 mm. Since in our standard technique the tight sutures (Fig 1) do prevent the stretched and fixed muscle fibers from slipping forward, the effect of a moderate slack, i.e. recession of the posterior segment arises (20). This mechanical effect is different from a myosensory "stretch effect" discussed by Ishikawa(16). It explains the high "correction rate" by "Faden only" reported by de Decker (14). The original technique(15),(4) allows the stretch to disappear more or less. Having learned to govern the stretch effect (Fig 8),(20), we have the choice: zero static component of efficacy as postulated by Cuppers(1,15) and by Muhlendyck(4) from the theoretical point of view-or the marked static effect which de Decker(10) produced practically, and which Muhlendyck (see chapter "variable angles") seemingly had.

Physiological Considerations

The "static" effect or the effect in primary position, at far, on minimum angles is explained by the stretch of the anterior segment (Fig 11) of the muscle at the time of suturing (Fig 1). This creates a recession of the posterior segment. Hence its tension is reduced. Our assumption of an inherent paretic component due to the inactivation of the anterior 13 mm (17) must be refuted: The force at a given innervation and cross section of the muscle depends solely on its extension(19). None of these factors is influenced by a pure Fadenoperation. This hypotheses explains all clinical experiences. We could prove it(20) by frog muscle experiments, "disc and rubber band" models, and by operating with our unstretch technique, which allows a wanted zero static effect.

This stretch effect aims at: all positions; concomitant components; any distance of fixation; and minimum ET angle ("static" component, "basic"/"constant" deviation).

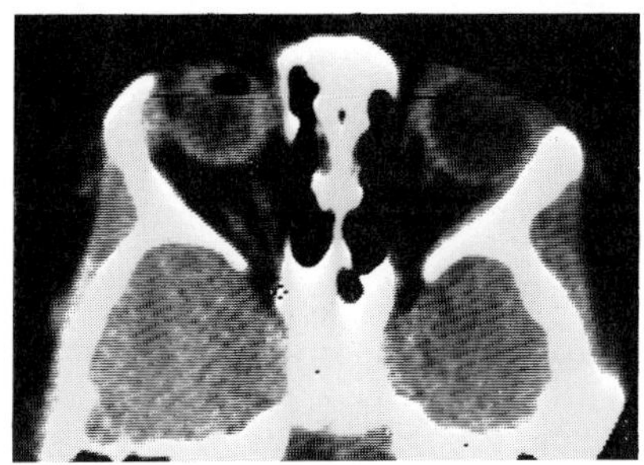

Figure 12. CT scan records (2-mm-layers, exposure time 3 sec.) from the Radiologische Klinik, University Kiel, Director Prof. Dr. med. H. Gremmel. (We are indebted to our colleagues A. Frank and A. Ahlendorf.) Preop. ET + 50°, postop. ET + 20° (glasses taken off). Bilateral 13 mm Fadenoperation, standard technique with stretch effect. Preop. the medial rectus muscle lies tangentially whether eye is adducted or straight. Like the abducted right eye, the path of the medial rectus to its origin is straight back or even a bit in the medial direction. Post op. the posterior segment of the left muscle aims at a point close to the middle of the globe when the eye is adducted. This illustrates that the torque has vanished exponentially according to the decreasing lever arm. The muscle contracts by 8 - 9 mm preop., but only 3 - 4 post op.

The "dynamic" effect of the Fadenoperation depends solely on the length of the lever arm (See figure 12). For the adducted position Conrad and Treumer(1) (18) assumed an accelerated decrease of extension of the posterior muscle segment alone and consequently of muscle forces. This must be refuted, too. If the arm of contact is fixed, the posterior segment contracts by only few millimeters because it pulls a short lever arm. This can be demonstrated in a disc-and-rubber-band model, and from CT scan measurements (Fig 12)(20). Hence the length-tension characteristics (19) point to increased rather than decreased forces.

The decrease of the lever arm aims at: lateral gaze; incomitant yoke muscle disorders; convergence (excess); maximum ET angle, ("dynamic" components/"variable" angles); eccentric fixation(21); improving in extreme; and adduction, but ET angle only moderate.

The slight exponential curve of angle reduction (Fig 2) appears flat(22) as compared with the steep reduction of torque calculated by Cuppers(1) as consequence of the shortening lever arm. But in fact it adds up with the slight exponential increase of muscle forces (and consequently of torque) required in extreme adduction(19).

Further comments on the Fadenoperation

1. (Over) adduction (excursion) is reduced by 2-3 mm.

2. Alphabetic patterns are reduced like variable angles.

3 Upshoot or downshoot is leassened if manifest with extreme adduction.

4. There are no vertical side effects (unless the muscle slipped up or down).

5. Postop forced duction usually is free.

6. Four muscle Fadenprocedures reduce large nystagmus amplitudes or bring exhaustable, and therefore alternating, contrary neutral zones of nystagmus into the practical field of fixation.

7. The shift of a gaze directed neutral zone of nystagmus by Fadenoperations is indicated, if the extent varies.

8. The Fadenoperation overcomes the contradiction: Small angle of squint in primary position but extreme eccentricity of nystagmus null-points of the fixating eyes (cross fixator).

9. The Fadenoperation of a yoke muscle sometimes leaves slight diplopia at small versions, and causes overcorrection of the extreme version, because the profile is too flat at tis beginning and too steep at its end. A resect-recess operation would overcorrect the primary position.

10. Instead of resection plus Fadenoperation(23) in cases with XT at far and ET at near, we might exaggerate the unstretch principle and stretch the posterior segment.

11. If the spring back balance test(24) reveals a marked contracture or a strabismus fixus, a recession is needed since the static angle will not be overcome if the muscle cannot be stretched at the time of locking the Faden.

12. If horizontal and vertical recti are to be operated, the Fadenoperation without dissection of the insertion saves ciliary blood vessels.

REFERENCES

1. Cuppers C: The so-called "Fadenoperation". Surgical corrections by well-defined changes of the arm of contact. In Fells P (ed), II Congr ISA, Marseilles 1974, pp. 395, 1976.

2. de Decker W, Conrad HG: Fadenoperation nach Cuppers bei komplizierten Augenmuskelstorungen and nichtakkommodativem Konvergenzexzeb. Klin Mbl Augenheilk 167:217-226, 1975.

3. Conrad HG, de Decker W: Zur Technik der Fadenoperation. 133 Vers Rhein Westf Augenarzte, Pro p. 73, 1977.

4. Muhlendyck H: Diagnosis of convergent strabismus with nystagmus and its treatment with Cuppers´ "Fadenoperation". III Internat Orthoptic Congress, Boston 1975, Trans 1976, p. 143.

5. Conrad HG: Fotografische Erfassung des schwankenden Schielwinkels. Arbeitskreis Schielbehandlung BVA 1980, 13:87, 1982.

6. Seitz E, Zehender W: Handbuch der gesamten Augenheilkunde, 2nd ed, p. 924 f Enk, Erlangen 1869.

7. Muhlendyck H, Linnen HJ: Die operative Behandlung nystagmusbedingter schwankender Scghielwinkel mit der Fadenoperation nach Cuppers. Klin Mbl Augenheilk 167:273-290, 1975.

8. Burian HM, von Noorden GK: Binocular vision and ocular motility, 2nd ed. p. 185 & 448, C V Mosby, St. Louis, 1980.

9. von Noorden GK: Personal communication, Hamburg 1982.

10. de Decker W: Gibt es einen statischen und einen hynamischen Schielwinkelanteil? (Beobachtungen nach Fadenoperation trotz stabil scheinendem Schielwinkel). Vortrag, BVA-Strabolog. Seminarwoche 1980 (Eifel).

11. Muhlendyck H: Personal communication, Gottingen 1982.

12. Knapp P: Personal communication, Kyoto 1978.

13. Baenge J: unpublished observations, Kiel 1979.

14. de Decker W: The Fadenoperation. When and hot to do to. Trans Ophthalmol Soc UK 101:264, 1981.

15. Cuppers C: Kommentar zum Film: Bernardini D, Raspiller: Die Fadenoperation - Bilanz und Ausblick. Arbeitskreis Schielen BVA 1979, 12:11, 1980.

16. Ishikawa S: Personal communication, Kyoto 1978.

17. Conrad HG, Treumer H: Inkomitanzen nach Fadenoperation. Arbeitskreis Schielbehandlung 1977, Bd. 10:71-77, 1978.

18. Conrad HG, Treumer H: Zum Wirkungsprofil der Fadenoperation. Klin Mbl Augenheilk 178:174-179, 1981.

19. Bach-Y-Rita P, Collin CC, Hyde JE: The control of eye movements. Academic Press, New York 1971.

20. Kluge G: Unpublished investigations for an Inauguraldissertation at Faculty of medicine, Kiel 1982.

21. Thomas C, Spielman A, Bernardini D: Erfahrugen bei der Behandlung der Amblyopia mit exzentrischer Fixation durch Veranderungen des Innervationsimpulses auBerer Augenmuskeln

mittels Prismen und chirurgischen Eingriffen nach den von Cuppers aufgestellten Prinzipien. Klin Mbl Augenheilk 167:157-162, 1975.

22. Scott AB: The Faden operation: Mechanical effects. Am Orthopt J 27:44-47, 1977.

23. Spielmann A, Laulan J: Action of recessions and resections when associated with Cuppers´ Fadenoperation in esotropia. Statistical results. In (Ed) Reinecke RD: Strabismus Proc III Meeting ISA, Kyoto 1978. Grune & Stratton, New York 1978, pp. 355-369.

24. Jampolsky A: Spring-back balance test in strabismus surgery. Trans New Orleans Academy Ophthalmol, C V Mosby, St. Louis 1978, p. 104-111.

EVALUATION OF THE POSTERIOR FIXATION OPERATION WITH SACCACIC VELOCITIES

B. J. Kushner

ABSTRACT

I performed a posterior fixation of the medial rectus in 7 patients with convergence excess esotropia and successfully reduced their esotropia at near. Postoperative saccadic velocity testing did not reveal the expected decrease in saccadic velocity as the eye moved increasingly into the field of action of the operated muscle. Posterior fixation of a rectus muscle may enhance the effect of the standard recession operation by increasing the amount of slack created in the functional part of the muscle after recession. Also, it may make a large percentage of the muscle fibers ineffective.

INTRODUCTION

The Faden operation was described by Cuppers(1) as a new way of weakening an extraocular muscle. von Noorden(2) suggested the English term "posterior fixation" as more appropriately describing the surgical procedure. The operation consists of suturing part of a rectus muscle to the sclera posterior to the equator creating a second functional insertion. It may be combined with a recession operation. The posterior fixation operation ws initially described as a treatment for the nystagmus blockage syndrome of Cuppers.(3) More recently, posterior fixation surgery has been recommended for treating dissociated vertical divergence, convergence excess esotropia, Duane's syndrome, Brown's syndrome, double elevator palsy, and face turns associated with nystagmus.(4,5,6,7) Scott(7) described the changes in torque that would theoretically occur as the medial rectus was recessed various amounts combined with a posterior fixation. He theorized that a posterior fixation of a rectus muscle should result in a decreased torque exerted by that muscle as the eye moved into the field of action of the muscle.

The purpose of this paper is to investigate the forces generated by muscles having undergone posterior fixation in various fields of gaze postoperatively using saccadic velocities, and to suggest several other mechanisms by which the posterior fixation operation may enhance the effect of a recession operation.

STRABISMUS II
ISBN 0-8089-1424-3

SUBJECTS AND METHODS

This series consists of 7 patients treated by me with a posterior fixation of a medial rectus 14 mm. from the insertion combined with a recession ranging from 2 to 7 mm. for convergence excess esotropia. All were adults with either strabismic, refractive, or organic amblyopia in the deviating eye and were bothered cosmetically by an esotropia at near. Although many of them demonstrated a high accommodative convergence to accommodation ratio, the presence of amblyopia and the absence of good fusion made bifocals an unsatisfactory treatment modality. Measurements were made using the prism and cover test at 6 meters and at 1/3 meter with appropriate spectacle corrections. All patients had central fixation in their amblyopic eye.

Surgical technique consisted of isolating the medial rectus through a limbal opening. Prior to disinserting the medial rectus a point in the muscle 14 mm. posterior to the insertion minus the planned amount of recession was tagged with a 5-0 nonabsorbable suture, either dacron or supramid. The muscle wa then disinserted and one arm of the tagging suture was placed in the sclera 14 mm. posterior to the insertion as measured along the curve of the globe in a manner previously described.(8) The suture was then brought up through the undersurface of the medial rectus opposite the original entry site of the suture placed so approximately 50% of the fibers of the medial rectus were between the two arms of the posterior fixation suture. The muscle was then recessed the desired amount and the posterior fixation suture tied on the anterior surface of the medial rectus. In some patients surgery was performed on other extraocular muscles simultaneously.

Saccadic velocities were performed using our standard electro-oculogram apparatus in a manner previously described.(9) The saccadic velocity of the eye undergoing the posterior fixation operation was tested for a series of saccades of 20 degrees, each starting with the eye moving from 40 degrees temporal to 20 degrees temporal. Velocities generated during adducting saccades of 20 degrees were consecutively repeated as the starting point for the saccade was shifted in 10 degrees increments nasally. This resulted in a total of 6 saccadic velocity determinations of 20 degrees each beginning with 40 degrees temporal to 20 degrees temporal and ending with a recording from 20 degrees nasal to 40 degrees nasal.

In 5 of the subjects the operated eye was used for fixation during saccadic velocity testing. In two of the subjects their visual acuity was not satisfactory in the operated eye to allow for accurate fixation. It is noteworthy that these two patients had no measureable horizontal incomitance in their ocular alignment postoperatively as determined with prism and cover testing.

RESULTS

One patient will be described in detail.

A 28-year-old woman was evaluated for a left esotropia. She had been born with a cataract in her left eye and reported that her left eye had been esotropic all her life. Her visual acuity was 6/6 in the right eye when wearing -1.75 + .75 x 50. Her left eye had a best corrected visual acuity of 6/60 with -3.50 +2.00 x 90. She demonstrated no horizontal strabismus at 6 meters with a left hypertropia of 5 prism diopters. At near there was 35 prism diopters of left esotropia with 5 prism diopters of left hypertropia. A +3.00 sphere in the front of her fixing eye eliminated the esotropia at near. A posterior lenticonus cataract was present in her left eye. A bifocal had been previously tried, however, she felt that she did not use the bifocal for near and her left esotropia was cosmetically unacceptable.

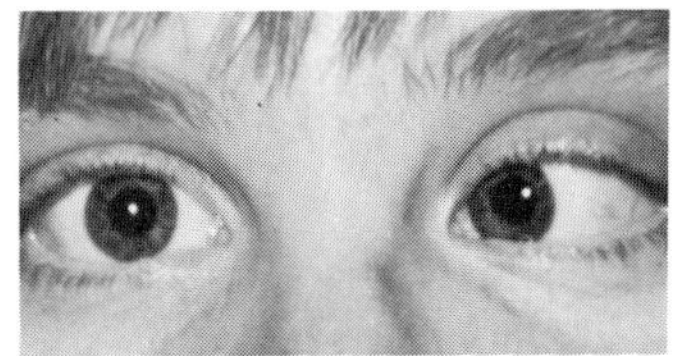

(Top)

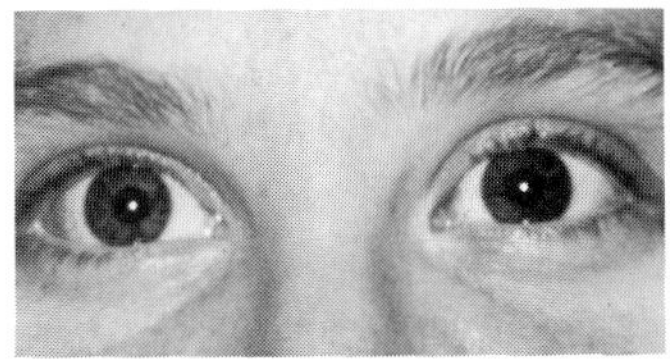

(Middle)

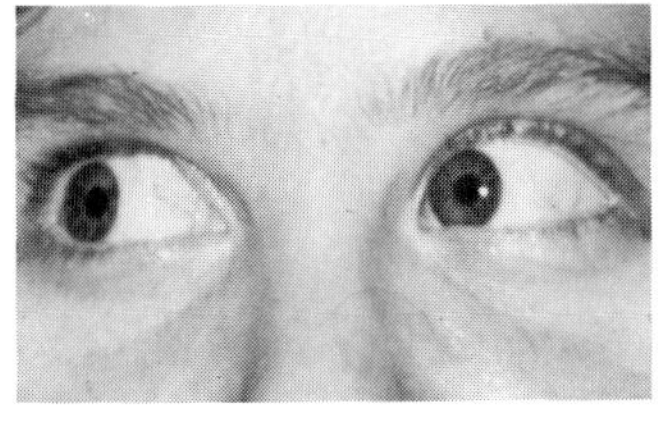

(Bottom)

Figure 1 (Kushner). Case 1 preoperatiely showing left esotropia at near fixation. (Top) Case 1 postoperatively demonstrating approximate orthophoria at near fixation. (Middle) Case 1 postoperatively showing no limitation of adduction of left eye (Bottom)

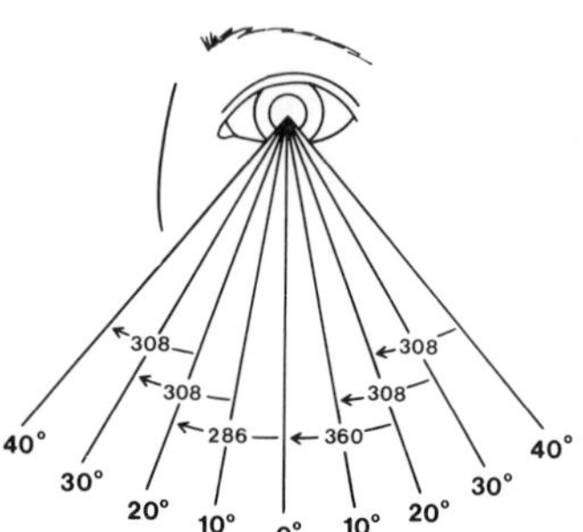

Figure 2 (Kushner). Diagram of saccadic velocities of Case 1, 14 months after surgery. There is no apparent decrease in saccadic velocities as the eyes are tested in fields of further adduction.

I performed a posterior fixation of the left medial rectus muscle 14mm. from the insertion combined with a recession of 3 mm. on an adjustable suture. No postoperative adjustment was made. Postoperatively, she demonstrated 5 prism diopters of left exotropia in the distance with a left hypertropia of 5 prism diopters. At near a 4 prism diopter left esotropia was present. Sixteen months after surgery, saccadic velocity testing was performed. Her ocular motility has remained stable for four years. No limitation of adduction was noted. (Figure 1) No decrease was noted in the saccadic velocity generated as the eye made 20 degrees saccades successively further into the field of adduction (Figure 2).

The clinical data on the remaining 6 patients and their postoperative saccadic velocities are summarized in Tables 1 and 2. In all 7 patients the saccadic velocity did not exhibit the expected progressive decrease as the eye was tested in fields that were successively further in adduction. Nevertheless, all 7 patients demonstrated postoperatively a greater decrease in the esotropia at near than one would expect from the amount of recession performed alone.

Table 1

Clinical Data, Cases 2 through 7

Case	Age at time of surgery (Years)	Ocular Findings	Preoperative Measurements	Surgery	Postoperative Measurements	Months between Surgery & Saccadic Velocities
2	29	OS Congenital cataract	Orthophoria distance variable LET' 18	Posterior fixation LMR 14 mm & recess 2 mm	LXT' 10	12
3	35	OS congenital cataract	45 LET 60 LET' & 10 L HYPO	Posterior fixation LMR 14 mm & recess LMR 7 mm resect LLR 8 mm	LXT 8 LET' 6	5
4	49	Anisometropia amblyopia OD	RET 10 RET' 30	Posterior fixation RMR 14 mm & recess RMR 2 mm	RET 5 RET' 5	10
5	61	Strabismic amblyopia OD	RET 20 RET' 40	Posterior fixation RMR 14 mm & recess RMR 4 mm adj	RXT 10 RET' 5	2
6	35	Corneal scar OS	LET 5 LET'40	Posterior fixation LMR 14 mm & recess LMR 2 mm	LET 5 LET' 10	2
7	41	Anisometropic amblyopia OS	LET 15 & LET'45	Posterior fixation LMR 14 mm & recess LMR 5 mm adj resect LLR 5 mm	LXT 5 & LXT' 5	8

adj = adjustable suture
ET = esotropia at 6 meters
ET' = ET at 1/3 meter
HYPO = hypotropia
RMR = right medial rectus
LMR = left medial rectus
LR = lateral rectus

Table 2

Saccadic Velocities Cases 2 through 7

Case #	40° Temporal to 20° Temporal	30° Temporal to 10° Temporal	20° Temporal to Primary	10° Temporal to 10° Nasal	Primary to 20° Nasal	10° Temporal to 30° Nasal	20° Temporal to 40° Nasal
2	278*	286	260	286	290	278	278
3	308	252	260	Not Tested	231	224	239
4	270	282	282	300	270	265	282
5	203	210	210	221	210	205	210
6	256	250	221	284	221	244	244
7	301	208	274	308	290	290	295

* All saccadic velocity measurements are in degrees per second.

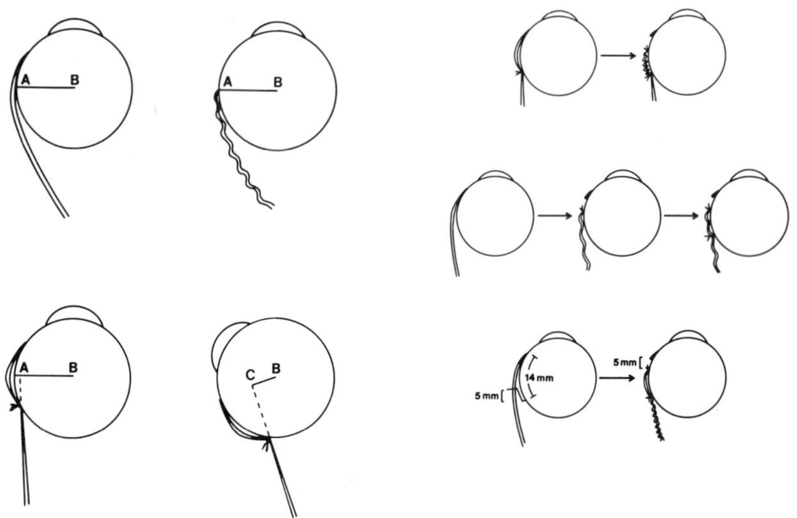

Figure 3

Figure 4

DISCUSSION

Figure 3 (Kushner). The effective lever arm of a medial rectus prior to recession runs from the equator to the center of rotation Line A-B (Top Left). If recession is carried out to the equator, the lever arm does change (Top right). With posterior fixation suture and the eye in the primary position, there is a negligible shortening of the lever arm (Bottom left). With posterior fixation as the eye moves into the field of action of the operated muscle, the lever arm is substantially shortened, Line C-B (Bottom right).

Figure 4 (Kushner). The different ways of placing the posterior fixation suture in the muscle. (Top) Posterior fixation is first carried out and then the muscle recessed, resulting in all of the shortening occurring anterior to the posterior fixation suture. (Middle) Muscle is recessed and then posterior fixation suture brought through the point of the muscle opposite the scleral site of the posterior fixation suture. This results in even distribution of slack. (Bottom) Posterior fixation suture brought through the muscle at a point posterior to the insertion equal to the distance of the posterior fixation suture (14 mm) minus the amount of recessing (5 mm). Thus placement of the suture in the muscle 9 mm posterior to the insertion results in all of the slack occurring posterior to the posterior fixation suture.

The torque that a muscle generates on an eye is a function of the force generated by the muscle and the lever arm with which the muscle is turning the eye. The medial rectus normally inserts anterior to the equator. Therefore, the functional end of the lever arm of the medial rectus is where the muscle is furthest away from the center of rotation of the globe, the equator, Figure 3. As the medial rectus is recessed increasing amounts, but not posterior to the equator, this lever arm does not change. If the recession is carried out so as to put the medial rectus posterior to the equator, the lever arm is shortened and the torque generated by the medial rectus is reduced. If a posterior fixation suture is used far posterior to the equator, the lever arm of the medial rectus is not substantially altered when the eye is in the primary position. As the eye rotates into the field of action of the medial rectus, the point of posterior fixation starts moving temporally and shortens the lever arm thereby reducing torque. Scott(8) calculated that the posterior fixation at 10 mm. will exert essentially no effect in decreasing the torque exerted by a medial rectus until the eye is adducted 15 degrees. This mechanism of action, therefore, cannot explain the apparent effect of the posterior fixation suture in enhancing the effect of a recession. If a patient having undergone a posterior fixation operation manifests a small deviation of only several diopters postoperatively, the posterior fixation suture would not be contributing anything to altering the torque generated on the eye, if in fact the eye is close to straight. Based on Scott's calculations the posterior fixation suture might decrease a deviation to 15 degrees from a larger amount. If however, the eye is less than 15 degrees misaligned the posterior fixation suture is not altering substantially to the torque that the muscle generates.

Also, in my experience, one typically does not see a significant limitation of rotation of an eye having undergone a posterior fixation operation as one would expect based on the theoretical calculations.

Reports with posterior fixation surgery, do suggest that a greater surgical correction is obtained than if one performed a recession alone.(4,6) Other possible mechanisms of action of the posterior fixation operation deserves investigation.

Scott(8) has pointed out that when a muscle is recessed, slack is produced in the muscle as when one relaxes a spring. The force a muscle can generate is related to its length. As a muscle is shortened, the tension it generates decreases.(10) The use of a posterior fixation suture can alter the amount of slack in the effective fibers of a recessed muscle depending on how the posterior fixation suture is placed in the muscle.

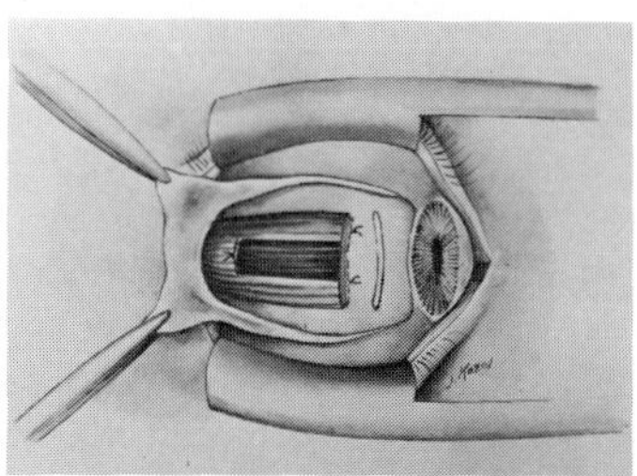

Figure 5 (Kushner). Fibers of muscle that are between the posterior fixation suture and the insertion of the muscle (dark shaded area) are incapable of exerting torque on the eye.

When a posterior fixation suture is combined with a recession, there are three basic alternative ways of determining where in the muscle the posterior fixation suture is placed, Figure 5. As Scott pointed out,(8) if one assumes the medial rectus to be approximately 28 mm. in length, and the posterior fixation suture is placed 14 mm. posterior to the insertion of the muscle, placement of the posterior fixation suture so that all of the slack in the medial rectus occurs posterior to the posterior fixation suture will double the amount of slack induced in the muscle posterior to the posterior fixation suture as compared to the standard recession operation. Thus, with a 5 mm. medial rectus recession one can obtain the amount of slack in the muscle that would otherwise require a 10 mm. recession, which would cripple the action of the medial rectus.

Alternatively, the posterior fixation suture could be placed in the muscle so that all of the shortening takes place between the new insertion of the muscle and the posterior fixation suture. This would appear less effective than the standard recession operation because none of the slack is occurring in the muscle between it origin and the posterior fixation suture. It is this part of the muscle that is effective in exerting torque on the eye. A third way of placing the posterior fixation suture in the muscle would allow the muscle to be recessed the desired amount and then to bring the posterior fixation suture through that part of the muscle which is opposite the posterior fixation suture as it leaves the sclera. This method would seem to distribute the slack evenly between the front and thė anterior and posterior part of the muscle and would seem les advantageous than the first method described, however, more effective than the second method.

Some authors are specific in describing where the posterior fixation suture is placed in the muscle,(1,4) and others are not specific.(3,6)

Clearly, different ways of placing the posterior fixation suture in the muscle would have different effects on ocular motility.

Another possible effect of the posterior fixation suture deserves mention. If the posterior fixation suture is firm enough that muscle fibers running between it and the insertion cannot slide under the suture, they have been made ineffective in exerting any torque on the eye. Thus, if the distance between the arms of a posterior fixation suture are approximately 50% of the width of the muscle, and if it is placed approximately midway along the length of the muscle (14 mm. from the insertion), 25% of the fibers of the muscle are in effect rendered inactive. If this mechanism of action is significant, then the number of sutures used to effect posterior fixation and the width of the bite of the muscle taken, would be important.

This study only attempts to determine whether muscles having undergone a posterior fixation in fact show a progressive decrease in saccadic velocity as the eye moves into the field of action of the operated muscle as would be expected on theoretical grounds. It does not attempt to describe the change in muscle function after posterior fixation surgery as compared to preoperative levels. Therefore, the fact that none of the patients in this study had preoperative saccadic velocities, or the fact that patients had posterior fixation combined with various amounts of recession, would not influence the conclusions in this article.

All of the patients were amblyopic in the eye being tested in this study. The possibility that the decreased reaction time of amblyopic eyes may have influenced the saccadic velocity results deserves discussion. Because this study compared the saccadic velocities of the same eye in different fields of gaze, one would expect that any error induced by the presence of amblyopia should be consistent in different fields of gaze. One would not expect the decreased reaction time of amblyopia to cause an artificially lower saccadic velocity only in the temporal fields of gaze. Also, two of the patients in this study had saccadic velocities measured with the non-amblyopic eye fixing as has been previously discussed.

Patients undergoing posterior fixation of a medial rectus muscle combined with an adjustable suture recession were excluded from this study if the amount of recession was in fact adjusted postoperatively. The two patients in this study who underwent an adjustable suture recession combined with posterior fixation (Cases 5 and 7) were not adjusted postoperatively, so the final amount of recession was known exactly. Postoperative adjustment to alter the point at which a muscle inserts on the sclera when it has been fixated posteriorly by a suture would not be expected to have the same effect on ocular muscle balance as postoperative adjustment of a muscle that had not been fixated posteriorly. Nevertheless, my experience with cases not included in this series who underwent postoperative adjustment of a recessed muscle combined with a posterior fixation suture indicates that one can change the postoperative alignment with adjustment. Therefore, altering the length-tension relationship and the muscle fibers anterior to the posterior fixation does affect ocular motility.

Theoretically, a posterior fixation suture should have resulted in a successive decrease in saccadic velocities as the operated eyes move into adduction. The reason this was not observed is not clear. Possibly because the posterior fixation encompassed only 50% of the muscle, the remaining 50% which continued to have their functional insertion at the anatommic insertion of the muscle, were sufficient to overcome any decrease in torque.

REFERENCES

1. Cuppers D: The so-called "Fadenoperation" (surgical correction by well-defined changes in the arc of contact). In Fells P (ed.): Second Congress of the International Strabismological Association. Marseilles, Diffusion Generale de Librairie, 1976, p. 395.

2. von Noorden GK: Indications of the posterior fixation operation in strabismus. Ophthalmology 85:512-520, 1978.

3. Muhlendych H: Diagnosis of convergent strabismus with nystagmus and its treatment with Cuppers Faden operation. In Moore S, Mein J, Stockbridge L (eds) Orthoptics: Past, Present, and Future, N.Y. Symposia Specialits, 1976, p. 143-154.

4. Sprague JB, Moore S, Eggers H, Knapp P: Dissociated vertical deviation. Arch Ophthalmol 98:465, 1980.

5. Schuckett EP, Hiles DA, Bigland AW, Evans DE: Posterior fixation suture operation (Fadenoperation). Ophthalmic Surgery 12:578-585, 1981.

6. Bedrossian EH: Recent advances in the surgical management of strabismus. J of Ocular Therapy & Surgery 1:(1A)25-30, 1982.

7. Scott AB: The Faden operation: mechanical effects. Am Orthopt J 27:44-47, 1977.

8. Kushner BJ: A measuring suture for large strabismus surgical measurements. Ophthalmic Surgery. 12:650-651 1981.

9. Jones RM, Stevens TS, Gould S: Normal EOG values of young subjects. In ERG, VER, and Psychophysics (14th ISCERG Symposium, May 1976, Louisville, Ky.) Lawwill T, editor, Doc Ophthalmol Proc Ser 1977, 13:93-97.

10. Hill AV: The mechanics of active muscle. Proc Roy Soc London. Series B. 141:104-117, 1953.

DISCUSSION BY G. KOMMERELL

Dr. Kushner aptly pointed out that the posterior fixation operation may work through several mechanisms, depending on the individual surgical technique. I certainly agree that after such procedures saccades are difficult to interpret.

PATTERN APPEARANCE - DISAPPEARANCE VEPS IN ANISOMETROPIC AMBLYOPIA

T. Ohzeki and E. Adachi-Usami

ABSTRACT

The amplitude of the appearance response of the pattern visual evoked potentials (VEPs) as a function of check sizes was studied in 32 anisometropic amblyopes with central fixation. In the poor visual acuity group, the amplitude vs. check sizes curve was remarkably depressed for all check sizes, while in the good visual acuity group the depression of the curve was observed only in small check sizes. In parallel to the improvement of the visual acuity, the maxima of the curves shifted to the smaller check sizes. It is assumed that the poor visual acuity group will reveal predominance of the parafoveal function, while the good visual acuity group will predominate in the foveal function.

INTRODUCTION

It is well known that uniocular hyperopia or astigmatism in early childhood is the major cause of amblyopia. If these anisometropic amblyopes receive occlusion therapy in the early stages, most amblyopes obtain good visual acuity, but hardly the same visual acuity as the healthy eye. Since a series of Wiesel's and Hubel works(9,10) suggested that in light deprived kittens there were functional and histological abnormalities in their higher visual pathways, pattern VEPs have been preferably used for studying human amblyopia. Lombroso et al(6), Spekreijse et al(7), Arden et al(2), reported that pattern VEPs of amblyopic eyes revealed reduction in amplitude. Recent works demonstrated that the amblyopic eye showed reduced sensitivity for high spatial frequencies and is affected by abnormal temporal tuning functions. However, in the majority of their amblyopes, fixation behaviors were not always central, and visual acuities were poor. We, therefore, studied spatial tuning activity using pattern appearance-disappearance VEPs, in anisometropic amblyopes with central fixation. Furthermore, following the visual acuity improvement, VEPs were evaluated.

STRABISMUS II
ISBN 0-8089-1424-3

METHODS

Checkerboard pattern stimuli of the appearance-disappearance mode, were employed.(7) Appearance and disappearance times were the same at 266ms. The mean luminance was 47.5cd/m(2) and the contrast of the pattern was 53%. Check sizes were 1 degrees 36', 48', 24' and 12'. The test field was circular subtending 12.6 degrees for the subjects sitting 1m from the surface of the T.V. monitor. The screen was viewed monocularly with central fixation. The VEPs were recorded by a silver/silver electrode placed at the inion and an indifferent electrode was attached to the earlobes. The time constant was 0.3 and a high cut filter of 25Hz was used. Sixty-four or 128 responses were averaged and written out by an X-Y recorder. When the fixation was moved from a fixation point, recording was stopped immediately. An artificial pupil was not used. Subjects were asked to fixate on the center of a pattern field monocularly. Cycloplegia was obtained with 1% cyclopentrate and the refractive error was corrected. Thirteen normal subjects from 4 to 14 years were examined for the controls. Thirty-two anisometroic amblyopes from 5 to 14 years were studied. All were hypermetropic anisometropes of more than 1.75D. with central fixation. The amplitude of the first negative trough, N1, to the first positive, P1, and peak implicit time of N1, P1 and second positive, P2, were measured.

RESULTS

Pattern appearance-disappearance VEPs were examined in the anisometropic amblyopes in order to investigate the central function of clinical amblyopes. One example of anisometropic amblyopia had visual acuity of 0.3. The normal eye showed prominent appearance VEPs (negative N1 and positive P1) on all check sizes from 1 degrees 36' to 12' tested, with rather small disappearance VEPs. The amblyopic eye showed M-shaped appearance VEPs (namely negative N1, N2 and positive P1, P2) with disappearance VEPs almost the same as the healthy eye. In this case the amplitude of N1 to P1 of the amblyopic eye showed marked attenuation compared to the amplitude of the healthy eye. While N1 peak implicit time (p.it.) was about 70ms. with both eyes,P1 p.i.t. was 157 ms. with the healthy eye and 100 ms. with the amblyopic eye, but P2 p.i.t. was 180ms only with the amblyopic eye. When the visual acuity was improved to 0.6, the amplitude of VEPs of the amblyopic eye showed marked increase and M-shaped appearance VEPs of the amblyopic eye changed to the same pattern as the healthy appearance VEPs. P1 p.i.t. of both eyes were almost the same. Fig 1 shows the relative amplitude vs. check size curve. When the visual acuity in the amblyopic eye was 0.3, the amplitude of VEPs was markedly attenuated in all check sizes, but in parallel to the improvement of the visual acuity, the amplitude showed marked increase with 2 check sizes (48' and 24'), but no amplitude change was found with the smallest check size (12').

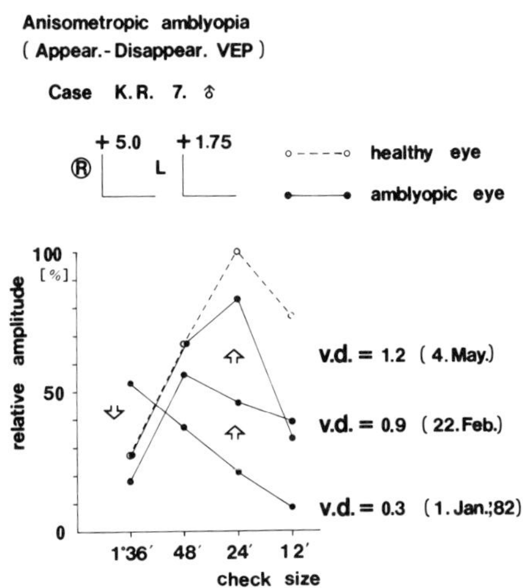

Figure 1 illustrates the amplitude vs. check sizes curves. The amplitude increased markedly with 2 check sizes (48' & 24'), but the smallest check size did not change. The maximum amplitude shifted from the largest to the smaller check sizes.

In parallel to the improvement in visual acuity, the amplitude of VEPs increased with small check sizes of 24' and 12', while contrary to the improvement of the visual acuity, the amplitude decreased with large check sizes of 1 degrees 36' and 48'. Fig 2 summarizes amplitude vs. check sizes curve. The ordinate represents relative amplitude of VEPs and the abscissa represents check sizes. Open circles connected by a broken line indicate healthy eyes and solid circles connected by a solid line, amblyopic eyes. The upper left-hand and right-hand and the lower left-hand and right-hand figures show amplitude vs. check sizes curve concerning visual acuity from 0.3 to 1.2, visual acuity from 0.3 to 0.5 (poor visual acuity group), respectively. The

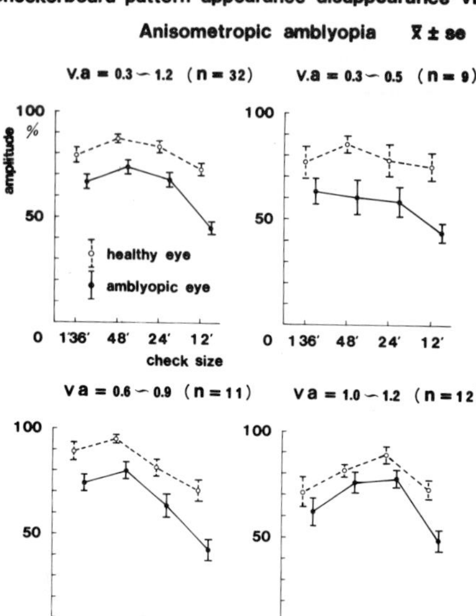

Fig 2. Top left graph shows the averaged curves of the 3 types of amplitude vs. check sizes curves obtained from poor, moderate and good visual acuity groups. The other 3 graphs show these groups individually. The amplitudes of the amblyopic eyes markedly decreased on all check sizes in poor visual acuity group. In parallel to improved visual acuity, the amplitude increased, while maximum amplitude shifted from largest to smaller check sizes.

amplitude vs. check sizes curve of the amblyopic eyes were decreased by approximately 25%, 15% and 5% for the poor visual acuity group, moderate visual acuity group and the good visual acuity group, respectively, compared to the healthy eyes. The maximum amplitude of the amblyopic eyes shifted on from the largest (1 degrees 36') to smaller check sizes (48',24') improving the visual acuity. Fig 3 shows the p.i.t. and check sizes curve with the moderate visual acuity group. No difference was found between the healthy and the amblyopic eyes with the N1 and P1 p.i.t. Fig 4 shows the p.i.t. and check sizes curve in the poor visual acuity group. N1 p.i.t. was similar to normal N1 p.i.t. Normal eyes showed a prominent P1 wave, but the amblyopic eyes showed and

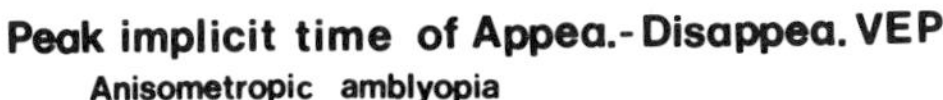

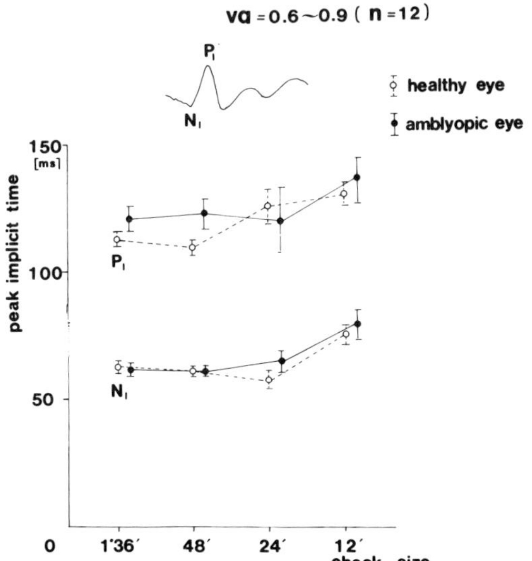

Figure 3 summarizes peak imlicit time and check sizes curve in the moderate visual acuity group. No difference was found in both eyes.

M-shaped wave, while the P1 p.i.t. of the healthy eyes were placed between P1 and P2 of the amblyopic eyes.

DISCUSSION

It is important that a subject fixate on the center of the stimulus field in the VEP recording, however, in the many reports of VEPs of amblyopia, the visual acuity of the amblyopes were poor and their fixation behaviors were not always central. Chiba et al(4) reported that the VEPs are not recordable when the fixation point is moved 3 degrees from the fovea. Adachi et al(1), reported when the normal eye moved freely within the stimulus field, amplitudes were markedly attenuated compared to the same eye fixated on the center of a pattern field. Therefore, in the present study

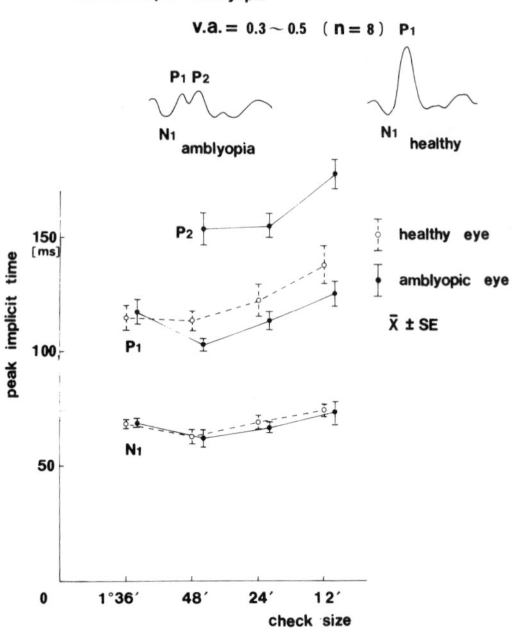

Figure 4. P1 peak implicit time of the healthy eye was placed between P1 and P2 peak implicit time of amblyopic eyes in the poor visual acuity group.

the anisometropic amblyopes with central fixation, were selected. VEPs were recorded on these subjects. The amplitudes were decreased markedly with all check sizes from 1 degrees 36' to 12' tested in the poor visual acuity group. The amplitude vs. check sizes curve revealed maximum amplitude with the largest check size. As the visual acuity of the amblyopic eye improved, the maximum amplitude shifted to smaller check sizes. If the assumption proposed by Behrman et al(3), can be made that the larger check sizes represent parafoveal function, and smaller check sizes represent foveal function, it is supposed that the poor visual acuity group reveals predominance of the parafoveal function, while the good visual acuity group predominates in the foveal function.

It was noteworthy that the amblyopes whose visual acuity improved to the level of normal acuity showed amplitude reduction in the smallest check size of 12'. It was thus, suggested that the amblyope had irreversible functional abnormality for defining fine pictures.

REFERENCES

1. Adachi-Usami E, Chiba, J: Influence of freely moved fixation in the pattern field on VECP amplitudes. Nippon Ganka Gakkai Zasshi 86:333-336, 1982

2. Arden GB, Barnard WM, Mushin AS: Visually evoked responses in amblyopia. Br J Ophthalmol, 58:183-192, 1974

3. Behrman J, Nissim S, Arden GB: A clinical method for obtaining pattern visual evoked responses. In Arden GB (ed): The Visual System, Neurophysiology, Biophysics and Their Clinical Applications. Proceedings of the Ninth ISCERG Symposium, 1971. Plenum Press, N.Y., p. 199-206, 1972.

4. Chiba Y, Kanaizuka DD, Adachi-Usami E: Psychophysical and VECP examinations of emmetropia, myopia, hypermetopia and aphacia. In Lawwill T, Doc. Ophthalmol Proceeding Series. 14th I.S.C.E.R.G. Symposium, Louisville, Kentucky, USA, 47-55, 1976.

5. Ikeda H: Is amblyopia a peripheral defect? Trans Ophthalmol Soc UK 99:347-352, 1979.

6. Lombroso CT, Duffy FH, Robb RM: Selective suppression of cerebral evoked potentials to patterened light in amblyopia ex anopsia. Electroenceph. Clin. Neurophysiol., 27:238-247, 1969.

7. Spekreijse H, Khoe LH, Van der Tweel LH: A case of amblyopia, electrophysiology and psychophysics of luminance and contrast. The visual system, neurophyiology, biophysics, and their clinical application. In Arden GB: Proceedings of the Ninth ISCERG Symposium, 1971. New York, Pleunum Press, 141-156, 1972.

8. Spekreijse H, Van der Tweel LH, Zuidema Th.: Contrast evoked responses in man. Vision Res., 13:1577-1601, 1973.

9. Wiesel TN, Hubel DH: Effects of visual deprivation on morphology and physiology of cells in the cat's lateral geniculate body. J. Neurophysiol. 26:979-993, 1963.

10. Wiesel T, Hubel DH: Single-cell responses in striate cortex of kittens deprived of vision in one eye. J Neurophysiol 26:1003-1017, 1963.

OBJECTIVE EVALUATION OF BINOCULARITY IN STRABISMUS WITH VER

E. C. Campos, C. Chiesi,
A. D. Sargentini and V. Macellari

ABSTRACT

In the present study pattern VERs were recorded monocularly and binocularly from 20 small-angle esotropia patients. Patients exhibiting either ARC or suppression at Bagolini's lenses were examined. The influence of the following parameters was investigated: spatial frequency, contrast and size of the stimulus and amount of the deviation. It is concluded that: (1) cortical binocularity can be shown with pattern VER in patients with small-angle strabismus and ARC; (2) the size of the stimulus and the spatial frequency strongly influence the results. No significant effect is attributed to the contrast; (3) the reduced summation is proportional to the amount of deviation and in some cases it is not significantly different from that of normals; and (4) no summation is detectable in patients with suppression with Bagolini's lenses. In small-angle strabismus with ARC there is evidence for a cortical rearrangement with features which appear to be an exaggeration of physiological phenomena at least as can be seen with VER. VER may be potentially useful for differentiating binocular vision from large suppression scotomas of the deviated eye in non-cooperative patients.

INTRODUCTION

In a previous publication, one of us showed that flashed visual evoked responses (VER) obtained in a binocular condition are larger than the monocular ones in strabismics with small- angle esotropia and anomalous retinal correspondence (ARC) with Bagolini's lenses. This enlargement, defined as summation, has been considered as an electrophysiological correlate to sensory fusion.(1-12) It was not detected in strabismics with suppression. Therefore, it was possible to objectively prove the existence of an anomalous binocular vision (ABV) in strabismics with ARC. However, this method did not appear to provide a reliable way to differentiate normals with normal binocular vision from strabismics with ABV.

The aim of this paper is: (1) to confirm the flashed VER results with pattern stimuli; (2) to evaluate the parameters which could influence the VER results; and (3) to design a test which could differentiate normals from strabismics by means of VER.

MATERIALS AND METHODS

Twenty patients with small-angle esotropia (no more than 15 prism diopters) were examined. Fourteen exhibited ARC with Bagolini's lenses, whereas six had suppression of the deviated eye. Eleven normals served as controls.

A suitably modified TV apparatus provided an alternating black and white pattern stimulus position 1 m in front of the patient. VERs were recorded with bipolar electrodes. Each recording was the sum of 128 averaged signals amplified of a factor of 104.

Monocular and binocular recordings were made in all the subjects. The influence of the following stimulus parameters was studied: (a) temporal frequency; (b) spatial frequency; (c) contrast.

As far as the subjects were concerned, a possible relationship between VER summation and amount of the angle of deviation was evaluated. Also, neutral filters of increasing density were placed in front of the fixing eye in order to establish the influence of such an obstacle to fusion on the VER summation.

RESULTS

1. With pattern VER it was possible to show a summation in patients with small-angle strabismus and ARC (Figure 1). These results confirmed the flashed VER results.

2. The amount of summation found in normals was not significantly different from that present in strabismics in ARC and seemed independent from the amount of the deviation (Figure 2).

3. Patients with large or small-angle strabismus and suppression with Bagolini's lenses did not show a VER summation (Figure 3).

4. The optimal frequency of alternation for the stimulus was of 7 Hz. High spatial frequencies are best to show VER summation. Low frequencies saturate the system; i.e., the monocular signal is already so large that summation is cancelled by the averaging device. The contrast of the

stimulus did not appear to be crucial for obtaining optimal summation.

5. VER summation disappeared in normals when a neutral density filter of at least 1.6 Log U was interposed on the fixing eye. In strabismics and in subjects with easily disruptable heterophoria, summation was cancelled by a much weaker filter; i.e., no more than 0.4 Log U (Figure 4).

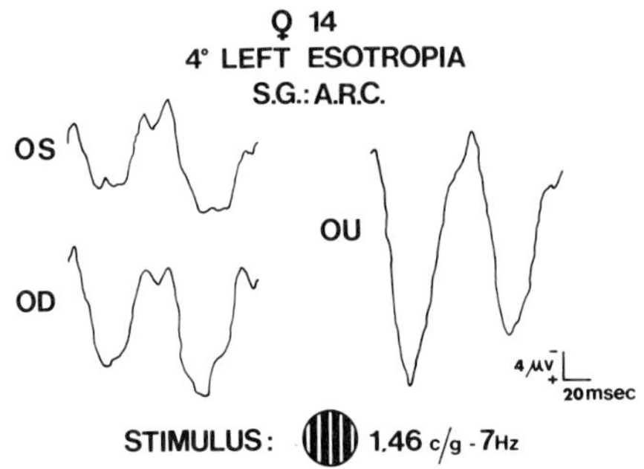

Figure 1. VER summation in a patient with small-angle esotropia. The binocular signal (OU) is definitely larger than the two monocular ones (OD and OS).

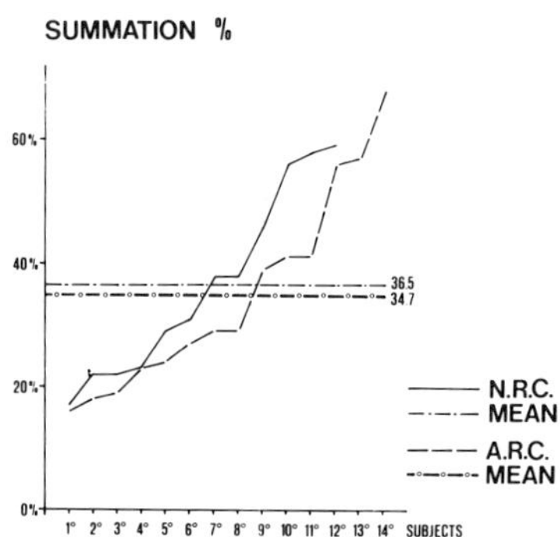

Figure 2. Percentage of VER summation found in normal subjects (continuous line) and in patients with small-angle strabismus and anomalous binocular vision (dotted line). The mean summation found in normals (36.5%) is not significantly different from that of strabismics (34.7%).

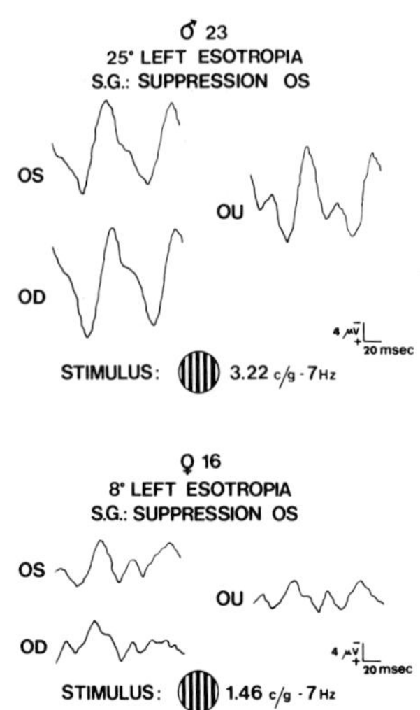

Figure 3. No VER summation is present in patients with strabismus who exhibit suppression of the deviated eye, independently from the amount of the angle of deviation. VER amplitude (UV) versus density of neutral filters.

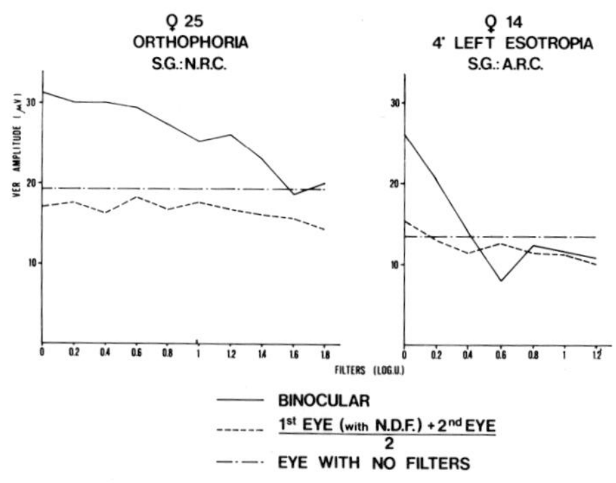

Figure 4. In a normal subject (left part of the figure) summation disappears with a filter of about 1.6 Log U in front of one eye. In a patient with small-angle strabismus, summation is interrupted with a 0.4 Log U filter in front of one eye (right part of the graph).

DISCUSSION AND CONCLUSIONS

VER summation was shown to be present when pattern stimuli were used in strabismics with ARC. In normals, summation is related to binocularity. Hence, the binocular vision of anomalous type previously described with psychophysical techniques(13-17) can be objectively assessed by means of VER. Interestingly, VER summation is absent in strabismics with suppression of the deviated eye and is independent from the amount of the angle of deviation. Lack of summation should, therefore, not be related to an eccentric presentation of the stimulus per se.

Obviously, a differentation between normals and strabismics with VER seems tempting. Nevertheless, such differentation cannot be made on the basis of the entity of summation. In fact, as stated previously(10), summation varies on a wide range even in normals. However, the use of neural density filters interposed on the fixing eye may determine whether a subject is normal or if he is at risk (easily disruptable heterophoria) and/or if he has strabismus with ARC.

In conclusion binocular VER allows us to classify subjects according to the following Table.

We hoped that the method proposed here could be used to evaluate non-cooperative children. If so, it will be possible to diagnose strabismus early or to identify subjects at risk, considering that in normals VER summation is present as early as at ten weeks of life(18-21).

TABLE 1

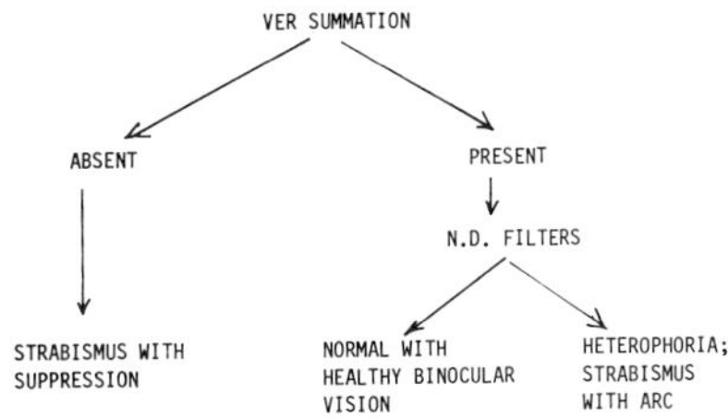

REFERENCES

1. Campos EC: Anomalous retinal correspondence. Monocular and binocular visual evoked responses. Arch Ophthalmol 98:299-302, 1980.

2. Cobb WA, Morton HB, Ettlinger G: Cerebral potentials evoked by pattern reversal and their suppression in visual rivalry. Nature 216:1123-1125, 1967.

3. Fiorentini A, Maffei L: Electrophysiological evidence for binocular disparity detectors in human visual system. Science 169:208-209, 1970.

4. Harter MR, Seiple WH, Salmon L: Binocular summation of visually evoked responses to pattern stimuli in humans. Vision Res 13:1433-1446, 1973.

5. Harter MR, Towle VL, Zakrzewski M, Moyer SM: An objective indicant of binocular vision in humans: Size-specific interocular suppression of visual evoked potentials. Electroencephalogr Clin Neurophysiol 43:825-836, 1977.

6. Lennerstrand G: Some observations on visual evoked responses (VER) to dichoptic stimulation. Acta Ophthalmol 56:638-647, 1978.

7. Srebro R: The visually evoked response: binocular facilitation and failure when binocular vision is disturbed. Arch Ophthalmol 96:839-844, 1978.

8. Apkarian PA, Nakayama K, Tyler CW: Binocularity in the human visuial evoked potential: facilitation, summation and suppression. Electroencephalogr Clin Neurophysiol 51:32-40, 1981.

9. Apkarian P, Tyler CM: Binocular facilitation in the VEP of normal observers and strabismic amblyopes. Doc Ophthalmol Proc Series 27:323-335, 1981.

10. Apkarian P, Levi D, Tyler CW: Binocular facilitation in the visual evoked potential of strabismic amblyopes. Am J Optom Physiol Optics 58:820-830, 1981.

11. Groneberg A, Teping C: Pattern evoked cortical potentials to simultaneous stimulation of both eyes. Doc Ophthalmol Proc Series 27:313-322, 1981.

12. Jacobson P, Lennerstrand G: A comparison of different VEP methods for the assessment of binocular vision. Doc Ophthalmol Proc Series 27:337-344, 1981.

13. Bagolini B: Anomalous retinal correspondence: definition and diagnostic methods. Doc Ophthalmol 23:346-398, 1967.

14. Bagolini B: Sensorial anomalies in strabismus (suppression, anomalous correspondence, amblyopia). Doc Ophthalmol 41:1-22, 1976.

15. Bagolini B, Campos EC: Binocular campimetry in small-angle concomitant esotropia. Doc Ophthalmol Proc Series 14:405-409, 1977.

16. Campos EC, Chiesi C: Perimetrie dans l´exotropie concomitant. Bull et mem Soc Francaise d´Ophthalmol 92° annee, Paris, Masson, 1981, p. 301.

17. Campos EC: Binocularity in comitant strabismus: binocular visual field studies. Doc Ophthalmol, in press.

18. Julesz B, Kropfl W, Petrig B: Large evoked potentials to dynamic random-dot correlograms and stereograms permit quick determination of stereopsis. Proc Nat Acad Sci USA-Psychology 77:2348-2351, 1980.

19. Braddick O, Atkinson J, Julesz B, Kropfl W, Bodis-Wollner I, Raab E: Cortical binocularity in infants. Nature 288:363-365, 1980.

20. Petrig B, Julesz B, Kropfl W, Baumgartner G, Anliker M: Development of stereopsis and cortical binocularity in human infants: electrophysiological evidence. Science 213:1402-1405, 1981.

21. Baraldi P, Penne A: Personal communication. Work in progress.

A NEW APPROACH TO THE OBJECTIVE EVALUATION OF BINOCULAR FUNCTION

Y. Uemura and O. Katsumi

ABSTRACT

A new of measuring binocular function using the pattern reversal VEP and the Fast Fourier Transfer program in the microcomputer is introduced. By using this method the separation of activity of each eye during the binocular condition was possible. Additionally, we found the intermediate element on the power spectrum only in the state of fusion and at the same time the subjective change of stimulus frequency. As these phenomenon were never recognized when the fusion was broken or in the cases with abnormal binocular vision, we speculate that these phenomenon are strongly related with the binocular function.

INTRODUCTION

In the field of strabismology, the evaluation of binocular function, retinal correspondence, and stereopsis are usually determined with subjective methods such as the major amblyoscope, the phase difference haploscope, Bagolini striated glasses and others. These methods of examination are sometimes difficult to perform on young children and reliable responses can be obtained only at a later age. For this reason, the development of an objective method of examination of binocular function is important.

Recently, attempts to evaluate the binocular function using pattern reversal visually evoked responses (VEP) have been made. Most of these attempts, however, used either binocular summation or interocular suppression. They are the indirect method of evaluation and activity of the individual eye cannot be determined with these methods. We have recently developed a system using the pattern reversal VEP and Fast Fourier Transfer (FFT) that enables us to evaluate the binocular activity in more natural visual conditions. The purpose of this report is to introduce the system, the apparatus, and the records obtained from normals and patients with abnormal binocular vision.

STRABISMUS II
ISBN 0-8089-1424-3

SUBJECTS AND METHODS

Controls were 12 adults (3 males and 9 females) ages ranging from 20 to 42 years old. Two esotropic patients aged 11 and 20 year old also participated in this study. Fig 1 shows the block diagram of the system for producing the stimulus and recording the binocular VEP. The method of presentation of stimulus was a pattern generator (Visual Stimulator Medelec, England).

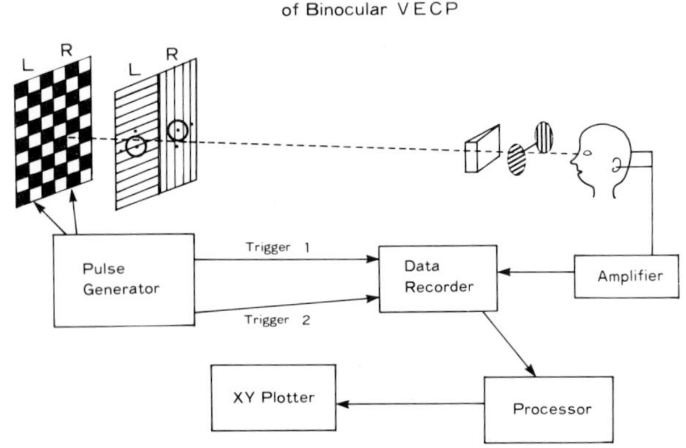

Figure 1. Block diagram of stimulus apparatus and recording of binocular VEP

In front of the TV screen, two polaroid filters were placed with the axis of each, orthogonal to the other and the border of each filter coincident with the center of the TV screen. On the center of each TV hemiscreen, an additional pair of fusional targets (Paramacular size, AFIM 118a and 118b) were positioned. The subject wore polaroid spectacles whose axis of filters coincides with the axis of the filters of each hemifield. Thus when he saw through the polaroid spectacles, his right eye saw the right hemifield and his left eye saw the left hemifield only. Fig 2 shows the target as seen by the controls when the targets are completely fused. Some subjects can fuse the targets, but others need base-out prisms to keep fusion stable. Once the state of fusion is achieved, it is easy to maintain for an hour or so. Subjects were asked to concentrate on the fused target. If suppression occurs, the number of small dots outside of the ring become 2 instead of 4. As a stimulus pattern, we employed the checkerboard pattern. By selecting vertical splitting mode on the pattern generator, it is possible to send dichoptic stimulation (different in temporal frequency but same in spatial frequency) to each hemifield of the TV screen. When fusion is complete, each check is completely superimposed to each other. The mean luminosity of the surface of the TV screen is around 50 Cd/m2, however, with the use of two pairs of polaroid filters, the mean luminosity drops to about one tenth of the stimulus surface. The check size of each pattern was 20 min of arc (1.5 CPD) and the contrast ratio of the pattern was kept at 30%. The VEP was derived monopolarly from 5% and 15% above the inion in the midline. The evoked potentials were amplified (Nihon Kohden VC-9, biophysical amplifier) and recorded by a data recorder (SONY 3515 DFR) with trigger 1 and trigger 2 from the pulse generator. The data of evoked potentials on a magnetic tape were analyzed with a FFT program of the microcomputer (Nihon Kohden ATAC 450). The analog data was sampled for each 20 msec. Power spectrum was calculated by the data for about 5 sec (20 msec x 256 points). The calculation of power spectrum was performed by the FFT program by the data processor (Nihon Kohden, ATAC 450). The power spectrum was added 15 times. The power spectrum obtained from FFT was recorded on a X-Y plotter (Watanabe). The evoked potentials on a magnetic tape were averaged by the trigger 1 and trigger 2 respectively. These averaged VEP were recorded on a X-Y recorder. (Yokogawa Electric, Type 3077)

RESULTS

I. Controls

Of the 12 normal subjects who participated in this investigation, we will detail the results of 2 subjects. Fig 3 shows the result of binocular VEP when both eyes were stimulated with 11.7 Hz, the dioptic stimulation. As shown in Fig 3, the large element is recognized at 11.7 Hz, which corresponds to the stimulus frequency. The large element around 8 to 8.5 Hz is believed to be the alpha activity. Fig 4 shows the result of examination when the dichoptic stimulation, that is 12.6 Hz to the right eye and 9.5 Hz to the left eye were sent and recording was made in complete fusion. On the power spectrum, three major elements were recognized. Two major elements at 9.5 Hz and 12.6 Hz correspond to the stimulus frequency respectively. In complete fusion one additional element was observed at the frequency of 11.3 Hz which is just in the intermediate position of two previous elements. In complete fusion one remarkable psychophysical phenomenon was observed in all subjects. That is the "subjective" change of the stimulus frequency. Suppose, a stimulus frequency of 12.6 Hz was sent to right eye and 9.5 Hz was sent to left eye, in complete fusion, the subjective frequency that he "feels" is neither 12.6 Hz nor 9.5 Hz. The speed of frequency that he feels in binocular seeing condition, is faster than 9.5 but slower than 12.6 Hz. This subjective change of frequency can be recognized easily. If one eye is suddenly covered in complete fusion, the change of stimulus frequency is easily noticable. One will feel that the speed of stimlus pattern becomes faster by closing left eye and will feel slower by closing the right eye. This subjective change of stimulus frequency in complete fusion occurred only in subjects with normal binocular vision and was never recognized in the subjects with abnormal binocular vision.

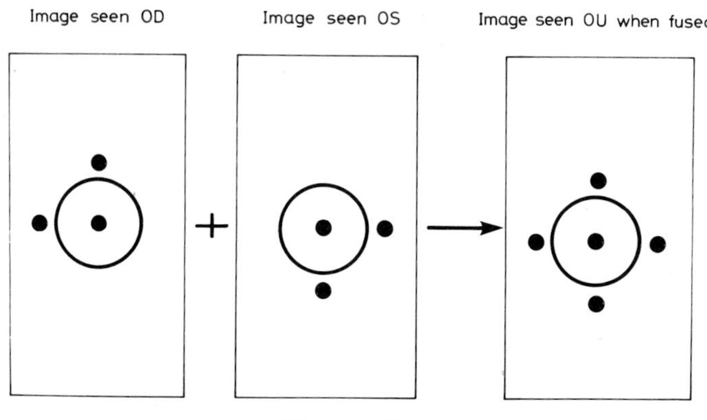

Figure 2

Figure 5 shows the result of binocular VEP on the same subject in similar recording conditions except the fusion is broken with the base-in prism instead of base-out. In the power spectrum, two major elements which corresponds to each stimulus frequency is observed. However, the power element which was recognized in the intermediate position in the state of fusion was not recognized.

Figure 6 shows the result of binocular VEP in 32-year-old woman with normal binocular function. 12.6 Hz was sent to her right eye and 16.9 Hz was sent to her left eye. The recording was made in complete fusion. As was the same with the previous recording, three major elements which

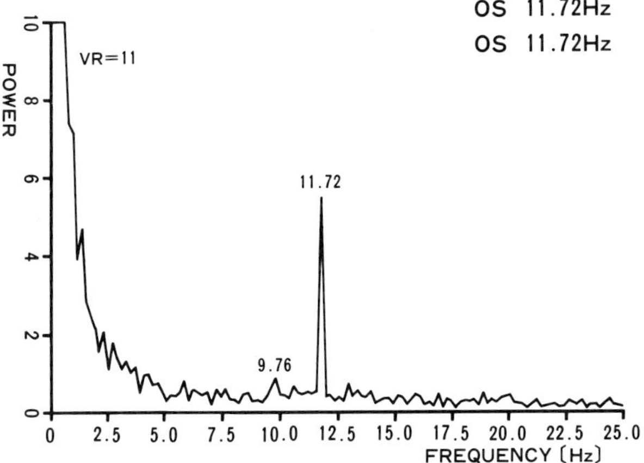

Figure 3. Result of binocular VEP in 28-year-old woman with normal binocular vision. Both eyes were stimulated with 11.7 Hz. On the power spectrum a large component is recognized at 11.7 Hz. Abcissa shows the spatial frequency and ordinate shows the power of the response.

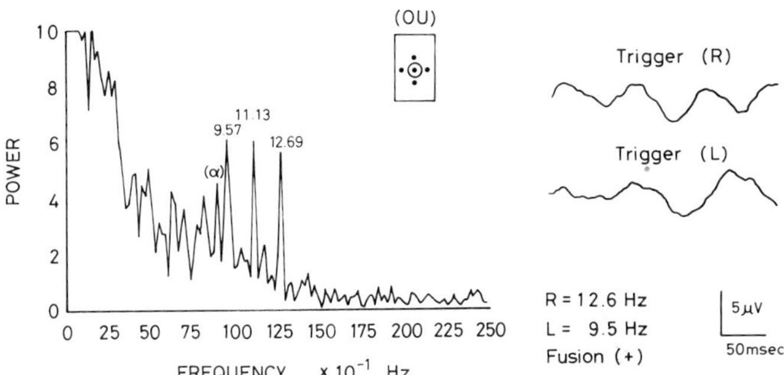

Figure 4. Result of binocular VEP in a 20-year-old woman with normal binocular vision. Right eye was stimulated with 12.6 Hz and left eye was stimulated with 9.5 Hz. The VEP was recorded in complete fusion. There are three major component on power spectrum. Two of them correspond to the stimulus frequency presented to each eye. One additional component is recognized in approximately intermediate position between these two components.

would correspond to each stimulus frequency and intermediate component were recognized in the power spectrum. Fig 7 shows the recording of the same subject when the fusion is broken with base-in prism. In this power spectrum, the two major elements which correspond to each stimulus frequency were observed, however, the intermediate component which was observed in fusion was not recognized in the power spectrum.

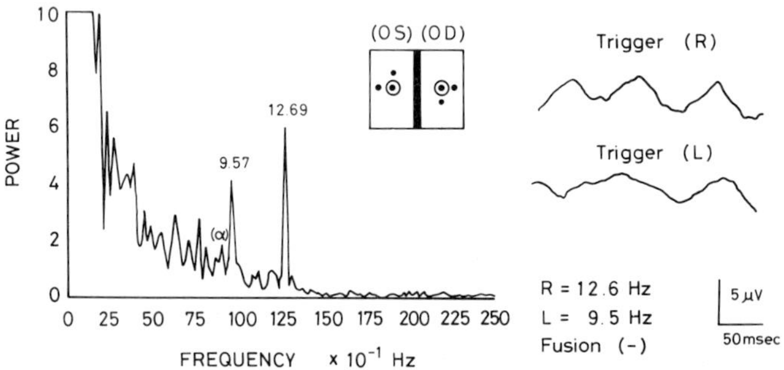

Figure 5. Result of binocular VEP in the same subject as in Fig 4. Recording conditions were the same except the fusion is broken with the base-in prism. On the power spectrum, there are only two major components which correspond to each eye. The intermediate component which was recognized in complete fusion was absent in this condition.

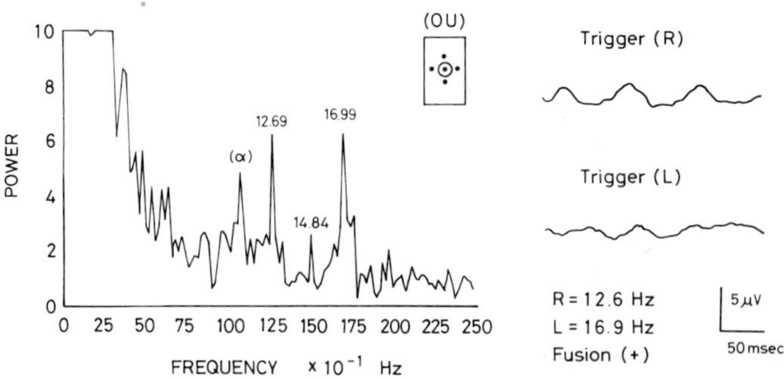

Figure 6. Result of binocular VEP in 32-year-old woman with normal binocular vision. Recording was made in complete fusion. On the power spectrum, there are three major components, two components which corresponds to each eye and the intermediate component.

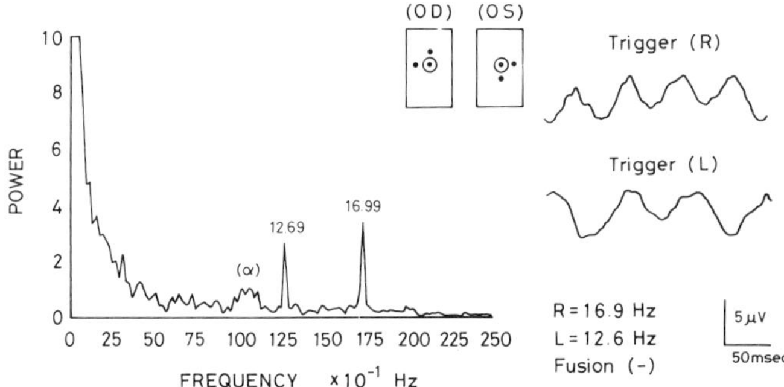

Figure 7. Result of binocular VEP in the same subject as in Fig 6. Recording was made in the condition which fusion was disrupted with base-in prism. On the power spectrum, there are only two major components and the intermediate component is not recognized.

II. Cases with esotropia

We employed this new system with a few esotropes with and without normal binocular vision. Although the cases are few, we will introduce some of the results. Fig 8 shows the result of binocular VEP in 20-year-old woman with residual esotropia. She responded as unharmonious ARC on the major amblyoscope. In the power spectrum, the power element from the fixating eye was prominent. The power element from the deviated eye was suppressed and the intermediate component was not recognized. She was not able to perceive the subjective change of the stimulus frequency in the state of fusion. Fig 9 shows the result of binocular VEP of an 11 year old girl with late onset esotropia. She showed NRC on the major amblyoscope. This recording was taken without correcting the deviation. The element recognized in the power spectrum was the element from the fixating eye. Fig 10 shows the result of the binocular VEP of the same patients but in this recording the deviation was corrected with base-out prisms. In this recording, though rather noisy, the element from each eye and intermediate element were recognizable, and she was able to perceive the subjective change of stimulus frequency.

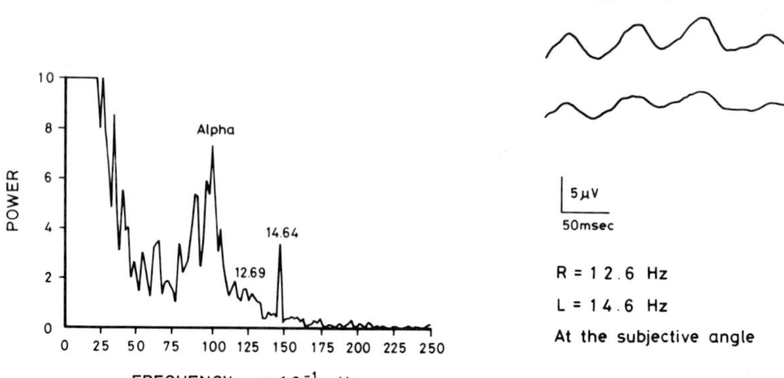

Figure 8. Result of binocular VEP in a 20-year-old woman with esotropia with unharmonious ARC. On the power spectrum, the only major component recognizable was from the fixating eye. The power from the deviating eye and the intermediate component were absent.

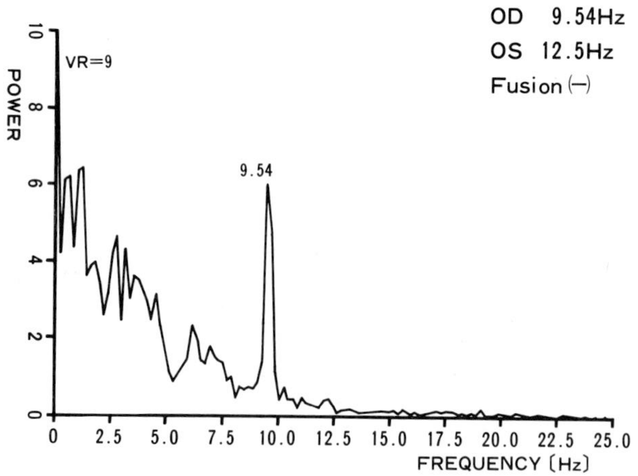

Figure 9. Result of binocular VEP in a 11-year-old girl with late onset' esotropia with NRC. Recording was made without correcting the deviation angle. On the power spectrum only component recognizable was the one from her fixating eye.

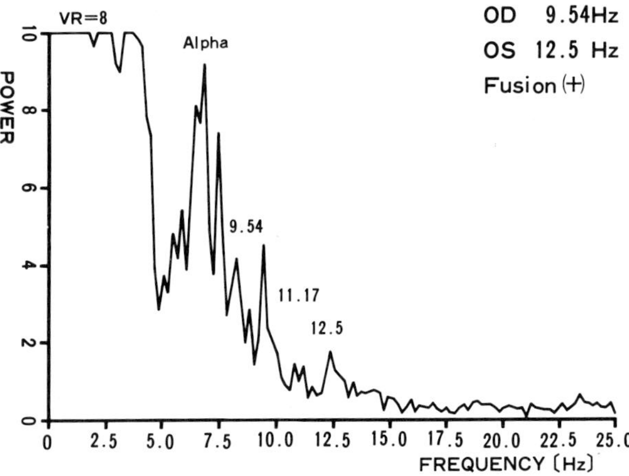

Figure 10. Result of binocular VEP in the same subject as in Fig 9. This time recording was made with correction of her deviation angle with prism. On the power spectrum, two components which correspond to the stimulus frequency to each eye and the intermediate component were recognized.

DISCUSSION

Many investigators have reported that the amplitude of VEP response becomes larger when recorded with binocular stimulation as opposed to monocular stimulation.1-4 This phenomenon is called as the binocular summation or binocular addition. In normals, the binocular summations are from 30% to 50%. This method of evaluation is rather easy to perform, however, the results are inconsistent. The results are considerably influenced by numerous stimulus parameters such as spatial frequency, temporal frequency, contrast ratio, stimulus field size and so on. As some investigators note, it may be misleading to evaluate the binocular fusion only with this method. If one want to be more reliable, multiple number of examinations will be necessary. Recently, Fukai and Tsutusi5 developed the method which utilize the dispartity sensitive stimulus target using the liquid crystal phase difference haploscope. They maintain that the purely binocular sensitive responses will be detected if there is a binocular summation of more than 100%. The method of binocular summation has many merits, however, their evaluation is based upon the indirect evaluation and the activity or response of each eye during the binocular vision is not possible.

As to the experiments using the dichoptic stimulation, where a different stimulus is sent to each eye, investigations by Lennerstrand and Hansen,6 Lehmann and Fender7 are found in the literature. Their methods are advanced, one using the theory of interocular suppression. The evaluation of activity of each eye seems to be difficult with their method.

In our method there are two key features of our apparatus. One is the use of Fast Fourier Transformation program in the microcomputer and the second is use of the fusional targets. By using the FFT program, it is possible to separately visualize, on the power spectrum, the individual activity of each eye during binocular viewing. The role of fusional targets is to make the state of fusion stable during the examination. By watching the fusional targets one can easily monitor the state of fusion. In the normal subjects, we could separate the power element on the power spectrum. Thus we can decide the individual activity of each eye during binocular viewing. This method will be valuable to determine the dominancy of the individual eye in the pathological cases. As to the intermediate element which appeared during the recording, this element never appeared when the fusion was broken or in cases of defective binocular function. We suggest that intermediate element is strongly correlated with the binocular function. As to the subjective change of the stimulus frequency, we reasoned as follows. When the dichoptic stimulation enters each eye, disparity of temporal frequency will stimulate the binocular sensitive neurones and they will compensate the time lag and as a resultant stimulus appears as harmonics in the binocular state. In cases with defective binocular function, the dysfunctioning binocular sensitive neurones will not compensate, and no subjective change will be perceived. As to the nature of the intermediate element which appeared only in the fused state and the subjective change of the stimulus frequency, further investigation will be necessary. However, we strongly suggest that these phenomenon are correlated with the binocular function and this new method will have a potential to objectively evaluate binocular functions in the near future.

ACKNOWLEDGEMENT

We are grateful to Prof. L.H. van der Tweel of the University of Amsterdam for his valuable suggestions and discussions for this investigations. We owe a great deal to Yoshihisa Oguchi, M.D., of the University of Keio and to Tetsuo Kawara, D. Sci. for the collaboration in this investigation.

REFERENCES

1. Spekreijse H: Analysis of EEG responses in man. The Hague, Netherlands. Dr. W. Junk, 1966, pp. 129-143.

2. Tsutsui J: Binocular VECP. Acta Soc Ophthalmol Jap 71:785-790, 1967.

3. Perry NW, Childers DG: Cortical potentials in normal and amblyopic binocular vision, in Schmoger E (ed): Advances in electrophysiology and-pathology of the visual system. Proceedings of the 6th ISCERG Symposium Leipzig, Thieme, 1968, pp 151-161.

4. Srebro R: The visually evoked response. Binocular fascilitation and failure when binocular vision is disturbed. Arch Ophthalmol 96:839-844, 1978.

5. Fukai S, Abe T, Tsutsui J: Studies on the binocular disparity sensitive VECP (preliminary report). Nippon Ganka Gakkai Zasshi 84:1629-1633, 1980.

6. Lennerstrand G: Binocular interaction studied with visual evoked responses (VER) in humans with normal or impaired binocular vision. Acta Ophthalmol 56:628-637, 1978.

7. Lehman D, Fender DH: Averaged visual evoked potentials in humans: mechanism of dichotpic interaction studied in a subject with split chiasma. Electrencephalogr Clin Neurophysiol 27:142-145, 1969.

OBSERVATION OF ABNORMAL RETINAL CORRESPONDENCE BY INFRARED TELEVISION FUNDUS HAPLOSCOPE

E. Ohmi and K. Kani

ABSTRACT

Among 1754 cases of strabismus patients examined by direct observation through an infrared television haploscope, only 18 cases were found to have abnormal retinal correspondence. The site of correspondence was the central fovea in all dominant eyes and parafoveal points in all non-dominant eyes. In 15 non-dominant eyes, the corresponding point was on the nasal side. In the remaining three cases, it was on the temporal side in one, downward in another, and upward in the last.

Central fixation was found in 13 cases and eccentric fixation in five cases. All eccentric fixation points corresponded to the point of abnormal retinal correspondence and they were located inside the macular ring.

INTRODUCTION

Abnormal retinal correspondence (ARC) is an important phenomenon occasionally observed in strabismic patients.(1-5) Past discussions have been based on the findings exclusively obtained by indirect observation.

One of the authors (Kani) has devised an haploscope on which a pair of infrared television cameras were mounted permitting direct and simultaneous observation of the ocular fundi during examination. This paper details the results obtained from a number of strabismic patients examined with this haploscopic instrument.

METHODS

An infrared television haploscope (Konan Camera Research Institute, Inc.) was used in the study. The instrument featured a pair of infrared television cameras mounted on the haploscope. No pupil dilation was required and the system was capable of displaying the ocular fundus and the visual target simultaneously (Fig 1).

STRABISMUS II
ISBN 0-8089-1424-3

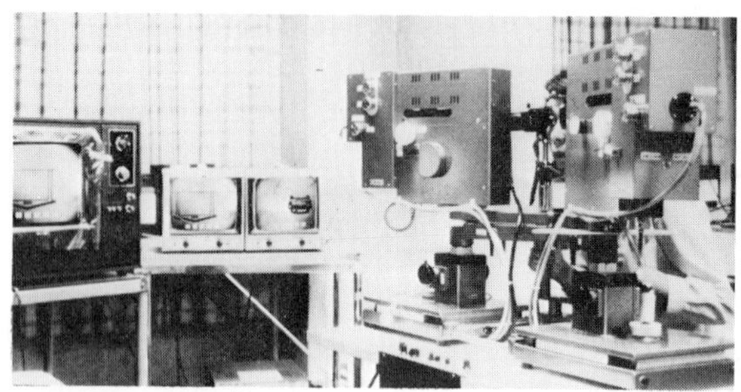

Figure 1. Infrared television fundus haploscope.

The binocular visual functions were examined by direct observation of the central fovea and the target on the same television screen along with patient's subjective perception. Two sets of television were necessary to display both eyes. A pair of video tape recorders were used for the magnetic recording of television pictures for more specific observations by playback.

The retinal sensitivity also was measured by using the light source unit attached to the haploscope which was originally designed for the purpose of plotting the visual field while directly observing the ocular fundus. The target size was 8 minutes and the background luminance was set at 10 asb. Target presentation was 200 msec and on 0.1 log steps (Fig 2).

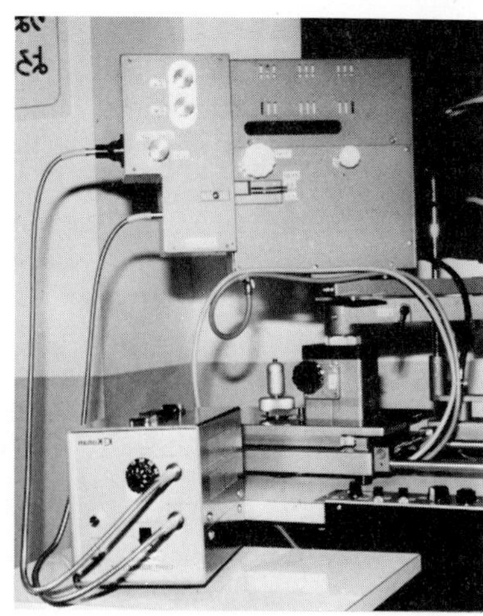

Figure 2. Light source unit attached to the haploscope.

Observations were made on 1754 strabismus patients which consisted of 1051 exotropes, 498 of esotropes, 158 of overactions of the inferior oblique muscle, and 47 of hypertropes (Table 1).

		ARC	
Exotropia	1051	6	(0.57%)
Esotropia	498	10	(2.01%)
Overaction I.O.	158	0	
Hypertropia	47	2	(4.26%)
Total	1754	18 cases (1.02%)	

Table 1: The proportion of true abnormal retinal correspondence.

RESULTS

Abnormal retinal correspondence: Among those patients examined by the infrared television haploscope, 18 cases were found to have an abnormal retinal correspondence of which 10 were esotropes, 6 exotropes, and 2 hypertropes (Table 2). Sites of retinal correspondence under the direct observation with the instrument were found to be central in all dominant eyes and parafoveal in all non-dominant eyes. In 15 patients the abnormal corresponding point was located on the nasal side of fovea. In the remaining 3 cases, it was on the temporal side in one case, down in another, and above in the last.

Central fixation was observed in 13 cases and eccentric fixation was found in five cases. All eccentric fixation points corresponded to those of ARC and they were located within the macular ring.

In those patients with esotropia, the ARC point was located on the nasal side of fovea and the central fixation was observed in eight cases while the eccentric fixation was seen in two patients.

Out of six cases with exotropia, the ARC point located on the nasal side of fovea was seen in five patients. The remaining one showed the point on the temporal side. Central

No.					
1	19 Y.f.	ET	RV:0.8 LV:1.2	c	L
2	7 Y.f.	ET	RV:1.0 LV:1.0	c	L
3	19 Y.f.	ET	RV:(2.0) LV:(1.2)	c	L
4	7 Y.f.	ET	RV:(0.4) LV:(0.4)	c	L
5	21 Y.m.	ET	RV:(1.0) LV:(1.0)	c	L
6	9 Y.m.	ET	RV:1.2 LV:1.5	c	R
7	10 Y.f.	ET	RV:(1.5) LV:(0.2)	c	L
8	11 Y.m.	ET	RV:1.2 LV:1.2	c	R
9	5 Y.f.	ET	RV:(1.2) LV:(0.2)	e	L
10	7 Y.f.	ET	RV:(0.3) LV: 1.2	e	R
11	11 Y.m.	XT	RV:(1.2) LV:(1.0)	c	L
12	20 Y.m.	XT	RV:1.2 LV:1.2	c	L
13	28 Y.m.	XT	RV:(1.0) LV:(1.0)	c	L
14	11 Y.m.	XT	RV:1.0 LV:1.0	c	L
15	22 Y.f.	XT	RV:(1.5) LV:(0.15)	e	L
16	8 Y.m.	XT	RV:(0.3) LV:(1.2)	e	R
17	12 Y.m.	Hyper tropia	RV:(0.1) LV:(1.2)	e	R
18	7 Y.f.	Hyper tropia	RV:(1.0) LV:(1.0)	c	R
Total	18				

c : central fixation
e : eccentric fixation

fixation was observed in four cases and eccentric fixation in two cases.

In the two patients with hypertropia, the ARC point was seen on the superior side of fovea in one and inferiorly in the other. An eccentric fixation was observed in the latter case (Fig 3,4).

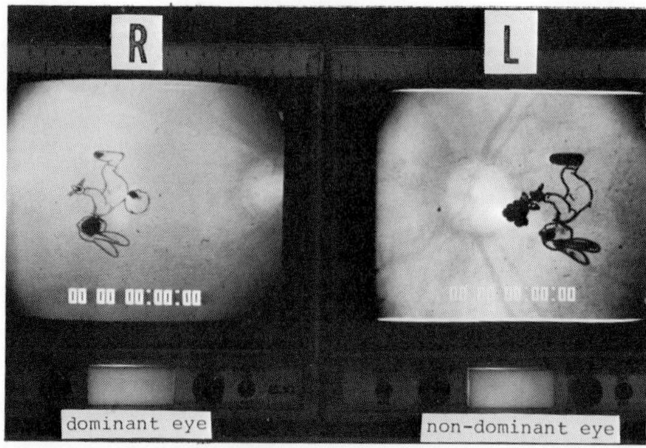

Figure 3. The ocular fundus of abnormal retinal correspondence. The site of correspondence under the direct observation. It was in the central fovea in the dominant eye and was in parafoveal in the non- dominant eye.

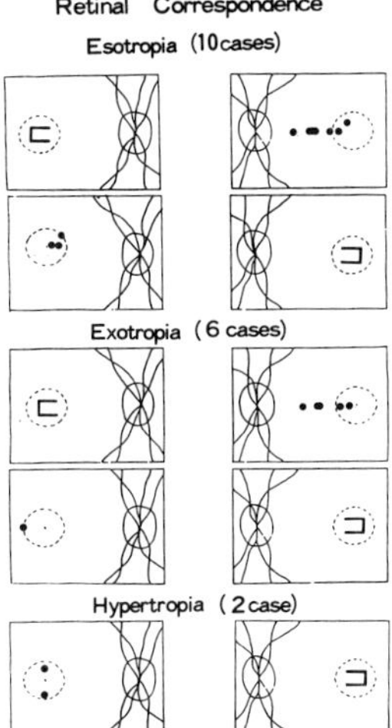

Figure 4. The site of correspondence. Simultaneous perception, fusion and stereoscopic vision are in the same site.

Retinal visual sensitivity:

Retinal visual sensitivity was measured in 15 cases on both the central fovea and the ARC point along with an area of the dominant eye which corresponded to the ARC point of the non-dominant eye.

In non-dominant eye, the retinal visual sensitivity of the ARC point was approximately equivalent to that of the central fovea of the dominant eye and was even higher than that of the corresponding area of the dominant eye. The central fovea of the non-dominant eye showed the sensitivity 2.4 log units above background luminance while it was 2.5 log units above the level at the ARC point.

In the dominant eye, the sensitivity of fovea was found to be 2.5 log units above the background luminance level and the area corresponding to the ARC point showed the sensitivity of 2.3 log units above the level (Table 3).

The sensitivity curve of a strabismic eye appeared to improve after surgical correction in that the distribution pattern of sensitivity at the ARC area became similar to that of the dominant eye (Fig 5, 6).

RETINAL VISUAL SENSITIVITY

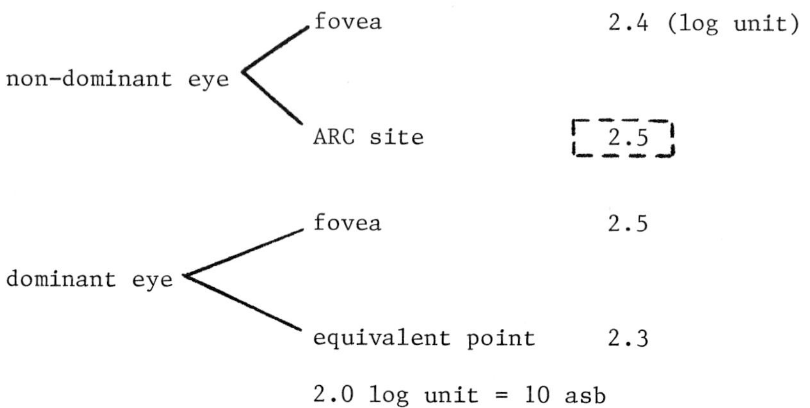

non-dominant eye	fovea	2.4 (log unit)
	ARC site	2.5
dominant eye	fovea	2.5
	equivalent point	2.3

2.0 log unit = 10 asb

Table 3: Retinal visual sensitivity

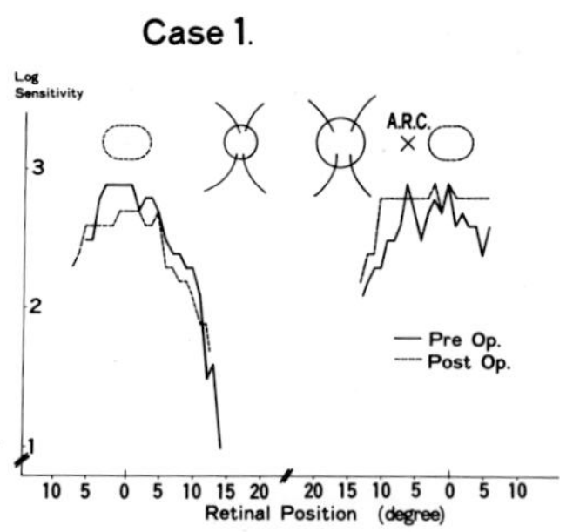

Figure 5: The sensitivity curve.

Pre-op. In non-dominant eye, the retinal visual sensitivity of the ARC point was approximately equivalent to that of the central fovea.

Post-op. The sensitivity curve of a strabismic eye appeared to improve.

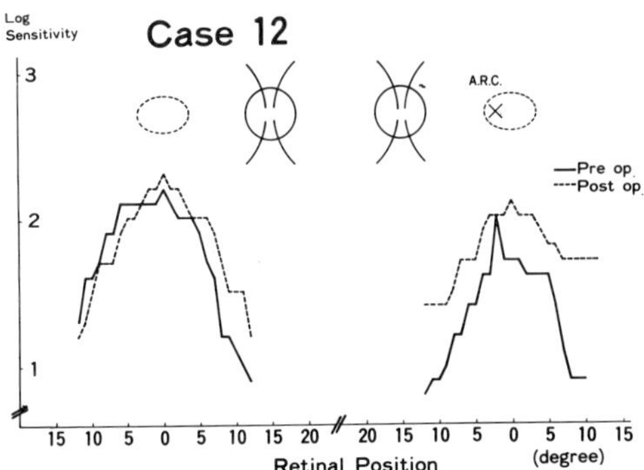

Figure 6: The sensitivity curve. The distribution pattern of sensitivity at the ARC area became similar to that of the dominant eye after surgery.

DISCUSSION

Many papers(1-5) have dealt with ARC, most hold to the view that there is a moderate incidence of ARC among the strabismic eyes. The direct observation which is now feasible by means of infrared television haploscopem reveals that among 1754 strabismus patients only 18 cases were found to have ARC. They represented one percent of the total sum.

Yuge (1963)(6) described and defined ARC in that there was no correspondence of central fovea between fellow eyes and that the fovea of the dominant eye corresponded to the psuedofovea of the non-dominant eye. He stated further that the incidence of true ARC was rare.

The localization of the ARC point in the ocular fundus examined by the present instrument(7-11) was in the area as expected in esotropia and of hypertropia. In exotropic patients, however, the ARC point was found on the nasal side of the fovea in five out of six cases. Three of them had strabismus surgery in childhood to correct an esotropia, one esotropic in his early infancy, and the remaining one was suspected to possibly develop an ARC when his eye position was still unstable after birth.

The majority of ARC patients (13 out of 18) in this series showed central fixation. An eccentric fixation was found in the remaining five cases in which the fixation point corresponded to that of ARC in all of five cases and it was located inside the macular ring.

All those with the eccentric fixation had a small angle strabismus accompanied by an amblyopia which might be considered as those with the microstrabismus through the findings obtained by the direct observation.

REFERENCES

1. Parks MM: Small angle esodeviations. Amer Orthopt J 12:32-39, 1962.

2. Helveston EM, GK von Noorden: Microtropia, a new defined entity. Arch Ophthalmol 78:272-281, 1967.

3. Lang J: Microtropia. Arch Ophthalmol 81:758-762, 1969.

4. Uemura Y: Abnormal retinal correspondence and Microtropia. Ophthalmology J Tokyo 12:198-206, 1970.

5. Watanabe Y: Microtropia amblyopia. Ophthalmology 19:1381, 1977.

6. Yuge T: II. 6. Anomaly of binocular vision. Strabismus and Amblyopia 101, Nanzando Tokyo, 1963.

7. Ohmi E, Kani K: Observation of Retinal Correspondence by Infrared Television Fundus Haploscope. The 1st Report, Orthophoria, esotropia and exotropia. Japanese Review of Clinical Ophthalmol 74:1575, 1980.

8. Ohmi E, Kani K: Observation of Retinal Correspondence by Infrared Television Fundus Haploscope, 2nd Report, Abnormal Retinal Correspondence. Folia Ophthalmol Jpn 32:1265, 1981.

9. Ohmi E: Observation of Retinal Correspondence by Infrared Television Fundus Haploscope, 3rd Report, Abnormal Retinal Correspondence. Nippon Ganka Zasshi 85:959-964, 1981.

10. Ohmi E: Observation of Retinal Correspondence by Infrared Television Fundus Haploscope, 4th Report, Binocular Vision of ARC. Japanese Review of Clinical Ophthalmology 75:2007, 1981.

11. Ohmi E: Observation of Retinal Correspondence by Infrared Television Fundus Haploscope, 5th Report, Retinal Visual Sensitivity of Dominant Eye and Non-Dominant Eye. Jpn J Clin Ophthalmol 36:504, 1982.

A NEW INSTRUMENT FOR THE STUDY OF BINOCULAR VISION AND THE CORRECTION OF ITS ANOMALIES

L. Mawas, E. Mawas, and J.B. Weiss

ABSTRACT

Physiological diplopia was discovered by Al Hazen in the Xth century and demonstrated with a fairly complicated tool. The analysis of this forgotten instrument shows that it can be reduced to a rectangular tablet (42 x 10 cm) or rule with an anteroposterior central line. This simplified "Plaquette" or "Diplometer" shows at a glance the type and degree of binocular single vision or its absence. The result is achieved by the separation of the retinocortical projections of the middle line which is seen as two oblique lines, crossing at a variable distance. Further one or two magnetic objects and/or stereograms can be moved along the medial line. We measure the amplitude of convergence or divergence and we may deneutralise the temporal (near) or nasal (distal) retina.

INTRODUCTION

Herein is described a new simple instrument which allows instant diagnosis of binocular vision and its anomalies. It may be used from early childhood to adult age. Physiological diplopia is the basis of this method (Fig. 1).

Figure 1

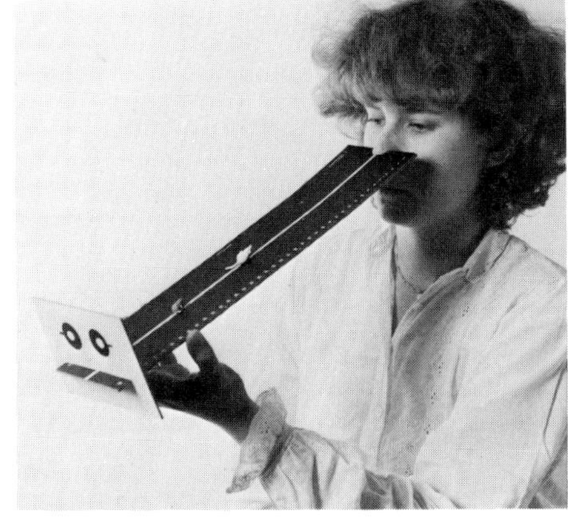

INSTRUMENTATION

Our instrument, the "PLAQUETTE", is a cardboard of 10 cm x 42 cm, carrying one medial sagittal line on each side and two lateral graduations, one in degrees, the other in decimals and a slot for the nose. Mobile magnetic objects attractive for children, and colored as well as variable stereograms, are moved along the medial line. In few minutes, with two questions, we can detect if binocular vision is absent or present, its type and/or the existence of suppression.

1st Question: "HOW MANY LINES CAN YOU SEE ON THE PLAQUETTE?"

The normal subject sees two lines. The main feature is the disappearance of the objective medial line and its transformation into two diagonal lines crossing in an "X" figure. This transformation is obvious, inevitable, nearly instant, and can be expressed even by small children (Fig. 2). This crossing point corresponds to CENTRAL FUSION as well as to the crossing of the visual axes. It determines the angle of convergence in a normal subject and the objective angle of the strabismus measured by the lateral graduation in degrees. The right "virtual line" corresponds to a peripheral retinal area of the left eye. The left "virtual line" to a peripheral area of the right eye. The section of the medial line far away from the the eyes in relation to the fixation point is perceived by nasal retina and constitutes the "V" legs of the "X" and stimulates the opposite hemi-cortex (homonymous diplopia) (Fig. 3).

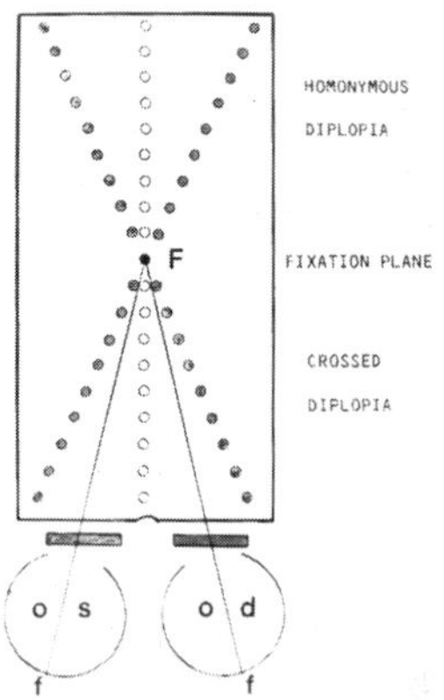

Figure 2

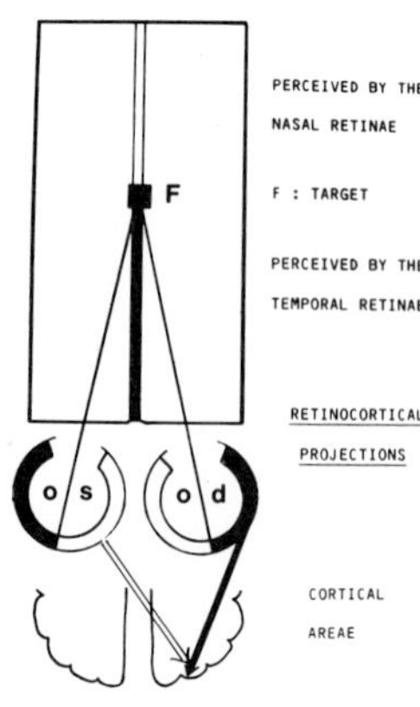

Figure 3

The section of medial line close to the eyes is perceived by the temporal retina and constitutes the "A" legs of "X" and stimulates the homonymous hemi-cortex (crossed diplopia).

Diagnostic Use of the "Plaquette" in Anomalies of Binocular Vision (A.B.V.)

With the plaquette set in horizontal plane, upwards and then downwards, the diagnosis os A.B.V. is made.

Abnormal Binocular Vision Responses

1. The patient sees only one line. Total suppression of one eye and no A.B.V. is diagnosed. This usually occurs in untreated strabismus (Fig. 4) (and in organic lesions which are outside the scope of our paper).

2. The patient sees a crossing in only one specific position: e.g., the second line appearing when "PLAQUETTE" is held: a) downwards or b) upwards: a) esotropia with A pattern or exotropia with V pattern, b) esotropia with V pattern or exotropia with A pattern (Fig. 5).

3. The subject locates one line less clearly than the other = partial suppression or peripheral amblyopia. A RYSER ruler or BAGOLINI'S colored filter ruler placed in front of the fixating eye allows an evaluation of peripheral visual acuity. A partial suppression may appear in the case of wrong lens in front of one eye, anisometropia, reeducated strabismus or strong dominance of one eye (Fig. 4).

4. The patient does not perceive the "V" legs of the "X". This is a manifestation of the suppression in cases of exophoria-tropia. It is rarely the manifestation of a bitemporal hemianopsia. If the patient does not perceive the "A" legs of the "X", it is a manifestation of exophoria-tropia (Fig. 6).

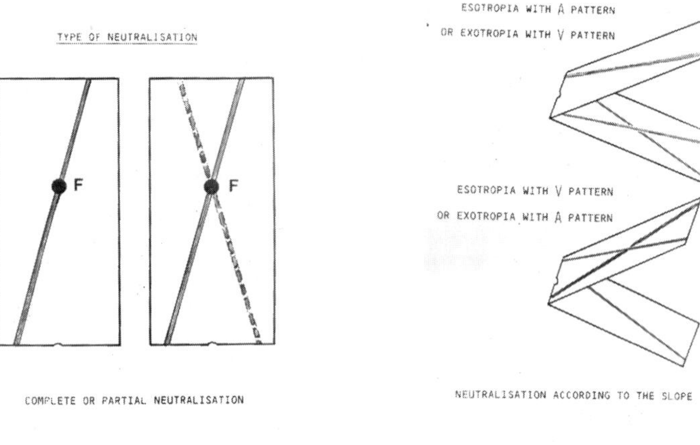

Figure 4

Figure 5

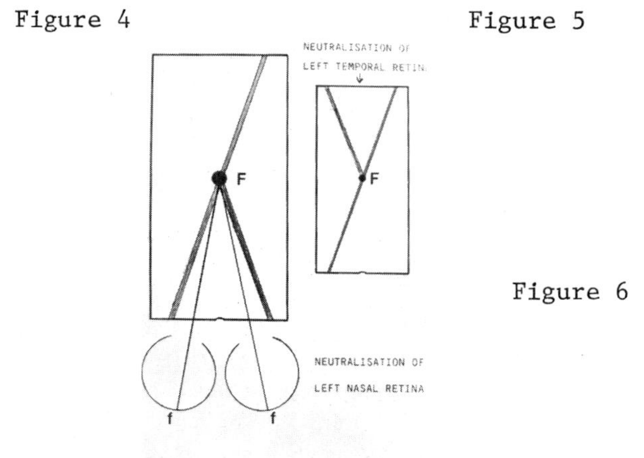

Figure 6

2nd Question: "CAN YOU PUT YOUR FINGER ON THE CROSSING OF THE LINES?"

The answer gives us the diagnosis of the type of PHORIA according to the crossings' position: A crossing situated between 20-25 cm corresponds to ORTHOPHORIA, betweem 25-42 cm to EXOPHORIA and between 20-7 cm to ESOPHORIA (Fig. 7 - Fig. 8). These findings were confirmed in a study of 558 patients in an ophthalmological outpatient clinic. Subjects perceiving only one line or a vague second line on the "PLAQUETTE" were excluded. The patient was fitted with the most adequate nearsight corrective lenses and asked to look calmly into the "PLAQUETTE" slightly slanted downwards. He points, with his finger, to the crossing point and the distance is read on the decimal line. With the patient's head in the same position, the MADDOX ROD test and the WING TEST are performed. In all cases the Titmus test gave a stereoscopic answer of 40" to 100" (Fig. 9 - Fig. 10). The PULFRICH phenomenon was always found positive.

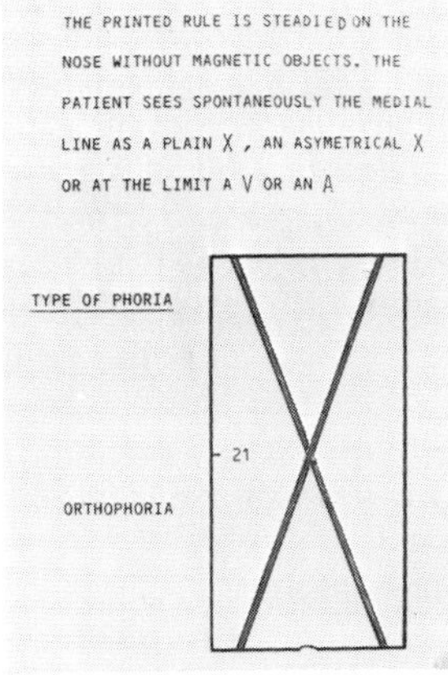

Figure 7

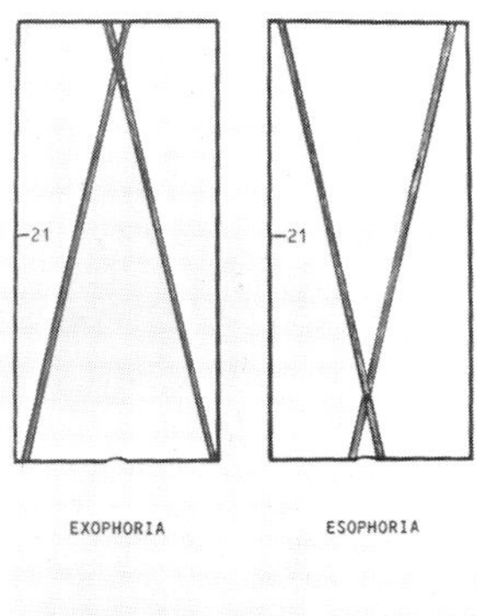

Figure 8

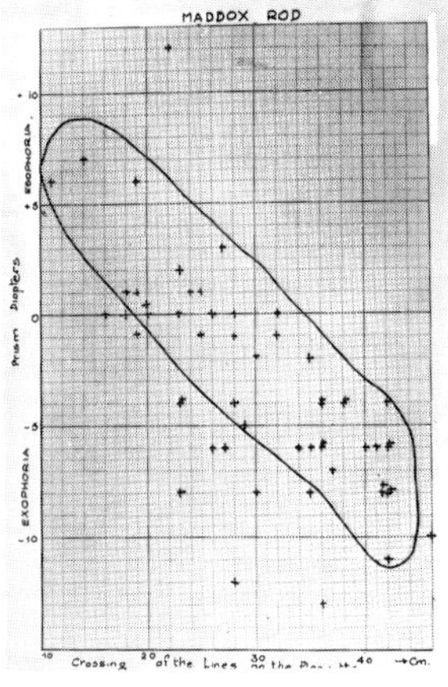

Figure 9

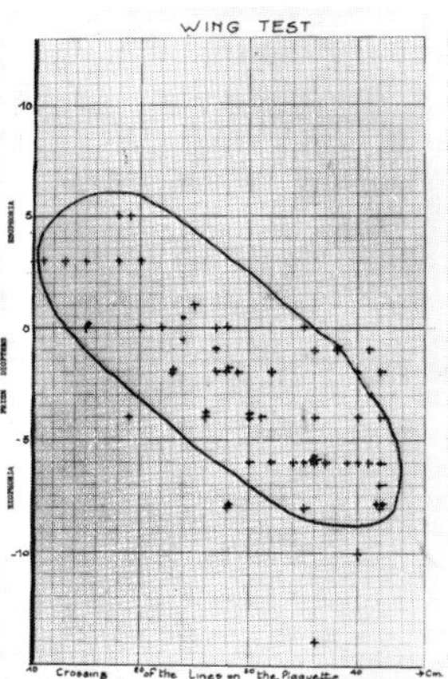

Figure 10

A. The most heterogenous group (group A) includes patients with crossings situated between 20-32 cm--210 cases (37.6%). Studied with M.R. and W.T. we found orthophoria between 22-25 cm; small exophorias between 25-32 cm (or 1 to 4 prism diopters) and small esophorias between 23-20 cm (or 1 to 4 prism diopters).

B. The most homogenous group (group B) includes patients with crossings between 32-42 cm and beyond that limit (outside the "PLAQUETTE") 235 cases (42.11%). These cases as tested with the M.R. and the W.T. show 4 to 16 prism diopters of exophoria, confirmed also by the cover test.

C. Group C includes 113 cases of crossings between 20-7 cm. Most of the group comprises esophorias of 1 to 14 prism diopters. However, a few orthophorias are found with the M.R. (7.5%) and even less with the W.T. (1.6%).

D. If one line is higher than the other, there is an Hyperphoria.

Further Uses of the Plaquette

A. Measurement of the N.P.C. and the N.P.A.: the N.P.C. is the nearest point where the subject may see an object in a single form on the crossing of the lines. The N.P.A. is the nearest point where this object can be seen distinctly (Fig. 11).

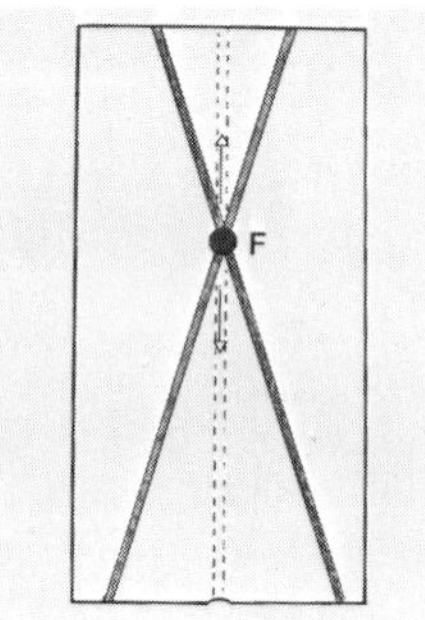

THE PATIENT MOVES THE TARGET ALONG THE MEDIAL LINE MEANWHILE HE ALWAYS SEES THE TWO LINES CROSSING UNDER F. DENEUTRALISATION OF WHOLE RETINA IS OBTAINED BY THE CROSSED LINES.

Figure 11

B. Measurement of amplitude of fusion: we ask the patient to follow the medial line with his eyes, from far to near and vice versa. In the case of binocular vision he will see the crossing travelling up and down the tablet (Fig. 11).

C. Variation of the position of the crossing with correcting glasses: First we note the number on the decimal line corresponding to the crossing. Then add a convex glass +1.D. on the trial frame and the new number is read. The difference between both numbers shows the decrease in convergence due to relaxation of accommodation and in the represents the AC:A.

D. Treatment of minor suppression: one magnetic target is moved along the medial line a number of times; this overcomes suppression of temporal and nasal retinae of both eyes (Fig. 1).

E. Evaluation and treatment of deep suppression: the treatment aims at overcoming suppression. Areas of suppression are recorded (Fig. 12 - Fig. 13). Treatment uses 2 or 3 magnetic objects which are moved in those areas (Fig. 14).

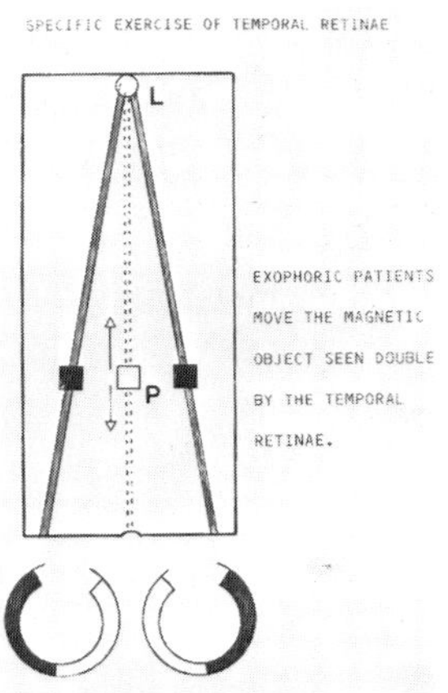

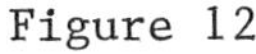

Figure 12

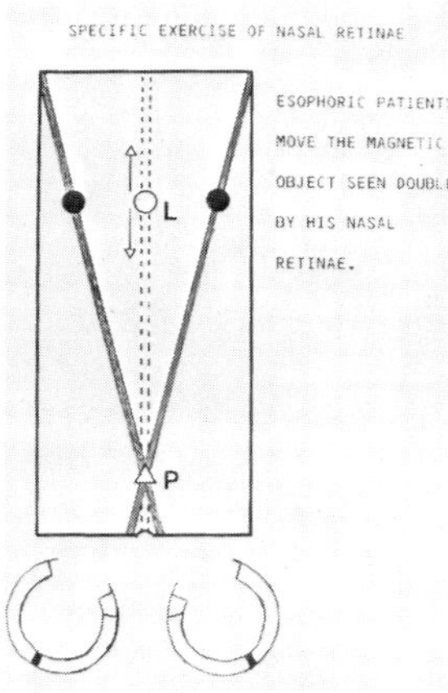

Figure 13

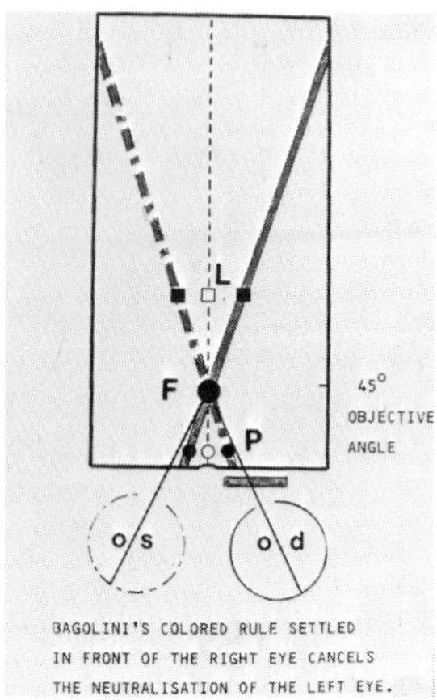

Figure 14

CONCLUSION

Although the instrument we have described is simple, fast, cheap and easy to manage, it can give a great deal of practical information, and may be used for treatment.

REFERENCES

1. Mawas LJ, Mawas E, Weiss JB: Dix siecles de diplopie physiologique d'Al-Hazen a nos jours. Bull Soc Ophthalmol Fr 81(3):281-286, 1981.

2. Mawas LJ, Mawas E, Weiss JB: Interet en strabologie de la plaquette modifiee de Al Hazen. Bull Soc Belge Ophthalmol 196:53-65, 1981.

DISPARITY IN STEREOTESTS

L. L. K. Lin and S. Jeng

ABSTRACT

The TNO random-dot stereogram and the Titmus stereotest were performed on 120 small-angle eso-strabismics, 112 intermittent esotropes and 123 anisometropic amblyopes. We found a significant discrepancy between the results of Titmus and TNO stereotests in patients with small-angle esodeviations. Intermittent exotropes and anisometropic amblyopes showed no substantial difference between Titmus and TNO stereoscores. The discrepancy was explained on the basis of abnormal retinal correspondence and fusional vergence ability.

INTRODUCTION

The two eyes of humans ensure a good sense of depth, in addition to length and width. Strabismics and amblyopes who suffer from defective ability of depth perception. Although the three-rod test is a standardized method in the assessment of stereopsis, the Titmus stereotest, which employs the Polaroid-vectographic system, has been commonly used by ophthalmologists.

The random-dot stereogram, introduced by Julesz in 1971, has become popular. The most impressive advantage of the random-dot stereogram is its lack of monocular clues, thus giving us reliable means of detecting binocular dysfunctions. Reinecke and Simons have recommended their random-dot E stereogram as a screening device for amblyopia and strabismus.

Upon study, ophthalmologists have begun to find discrepancies between the results of different stereotests. Okuda et al. noticed a significant difference between the Titmus and TNO stereotest in strabismic patients. To elucidate the descrepancies between stereotests, we compared the Titmus with TNO test in our patients with small-angle esodeviation, intermittent exotropia and anisometropic amblyopia. The results are analyzed in respect to abnormal retinal correspondence and fusional amplitudes.

STRABISMUS II
ISBN 0-8089-1424-3

MATERIALS AND METHODS

All the patients were from the Muscle Clinic of National Taiwan University Hospital in the past four years, and were divided into three groups. The first group comprised 120 esotropes with deviation less than 16 prism-diopters. The majority were postoperative residual esotropes, with ages from four to 24 years (mean 11.5 years). The second group consisted of 112 intermittent exotropes whose angles exceeded 20 prism diopters. Their ages ranged from four to 44 years, with a mean of 14.8 years. The last group of 123 anisometropic amblyopes had amblyopic vision of 0.2 to 0.6 and a mean age of 13.5 years (from six to 33 years).

The examinations included visual acuity, retinoscopy, prism cover test, Worth 4-dots, after-image test, Titmus, TNO and Frisby stereotests, etc. Major amblyoscopy was done on some patients where indicated. All the patients wore their spectacles. The Titmus tester was held at a distance of 35-40 cm and the TNO at 30-35 cm. The Frisby test was performed as instructed. While the scores of Frisby are based on testing distances, the Titmus and the TNO are tested with a fixed distance. The stereoscores obtained with Titmus and TNO are graded differently, hence they cannot be treated as the precise stereoacuities and subjected to statistics. Our modification was to arbitrarily divide the scores of Titmus and TNO stereotests into a series of 3000-800", 480-400", 240-200", 140-80" and 60" or better. Only those with some degree of binocularity were enrolled in this study. The results on small-angle esotropia, intermittent exotropia and anisometropic amblyopia are tabulated separately (see Tables 1-3).

RESULTS

Because the number tested in our study was high, the results in Tables 1 to 3 were treated as groups of rank-order, and subjected to statistical analysis. The paired-t test in Table 1 demonstrated a significant difference ($p<0.001$) between Titmus and TNO stereotests, indicating that in small-angle esodeviations, the measured stereoscores of Titmus test exceeded those with TNO stereogram.

With intermittent exotropes in Table 2, the correlation coefficient between results of the Titmus and TNO stereotests was high ($r = 0.09$), and the paired-t test between them showed non-significant difference ($p > 0.1$). This means

TABLE 1

Stereoacuities in Small-Angled Esodeviations (N=120)

TNO Titmus	60"	80"- 140"	200"- 240"	400"- 480"	800"- 3000"	no stereo
60"	12	2	3	6	3	3
80"-140"	2	7	9	3	14	7
200"-240"			5	2	17	3
400"-480"				2	3	7
800"-3000"					1	9
no stereo						

paired-t test $p < 0.001$

TABLE 2

Stereoacuities in Intermittent Exotropia (N=112)

TNO Titmus	60"	80"- 140"	200"- 240"	400"- 480"	800"- 3000"	no stereo
60"	42	3				
80"-140"	4	26	2			
200"-240"		4	14	1	1	
400"-480"		1	3	5	1	1
800"-3000"				1	2	1
no stereo						

Correlation coefficient V = 0.90
Paired-t test $p > 0.1$

TABLE 3

Stereoacuities in Anisometropia Amblyopia (N=123)

TNO Titmus	60"	80"- 140"	200"- 240"	400"- 480"	800"- 3000"	no stereo
60"	11	2				
80"-140"	3	40	4			
200"-240"		6	32	2		
400"-480"			1	6	2	
800"-3000"				3	9	2
no stereo						

Correlation coefficient V = 0.92
Paired-t test $p > 0.1$

that, for most patients with intermittent exotropia, the Titmus and the TNO stereotests will give the same results.

In Table 3, there was no statistically significant difference ($p > 0.1$) between the scores of the Titmus and TNO stereotests with anisometropic amblyopes. And the correlation coefficient between them was high ($r = 0.92$).

DISCUSSION

Our results demonstrate that, in patients with small-angled deviations, the scores of TNO stereogram were invaribly poorer than those of Titmus stereotest. Which scores were more correct or closer to the true stereopsis? With the Frisby test, the measured stereoscores in small-angle esotropes seemed to be the same or better than those with the Titmus test, suggesting that the patients might actually have good stereopsis, in spite of poor TNO scores. In fact, some of them did play basketball well. Without some binocular depth perception, they could not have had such a good sense of depth through practice on monocular clues. In one study by Henson and Williams, both the Titmus and Frisby tests correlated fairly well with the modified Howard-Dolman test in that all of the small-angled strabismic subjects with significant better binocular thresholds than monocular ones obtained fairly good stereoacuities as measured with both the Titmus and Frisby test.(3)

Most of our patients with small-angle esodeviations were either esophoric-esotropic or esotropic of minimal to mild degrees following surgery. Many of them had strabismic amblyopia of varying extents. Was it the amblyopia that caused esotropes to have difficulty in seeing binocularly through red-green glasses? In Table 3 we see no substantial difference between the Titmus and the TNO stereotests among the amblyopes due to anisometropia, from whom the strabismic amblyopes did have different sensory adaptations. Many of the small-angle esotropes would develop abnormal retinal correspondence to obtain gross peripheral binocular single vision. And this abnormal retinal correspondence can be detected with devices of graded dissociating effects.(4) In intermittent exotropia, while there is a hemi-retinal suppression during the exotropic phase, most will have varying degrees of stereopsis on near fusion. And our results with both Titmus and TNO stereotests showed the same good binocularity. The stereoscores with either test were not different, whether the intermittent exotropes had, on after-image test, normal retinal correspondence or not. On the other hand, the abnormal retinal correspondence enabled the patients with small-angled esotropia to see binocularly. Since the red-green glasses have more dissociating effect than Polaroid ones, the different stereoscores with TNO in comparison with Titmus in small-angle esotropia might be due to abnormal retinal correspondence.

As has been noted, the random-dot stereograms need vergence movement to see the figure among the anaglyphs.(5,6) That is to say, the TNO stereotest needs the motor component of fusion and stereopsis in addition to sensory fusion and stereopsis. And this is why it always took longer for the patients to see the TNO pictures than the Titmus ones which employ the Polaroid-vectographic system. Most of our cases with intermittent exotropia and anisometropic amblyopia possessed sufficient fusional amplitudes to allow them to pass the TNO as wll as the Titmus stereotest. Detailed major amblyoscopic examination was done on 70 small-angle esotropes. After correlating their fusional amplitudes with the results of TNO stereoscores, we found a positive relationship between them (see Table 4). In other words, an esotrope lacking vergence ability would fail TNO random-dot stereograms, while an intermittent esotrope, or a small-angled esotrope with good range of fusional amplitudes covering both convergence and divergence would have the motor, in addition to sensory, fusion to get a better score on random-dot stereograms.

TABLE 4 RELATIONSHIP BETWEEN TNO STEREOSCORES AND FUSIONAL AMPLITUDES ON MAJOR AMBLYOSCOPY

TNO	no stereo	33'	480"-60"
mean ± SD fusional amplitude (p.d.)	6.4 ± 5.8 (N = 11)	#19.0 ± 11.7 (N = 24)	#24.5 ± 12.0 (N = 35)

#Significant difference (t-test, 0 < 0.05)

Two other things are noteworthy. The first is that neither the Titmus nor the TNO stereotest alone is a good device in screening for intermittent exotropia. In our experience, more than 80% of exotropes will pass the 240"-criterion. The cover test for distance and near fixation with a penlight would be the best way to screen for intermittent exotropia of any degree. Secondly, while most uncorrected anisometropes might fail the screening test,(7,8) many of our patients, though from a biased selection, after spectacle correction, passed the 200/240" criteria.

In conclusion, the TNO random-dot stereogram is good in screening children for strabismus with poor fusional ability. But in daily clinic, the assessment of the patient's stereoacuity should be carefully evaluated with TNO, Titmus and other available tests.

REFERENCES

1. Reinecke RD, Simons K: A new stereoscopic test for amblyopia screening. Am J Ophthalmol 78:714-721, 1974

2. Okuda FC, Apt L, Wanter BS: Evaluation of the TNO random-dot stereogram test. Am Orthopt J 27:124-130, 1977

3. Henson DB, Williams DE: Depth perception in strabismus. Br J Ophthalmol 64:349-353, 1980

4. Bagolini B: Diagnostic errors in the evaluation of retinal correspondence by various tests in squints, in Arruga A (ed): International Strabismus Symposium Giessen, August 1966, Basel, Karger 1968, p. 163-174.

5. Frisby JP, Mein J, Saye A, Stanworth A: Use of random-dot stereograms in the clinical assessment of strabismic patients. Br J Ophthalmol 59:545-552, 1975

6. Westheimer G, McKee SP: Stereogram design for testing local stereopsis. Invest Ophthalmol 19:802-809, 1980

7. Kani W: Stereopsis and spatial perception in amblyopes and uncorrected ametropes. Br J Ophthalmol 62:756-762, 1978

8. Marsh WR, Rawlings SC, Mumma JV: Evaluation of clinical stereoacuity tests. Ophthalmology 87:1265-1272, 1980 (discussion by Dr. Reinecke) p. 1272.

DISCUSSION BY R. A. CRONE

Lin and Jeng found that small-angle esotropia has significantly more difficulties with the TNO test than with other stereotests. I have the same experience. Of 30 patients with micro-esotropia and good fusion examined in my clinic, many had coarse stereopsis but only 2 could read the TNO charts. Surely ARC together with red-green dissociation are the cause of the discrepancy between TNO and other tests.

Vergency power has little to do with stereopsis. There is no such thing as sensory and motor stereopsis. Every disparity, produced in any stereotest, is a stimulus to vergency, whether executed or suppressed.

It is interesting that the only 2 patients in my series who could read the TNO charts had a large amplitude of sensory fusion, but poor vergence. This does not conform to the expectations of Drs. Lin and Jeng.

STUDIES ON ANISEIKONIA AND STEREOPSIS WITH THE "NEW ANISEIKONIA TESTS"

S. Awaya, M. Sugawara, F. Horibe, and M. Miura

ABSTRACT

The "New Aniseikonia Tests" (NAT) developed by the authors and now commercially available have been introduced and the measurements of aniseikonia given for various refractive errors. The comparison of the data with those of the phase difference haploscope (PDH) validated this new test. Since each case shows an unpredictable amount of aniseikonia in the correction of the refractive errors, it is of vital importance to actually measure the aniseikonia in each individual routinely before the correction is given.

The aniseikonia tolerance for stereopsis is approximately 7% for 40" stereoacuity, 13% for 100" stereoacuity in the Titmus Stereo Test, and 7% for 60" stereoacuity, and 12% for 120" stereoacuity in the TNO Stereo Test.

INTRODUCTION

Aniseikonia is defined as differences of the two retinal images. It has a close relationship to the amount of refractive error and the optical correction. However, the aniseikonia is variably modified through the complicated neurophysological processes in the formation of "ocular image" or mental image by which we measure the size of aniseikonia. A certain amount of aniseikonia exceeding the tolerance threshhold may result in asthenopia or a disturbance of binocular fusion (Figure 1).

Aniseikonia is of clinical significance and of academic interest to quantitate the aniseikonia in refractive errors. It has been routinely measured in the clinical examination, partly due to the variable responses modified by the various optical and neurophysiological factors and partly due to the complexity of the testing equipment.

Our new method, the "New Aniseikonia Tests" permits us to measure easily the size of aniseikonia. We present studies herein which have been made with New Aniseikonia Tests on patients with various refractive errors.

STRABISMUS II
ISBN 0-8089-1424-3

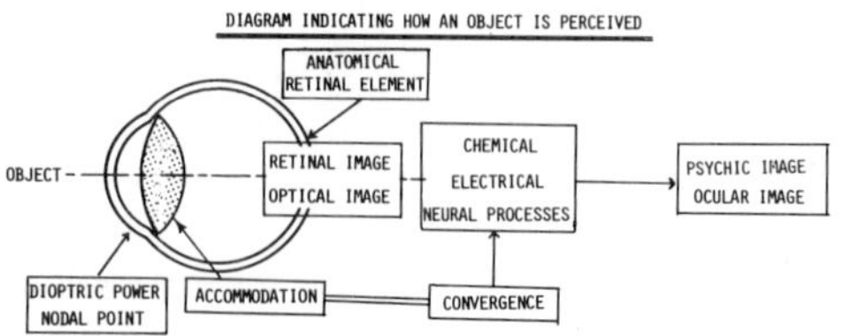

Figure 1. Diagram of indicating several factors influencing the size of retinal image and ocular image.

MATERIALS AND METHODS

The validity of the New Aniseikonia Tests (NAT) was confirmed by the artificial aniseikonia produced by size lenses of four different powers on one eye of the 20 normal subjects and compared with those measured by the Aulhorn phase difference haploscope (PHD).

The New Aniseikonia Tests were applied for measuring the aniseikonia observed under three optical situations; no correction, spectacle lens correction and contact lens correction in 22 cases of hyperopic anisometropia, 11 cases of myopic anisometropia and 20 cases of unilateral aphakia.

Furthermore, in order to clarify the aniseikonia tolerance for stereopsis in normal subjects, in whom aniseikonia of various sizes was produced by the size lenses, stereoacuity was measured by the Titmus Stereo Tests and TNO Stereo Test

A pair of halfmoons, one red and the other one green is placed, facing each other at their rectilinear edges with a small cross mark in center of the interval between the two halfmoons. When viewed through a pair of red-green glasses, the red halfmoon is visible to the eye with the green glass, while the green halfmoon is seen by the eye with the red glass. In figure 2, No. 0 presents a pair of halfmoons of equal size and No. 1 shows a pair of halfmoons in which the green one is 1% smaller than the red one. No. 2 shows 2% difference and the greeen halfmoon is further decreased by 1% in a stepwise fashion in each of the following nos. through 6. Thus, the number of the figures coincides with the difference in percent between the two halfmoons. In the acutal series, the stepwise 1% increase of the green halfmoon continues until a difference of 24% is reached in no. 24. For example, in Figure No. 5, the green halfmoon is 5% larger than the red halfmoon (Figures 2 and 5). When measurement of

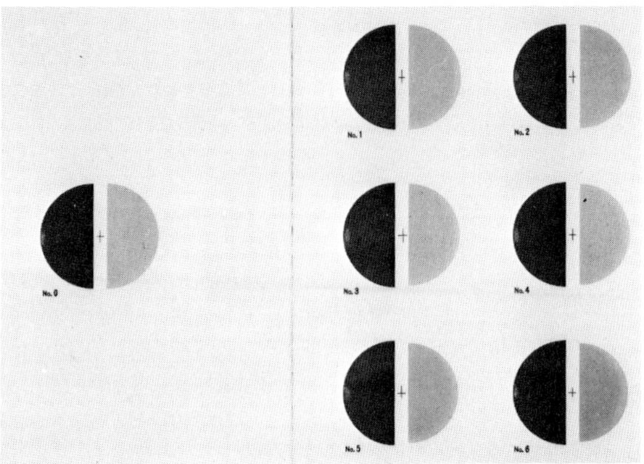

Figure 2

aniseikonia in the horizontal or oblique meridian is required, the test book is tilted so that the rectilinear edges of the halfmoon coincides witht he meridian to be examined. This cannot be accomplished by the polaroid system.

RESULTS

1. Artificial aniseikonia produced by the size-lenses in 20 normal subjects.

A normal 27-year-old female presented four different amounts of aniseikonia produced by the size-lenses of four different powers. The measurements by the N.A.T. were in good accordance with those by the P.D.H. (Table 1). The mean value of the 20 normal cases examined revealed a tendency of slightly smaller aniseikonia measured by the N.A.T. as compared with that measured by the P.D.H. (Table 2).

2. Aniseikonia in hyperopic anisometropia.

This 13-year-old male with hyperopic anisometropia demonstrated a small aniseikonia with spectacle lens correction as compared to contact lens correction. This is likely to be a case of axial anisometropia in which the Knapp's Law(2,3) holds true (Table 3).

An 11-year-old female with hyperopic anisometropia demonstraded a moderate amount of aniseikonia (+2.0 to +4.5%) with spectacle lens correction, while she showed an opposite aniseikonia, that is, reduction of image in the more hyperopic eye with contact lens correction. This may be a

NORMAL SUBJECT

Y.I. 27 YRS. F.

V R: 1.0
L: 1.0

METHOD	ANISEIKONIA (%)				
	SIZE LENS				
	(-)	NO. 1	NO. 2	NO. 3	NO. 4
N.A.T.	0	+4.5	+5.5	+11.5	+14.5
P.D.H.	+0.7	+3.7	+7.5	+12.0	+14.8

N.A.T.: NEW ANISEIKONIA TESTS
P.D.H.: PHASE DIFFERENCE HAPLOSCOPE

TABLE 1

MEAN SIZE OF ANISEIKONIA PRODUCED BY SIZE LENSES OF FOUR DIFFERENT POWERS IN 20 NORMAL SUBJECTS

	METHOD	SIZE LENSES(4 DIFFERENT POWERS)			
		NO. 1	NO. 2	NO. 3	NO. 4
MEAN SIZE OF ANISEIKONIA (%)	N. A. T.	3.09	5.71	9.98	13.58
	P. D. H.	4.62	8.19	12.43	14.90

N.A.T.:NEW ANISEIKONIA TESTS.
P.D.H.:PHASE DIFFERENCE HAPLOSCOPE

TABLE 2

HYPEROPIC ANISOMETROPIA

H.I. 13 YRS. M.

V R: 1.0(N.C.)
L: 0.2(1.0 x +2.5⊂CYL+2.0 90°)

METHOD	ANISEIKONIA (%)		
	WITHOUT CORRECTION	SPECTACLE LENSES	CONTACT LENSES
N.A.T.	-1.5	-1.5	-2.0
P.D.H.	-5.1	-0.3	-4.1

N.A.T.: NEW ANISEIKONIA TESTS
P.D.H.: PHASE DIFFERENCE HAPLOSCOPE

TABLE 3

case in which axial and refractive factors combined to be responsible for the formation of this anisometropia (Table 4).

When the size of aniseikonia of all 22 cases are plotted in three different situations: no correction, spectacle lens correction and contact lens correction, essentially all cases show minus aniseikonia in uncorrected condition. In spectacle lens correction, 8 cases showed almost no aniseikonia and the remaining 14 cases showed plus aniseikonia. However, in contact lens correction, all except for 6 cases showed minus aniseikonia (Figure 3).

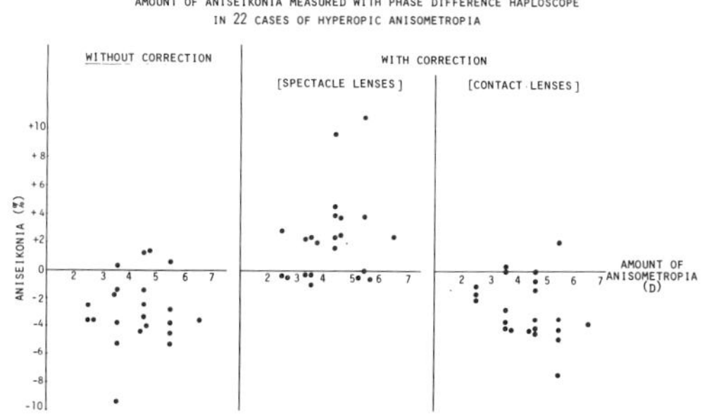

Figure 3. The New Aniseikonia Tests. There is a stepwise 1% increase of the green halfmoon in each figure from Figure No. 1 to Figure No. 24 (Minus Aniseikonia Series).

HYPEROPIC ANISOMETROPIA

R.T. 11 YRS. F.

V R: 1.0(1.0 x+5.5)
L: 1.0(1.0 x+0.5)

METHOD	ANISEIKONIA (%)		
	WITHOUT CORRECTION	SPECTACLE LENSES	CONTACT LENSES
N.A.T.	R-SUPP.	+2.0	-3.0
P.D.H.	-4.0	+4.5	-3.3

N.A.T.: NEW ANISEIKONIA TESTS
P.D.H.: PHASE DIFFERENCE HAPLOSCOPE

TABLE 4

3. Myopic anisometropia.

A 51-year-old female with myopic anisometropia presented a larger aniseikonia with spectacle lens correction (-5.5%) than that with contact lens correction (+1.45%), indicating that a refractive factor was more responsible than an axial one in the formation of this anisometropia (Table 5). Conversely, a 51-year-old male with myopic anisometropia presented essentially no aniseikonia with spectacle lens correction, but some demonstrable aniseikonia with contact lens correction. This case is likely to be the so-called "axial myopic anisometropia" in which Knapp's law holds true (Table 6).

When the size of aniseikonia observed in 11 cases was compared, all but one case showed some amount of aniseikonia, which became more evident as the amount of anisometropia increased without any correcting lens, and 10 cases except for only one showed an aniseikonia of -4% or smaller with spectacle lens correction. However, contact lens correction made the retinal image, hence ocular image too, slightly larger up to +4% in 9 cases and larger amount of aniseikonia in two other cases; +8.0% in one case and +9.0% in another case (Figure 4).

MYOPIC ANISOMETROPIA

N.M. 51 YRS. F.

V R: 0.3(0.8 x -2.5⊃CYL-1.5 90°)
L: 0.7(0.8 x +0.5⊃CYL-1.0 90°)

METHOD	ANISEIKONIA (%)		
	WITHOUT CORRECTION	SPECTACLE LENSES	CONTACT LENSES
N.A.T.	R-SUPP.	-7.0	+1.0
P.D.H.	+3.5	-4.1	+1.9

N.A.T.: NEW ANISEIKONIA TESTS
P.D.H.: PHASE DIFFERENCE HAPLOSCOPE

TABLE 5

When we compared the size of aniseikonia with respect to the correction with spectacle lens and contact lens in hyperopic anisometropia and myopic anisometropia, slightly more than a half of the cases in both groups of anisometropia demonstrated smaller amount of aniseikonia by spectacle lens than contact lens correction.

MYOPIC ANISOMETROPIA

M.K. 51 YRS. M.

V R: 0.1(0.8 x-3.5⊃CYL-1.0 90°)
L: 0.8(1.0 x CYL-1.0 70°)

METHOD	ANISEIKONIA (%)		
	WITHOUT CORRECTION	SPECTACLE LENSES	CONTACT LENSES
N.A.T.	R-SUPP.	+0.5	+3.0
P.D.H.	+6.5	-0.7	+3.7

N.A.T.: NEW ANISEIKONIA TESTS
P.D.H.: PHASE DIFFERENCE HAPLOSCOPE

TABLE 6

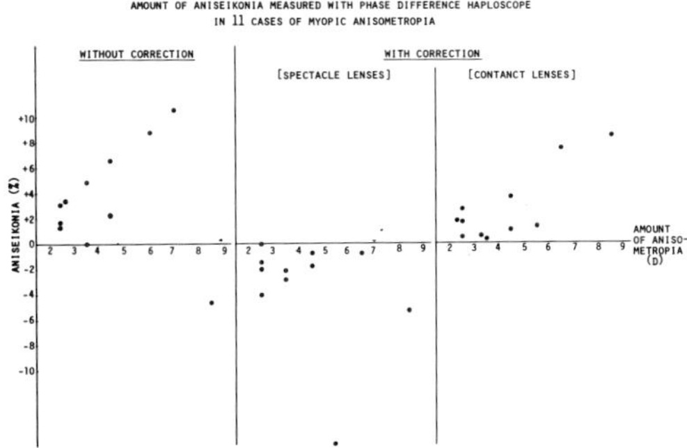

Figure 4. Amount of aniseikonia measured with phase difference haploscope in 22 cases of hyperopic anisometropia.

4. Unilateral aphakia

A 65-year-old female with unilateral aphakia presented a +23.8% aniseikonia with spectacle lens correction, but only +2.4% aniseikonia with contact lens correction. While without correction the aphakic eye was suppressed with the N.A.T., while +15% aniseikonia was demonstrated by the P.D.H. (Table 7). The total of 20 cases examined showed a relatively large amount of aniseikonia without any correction, and aniseikonia of +12% to +37% was demonstrated by spectacle lens correction, while less than +7% aniseikonia was found by contact lens correction (Figure 5).

UNILATERAL APHAKIA

H.F. 65 YRS. F.

V R: 0.01(0.9 x +14.0⊂CYL+3.0 110°)
L: 0.1 (1.0 x +5.75)

METHOD	ANISEIKONIA (%)		
	WITHOUT CORRECTION	SPECTACLE LENSES	CONTACT LENSES
N.A.T.	R-SUPP.	+23.0	+1.5
P.D.H.	+15.0	+24.5	+3.2

N.A.T.: NEW ANISEIKONIA TESTS
P.D.H.: PHASE DIFFERENCE HAPLOSCOPE

TABLE 7

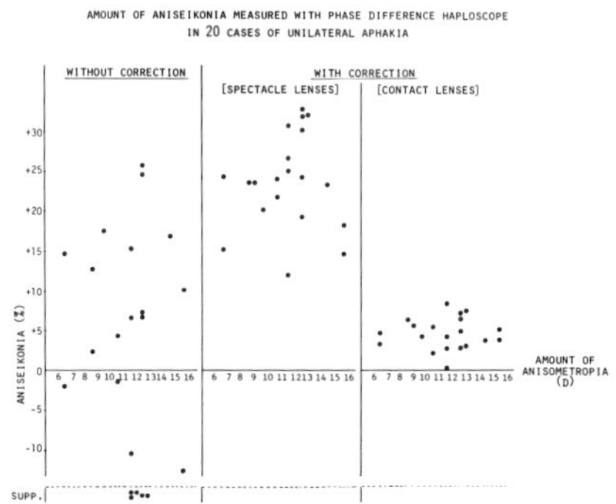

Figure 5. Amount of aniseikonia measured with phase difference haploscope in 11 cases of myopic anisometropia.

5. By producing various sizes of artificial aniseikonia by the sizelenses of four different powers, we analyzed the relationship between the size of aniseikonia and stereoacuity which is assessed by the Titmus Stereo Tests and TNO Stereo Test. The aniseikonia tolerance for stereopsis is 7% to pass the Titmus No. 9 Circle Test (40 sec. of arc) and 13% of aniseikonia to pass Titmus No. 5 Circle Test (100 sec. of arc) and 7% to pass 30" chart and 12% to pass the 120" chart of the TNO Stereo Test (Tables 8 & 9).

Aniseikonia tolerance for the Titmus Stereo Tests in 20 normal subjects

Circle No.	Stereoacuity (Sec. of Arc)	Aniseikonia Tolerance	
		Mean	Standard Deviation
9	40"	7%	2.3
8	50"	11%	2.4
7	60"	12%	1.3
6	80"	13%	1.9
5	100"	13%	1.5

TABLE 8

Aniseikonia tolerance for the TNO Stereo Test in 20 normal subjects

Stereoacuity (sec. of Arc)	Aniseikonia Tolerance	
	Mean	Standard Deviation
15"	2%	2.8
30"	7%	3.2
60"	9%	2.2
120"	12%	1.7

TABLE 9

DISCUSSION

Several instruments are available for measuring aniseikonia, such as the standard eikonometer, space eikonometer, synoptophore, Pola-Test and phase difference haploscope, among which the Aulhorn phase difference haploscope(4,5) is the most sophisticated, accurate, and reliable. However, all of these instruments require a relatively large testing space. The New Aniseikonia Test as studied herein is an entirely new "test chart" which enables us to measure aniseikonia easily in a routine clinical examination.

Essentially similar results of aniseikonia measurement have been obtained in many clinical conditions with the New Aniseikonia Tests and the phase difference haploscope, indicating validity of these new tests. One small difference between the two measurements is that a smaller aniseikonia is often observed by the New Aniseikonia Tests than by the phase difference haploscope. This may be because this test elicits more fusional capacity with such a cross mark in the center or numerals printed below the halfmoons. Under these least dissociating conditions some innervational mechanism may intervene to minimize the image size difference between the two eyes. This assumption may be correct in that suppression of one image sometimes occurs with the New Aniseikonia Tests.

The difference of colors, red and green of each halfmoon is unlikely to cause much disturbance in chromatic aberation in the optical structure of the eye, for these two different colors appear as similar greys when viewed through green and red filters, respectively.

Regarding aniseikonia tolerance for stereopsis, it is generally known that a 5% aniseikonia is a tolerance threshold for binocular fusion and that approximately two diopters difference between the correcting lenses for the two eyes is likely to be the amount to cause this much aniseikonia.(6) We have been of opinion that this concept is not always correct, for the influence of the correcting lens on the size of the retinal image is not always uniform from patient to patient and may not be proportional to the power of correcting lens. The image size difference may depend on the cause of the anisometropia being axial or refractive or both. Several other investigators advocated different values of the aniseikonia tolerance thresholds. Among them are Ogle (1.5%),(7) Crone (5-8%),(8) Julesz (15%),(9) and Berger (18%).(10) The results of our studies have shown that aniseikonia larger than 5%, that is, 7% to 13% of aniseikonia permits binocular fusion. However, both in the Titmus Stereo Tests and TNO Stereo Test, a smaller amount of aniseikonia tolerance is necessary for higher stereoacuity.

REFERENCES

1. Awaya S, Sugawara M, Horibe F, Torii F: The "New Aniseikonia Tests" and its clinical applications. Nippon Ganka Gakkai Zasshi 86:217-222, 1982.

2. Linksz A: Physiology of the Eye. Vol 1: Optics. New York: Grune & Stratton, 1950, p 299

3. Ogle KN: Optics, 2nd ed. Springfield, Ill: CC Thomas, 1971, p 205

4. Aulhorn E: Phasen differenz-haploskopie. Klin Monatsbl Augenheilkd 148:540-544, 1966

5. Awaya S, von Noorden GK: Aniseikonia measurement by phase difference haploscope in myopic anisometropia and unilateral aphakia. J Jap Contact Lens Soc Dec 71:13(12):131-139.

6. Duke-Elder: System of Ophthalmology, Vol 5. London: Henry Kimpton, 1970, p 507

7. Ogle KN, Burian HM, Bannon RE: On the correction of unilateral aphakia with contact lenses. AMA Arch Ophthalmol 59:639-652, 1958

8. Crone RA, Leuridan OMA: Tolerance of aniseikonia. Albrecht von Graefe Arch Klin Exp Ophthalmol 188:1-16, 1973

9. Julesz B: Foundations of Cyclopean Perception. Chicago: University of Chicago Press, 1971

10. Berger A, Monje M: Uber den Einfluss der Aniseikonie auf Tiefensehen. Albrecht von Graefe Arch Klin Exp Ophthalmol 148:515-528, 1948

DISCUSSION BY R. A. CRONE

The new aniseikonia test of Awaya and co-workers should be warmly recommended because it is cheap and simple and will make ophthalmologists familiar with aniseikonia. Too often - at least in Europe - it is thought that anisometropia and aniseikonia are parallel phenomena. Clearly, because of Knapp's law, that is not the case. Aniseikonia should not be inferred but measured.

I am not quite convinced that the authors have found a real influence of aniseikonia on stereopsis. Personally I did not find much correlation. In any case the size effect on stereopsis will not easily be demonstrable. Julesz showed that large field targets with 15% size differences could be seen stereoscopically. In the central field the relative diplopia threshhold is high. Difficulties with small stereo-targets, such as the Titmus rings, are, therefore, possible, but not very likely.

USEFULNESS OF FILTERS OF PROGRESSIVE DENSITY AS A DIAGNOSTIC TOOL FOR SOME STRABISMIC PROBLEMS

B. Bagolini

ABSTRACT

A bar of red filters of progressive density is useful for the diagnosis of the intensity of a suppression scotoma and diagnosis of the intensity of normal and anomalous retinal correspondence. For these two diagnostic modalities the bar has to be used in combination with the striated glasses. The bar is also useful for prediction of the likelihood of occurrence of diplopia during treatment of strabismic or anisometropic amblyopia in patients older than 8-10 years and for the prediction of postoperative diplopia in adult-patients with childhood onset comitant strabismus. The progressive filters assist in evaluation of the strength of the power that keeps the eyes undissociated in "dissociated vertical divergences" and give some implications on the choice of surgery. Theoretical as well as practical implications for each testing condition are discussed.

INTRODUCTION

A bar of filters of increasing density may be useful in studying various reactions to dissociation in strabismic subjects.(1) The bar of filters here described is made up of 17 red filters numbered with conventional numbers (Fig 1). Eight uses of the bar filter are reviewed.

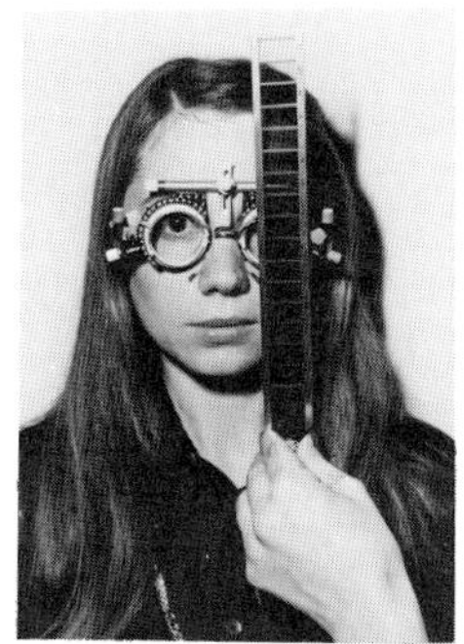

Figure 1. The striated lenses are in the trial frame.

STRABISMUS II
ISBN 0-8089-1424-3

METHODS

1. Evaluation of the intensity of suppression. In heterotropia, suppression may be the prevalent feature of the deviated eye. This is particularly true in large angles of strabismus as can be demonstrated in casual seeing with striated glasses. The test is performed in the following way.

Striated glasses are mounted on a trial frame to judge if the patient sees one or two stripes crossing the fixation light. If there is suppression he will see only one stripe corresponding to the fixing eye (Fig 2). (He may occasionally see parts of the other strips not reaching the fixation light.) The bar of filters is slowly slid in front of the deviated eye from the weaker toward the denser filters. When the patient sees two lights with the less denser filters the intensity of suppression is weak. The intensity of suppression will be more and more important when denser filters are necessary to make the strabismic subjects see double. It is convenient to slide the bar of filters in front of the deviated eye. This in order to avoid a change of the fixing eye that frequently occurs if we put the bar of filters in front of the fixing eye.

2. Evaluation of the intensity of anomalous retinal correspondence (ARC). In heterotropia, ARC may be the prevalent feature and areas of suppression may be disregardable or even absent. Diplopia may be avoided by the change in spatial value of the retinal elements of the deviated eye and a sort of binocular vision is created with the deviated eye. This feature is commonly found in small angles of esotropia.(2-5) With the striated glasses (Fig 2), the patient will see two stripes crossing the fixation light like a normal subject in spite of a deviated eye. By sliding the filter bar in front of the deviated eye we can measure the strength of the anomalous vision supported by ARC. The darker the filter to evoke diplopia (by dissociated this anomalous vision the stronger the ARC be. Obviously, if the ARC is strong it will be difficult to acquire a normal retinal correspondence.

3. Elimination of suppression. The filter bar can be slid in front of either eye until a filter makes the patient aware of diplopia. By repeating this manuever several times in front of the fixing eye, diplopia will appear with progressively lighter filters, until it persists without filters. This manuever has to be used only when we are sure

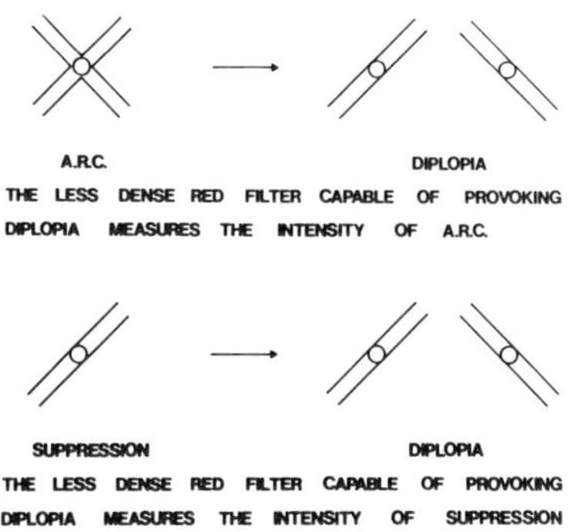

Figure 2.

that a normal correspondence is present and normal fusional movements can be restored. It is, however, a type of orthoptic exercise which is seldom necessary because suppression in casual seeing is rare in these cases.

4. Reinforcement of fusional ability. Some patients have weak normal binocular vision. This may occur in previously strabismic subjects who are regaining normal binocularity, or heterophoric subjects with weak binocularity and tendency to become heterotropic. Exercises at the major amblyoscope to enlarge motorial fusional abilities may be indicated. It is useful in these cases to exercise the patients in casual seeing. The patient must learn to fuse with progressively darker filters. He should maintain the ability of seeing only one light even with the darkest filters.

5. Prediction of diplopia when treating amblyopia. When amblyopia must be treated in relatively adult subjects (more than 10 years of age) by occlusion or penalization techniques, diplopia may be a danger. Before starting such treatment and throughout the treatment, the intensity of suppression should be measured. If the latter is eliminated and diplopia is reached with light filters (n degrees 1 to 5), a real danger of diplopia exists.

6. Prediction of postoperative diplopia in adult subjects. When operating on an adult subject for cosmetic reasons, the possibility of postoperative diplopia frequently exists. Prismatic correction gives a reasonable preoperative idea of this possibility. Further information can be gathered

by testing the intensity of suppresion while strabismus is corrected by prisms. If diplopia can be elicited only by rather dense filters, danger of postoperative diplopia is slight.

7. Judgement on the operability of an heterophoria. We refer here only to exophoria. Operation is not indicated if the angle is small, if it does not decompensate to exotropia, and no asthenopic complaints are present. When the angle is large and the patient intermittently exhibits this large exotropia, there may be the tendency for this patient to acquire a constant exotropia with the passing of time. This may be evaluated with the filter ladder. When the patient in repeat examinations shows a tendency to let the eye deviate with progressively lighter filters, it is an indication that his sensorial status is deteriorating and surgery becomes mandatory. If the dissociation occurs only with dense filters this means that the exophoria is seldom intermittent and surgery will be successful even if the angle of deviation will not be fully corrected. The chances are that such patients will remain purely heterophoric. If the exophoria is dissociated by light filters the surgical correction needs to be more precise and it is more important that the angle be fully corrected. The evaluation of the filter necessary to dissociate an exophoria is more important for distant vision. Care must be taken to assure that repeat measurements are done with the same conditions of illumination and of fixation light intensity.

8. Judgement on the operability of a dissociated vertical divergence (DVD). The density of the filter necessary to elevate the eye covered by the filter in a DVD indicates the ease of dissociation. If a dense filter is necessary to dissociate it, a small recession of the superior rectus will probably correct the situation. If light filters provoke a dissociation the recession has to be more generous. The amount of vertical deviation must also obviously influence the amount of recession necessary and the utility of an additional "faden".

It is important to have light filters in the ladder; much lighter than the red filters commonly supplied with lens boxes. The filter ladder described by Capobianco starts with too dense filters.(6) An evaluation of the sensorial status can be done with these filters only by starting from a too great dissociating level and they are of little utility in studying the sensorial status with striated glasses. These in fact are particularly useful in evaluating weak sensorial statuses. Furthermore, the filter ladder described by me is standardized and filters have the same density in different manufactured bars.

REFERENCES

1. Bagolini B: Diagnostic et possibilite de traitement de l'etat sensoriel du strabisme concomitant avec des instruments peu dissociants. (Test du vere strie et barre de filtres). Ann Ocul 194: 236-258, 1961.

2. Bagolini B: Anomalous correspondence: Definition and diagnositc methods. Doc Ophthalmol 23:346-386, 1967.

3. Bagolini B: Part I: Sensorial anomalies in strabismus. (Suppression, anomalous correspondence, amblyopia). Doc Ophthalmol 41:1-22, 1976.

4. Bagolini B, Capobianco NM: Subjective space in comitant squint. Amer J Ophthalmol 59:430-442, 1965.

5. Campos EC: Binocularity in comitant strabismus. Binocular visual field studies. Doc Ophthalmol, 53:249-281, 1982.

6. Capobianco NM: The subjective measurement of the near point of convergence and its significance in the diagnosis of convergence insufficiency. Am Orthopt J 2:40-42, 1952.

DISCUSSION BY R. A. CRONE

Bagolini discussed the usefulness of his filter bar. The principle of this bar is quite sound. So why has Bagolini's filter bar never attained the popularity of his striated glasses? Probably because the invention of a minimally dissociating test was a major achievement while we had a multitude of dissociation tests already.

Bagolini mentioned 8 indications for the use of the filter bar. Very attractive seems the use of the bar to judge the depth of suppression before strating amblyopia treatment in older children. The same can be done before deciding to do a cosmetic operation in an adult. The measurement of the extension of the suppression scotoma with a prism bar, however, is in my view more important as a preoperative measurement.

The other indications seem less urgent. The result of the filter bar in micro-strabismus is difficult to interpret. Does diplopia mean a change in the objective angle or in the angle of anomaly?

Finally, the use of the filter bar is questionable in the last mentioned indications. Cases of heterophoria, intermittent exotropia and DVD should only be operated upon when there are manifest clinical symptoms, not when symptoms can only be provoked by filters.

A COMPARATIVE STUDY OF DENERVATION AND EXTIRPATION FOR MARKED INFERIOR OBLIQUE OVERACTION

M. A. Del Monte and M. M. Parks

ABSTRACT

Parks(1) demonstrated that recession was more effective than myectomy at insertion or origin, or disinsertion for eliminating inferior oblique overaction. This study simultaneously compares an improved procedure, denervation and extirpation of the inferior oblique, to 14 mm recession in a prospective, consecutive series of 16 patients with symmetrical marked overaction of the inferior oblique; one technique (denervation and extirpation) performed on the right eye, and the other 14 mm recession) on the left. Mean duration of followup was 20.8 months (range 17 to 34 months). Denervation and extirpation resulted in 100% normal action, without residual overaction or underaction. Recession, however, resulted in mild to moderate residual overaction in 75% of patients and marked overaction requiring reoperation in 13%. It appears that denervation and extirpation of the inferior oblique is far superior to 14 mm recession for treatment of marked overaction of the inferior oblique.

INTRODUCTION

There continues to be some controversy concerning the ideal technique for weakening the markedly overaction inferior oblique muscle. Parks,(1,2) Dyer,(3) and Dyer and Duke(4) have nicely reviewed the development of inferior oblique weakening procedures from the historical perspective. In summary, the inferior oblique can be weakened by (1) disinseration at origin or insertion, (2) myectomy at origin or insertion, (3) recession, (4) denervation, and more recently described (5) denervation and partial or total myectomy, as well as (6) myotomy. Each technique has its advocates, however, there have been few prospective, controlled studies comparing the advantages, disadvantages, and results of one technique with the others. Parks(1) demonstrated in a controlled, prospective study of 306 patients that a 10 mm recession was more effective than myectomy at insertion, myectomy at origin, or disinsertion, for eliminating inferior oblique overaction. In addition,

STRABISMUS II
ISBN 0-8089-1424-3

further study by Parks(5) in a larger series convinced him that the 14 mm recession was superior to the 10 mm recession. Gonzalez(6) first described isolated denervation of the inferior oblique as a weakening procedure. Although initial results were good, 100% recurrence of overaction was noted within 2-1/2 to 8 months with the post-operative overaction more marked than pre-operative. He later found that denervation together with either myectomy of the middle 1/3 or even the "whole muscle" was much more effective than denervation alone. There have been, however, no large studies comparing his procedure to other inferior oblique weakening procedures. This study simultaneously compares an improved procedure, denervation and extirpation of the inferior oblique, with the 14 mm recession in a prospective, consecutive series of patients with symmetrical marked overaction.

METHODS

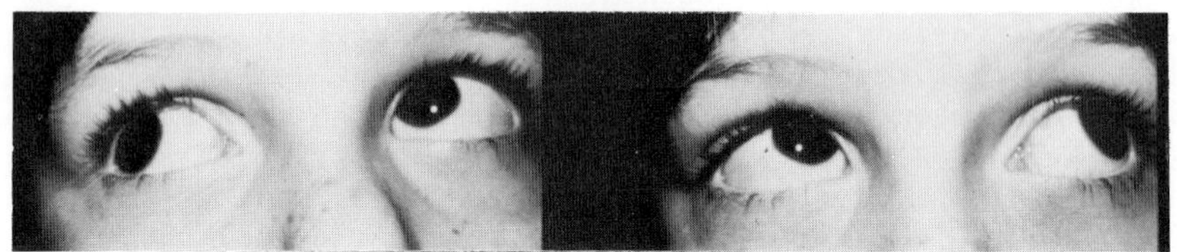

Figure 1: A six-year-old child demonstrating the typical symmetrical symmetrical marked (+4) overaction of the inferior oblique in both eyes.

Sixteen consecutive patients with symmetrical marked (+4) overaction of the inferior oblique operated on between April 18, 1979, and September 17, 1980, were entered into the study. Figure 1 shows the typical marked preoperative overaction in all our patients. In all patients, the right eye underwent extirpation and denervation while the left eye received a 14 mm recession of the inferior oblique. The mean age at diagnosis for the patients in this study was 5-2/12 years (range 1-8/12 to 11-3/12 years). The mean age at surgery was 5-5/12 years (range 1-9/12 to 11-8/12 years). Mean followup from time of initial oblique surgery was 20.8 months with a minimum of 17 months and a maximum of 34 months. Table 1 illustrates the major preoperative diagnoses of the patients in this study. Eighty-one percent had primary esotropia (50% congenital esotropia and 31% accommodative esotropia), 19% had primary overaction inferior obliques and 6% had intermittent exotropia. As illustrated in Table 2, 10/16 (62.5%) of the patients underwent separate inferior oblique surgery while the remaining 37.5% had their inferior oblique surgery combined with horizontal rectus surgery. Only those patients having had symmetrical horizontal recti muscle surgery were included in the study. None were included who had vertical displacement of their horizontal recti, vertical rectus muscle surgery, superior oblique muscle surgery, or previous inferior oblique muscle surgery. All pre-operative and post-operative examinations were made by the same observer (MMP) and all surgery was performed by the same surgeon, thus insuring no variation in surgical technique. Oblique overaction was graded according to the degree of over or under elevation of the eye in adduction using a scale ranging from -2 under-elevation to +4 over-elevation.

Table 1: Associated diagnoses in the 16 patients included in this study

DIAGNOSIS

Diagnosis	No. of Patients	Percentage
Congenital Esotropia	8/16	50%
Alternating hypertropia or overacting inferior obliques	3/16	19%
Accommodative Esotropia	5/16	31%
Intermittent Exotropia	1/16	6%
Monofixation	15/16	94%
Amblyopia	3/16	19%
Dissociated Vertical Deviation	2/16	13%

SURGICAL TECHNIQUE

The technique for 14 mm recession of the inferior oblique has been previously described by Parks.(7) The technique used for the denervation and extirpation operation is illustrated in Figures 2 thru 8. An 8 mm conjunctival incision is made 1 mm to 2 mm to the bulbar side of the inferotemporal cul-de-sac, arching on a course parallel to the cul-de-sac. Through the conjunctival incision, Tenon's capsule is incised perpendicualarly down to bare sclera. The lateral rectus is secured on a muscle hook, and a 4-0 black silk stay suture (Figure 2, inset) is passed beneath the muscle and secured to the drape holding the eye in a position

SURGICAL PROCEDURES

Type	No. of Patients
I. Separate inferior oblique surgery	10/16 (62.5%)
a) prior or subsequent horizontal rectus surgery	5/16 (31.2%)
b) no rectus surgery	5/16 (31.2%)
II. Combined horizontal rectus and inferior oblique surgery	6/16 (37.5%)

Table 2: Association of horizontal rectus surgery with inferior oblique surgery in the 16 patients of this study.

of elevation and adduction and giving the surgeon an inferior and temporal view around the surface of the globe through the retracted incision. The wound is held open by the assistant with a large Von Graefe hook inferiorly and a small Steven's hook temporally. With the eye held in this position, the distal portion of the inferior oblique muscle can be directly viewed and its anterior and posterior margins identified with a small Steven's hook and iris spatula (Figure 2). When the posterior margin is clearly seen and the inferotemporal vortex vein identified so it can be avoided, the inferior oblique is hooked with the Steven's hook and pulled up into the wound. A small incision is made at the tip of the hook separating the posterolaterlal margin of the muscle as identified by the sharp division between the red muscle and creamy fat within Tenon's space that is brought forward by the hood (Figure 3). Great care must be taken to separate inferior oblique muscle capsule from surrounding Tenon's capsule without entering the fat pad, which could result in an adherence syndrome. A large Green muscle hook is then placed around the muscle which is pulled up out of the wound allowing the distal muscle insertion to be completely cleared of intermusclar septum (Figure 4). The muscle is then cross-clamped with a small Harmon clamp and severed flush with the sclera at its insertion (Figure 5). The terminal portion of the muscle is then pulled up gently into the wound so that the fusiform enlargement of the muscle belly where the nerve enters becomes apparent (Figure 6). The nerve enters the muscle from the lateral border of the inferior rectus onto the superior surface of the inferior rectus at a point approximately 2/3 of the way from the nasal border and

1/3 from the temporal border of the inferior oblique at the point of fusiform enlargement. Knowing this location, the nerve and its associated vascular plexus can be gently isolated with a Steven's muscle hook as seen in Figure 6. A second small Steven's hook is then placed around the nerve to further isolate it and allow transection between the two hooks very carefully with electrocautery (Figure 6, inset). Great care must be taken to adequately cauterize the vascular plexus around the nerve, as significant bleeding can occur from this site. After transection of the nerve, the distal muscle prolapses 30% to 50% further into the wound allowing easy visualization of the site where its muscle capsule penetrates through Tenon's capsule (Figure 7). A 4-0 chromic ligature is placed around the muscle and tied tightly after being pushed as far proximally as possible to the site where the muscle penetrates Tenon's capsule (Figure 7). All muscle distal to the ligature is transected with hot cautery and removed. The small remaining cauterized stump is forced with the blunt end of a small muscle hook out through its sleeve of Tenon's capsule away from the globe. Finally, Tenon's capsule is closed with several interrupted sutures of 6-0 vicryl to completely isolate it from the globe and prevent any chance of its reattachment to the sclera, lower lid, or the proximal portion of its nerve (Figure 8). Conjunctiva and Tenon's capsule at the inferotemporal fornix incision are then massaged gently together closing the fornix incision, generally, without the need for sutures.

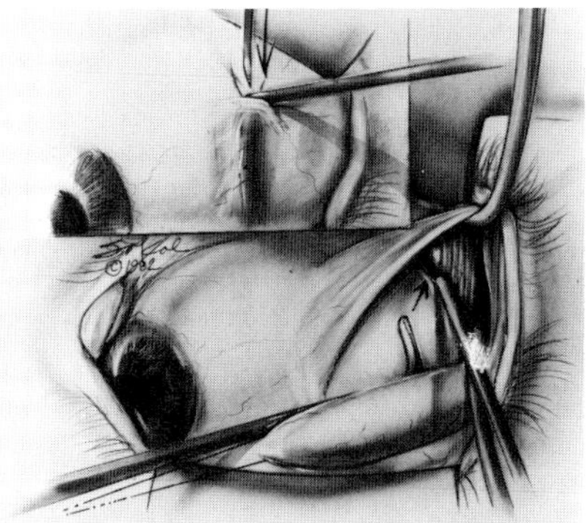

Figure 2. With the eye held in adduction and elevation by a 4-0 silk suture placed beneath the lateral rectus (inset) and clamped across the bridge of the nose, the inferior oblique is identified with a Steven's hook and iris spatula.

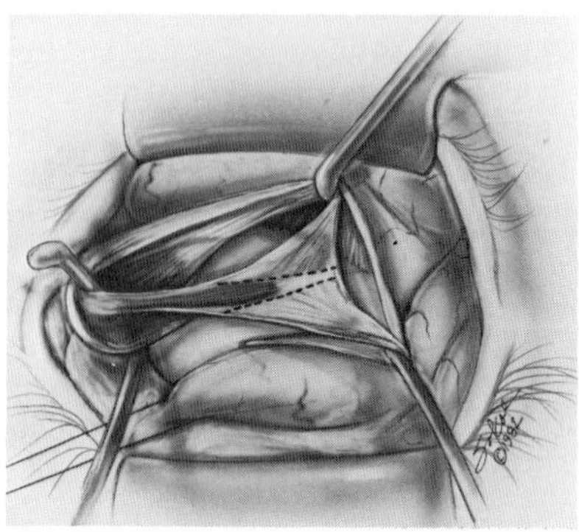

Figure 3. After direct visualization of its anterior and posterior borders, the inferior oblique is hooked with the small Steven's hook and pulled up into the wound. A small incision at the tip of the hook frees posterior tenons.

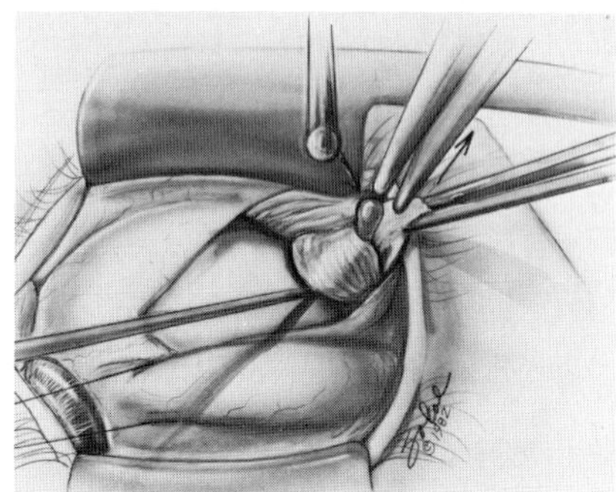

Figure 4. The entire inferior oblique insertion is exposed and the intermuscular septum removed along dotted lines above.

Table 3 shows the early postoperative results four to six weeks following denervation and extirpation as well as 14 mm recession. Extirpation resulted in significant underaction in four of the sixteen eyes (26%), normal oblique action in 11 or 16 eyes (68%), and slight overaction in one of 16 eyes (6%). Fourteen millimeters recessions resulted in significantly less weakening with no underactions, 5 of 16 eyes with normal action (31%) and 11 or 16 eyes with some overaction (69%). By the 12 to 18 month followup visit, Table 4, nearly all of the underaction associated with extirpation had disappeared, resulting in 15 of 16 eyes

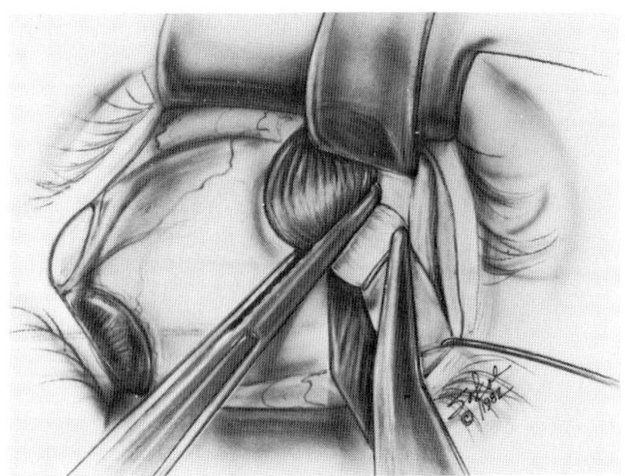

Figure 5. The insertion is cross-clamped with a Hartman clamp and excised from the sclera.

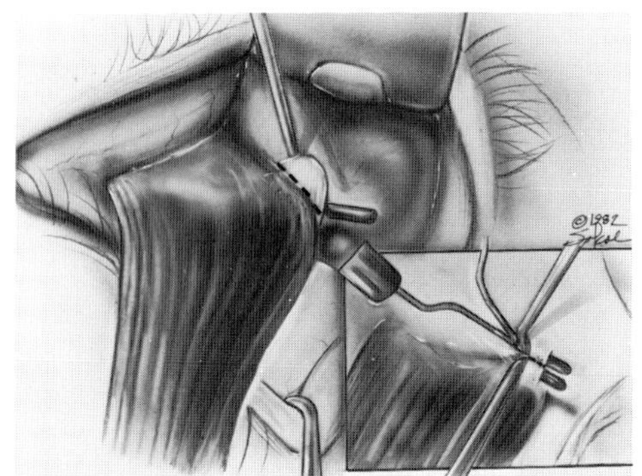

Figure 6. With the free distal muscle end lifted gently out of the wound, the nerve is identified (see text) and secured on two Steven's hooks for transection with hot cautery (inset).

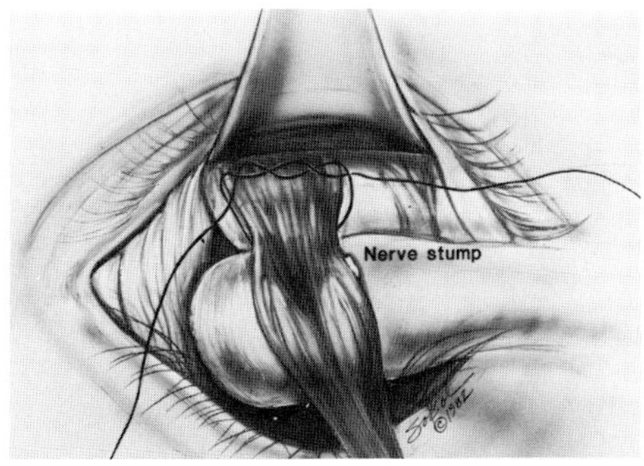

Figure 7. A 4-0 chromic ligature is secured tightly around the muscle as near its penetration through Tenon's capsule as possible in preparation for removing the distal muscle with hot cautery.

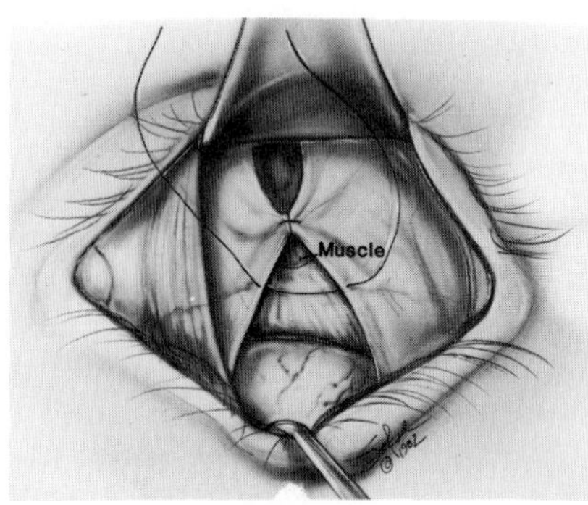

Figure 8. The tiny residual muscle stump is forced outside Tenon's capsule and the capsule is closed over it with interrupted 6-0 vicryl.

INFERIOR OBLIQUE ACTION

4-6 week follow-up

	-2	-1	0	+1	+2 (reoperation)	+3	+4
Rt inferior oblique (Extirpation)	2/16 (13%)	2/16 (13%)	11/16 (68%)	1/16 (6%)			
Lt inferior oblique (14mm recession)			5/16 (31%)	7/16 (44%)	4/16 (25%)		

Table 3: The inferior oblique action assessed in adduction and elevation at four to six weeks following surgery. Scale: -4 underaction to 0 normal to +4 overaction

graded as normal inferior oblique action. Those eyes that had undergone 14 mm recession, however, demonstrated significant return of overaction during this period. Only 4 of 16 eyes (25%) were graded as normal oblique action whereas 10 of 16 eyes had returned to slight to moderate overaction, 1 of 16 to moderate to severe overaction and 1 of 16 to marked (+4) overaction which necessiated reoperation, at which time denervation and extirpation was performed. This second procedure was curative in this patient with symmetrical, normal inferior oblique action which has persisted now for nearly twelve months.

INFERIOR OBLIQUE ACTION

12-18 month follow-up

	-2	-1	0	+1	+2	(reoperation) +3	+4
Rt inferior oblique (Extirpation)		1/16 (6%)	15/16 (94%)				
Lt inferior oblique (14mm recession)			4/16 (25%)	4/16 (25%)	6/16 (38%)	1/16 (6%)	1/16 (6%)

Table 4: The inferior oblique action assessed in adduction and elevation at 12-18 months following surgery. Scale: -4 underaction to 0 normal to +4 overaction

FINAL INFERIOR OBLIQUE ACTION

	-2	-1	0	+1	+2	+3	(reoperation) +4
Rt inferior oblique (Extirpation)			16/16 (100%)				
Lt inferior oblique (Recession)			2/16 (12%)	6/16 (38%)	6/16 (38%)		2/16 (12%)

Table 5: The inferior oblique action assessed in adduction and elevation at the final follow-up visit (17 - 34 months following surgery). Scale: -4 underaction to 0 normal to +4 overaction

Table 5 shows the final inferior oblique action measured in each patient at the most recent office visit from 17 to 34 months postoperatively (mean 20.8 months). At this last visit, all inferior oblique underaction had disappeared from the extirpated eyes resulting in 100% graded as normal action. On the other hand, only 2 of 16 (12%) of eyes undergoing 14 mm recession were graded as having normal inferior oblique action at the end of the followup period. Twelve of 16 eyes (76%) showed a return of slight to moderate overaction and 2 eyes (12%) had returned to marked overaction requiring re-operation with subsequent denervation and extirpation. Both of these eyes now demonstrate relatively normal, symmetrical inferior oblique action after a followup period of 6 to 11 months.

Operative time and simplicity are comparable for both denervation with extirpation and 14 mm recession. There were no significant early complications in any of the patients. Late complications were limited to one patient with mild hypotropia (less than 5 prism diopters) in the right eye which had undergone denervation with extirpation as compared to the eye which had undergone a 14 mm recession. This hypotropia appeared to be resolving slowly at the last office visit, 22 months postoperatively.

DISCUSSION

It is disconcerting to perform any strabismus operation only to have the original abnormality recur in a short time. There is probably no strabismus operation that has been plagued by this problem more than the marked overaction of the inferior obliques. Although many surgical procedures have been proposed, each with its strong supports, no concensus has developed to date as to the best surgical approach. The study by Parks(1) was the largest case-controlled, prospective study comparing several of the major operative techniques performed by one surgeon on the same patients. In this study the 10 mm recession operation was the most effective and predictable surgical approach for eliminating overaction of the inferior oblique. Further studies in his patients have demonstrated the slightly large 14 mm recession operation to be superior to the 10 mm recession. However, even with this procedure there was a small but significant recurrence of overaction.

In 1973, Gonzalez(6) presented 15 patients who underwent pure denervation of the inferior oblique alone for treatment of marked overaction. An additional three patients had denervation and total myectomy and two had denervation plus myectomy of the middle 1/3 of the muscle. Although all three techniques were initially successful, later elegant studies by Gonzalez(8,9) demonstrated that reinnervation of the nerve to the inferior oblique occurred in all patients treated with denervation alone with 2-1/2 to 8 months. Even removing a segment of distal nerve, surrounding the middle 1/3 of the muscle with Supramid Extra and the use of hemoclips on the cut proximal and distal nerve stumps to act as a surgical barrier, proved ineffective. His studies did indicate, however, that the addition of "total myectomy" as well as myectomy of the middle 1/3 of the muscle, when associated with denervation, were effective in long term elimination of marked overaction of the inferior oblique.

We felt that a prospective case-controlled study comparing denervation and extirpation of a large portion of the inferior oblique muscle to the favored 14 mm recession operation was important in establishing the optimal technique. This study reports such a comparison between the technique developed by one of us (MMP) for denervation with extirpation of the entire sub-Tenon's portion of the inferior oblique muscle and the 14 mm recession operation. As demonstrated above, denervation with extirpation proved to be significantly more effective than recession for marked overaction. The technique as described is simple, and no more time consuming than the recession operation. Its other advantages over previously described techniques include access to the muscle entirely within the sub-Tenon's space, thereby avoiding significant hemorrhage as well as invasion of the orbital fat pad. No loose distal muscle stump is left attached to sclera which may reattach to the lower lid or some other intraorbital site, thereby either restricting movement of the globe or producing actual secondary deviation. All steps are performed under excellent direct vision of all anatomical structures, thereby preventing "blind sweeping" with possible damage to the orbital fat pad or inferotemporal vortex vein. The procedure allows gentle, direct access to the nerve to the inferior oblique without significant tugging. This may prevent damage to the proximal nerve and ganglia which results in internal ophthalmoplegia as reported by Bajart and Robb.(10) In addition, we feel that by isolating the small proximal muscle stump outside Tenon's capsule, any possible chance of either reattachment to sclera or other significant periocular structure, or of regrowth or reinnervation of the small residual muscle stump, will be prevented.

In summary, we have presented a simple technique developed for denervation with extirpation of the inferior oblique which proved more effective than the previously preferred procedure (14 mm recession) for treatment of marked overaction of the inferior oblique. No significant complications were encountered with this new technique; therefore, it has become our procedure of choice for marked overaction. Current studies are in progress to determine whether it is equally effective and complication-free in patients with less marked overaction of the inferior oblique.

REFERENCES

1. Parks MM. The weakening surgical procedures for eliminating overaction of the inferior oblique muscle. Am J Ophthalmol 73:107-122, 1972.

2. Parks MM: The overacting inferior oblique muscle. Am J Ophthalmol 77:787-797, 1974.

3. Dyer JA: Tenotomy of the inferior oblique muscle at its scleral insertion. Arch Ophthalmol 68:176-181, 1962.

4. Dyer JA, Duke DG: Inferior oblique weakening procedures. In: Little F (ed). Internat Ophthalmol Clinics 16(3): Strabismus Surgery. Boston, Little, Brown and Co., 1976, pp 103-113.

5. Parks MM: personal communication.

6. Gonzalez C: Denervation of the inferior oblique (as a weakening surgical procedure). Trans Amer Acad Ophthalmol Otolaryngol 78:816-823, 1974.

7. Parks MM: Inferior oblique muscle surgery. In: Parks MM (ed): Atlas of Strabismus Surgery. Philadelphia: Harper and Row Publishers, 1982, pp 182-183.

8. Gonzalez C: Denervation of the inferior oblique: Current status and long-term results. Trans Amer Acad Ophthalmol Otolaryngol 81:899-906, 1976.

9. Gonzalez C: Reinnervation of the nerve to the inferior oblique after iatrogenic denervation. J Ped Ophthalmol and Strab 18:21-24, 1981.

10. Bajart AM, Robb RM: Internal ophthalmoplegia following inferior oblique myectomy: A report of three cases. Ophthalmology 86:1401-1406, 1979.

DISCUSSION BY R. A. CRONE

Delmonte and Parks demonstrated that denervation and exstirpation of the inferior oblique is more efficient than a large recession. Their data are convincing but it should be stressed that the procedure is radical and hypotropia after a longer period of observation is not impossible. In my view the procedure should be limited to cases of suppression. In cases of diplopia I would prefer a procedure which can be undone in case of overcorrection.

MUSCLE IMBALANCE IN RETINOBLASTOMA: A STUDY OF 104 PATIENTS

U. M. Carbajal and T. Sison-Diego

ABSTRACT

In this study, 104 children were brought in for consultation primarily because of the presence of a peculiar eye reflex in one or both eyes. Muscle imbalance was observed and recorded by the examining ophthalmologists and occasionally by the parents. In fact, a six-year old Caucasian girl with bilateral retinoblastoma was brought to the senior author for muscle correction.

The type of muscle imbalance is classified in each patient. Of the 104 patients, there was gross muscle imbalance in only 25 patients (as gathered from the hospital records in Childrens Hospital in Los Angeles and in the Manila Sanitarium & Hospital in the Philippines as well as in my own files). Esotropia was observed in 8; exotropia in 11 but in 6 patients, the type of muscle imbalance was not indicated in the records.

An attempt is also made to see the relationship of the type of muscle imbalance to that of bilaterality of disease; type of muscle disparity to that of size or extent of macular involvement; type of muscle imbalance to that of age of onset and duration of the disease.

The authors conclude that in all cases of muscle imbalance among young children a dilatated study of the fundus using indirect ophthalmoscopy should be done to rule out retinoblastoma.

STRABISMUS II
ISBN 0-8089-1424-3

DISCUSSION BY R. A. CRONE

Dr. Carbajal and Sison-Diego reported on strabismus and nystagmus in retinoblastoma. They remind us of the ancient truth that every case of strabismus should be referred to an ophthalmologist without delay. Since only posterior pole tumors can cause ordinary-looking convergent strabismus, a perfunctory inspection of the posterior poles is enough. With dilated pupils and indirect ophthalmoscopy a quick inspection during just a few seconds is possible. I have never felt the need for general anesthesia.

THE FACTORS DETERMINING THE SURGICAL STRATEGY FOR STRABISMUS

A. Roth, A. B. Safran, and B. Rapp

ABSTRACT

Measurements of the strabismus angle give values for the deviation which depend on the conditions of examination. The extent of the surgery must be based on the minimal and maximal values of the deviation or, in other words, on the minimal value and the variability. The eye showing the greater motor disturbance must also be determined.

The position of the eyes under general anesthesia, which is deep and stable, and the tests of muscular elongation measuring the extensibility of each muscle on which to be operated, furnish further significant information. Correctly interpretated, these data determine several adjustments of the surgical plan.

Finally, the manner in which the operation is performed may in itself influence the amount of surgery. The various factors involved in this, can, however, be standardized so as to reduce the variability of the results.

INTRODUCTION

In the last ten years, the range of surgical solutions for the correction of strabismus has expanded. Surgeons can choose the procedures that are best adapted to the motor dysfunction to be corrected, basing their choice not only on the clinical examination, but also on the position of the eyes under anesthesia and the degree of muscular extensibility.

METHODS

The Clinical Steps

The clinical sensorimotor evaluation remains the first and most important step in the preparation of the operatory plan. Four essential questions must be answered:

STRABISMUS II
ISBN 0-8089-1424-3

1. What are the values for the minimum angle in the case of esotropia or the maximum angle in the case of exotropia, i.e. what are the values reflecting the degree of dystonia which must be corrected by the classical surgery of recession and resection?

2. In the case of esotropia, is there a difference between the minimum and the maximum of the strabismic angle, and/or a variability of the angle in the course of the version movements, i.e., a dyskinesia justifying a Cuppers posterior fixation suture?

3. Is there, in addition, a vertical and/or and alphabetical incomitance justifying appropriate surgery on the oblique muscles or the horizontal recti?

4. Which eye deviates most when the other eye fixes, i.e., which is the side in which the motor dysfunction probably predominates and should be operated preferentially?

The answers to these question define the surgical plan and the calculation of the extent of surgery necessary.(11) The preoperatory data are important, however, as established by the Eye Clinic of Nantes(4-6) which has systematically classified them with regard to position of the eyes under anesthesia and degree of muscular elongation. By means of these data, it is possible to determine with a greater degree of certainty, the extent to which the strabismic deviation is of innervational or musculo-aponeurotic origin and the muscle or muscles in which the motor dysfunction is principally located. The surgical plan can then be modified accordingly.

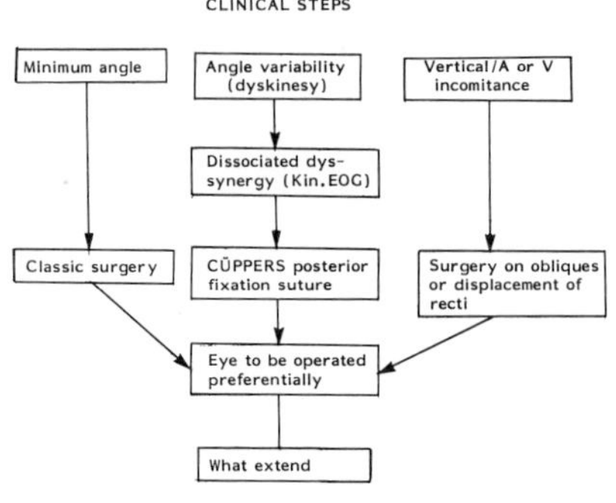

Figure 1

The Position of the Eyes Under Anesthesia

Deep stabilized general anesthesia necessary for surgery on oculo-motor muscles reduces by about 75% the innervational influx to the striated muscles. Because of this reduction, the musculo-aponeurotic equilibrium (or dysequilibrium) which depends on the visco-elasticity of the muscles and their sheaths will predominate over the equilibrium of innervational origin . (In normal patients the eye position is slightly divergent under anesthesia.) The position of the eyes thus reveals the state of musculo-aponeurotic equilibrium between the lateral and medial recti (and possibly also among the vertical-acting muscles) for each eye.

The eye with the greater deivation, whether it is the dominant or the non-dominant eye, is usually the same regardless of whether the patient is under anesthesia or conscious. Sometimes, however, this is not the case, possibly for the following reason: the horizontal muscle needed for fixation must make a greater effort in the disturbed eye; this increased effort could, by the mechanism of Hering's law, cause hyperactivity of the agonist muscle of the opposite eye, which would increase the strabismic angle. The position of the eyes under anesthesia would then be determinant and the eye most deviated under anesthesia would be chosen for surgery.

In the case of esotropia, a decrease of the strabismic anbgle under anesthesia would indicate that the ocular-motor dysfunction is mainly due to innervational hypertonia of the medial rectus as compared to the lateral rectus. Resection of the lateral rectus, which would compensate for the excessive innervational tonus of the medial rectus, is essential, even if, depending on the minimum strabismic angle value, a recession of the medial rectus should also prove necessary. If, in addition, there is evidence of clinical dyskinesia, associated with the decreased strabismic angle, a posterior fixation suture is especially indicated. Conversely, if the strabismic angle remains unchanged under anesthesia, the recession of the medial rectus, reducing the effect of its musculo-aponeurotic hypertonia as compared with that of the lateral rectus, assumes greater importance than the resection of the lateral rectus.

Similarly, in the case of exotropia, a decrease of the strabismic angle under anesthesia indicates innervational hypertonia of the lateral rectus as compared to the medial rectus. Recession of the lateral rectus, to compensate for the insufficient innervational tonus of the medial rectus, is essential. Conversely, if the strabismic angle remains unchanged under anesthesia, the resection of the medial rectus, reducing the effect of its musculo-aponeurotic hypotonia as compared with the lateral rectus, becomes more important than recession of the lateral rectus.

It is thus possible to assume that, in general, regardless of the type of strabismus involved, if under general anesthesia, the angle is decreased or even reversed, it is necessary to operate more on the lateral rectus and less on the medial rectus. Conversely, if the angle remains unchanged or increases, it is necessary to operate more on the medial rectus and less on the lateral rectus. In the case of further surgery, however, it is essential that what has been done previously be taken into account.

The position of the eyes under anesthesia can thus provide an accurate indication of the eye to be operated preferentially and the proportions of surgery to be performed on the medial and lateral recti.

Muscle Elongation Test (MET)

The variability of the degree of muscular extensibility is common knowledge among ophthalmologists. Muscular extensibility is an index of visco-elastic forces; it is an

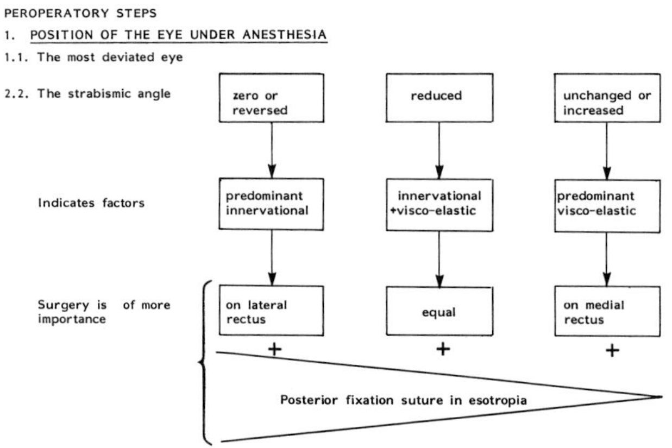

Figure 2

inverse function of the resistance to extension that is normally compensated for by the action of the antagonist muscle.(2) For Quere et al,(5,6) the measurement of muscular extensibility has become a routine operative test for which they have proposed the term "Muscle Elongation Test" in order to distinguish it from the Passive Duction or Traction Test.

If a purely manual evaluation of the visco-elastic force is considered insufficient and if there is no possibility of determining the length/tension curves for active and passive forces according to Collins et al,(1) one of the following two methods could be used: (1) measurement (in mm) of the elongation for a given tension (50-60 gr, isotonic method), or, (2) measurement of the force required to obtain a given elongation (e.g., 10 mm, isometric method, which we used on the isolated muscle, before disinsertion.(7-10) A reference marker (e.g., the tip of closed forceps, a muscle hook or a graduated blepharostat) was placed in contact with the center of the cornea with the eye held in primary position; the muscular insertion was then pulled, at a traction force of 50-60 gr, toward the marker which was held perfectly immobile, thus causing the ocular globe to turn. The traction was effected by means of a spring myodynamometer (derived from an instrument developed by H. Kaufmann, Giessen, W-Germany) with a strabismus hook at the end which was passed under the muscular insertion.

If the insertion can be brought into direct contact with the reference marker or one mm beyond, extensibility can be considered normal; the elongation distance is thus somewhat variable depending on the rectus muscles tested, since the average distance from the insertion ot the limbus is different for each of them. If the insertion cannot be brought into contact with the marker, the extensibility must be considered decreased; if the insertion can be pulled to a point more than 1 mm beyond the marker, the extensibility must be considered increased.

The results were expressed not in terms of the elongation distance, but rather in terms of the difference between the measured distance and the normal, i.e., the distance in mm separating the final position of the insertion from the position of the marker; thus the normal range of extensibility would be between 0 and 1 mm, decreased extensibility would be expressed by negative values, while increased extensibility would be expressed by positive values above 1. This manner of expressing the results is more striking and facilitates the calculation of the adjustment of the extent of surgery required. If a graduated blepharostat has been used as the marker, it will, in most cases, be possible to get a direct reading of the elongation distance.(3)

The MET values shown in Table 1 were obtained from a series of cases of unselected concomitant strabismuc during the first semester of 1982 at the Clinic of Ophthalmology of Geneva. The results, which relate to 74 muscles, show frequent decreased extensibility (11 out of 17) in cases of exotropia of the lateral rectus, and of the medial rectus (12 out of 20) in cases of esotropia. On the other hand, they show increased extensibility of the medial rectus (5 out of 13) in cases of exotropia and occasionally increased extensibility of the lateral rectus (4 out of 23) in cases of esotropia. In a pair of antagonists such as medial and lateral recti, the elongation distance can be abnormal for either only or for both muscles. When both muscles are involved, the abnornality can be greater for one than for the other or can be of the same magnitude for both (but in opposite directions). It should be noted, however, that occasionally, extensibility is abnormal in a direction that is opposite from what would be expected for the type of strabismus involved, e.g., reduced extensibility for the lateral rectus and/or increased extensibility for the medial rectus in cases of esotropia; similarly, paradoxical extensibility values have since been found for cases of exotropia.

Extensibility mm		Reduced		Normal	Increased		Average
		-3 to -6	-1 to -2	0 to +1	+2 to +4	≥+5	
Exotropia	Lateral recti (17 muscles)	4	7	6			-1,29
N = 19	Medial recti (13 muscles)			8	4	1	+1,71
Esotropia	Lateral recti (23 muscles)		4	15	4		+0,35
N = 26	Medial recti (21 muscles)	1	11	8	1		-0,69

Table 1 : Results of the MET (74 muscles) in cases of exotropia (19 cases) and of esotropia (26 cases).

TABLE 1

It is important that the variability of muscular extensibility be taken into account, no so much for determining the extent of the surgery but rather for adjusting it. It is obvious that for a given extent of surgery, the operatory effects would be different depending on the visco-elastic tonus of the muscle or muscles involved; i.e., greater for muscles with decreased extensibility and lesser for those with increased extensibility. Thus, when extensibility is normal, recession and resection are determined according to the usual accepted values. In cases of increased extensibility, these values must be proportionally increased. (For increased extensibility of from 2 mm to 4 mm, 2/3 of this increase must be added for increased extensibility in the range of 5 mm or more, 1/2 of the increased must be added.) In cases of reduced extensibility, these values must be decreased. (For decreased extensibility of from -1 to -2, 0.5 mm to 1 mm should be substracted; for reduction of extensibility that is greater than this, 2 mm should be subtracted.

It is also possible and sometimes advantageous, in cases of combined surgery, rather than reduce the extent of surgery on the muscle with reduced extensibility, to make the adjustment by reducing the extent of surgery on the antagonist; this is particularly indicated in cases where the extensibility of the latter is close to normal.

Experience with the MET indicates the importance of being wary of paradoxical abnormalities of extensibility which lead to resection of a muscle with decreased extensibility or recession of a muscle with increased extensibility; in the latter case in particular, the risk of overcorrection, either immediate or delayed, and the risk of limitation of motility in the direction of the recessed muscle and increased.

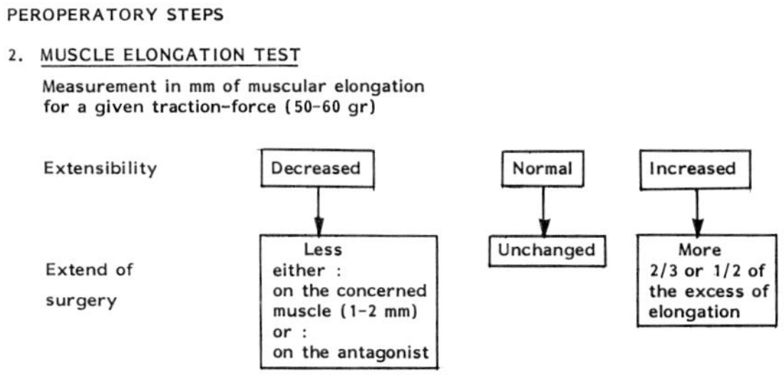

PEROPERATORY STEPS

2. MUSCLE ELONGATION TEST

Measurement in mm of muscular elongation
for a given traction-force (50-60 gr)

Extensibility	Decreased	Normal	Increased
Extend of surgery	Less either : on the concerned muscle (1-2 mm) or : on the antagonist	Unchanged	More 2/3 or 1/2 of the excess of elongation

Figure 3

Surgery

It is evident that the operatory result will depend to a great extent on the precision of the surgery itself. The use of magnifying optics, either microscope or glasses, is imperative. It is also essential to verify the precision of the measurement instruments. Finally, the variability of the operatory result can be minimized by precise definition and verification of the following factors: (1) the manner in which the muscles are separated, (2) the reference points chosen on the sclera (3) the degree of traction on the muscle being measured, (4) the position of the sutures placed in the muscle and (5) the tightness of the knots.

The use of this surgical strategy over a five-year period has made it possible to achieve more uniform and more lasting operatory results.

ACKNOWLEDGEMENTS

We are deeply indebted to Mrs. E. Gadelle-Barbier and Miss C. Tournier (Besancon), Mrs. F. Huguenin and Miss L. Bianchi (Geneva) for their collaboration in the orthoptic examination of the patients and to Mrs. Judith Noebels for her collaboration in the preparation of the English version of this paper.

REFERENCES

1. Collins CC, Jampolsky A: Objective calculation of strabismus surgery. In: Lennerstand G, et al (eds): Functional Basis of Ocular Motility Disorders. 1981, Pergamon Press, pp. 185-194.

2. Esslen E, Esslen D, Huber A: Elektromyographische innervationalyse des strabismus concomitans. Ueber die beim strabismus concomitans wirksamen muskelkrafte. Ophthalmologica 154:189-200, 1967.

3. Paliaga GP: Intraoperatory strabometry. Europ Symp on Strabismus, 1982 (in press).

4. Quere MA, Pechereau A, Clergeau G: La nouvelle chirurgie des esotropies fonctionnelles. I. Analyse des phenomenes mecaniques induits par les actions musculaires chirurgicales. II. Les dereglements moteurs fondamentaux et leur cure chirurgicale. III. Conclusions pratiques et plan operatoire. J Fr Ophthalmol 1:5-60, 151-162, 221-228, 1978.

5. Quere MA, Pechereau A, Clergeau G: The muscle elongation test in functional squints: History, basis and clinical features. Ophthalmolgica 182:81-89, 1981.

6. Quere MA, Pechereau A, Lavenant F: The muscle elongation test in functional esotropias: Statistical survey of 211 cases. Ophthalmologica 182:90-95, 1981.

7. Roth A, Montard M: Le test d'elongation musculaire sans desinsertion dans la chirurgie du strabisme. Bull Soc Ophthalmol Fr 81:707-709, 1981.

8. Roth A, Montard M, Gadelle-Barbier E, Tournier C: Approche d'une chirurgie differenciee du strabisme divergent primitif. Bull Mem Soc Fr Ophthalmol 93:224-229, 1981.

9. Roth A, Safran AB, Le niveau de precision dans la chirurgie des strabismes. Bull Mem Soc Fr Ophthalmol 94, 1982 (in press).

10. Roth A, Rapp B, Ilic J: La mesure et la signification de l'extensibilitie musculaire au cours de la chirurgie du strabisme. Klin Mbl Augenheilk 182:369-372, 1983.

11. Russman W: Microcomputer use in planning strabismus surgery. Europ Symp on Strabismus, 1982 (in press).

THE POSTERIOR FIXATION SUTURE FOR ABNORMAL DISTANCE/NEAR RELATIONSHIP ESOTROPIA

J. D. Reynolds and D. A. Hiles

ABSTRACT

A retrospective review of 34 consecutive patients with abnormal distance/near relationship or high accomodative convergence/accomodation (AC/A) esotropia treated with a posterior fixation suture operation was conducted. The surgery was combined with medial rectus muscle recessions or unilateral recess/resect operations. The indications for placement of the posterior fixation suture were an esotropia in a patient with a near measurement at least ten prism diopters (PD) greater than the distance deviation and failure of optical control. The patients were grouped according to the size of the abnormal distance/near ratio preoperatively. The patients achieved a mean reduction in the AC/A ratio of 13 PD. A normalization of the abnormal ratio occurred in 24 (70%) of patients. Eleven (85%) of the 13 bifocal wearing patients were able to discard their bifocals postoperatively. There was no difference in the success of the surgery when analyzed according to the type of distance refractive error or the presence or absence of amblyopia. There was a difference in the success rate among the surgical subgroups of the type of esotropia surgery aimed at the distance deviation. The greatest success was in the bilateral medial rectus muscle recessions combined with bilateral posterior fixation surgery and in the re-recessions of a single previously recessed medial rectus muscle and the placement of a posterior fixation suture combined with lateral rectus muscle resection.

The posterior fixation suture (fadenoperation) was first described by Cuppers in 1976.(1) The operation has been employed to correct esodeviations which include patients with abnormal distance/near relationships or high AC/A ratios.(1-5) It is the purpose of this paper to review a series of patients and to analyze the results obtained following the use of the posterior fixation suture in conjunction with esotropia surgery.

STRABISMUS II
ISBN 0-8089-1424-3

MATERIALS AND METHODS

The records of 34 consecutive patients with abnormal distance/near relationships treated between 1979 and 1981 with a posterior fixation suture operation were retrospectively reviewed. The surgery was combined with medial rectus muscle recessions or unilateral recess/resect operations through an inferior cul-de-sac approach. The posterior fixation suture was placed on the sclera 13-16 mm posterior to the medial rectus insertion.(1-3) We excluded cases of nystagmus blockage syndrome or patients with paretic components. The indication for placement of the posterior fixation suture was an esotropia measuring at least ten PD more at near than the distance esodeviation and not controlled with glasses including bifocals. The ages of the patients ranged from 2.5 years to 20 years with a mean of 11 years. The followup time ranged from two to 18 months with a mean of four months.

RESULTS

Preoperatively the patients were grouped according to the differences in the esotropic angle size between distance and near with accommodation controlled by the use of accommodative targets. Five (15%) patients had 30 PD or greater differences, 10 (29%) patients had 20-29 PD, and 19 (56%) patients had 10-19 PD. Sixteen (47%) patients had previous esotropia surgery and four of these patients also had inferior oblique muscle recessions. One patient had a Knapp procedure for a double elevator palsy.

Preoperatively 13 (25%) patients were wearing bifocals in an attempt to equalize the abnormal distance/near relationship.

Twelve (36%) patients had unilateral recess/resect operations for esotropia combined with a posterior fixation suture on the medial rectus. Nine (25%) patients had a re-recession of a previously recessed medial rectus muscle plus the placement of the posterior fixation suture combined with a resection of the lateral rectus. Nine (26%) patients had bilateral recessions of the medial recti combined with bilateral posterior fixation sutures and four (12%) patients had a re-recession of a previously recessed medial rectus muscle combined with a posterior fixation suture (Table 1).

Table I

Type of surgery vs. post operative result

	No.	%	D/N reduction (PD)	% Normalized
R&R	12	36	10	58
Re Rec MR & RES	9	26	15	89
MROU	9	26	17	78
Re Rec MR	4	12	8	50
Total	34	100	13	70

Postoperatively, the patients having a bilateral recession of the medial rectus muscles realized a mean reduction in the abnormal distance/near relationship of 17 PD and 78% were normalized to within 10 PD of the distance deviation. Patients with a recess/resect operation had a mean reduction of 10 PD and 58% were normalized to within 10 PD of the distance measurement. Of those patients undergoing a re-recession of the medical rectus combined with a resection of the lateral rectus, the mean reduction of the esodeviation was 15 Pd and 89% of these patients normalized their distance/near relationship. Four patients had a re-recession of the medial rectus combined with a posterior fixation suture and the mean reduction of the deviation was 8 PD and 50% normalized their AC/A ratios.

Postoperatively, 29 (85%) patients improved their abnormal distance/near relationship, with 24 (70%) normalizing their abnormal distance/near relationship. Six (18%) patients decreased by 21-30 PD, 12 (35%) patients decreased by 11-20 PD and 16 (47%) patients decreased 0-10 PD. The mean reduction in the distance/near relationship was 13 PD. Eleven (85%) of the 13 bifocal wearing patients were able to discard their bifocals postoperatively.

The distance sperical equivalent of the 34 patients revealed that eight eyes were emmetropic, 38 were hypermetropic, 20 were myopic and two patients were unilateral aphakes. The mean spherical equivalent of the hypermetropic eyes were +2.13 diopters and the mean for the myopic group was -3.00 diopters. The four emmetropic patients had a mean reduction in their distance/near ratio of six PD with one (25%) normalizing his ratio. The 19 hyperopic patients had a mean reduction in their ratio of 14 PD with 13 (70%) normalizing their ratio. The 11 myopic patients obtained a mean reduction in their ratio of 14 P.D. with nine (82%) patients achieving a normaliziation of their abnormal ratio.

Seven (21%) patients were amblyopic at the time of the posterior fixation suture operation. Four of these had associated ocular disease: two were unilaterally aphakic, one had toxoplasmic macular scars and one was brain damaged. These patients achieved a mean reduction in their abnormal ratios of 20 PD with six (86%) achieving a normalization of their abnormal ratio.

DISCUSSION

One of the more difficult problems facing the strabismologist is that of patients who have abnormal distance/near relationships. This includes patients who have poorly controlled near esodeviations with hypermetropic lenses, bifocals or miotics. Older patients frequently no longer require distance correction for visual acuity or ocular alignment and discard their glasses but remain with an esodeviation in the near range. The posterior fixation suture affords an additional parameter for the correction of this type of esodeviation in many of these patients.

The posterior fixation suture weakens a muscle in its field of gaze without affecting its action in the primary position by creating a new functional insertion 12 to 16 mm posterior to the original insertion site.(3,6) This principle may be applied to patients with abnormal distance/near relationships. The distance measurement represents the primary position deviation and the near measurement corresponds to the deviation in the field of action of the medial recti; hence, placement of a posterior fixation suture would theoretically alter the near measurement and not the distance measurement. The distance esotropia angle, when present, is corrected by medial rectus muscle recession or recess/resect operations. We have found, as have others,(3-4) that this theoretic effect of the posterior fixation sutures does occur and reduces the abnormal distance/near relationship. We achieved this result in 85% of our patients.

The success of this operation should be judged on the rate of normalization of the abnormal distance/near relationship, that is, the reduction of the near esodeviation to within 10 P.D. of the distance esodeviation. Normalization occurred in 24 (70%) of our patients when measured without a bifocal. We feel that this rate of normalization makes this a useful procedure for these diffcult patients. Additionally, we found that high ratios as well as small ones had an equal chance of normalization. That is, a patient with a distance/near measurement difference of 30 PD or more could be expected to normalize the distance/near relationship equally well as those patients with 10-20 PD differences. The size of the abnormal ratio is independent of the success or failure of the posterior fixation suture operation.

Another important criterion of success is the number of patients who are able to discard their bifocals. Eighty-five percent of patients in this series who were bifocal wearers preoperatively were able to discard them postoperatively. The patients who retained their bifocals were among the 30% who were considered not to have normalized their high AC/A ratios to an adequate degree.

The distance spherical equivalent, either hypermetropic or myopic, was independent of the success of the operation. The amblyopic patients also had a high success rate. Hence, both type of refractive error and amblyopia are independent of the success rate. No complications were noted in the series.

The authors feel that the posterior fixation suture operation is an effective addition to the treatment armanentarium for patients with abnormal distance/near relationships associated with esotropia.

ACKNOWLEDGEMENTS

This study was supported in part by grants to the Fight for Sight Children's Eye Clinic of the Eye and Ear Hospital, Pittsburg, PA, by Fight for Sight Inc., New York, NY.

REFERENCES

1. Cuppers C: The so-called "faden operation". Surgical considerations by well-defined changes of the arc of contact, in Fells P (ed): Transactions of the Second Congress International Strabismological Association. Marseilles, Diffusion General Libraire, 1976, pp. 395-400.

2. Von Noorden GK: Indications of the posterior fixation operation in strabismus. Ophthalmology 85:512-520, 1978.

3. Von Noorden GK: Posterior fixation suture in strabismus. In Transactions of the New Orleans Academy of Ophthalmology: Symposium on Strabismus. St. Louis, CV Mosby Co., 1978, pp. 307 320.

4. Spielmann A, Laulan J: Actions of recessions and resections when associated with Cuppers' Fadenoperation in esotropia. Statistical results, in Reinecke RD (ed): Strabismus. New York, Grune and Stratton, 1978, pp. 355-369.

5. Spielmann A: "L'operations du ful" de Cuppers: Princepe technique - applications. Read before the Conference de la Socete Flamande de Strabologe, Brussels, 1976.

6. Scott AB: The faden operation: Mechanical effects. Am Orthop J 27:44-47, 1977.

COMPLETE SUPERIOR AND INFERIOR RECTUS TRANSPOSITION WITH ADJUSTABLE MEDIAL RECTUS RECESSION FOR ABDUCENS PALSY

A. L. Rosenbaum, R. S. Foster, E. Ballard,
T. Rosales, P. Gruenberg, and A. Choy

ABSTRACT

Eight patients with acquired VI nerve palsy underwent transposition of the entire superior and inferior rectus muscle insertions to the lateral rectus insertions. Lateral rectus dysfunction was documented preoperatively by saccadic velocity analysis to eliminate any cases with residual significant abducting force. In the procedure the vertical recti was totally transposed, and the medial rectus (in 7) was recessed on an adjustable suture either primarily in the contralateral eye, or after at least a three-month interval as a second procedure in the ipsilateral eye. The adjustable medial rectus suture was used to maximize centration of the field of fusion, while minimizing limitation of adduction.

Binocular visual fields were used to assess the patient's pre- and postoperative diplopia-free field. Postoperatively the diplopia-free fields in abduction averaged 30 prism diopters (17 degrees), in adduction 47 prism diopters (37 degrees), for a total field of 77 prism diopters (44 degrees). Often the abduction and adduction fields of fusion were equal for the individual patient.

The results of the abduction diplopia-free fields were comparable to those reported in the Jensen procedure for monocular abduction alone. Binocular diplopia-free fields were used to follow the patients because they best characterize the patient's postoperative functional state.

It appears that the total transposition results in greater abduction diplopia-free field and therefore better centering of the patient's field of fusion.

INTRODUCTION

Following the work of Hummelschein in 1907, a variety of procedures have been described to increase muscle tone or force in the field of action of the lateral rectus muscle

STRABISMUS II
ISBN 0-8089-1424-3

following the occurrence of a VI nerve palsy.(1,3,5-7,10-12) The most popular techniques now performed in the United States are (a) partial transposition of the superior and inferior rectus muscle and (b) rectus muscle union commonly called the Jensen procedure.(6) The Jensen procedure was originally described as a technique to increase abduction tone but avoid the complication of anterior segment necrosis since the vertical rectus muscles were not disinserted. However, this complication has been reported by Von Noorden.(13)

To maximize abduction ability, we have studied the effectiveness of transposition of the entire superior and inferior rectus muscle to the lateral rectus muscle insertion in eight consecutive adult acquired VI nerve palsies. Either the ipsilateral or contralateral medial rectus muscle was recessed on an adjustable suture to provide optimum centration of the binocular visual field.

The comparison of the surgical treatment of VI nerve palsies is difficult because of the lack of diagnostically precise pre- and postoperative evaluation techniques. It is imperative to precisely quantitate the severity or density of the VI nerve palsy. The only previous study to analyze these factors is by William Scott et al on a series utilizing the Jensen procedure.(9)

Most reports have concluded that an inability to abduct the globe past the midline is evidence that the lateral rectus has little or no useful function.(1,4,6) However, the limitation of abduction may be the result of some degree of medial rectus restriction as well as compromised lateral rectus function. Recessing the medial rectus alone may relieve some of this restriction and confuse the analysis of the abduction force of any transposition procedure.

To better assess the efficacy of a transposition procedure, modern diagnostic techniques can be utilized including: (a) clinical saccadic velocity observation; (b) objective saccadic velocity measurement; (c) forced duction testing to assess medial rectus restriction; and (d) binocular visual fields to document the functional result.

Except for the Scott paper,(9) there is a total lack of data concerning the patient's binocular functional state following transposition procedures. Most surgeons have reported the results of their transposition technique by either estimating or measuring the degree of rotation in the field of action of the paralyzed muscle.(1,3,4,6,7,10-12) This type of assessment tends to exaggerate greatly the functional benefit to the patient since it stresses monocular ductional rotation with the paralyzed eye fixing.

In this situation, photos may demonstrate excellent monocular abducting ability due to excessive monocular innervation which is not present in the binocular state. This results in over-optimistic reporting and has little to do with the patient's binocular functional status.

The purpose of our study was to provide quantitative surgical information on evaluating and treating VI lesions by:

1. Differentiating partial from Total VI by saccadic velocity;

2. Performing total vertical rectus muscle transposition in order to provide the greatest active force in the field of the lateral rectus muscle;

3. Using an adjustable medial rectus muscle recession as a means of centering the binocular field; and

4. Assessing the functional result through pre- and postoperative binocular visual fields.

METHODS

Eight adults ranging in age from 17 to 63 who had bifoveal capability and good monocular visual acuity were treated. All patients were operated upon at least 6 months after the lateral rectus palsy had occurred, and after demonstrating stable deviations.

Preoperatively, lateral rectus dysfunction was documented by saccadic velocity measurements. Using EOG measurement techniques described by Metz,(9) 20 degrees horizontal saccades were generated from 30 degrees adduction to 10 degrees adduction, well out of the field of gaze limitation. The fellow eye was patched during testing. Four readings were averaged to determine mean velocity. A 40% or greater reduction in agonist to antagonist saccadic velocity was considered indicative of severely compromised lateral rectus function. In two cases the saccade was too slow to measure, but a floating saccade was observed clinically.

Binocular Goldmann visual fields were used to assess the patient's postoperative fusional range. The patient was positioned in the Goldmann perimeter and tested as decribed by Ferbel and Roper-Hall.(2,8) The patient's head was position in the Goldmann perimeter in line with the fixation target and the head strap was used to prevent any head rotation. The field was conducted with a III(e) test object, moving the test object from the central field peripherally until diplopia was reported.

Surgery consisted of a transposition of the entire superior and inferior rectus insertions to the area of the lateral rectus insertion. Either a primry contralateral medial rectus muscle recession on an adjustable suture, or a recession of the ipsilateral medial rectus muscle after a three-month interval was performed. In general, if forced duction analysis at the time of initial surgery indicated a contracted ipsilateral medial rectus muscle, it was recessed at a later date. If the medial rectus muscle was not contracted, the contralateral medial rectus muscle was recessed at the time of the transposition procedure. On the first postoperative morning, the medial rectus muscle recession was adjusted to obtain maximum centration of the binocular diplopia-free field wihout severely limiting adduction. Binocular visual field testing was performed at least three months following the last surgical procedure.

RESULTS

PATIENT	ETIOLOGY	DEVIATION 1° POSITION (Δ)	SACCADIC VELOCITY DEGREES/SEC ADD/ABD	MEDIAL RECTUS RECESSION (MM)	DIPLOPIA FREE FIELD (DEGREES)			VISUAL ACUITY		COMMENTS
					ABD	ADD	TOTAL	OD	OS	
1	CHORDOMA	50 R ET	509/109	6.5	15	45	60	20/20	20/20	RHT REQUIRED SURGERY
2	TRAUMA	40 R ET	FLOATING	6.0	15	30	45	20/25	20/20	
3	TRAUMA	50 L ET	150/50	6.0	18	35	53	--	--	
4	TRAUMA	50 L ET	FLOATING	6.5	25	20	45	20/50	20/50	
5	TRAUMA	75 L ET	177/54	7.5	15	15	30	20/20	20/25	
6	ACOUSTIC NEUROMA	30 L ET	184/77	NONE	8	30	38	20/20	20/30	PT. DECLINED MEDIAL RECTUS RECESSION
7	TRAUMA	55 R ET	230/146	6.0	18	19	37	20/25	20/25	
8	TRAUMA	30 L ET	230/120	6.5	18	20	38	20/25	20/25	

In our series of eight patients, seven underwent medial rectus muscle recession in addition to total vertical rectus muscle transposition. In these patients, the average diplopia-free field postoperatively was 17 degrees in abducton, and 27 degrees in adduction, for a total of 44 degrees of diplopia-free field. It should be emphasized that these results are in a patient group in whom severe VI paresis has been proven with saccadic velocity measurements, thereby excluding patients with any residual effective lateral rectus function.

When the primary contralateral rectus recession was performed, the average binocular field in abduction was 18 degrees. When the ipsilateral medial rectus recession was performed as a second procedure, the diplopia-free abduction ranged averaged 19 degrees.

One patient underwent transposition alone, declining later medial rectus recession as he was pleased with the results of the first procedure. One patient developed a hypertropia following the transposition which required further surgical correction.

DISCUSSION

The Jensen procedure has been the standard against which transposition procedures have been compared since 1964. This muscle union was designed to provide good abduction function without risking the complication of anterior segment necrosis.(6) However, this complication has been reported.(13)

Scott's series is the only other study to use saccadic velocity measurements to document the degree of lateral rectus muscle dysfunction, and binocular fields to assess surgical results.(9) In his series, 13 patients underwent Jensen procedures using the criteria of a 40% or greater difference between agonist and antagonist muscles as indication that the effective lateral rectus muscle force was minimal.

Three months postoperatively the total diplopia-free field averaged 34 degrees in his series, while our population averaged 44 degrees. Five of his 13 patients showed a significant esotropia in the primary position at least two months postoperatively. All had a significant face turn. None of our patients were esotropic in the primary position and no face turns were seen.

The Scott publication reports only the total diplopia-free field, and does not indicate the degree of abduction diplopia-free field obtained. However, since 6 of the 13 patients were esotropic in the primary position, we assume the diplopia-free field did not extend to the midline, or into abduction, in these patients. In our series of total vertical muscle transposition, all patients had diplopia-free fields in abduction. The average postoperative diplopia-free abduction field was 17 degrees in our patients, which even compares favorably to the results of previous series where only monocular abduction was measured.

While our series is not large, it appears that total vertical rectus muscle transposition combined with medial rectus muscle recession on an adjustable suture provides superior abducting force compared to muscle-splitting procedures. Having the medial rectus muscle on an adjustable suture allows optimal centering of the diplopia-free field, and minimizes the degree of medial rectus weakening. In our series, all patients had diplopia-free abduction, none were undercorrected and many had symmetric abduction and adduction fields, i.e., excellent centering of the field of fusion.

In our series there was no significant difference in the binocular visual field obtained when ipsilateral medial rectus muscle recession (19 degrees abduction) was performed at a subsequent procedure versus contralateral medial rectus muscle recession at the initial operation (18 degrees abduction). It thus appears that secondary ipsilateral recession affords no surgical benefit over a primary contralateral medial rectus muscle recession as long as medial rectus muscle restriction has been excluded. It is probably prudent to recess the contralateral medial rectus muscle at the same time in order to maximize the innervation in the field of the paretic lateral rectus muscle, and to perform an ipsilateral medial rectus recession at a later time, if needed.

ACKNOWLEDGEMENTS

Supported in part by Research to Prevent Blindness, Inc., (S770712) and the William Randolph Hearst Foundation.

REFERENCES

1. Berens C, Girard LJ: Transplantation of the superior and inferior rectus muscles for paralysis of the lateral rectus. Am J Ophthalmol 33:1041-1049, 1950.

2. Feibel RM, Roper-Hall G: Evaluation of the field of binocular single vision in incomitant strabismus. Am J Ophthalmol 78:800-805, 1974.

3. Frueh BR, Henderson JW: Rectus muscle union in sixth nerve paralysis. Arch Ophthalmol 85:191-196, 1971.

4. Girard LJ, Beltranena F: Early and late complications of extensive muscle surgery. Arch Ophthalmol 64:576-584, 1960.

5. Helveston EM: Muscle transposition procedures. Surv Ophthalmol 16:92-97, 1971.

6. Jensen CDF: Rectus muscle union: a new operation for paralysis of the rectus muscles. Trans Pac Coast Otoophthalmol Soc 45:359-387 , 1964.

7. Kushner BJ: Jensen procedure modified. Ann Ophthalmol 11 :1255-1257, 1979.

8. Lyle TK: Management of ocular palsies of traumatic origin. International Ophthalmology Clinics 11(4):146-176, 1971.

9. Metz HS, Scott AB, O'Meara D et al: Ocular saccades in lateral rectus palsy. Arch Ophthalmol 84:453-460, 1970.

10. Scott WE, Werner DB, Lennerson L: Evaluation of Jensen procedures by saccades and diplopic fields. Arch Ophthalmol 79:1886-1889, 1979.

11. Selezinka W, Sandall GS, Henderson JW: Rectus muscle union in sixth nerve paralysis. Arch Ophthalmol 92:382-386, 1974.

12. Uribe LE: Muscle transplantation in ocular paralysis. Am J Ophthalmol 65:600-607.

13. Vesey FA: Method of achieving functional correction of total abducens nerve paralysis. Br J Ophthalmol 56:892-895, 1972.

14. von Noorden GK: Anterior segment ischemia following the Jensen procedure. Arch Ophthalmol 94:845-847, 1976.

EFFECT OF PRISMS ON ANGLE OF STRABISMUS

S. Veronneau-Troutman

ABSTRACT

The horizontal and vertical angles of strabismus were neutralized carefully in 100 strabismus patients wearing their best optical correction. Alternate cover test and prisms were used at near and distance in up, down, to the right and left gazes. These measurements were compared with those obtained after the patient has been wearing Fresnel prisms for half an hour to neutralize their deviations.

The patients thus examined were grouped and analyzed according to their sensory and motor anomalies. It is well recognized that patients with ARC may show a quick and marked increase in the angle of strabismus - they "eat the prisms". This finding was duplicated. However, in patients with NRC there occurred statistically significant variations from their original measurements. This was found more often in patients with exotropia, and in patients with A and V patterns. For example, a patient with an exotropia much larger at distance may show at the end of the test an exotropia larger at near, or a V or an A pattern can become insignificant. The measurements obtained following the prism test are used preferentially to determine the surgical procedure to be done. Examples illustrating the improved surgical outcome were presented.

(No paper was submitted.)

STRABISMUS II
ISBN 0-8089-1424-3

DISCRIMINANT ANALYSIS OF ACQUIRED ESOTROPIA: PREDICTOR VARIABLES FOR SHORT AND LONG TERM SURGICAL OUTCOMES

J. B. Bateman, M. M. Parks and N. Wheeler

ABSTRACT

In a retrospective study, a computer-based stepwise discriminant analysis was used to create a biostatistical model of the results of surgery in acquired esotropia. 172 patients who had bilateral medial rectus muscle recession with at least 6 months postoperative follow-up were studied.

The outcome groups for the discriminant analysis were based on the ocular deviation 6 weeks after surgery and at the patient´s last visit, or the presence or absence of stereopsis at the last visit. With respect to the ocular deviation (esotropia or success) six weeks after surgery, 11 independent variables were analyzed; those dtermined to be prognostic of the outcome grouping were refractive error of the left eye and preoperative deviation, in that order. With respect to ocular deviation at last visit, 146 patients were followed for over two years and were last examined when over five years of age; of the 12 independent variables analyzed, postoperative deviation, refractive error of the right eye, and age of onset were predictive. With respect to stereopsis, 126 patients had similar follow up; of the 11 independent variables analyzed, only postoperative deviation was prognostic. The results indicate that in patients with acquired esotropia the postoperative deviation is the most important prognostic factor for both the maintenance of ocular alignment and the re-establishment of stereopsis; refractice error and the age of onset of the esotropia influence the ocular alignment at the last visit.

INTRODUCTION

Acquired esotropia, usually defined by an onset after 6 months of age, is a heterogeneous form of strabismus. Etiologic factors include the accommodative effort associated with hyperopia,(1) dyskinesis of the accommodative convergence and accommodation (AC/A) relationship,(2,3) primary defects in binocular function,(4,5) in many cases, multople factors are causative. The onset may be intermittent with a variable angle of deviation; the initial treatment is usually the full correction of refractive error with glasses if hyperopia is

STRABISMUS II
ISBN 0-8089-1424-3

evident. Miotics or bifocals may be useful in those cases with a high AC/A. If the deviation becomes or remains constant, surgical correction may be necessary. To further investigate those factors which promote ocular alignment and binocularity in patients with acquired esotropia, we used multivariate analysis to develop a biostatistical model of the surgnical outcome; parameters were identified which were predictive of ocular alignment six weeks postoperatively and at the last visit, and of stereopsis at the last visit.

MATERIALS AND METHODS

A retrospective study of patients with acquired esotropia (onset aftersix months of age) was undertaken by reviewing alphabetically the records of one of the authors, Dr. Marshall Parks. Selected parameters on 172 patients whose first surgery was performed by Dr. Parks as an isolated bilateral medical rectus muscle recession(12) were recorded and entered into a computer. All of Dr. Parks′s cases of concomitant esotopia underwent a symmetrical recession of both medial rectus muscles as the initial surgery except for patients with untreatable amblyopia; these patients had unilateral surgery. Excluded from the study were patients with neuroloical disease, paralytic strabismus, identifiable syndromes, or organic ocular disease. A minimum of six months follow-up after the surgery was required for inclusion.

Data obtained on each patient included sex, age of onset of the esodeviation (by history), age at the initial visit, refractive error of each eye at the initial visit, year of surgery, age at surgery, millimeters of recession of each medial rectus muscle, esodeviation preoperatively, heterotropia six weeks postoperatively, age at the last visit, heterotropia at the last visit, binocular status at the last visit, and total number of surgeries. Refractive error, in diopters, was determined by cycloplegic retinoscopy in young children and by cycloplegic refraction in cooperative children. Heterotropia, determined by the cover-uncover test and the alternate cover test, were expressed in prism diopters; all measurements, distance at 6 m and near at 0.33 m, were made with an accommodative target in the primary position. If ophthalmic lenses were prescribed, preoperative measurements were recorded with correction; if postoperative measurements were recorded both with and without correction, the smaller value was used. Demographic and chronologic summaries of the data base have been published previously.(13)

The computer-assisted analyses on the results of surgery were performed with the P-series (1981) of the BMDP Statistical Software.(14) The specific programs utilized were Description of Groups (Strata) with Histograms and Analysis of Variance (P7D) and Discriminant Analysis (P7M).

Discriminant analysis is a statistical method used to determine which quantitative, independent variables are predictive of an outcome group. Any number of variables, alone or in combination, may be entered as predictors into the linear function to best separate the groups. In this study, surgical success, either as ocular alignment or stereopsis, defined the outcome groups; prior probabilities were set equal to the actual percentages in each of the groups. In the BMDP discriminant analysis program, a stepwise analysis of variance is performed. At the initial step, an analysis of variance is performed on each variable; the usefulness of each in prdicting the outcome group is reflected in the F-statistic, a statistical measure obtained from the analysis of variance. The variable with the most significant F-statistic is used to determine the first coefficient in the linear (discriminant) function. Using this variable, a second analysis of variance is performed on the residual effect of each of the remaining independent variables; the most useful variable at this step (most statistically significant F-statistic) also is entered into the linear function. These analyses are repeated, using all previously slected variables at each step; the program is terminated when none of the available variables futher contributes to discrimination among the outcome groups at the designated statistical significance. In stepwise discriminant analysis, the usefulness reflected in the F statistic of a given variable changes at each step because of the effect of the previously entered variables. If the independent variables are correlated, the inclusion of one in the discriminant function will greatly reduce the predictive value of the others. The usefulness of the discriminant function lies in one possibility of predicting the most likely outcome group and the probability in the new case.

The discriminant function (for each outcome group) consists of a sum of mathematical terms, each of which is the product of the value of a significant variable in a given case and its coefficient; a constant term, calculated on the basis of prior probabilities, also is added. The coefficients weight and combine the useful variables in a way that best separates the outcome groups. The discriminant score for each case is computed by multiplying the numerical value of each significant variable by the respective outcome group coefficient; the sums for each outcome group are totaled and added to the appropriate constant; the highest value identifies the predicted group. The probability also is calculated. The accuracy of the model is based on percentage of correct classifications determined by comparing actual and biostatistically predicted outcomes.

The following surgical and sensory outcomes were seleced for discriminant analysis:

1) deviation six weeks postoperatively
2) deviation at the last visit
3) stereopsis at the last visit

The deviations were divided categorically into three groups: esotropia, exotropia, and success. Esotropia was defined as a deviation of 10 prism diopters or more of esotropia or esophoria; exotropia as 10 prism diopters or more of exotropia or exophoria; and success as 9 prism diopters or less of deviation. Binocularity was evaluated using the Titmus Stereotest (Titmus Optical Company) or Wirt Polariod vectograph test (copyright 1947 by S. Edgard Wirt, Ph.D.) and the Worth 4-dot test. Stereopsis was defined as a stereoacuity of 40 to 3000 seconds of arc; all other cases in which information was available were defined as No Stereopsis, including those with fusion on the Worth 4-dot test. Cases were excluded from the long term analyses of deviation and stereopsis (Dataset 1) if they had been followed for less than two years or if the last examination was prior to the age of five years. A second analysis (Dataset 2) of stereopsis was made on cases with two years or more of follow-up, the last examination after the age of five years, and the first surgery prior to five years of age.

The following (independent) variables for each case were selected for discriminant analysis:

1. sex
2. age of onset (years)
3. age at surgery (years)
4. interval (months) between onset of esotropia and surgery
5. preoperative esotropia, distance (prism diopters)
6. clinical relationship between accommodative convergence and accommodation (clinical AC/A; preoperative distance deviation minus near deviation in prism diopters)
7. refractive error, right eye, at initial examination

(spherical equivalent in diopters)
8. refractive error, left eye at initial examination (spherical equivalent in diopters)
9. anisometropia (refractive error of the right eye minus refractive error of the left eye in diopters)
10. millimeters of medial rectus muscle recession in each eye
11. year surgery was performed
12. postoperative deviaiton (6 m) at 6 weeks (prism diopters)

All 172 cases underwent analysis with respect to postoperative deviation at six weeks; 149 cases met the criteria for analysis of deviation at the last visit. The stereopsis status was evaluated in 126 cases for Dataset 1 and 83 cases for Dataset 2. The means of the age at the last visit (years) and the total number of surgeries for cases included in the long term studies of deviation and stereopsis underwent al analysis of variance.

RESULTS

The means and standard deviations of the independent variables for three analyses are set out in Tables 1, 2 and 3. The analysis of variance (testing the equality of the means) of each variable for the three six-weeks postoperative deviation outcome groups (Table 1) revealed that preoperative esotropia, refractive error of each eye, and millimeters of medical rectus muscle recession were significantly different at the 5% level; there was no difference among te groups with respect to sex. The analysis of variance of each variable, including sex, grouped according to the deviation at the last visit (Table 2) indicated that the means of anisometropia, refractive error of each eye, and postoperative deviation were statistically differenct (p´s 0.005). The analysis of variance of independent variables with respect to Stereopsis and No Stereopsis at the last visit (Table 3) indicated that the means of postoperative deviation were different ($p = .002$) in the two groups; additionally, there was a statistically significant predominance of males in the No Stereopsis group (p 0.05). The means and variance of the total number of surgeries were statistically different among the outcome groups based on either deviation or stereopsis at the last visit; there were no differences with respect to the age at the last visit for either group (Table 4).

Table 1

Means and Standard Deviations* for Independent Variables in Groups Defined by Deviation Six Weeks Postoperatively

Variable	ESOTROPIA	SUCCESS	EXOTROPIA
1. Age of onset (years)	2.4 (2.9)	2.8 (2.0)	2.0 (0.8)
2. Age at surgery (years)	4.8 (3.5)	4.5 (2.6)	3.2 (0.8)
3. Interval between onset and surgery (months)	28 (20)	22 (24)	14 (4)
4. Preoperative esotropia (prism diopters)	35 (20)	25 (11)	20 (6)
5. Clinical AC/A (prism diopters)	9 (9)	7 (9)	5 (6)
6. Medial rectus recession (mm each eye)	4.6 (0.7)	4.1 (0.6)	3.8 (0.8)
7. Refractive error, right eye (diopters)	+0.01 (4.45)	+2.08 (2.40)	+2.61 (1.50)
8. Refractive error, left eye (diopters)	+0.14 (4.10)	+2.21 (2.21)	+2.35 (1.50)
9. Anisometropia (diopters)	-0.13 (0.44)	-0.14 (1.14)	-0.25 (0.99)
10. Year surgery performed	1971 (4)	1970 (5)	1968 (5)
Cases	16	149	7

*Standard deviation is shown in parentheses

Table 2

Means and Standard Deviations* for Independent Variables in Groups Defined by Deviation at the Last Visit

Variable	ESOTROPIA	SUCCESS	EXOTROPIA
1. Age of onset (years)	2.2 (1.2)	2.8 (1.9)	3.4 (2.5)
2. Age at surgery (years)	4.7 (2.7)	4.7 (2.5)	4.0 (2.1)
3. Interval between onset and surgery (months)	32 (29)	24 (23)	6 (8)
4. Preoperative esotropia (prism diopters)	30 (17)	24 (11)	30 (10)
5. Clinical AC/A (prism diopters)	7 (8)	7 (9)	2 (3)
6. Medial rectus recession (mm each eye)	4.3 (0.5)	4.0 (0.6)	3.8 (0.8)
7. Refractive error, right eye (diopters)	+0.35 (4.28)	+2.35 (1.84)	-3.67 (6.36)
8. Refractive error, left eye (diopters)	+0.47 (4.11)	+2.38 (1.87)	+0.58 (1.04)
9. Anisometropia (diopters)	-0.12 (0.51)	-0.03 (0.50)	-4.25 (7.36)
10. Year surgery performed	1969 (5)	1970 (5)	1968 (3)
11. Postoperative deviation 6 weeks (prism diopters of esotropia)	8 (10)	1 (6)	2 (3)
Cases	25	121	3

* Standard deviation is shown in parentheses

Table 3

Means and Standard Deviations* for Independent Variables in Groups Defined by Stereopsis at the Last Visit

Variable	STEREOPSIS	NO STEREOPSIS
1. Age of onset (years)	2.9 (2.0)	2.0 (0.7)
2. Age at surgery (years)	4.8 (2.7)	4.1 (1.8)
3. Interval between onset and surgery (months)	25 (26)	25 (22)
4. Preoperative esotropia (prism diopters)	25 (11)	26 (12)
5. Clinical AC/A (prism diopters)	7 (8)	6 (10)
6. Medial rectus recession (mm each eye)	4.1 (0.6)	3.9 (0.7)
7. Refractive error, right eye (diopters)	+2.12 (1.67)	+2.15 (2.58)
8. Refractive error, left eye (diopters)	+2.13 (1.68)	+2.20 (2.54)
9. Anisometropia (diopters)	-0.01 (0.43)	-0.05 (0.72)
10. Postoperative deviation 6 weeks (prism diopters)	3** (6)	3*** (10)
Cases	111	15

* Standard deviation is shown is parentheses
** esotropia
*** exotropia

Table 4

Means and Standard Deviations for Age at Last Visit and Total Number of Surgeries

DEVIATION AT THE LAST VISIT

	ESOTROPIA	SUCCESS	EXOTROPIA
1. Age at last visit (years)	11.8 (3.9)	11.4 (4.3)	12.1 (4.3)
2. Total number of surgeries	1.3 (0.5)	1.3 (0.5)	2.3 (2.3)

STEREOPSIS AT THE LAST VISIT

	STEREOPSIS	NO STEREOPSIS
1. Age at last visit (years)	11.8 (4.1)	12.5 (4.2)
2. Total number of surgeries	1.3 (0.5)	1.9 (1.1)

Table 5

Discriminant Analysis of Ocular Deviation
Six Weeks Postoperatively and at Last Visit

6 WEEKS POSTOPERATIVE*			COEFFICIENTS	
Variables	F	P	Esotropia	Success
1. refractive error, left eye (diopters)	10.363	0.002	0.02489	0.37075
2. preoperative deviation (prism diopters)	8.338	0.005	0.23303	0.16873
Constant			-6.36043	-2.64099
LAST VISIT**				
Variables				
1. postoperative deviation (prism diopters)	17.934	<0.001	0.16423	0.04370
2. refractive error, right eye (diopters)	8.743	0.003	0.23040	0.55986
3. age of onset (years)	4.373	0.03	0.68852	0.97177
Constant			-3.18607	-2.20968

* 165 cases
** 146 cases

Table 6

Discriminant Analysis of Stereopsis at Last Visit

Dataset 1*			COEFFICIENT	
Variable	F	p	Stereopsis	No Stereopsis
1. Postoperative deviation (prism diopters)	10.887	0.001	0.06075	-0.07887
Constant			-0.20583	-2.25172
Dataset 2**				
Variables				
1. Postoperative deviation (prism diopters)	14.463	0.001	0.05832	-0.12763
2. Sex	3.706	0.06	6.24887	4.81360
Constant			-4.58735	-5.04872

* 126 cases
** 83 cases

In the studies of deviation as the basis of the outcome group, only seven cases (4%) were exotropic at the six-weeks postoperative visit and three cases at the final visit (2%). As multivariate analysis requires outcome groups considerably larger than seven for meaningful results, these exotropic cases were excluded from both analyses of deviation; the discriminant functions were determined only for the esotropia and success outcome groups. With the cases grouped into two six-weeks postoperative groups, esotropia and success (n = 165), the results of the analysis of variance were unchanged; again, the preoperative deviation, the refractive error of each eye, and the millimeters of medial rectus muscle recession were significantly different at the 5% level. With respect to esotropia or success at the last visit, postoperative deviation, the refractice error of each eye, the millimeters of medial rectus muscle recession, and the preoperative deviation were significantly different (p´s 0.05) between the two; anisometropia was not a predictive variable after cases which were exotropic at the last visit were eliminated.

The results of the three discriminant analyses are summarized in Tables 5 and 6. The outcome groups were esotropia or success six weeks postoperatively, esotropia or success at the last visit, or the presence or absence of stereopsis at the last visit. The descriptive statistics of the independent variables available to the program are in Tables 1, 2 and 3; those selected by the program and the statistical significance at each step are listed in order of entry. The coefficients for the variables, calculated by linear regression, and the constants for each outocme group are given. These coefficients and constants were used to classify each case in the data set; the percentages of correct classifications of the discriminant functions are summarized in Table 7.

Table 7

Accuracy of Discriminant Function in Classifying Cases Compared with Actual Outcome

Outcome Group	% Correct Classification
Deviation - 6 weeks postoperative	89.7
Deviation - last visit	84.9
Stereopsis - last visit	86.7

DISCUSSION

Discriminant analysis is a useful biostatistical tool for identifying quantitative variables predictive of outcome groups. Although the mathematical technique was developed in the mid-1930′s,(15) medical applications have been possible only recently as computers and the necessary biostatistical software have become more readily available. The method identifies those independent parameters that, in combination, discriminate among outcome groups. This multivariate approach has several advantages over univariate methods such as the t test. First, the stepwise progression of the analysis permits the identification of variables which alone may not discriminate among outcome groups. The significance of such factors may be overlooked by more traditional data analysis. For example, the separate dimensions of the head of the humerus in humans and chimpanzees are not statistically different and one cannot accurately identify the origin of a bone by inspection alone; however, if the dimensions are combined in a discriminant function, the differences are statistically significant and the origian of a given humerus may be correctly identified.(16) Second, the mathematical model, once develope, can be used to predict the result of surgical intervention or other modes of therapy in a new case. Identifying parameters which predict a "good" or "poor" result may permit the physician to prognosticate more accurately. This methodology has been useful in identifying risk factors in chronic simple glaucoma.(17-20) Third, because a statistical relationship exists between the predictive independent variables and the outcome groups, causal relationships may be explored. In interpreting the results, one cannot infer that the remaining variables do not influence the outcome; they are not included by the program if there is no increase in the accuracy of the function in discriminating amongst the outcome groups. Conclusions must be made carefully, however, as the model is a mathematical description of a system and not a mechanistic analysis.

In performing discriminant analysis on surgical outcomes in acquired esotropia, we set out to identify those parameters that were predictive of a desirable result. The definition of a "desirable result" is controversial and subject to value judgments and scientific interpretations. Previous studies have used differing criteria for success. Taylor(21,22) in advocating early surgery for patients with congenital esotropia, used the conversion of constant heterotropia to heterophoria in defining a successful result. Ing, Costenbader, Parks, and Albert(23) in a study of the sensory results in congenital esotropia defined a desirable result on the basis of binocularity on two or more sensory tests: fusional amplitudes on the amblyoscope, fusion on the Worth4-dot test (20 feet or 13 inches), or any stereopsis on the Wirt Stereotest; the same criteria were used by von Noorden and his colleagues(25) in a similar study. More recently, Ing(26) again used binocularity as the criterion for success, redefining it on the basis of one or more of the following sensory tests: Bagolini striated glasses, the Worth 4-dot at 0.33 m, and stereoacuity. As we believe that a desirable result would be the achievement and maintenance over a lifetime of properly aligned eyes, we defined success as orthotropia, or 9 prism diopters or less of esodeviation or exodeviation. The requisites for the maintenance of aligned eyes over a lifetime are more complicated; 40 or 50 years of follow-up would be desirable but this is difficult to achieve either prospectively or retrospectively. Biostatistical life-table analysis are useful in studies with cases of varying follo-up periods. Selection biases make this an unreliable method in the study of strabismus; the patient population returning to the ophthalmologist after the amblyogenic period is not representative as patients with straight eyes are much less likely to return than patients with residual deviations. As single binocular vision serves to stabilize ocular alignment, we elected to use the sensory status as an outcome that would reflect the long term stability of the ocular alignment. Although fusion on theWorth 4-dot test may be sufficiently stable to maintain ocular alignment, we selected stereopsis as both a stable and a more useful quality. We required a minimum postoperative follow-up of two years to allow for the status of stereopsis to be determined; the age at the last visit was set at over five years to assure that the patient was sufficiently mature to reliable undergo the stereopsis testing.

From the analysis of postoperative esotropic and success outocmes six weeks postoperatively, refractive error of the left eye and preoperative deviation, in that order, were prdictive. At the initial step, the means of the refractive error of each eye, preoperative deviaiton, and millimeters of medial rectus muscle recession were difference in the two groups. After the refractive error of the left eye was entered into the function, only the preoperative deviation and the millimeters of medial rectus muscle recession remained statistically significant; the refractive error of the right eye, a variable correlated to the refractiveerror of the left eye, was no longer discriminating. After the preoperative deviation was entered into the function, none of the remaining variables further contributed to the discrimination. Combined, the higher the hypermetropia and the smaller the angle of deviation, the greater were the chances for a success outcome at six-weeks postoperatively. The significance of the degree of hypermetropia probable reflects the surgeon´s ability to alter the corrective lenses to align the eyes postoperatively. The reasons for the influence of the preoperative deviation are more speculative. A discriminant analysis of congenital (infantile) esotropia showed that preoperative esotropia was also a significant predictor of the deviation six weeks postoperatively and at the last visit, and of the stereopsis at the last visit;(27) the authors speculated that the larger deviations were more difficult to correct in one surgical procedure. However, the mean preoperative deviation in this study for both outcome groups six weeks psotoperatively is 26 prism diopters, considerably less than the 54 prism diopters in the congenital esotropia study;(27) a similar explanation, although not plausible for the entire population with acquired esotropia, might apply for a subpopulation with a large angle esotropia.

In the discrimination between the outcome groups esotropia and success at the last visit, the useful variables in order of declining value were postoperative deviation at six weeks, refractive error of the right eye, and age of onset. The larger the esotropia at the six weeks postoverative visit, the lower the likelihood of rothotropia (+/- 9 prism diopters) at the last visit; the higher the hypermetropia, the greater were the chances for a success outcome. The probable explanation for the significance of these two variables is the surgeon´s ability to alter the corrective lenses to align the eyes in cases that are minimally esotropic or exotropic postoperatively. The third variable, which was not significant until the first two were entered, was the age of onset of the esotropia; a later age of onset increased the chances for success at the last visit. The usefulness of this variable is more difficult to explain; possibly, patients with a later onset are earier to measure preoperatively and have a greater likelihood for postoperative success; or alternately, a later onset may reflect the development of a more stable binocularity prior to the esotropia.

With the presence or absence of stereopsis (40 to 3000 seconds of arc) at the last visit defining the outcome groups, the analysis of variance at the initial step showed that only the postoperative deviation was statistically different. In Dataset 1, with all patients having 24 months of postoperative follow-up and being at least five years of age at the last examination, no other variables were entered at the subsequent step. The analysis of Dataset 2, in which all patients had surgery prior to the age of five years, the sex of the patient became statistically significan at step two. For reasons that are unclear, females were more likely to re-establish stereopsis than males. With either set of criteria, postoperative esotropia was predictive of no stereopsis.

Previous studies of acquired esotropia have implicated multiple factors influencing the long term deviation and sensory status. Esotropia without surgical intervention tends to decrease with time, particularly in cases with hypermetropia.(28-30) Conversely, deterioration may occur in cases with a high clinical AC/A.(31) Later onset, small deviation (less than 20 degrees), intermittency, and hypermetropia (over 4 diopters) have been found to be factors predictive of "successful treatment" with refractice correction; the clinical AC/A and anisometropia did not influence results.(32) The influence of surgical factors in acquired esotropia remains moot. Fletcher and Silverman(33) concluded that the timing of surgery did not influence the fusional results, as determined by prism and cover and prism and red-gladd test.(34) Uemura, however, found that fusion (as determined on the major amblyoscope or by prism test, stereotest, and Worth 4-dot test) was more liely to be present in individuals who had surgery prior to the age of three years. In this study, we found that the age at surgery played no role in predicting the results of treatment. Postoperative deviation was the only variable which was useful in predicting the sensory status (stereopsis) at the last visit. We found that a small degree of postoperative esotropia ranging to orthotropia increased the likelihood of re-establishing stereopsis. These findings contrast with those of Dankner, Mash, and Jampolsky,(36) who found that in the immediate posterative period in patients with acquired esotropia, surgical overcorrection increased the likelihood of fusion (determined by the cover/uncover and the 4 diopter base-out prism test).

A retrospective study such as this has inherent liminations. Acquired esotropia, which is applied to all non-syndromal cases of esotropia evident after the age of six months, may represent the final result of a mixture of neurological, anatomical, refractive, and genetic factors. As we are unable to quantitate the influence of these potentially causative factors, with the exception of the refractive error, the search for predictive parameters may be fruitless at best; the prognosis for ocular alignment and/or binocularity may correlate best with the etiology. The general lack of consensus in defining a satisfactory outcome complicates the interpretation of results and the comparison of studies. Although discriminant analysis is a multivariate approach which provides many advantages for the identification of trends, particularly in a data base that may be heterogeneous, the technique describes biostatistical, not causal, realtionships; the results should be interpreted cautiously. Discriminant analysis is based on linear functions; if the relationship between an independent parameter and the outcome is curvilinear, the program will create the best linear approximation. As an example, if there is no advantage to surgery at three months over eleven months of age in congenital esotropia but a sharp decrease in the likelihood of a desirable result during the second year of life, the function created by the program will be linear from birth on. Furthermore, the model is useful only within the range of the data set from which it was created. Lastly, the data base in this study was limited to patients operated on by a single surgeon. Although this reduces the variability associated with differing surgical criteria and techniques, we must be cautious in applying the results of this study to other surgeons.

During these limitations, we have shown in a series of cases in which the criteria for and the technique of surgery were consistent that certain quantitative variables are useful in predicting the outcome group. We have demonstrated that the modifiable factor, postoperative ocular alignment at six weeks, is predictive of the status of stereopsis.

ACKNOWLEDGEMENTS

Supported in part by a Research to Prevent Blindness Manpower Award CC810708 and NIH Grant EY 0331.

REFERENCES

1. Donders FC: On the Anomalies of Accomodation and Refraction of the Eye, with a preliminary essay on physiological dioptics, translated by WD Moore. London: The New Sydenham Society, 1864.

2. Costenbader FD: Clinical course and management of esotropia, in Allen JH (ed): Strabismus Ophthalmic Symposium

II. St. Louis: The C.V. Mosby, 325-353, 1958.

3. Parks MM: Abnormal accommodative convergence in squint. Arch Ophthalmol 59:364-380, 1958.

4. Jarval E: Manuel Theorique et Pratique du Strabisme. Paris, G. Masson, 1896.

5. Worth C: Squint: Its Causes, Pathology, and Treatment. Philadelphia: Blakiston, 59-62, 1903.

6. Scobee RG: Anatomic factors in the etiology of heterotropia. Am J Ophthalmol 31:781-795, 1948.

7. Nordlow W: Uber den Entstehungsmechanismus des Einwartsschielens, Goteborg, Elanders Boktryckeri Aktiebolag, 76-78, 1942.

8. Nordlow W: Permanent convergent squint-early operation and long-term follow-up. Arch Ophthalmol 55:87-100, 1956.

9. Francois J: Heredity in Ophthalmology. St. Louis: The C.V. Mosby Co., 255, 1966.

10. Smith D, Grutzner P, Colenbrander A, Hegmann JP, Spivey B: Selected ophthalmologic and orthoptic measurements in families. Arch Ophthalmol 87:278-282, 1972.

11. Richter S: Untersuchungen uber die Hereditat des Strabismus concomitans. Sammlung zwangloser Abhandlungen auf dem Gebiet Augenheil kunds. Leipzig: Threme, 1966.

12. Parks MM: Fornix incision for horizontal rectus muscle surgery. Am J Ophthalmol 65:907-915, 1968.

13. Bateman J, Parks MM: Clinical and computer-assisted analyses of preoperative and postoperative accommodative convergence and accommodation relationships. Ophthalmology 88:1024-1030, 1981.

14. Dixon WJ, Brown MB, Engelman L, Frane JW, Hill MA, Jennrich RI, Toporek JD (eds): BMDP Statistical Software 1981. Berkeley: University of California Press, 1981.

15. Fisher RA: The use of multiple measurements in taxonomic problems. Ann Eugen 7:179-188, 1936.

16. Howells WW: The importance of being human, in Tanur JM,

Mosteller F, Kruskal WH, Link RF, Pieters RS, Rising GR, (eds): Statistics: A Guide to the Unknown. San Francisco: Holden-Day, 92-100, 1972.

17. Drance SM: Correlation of optic nerve and visual field defects in simple glaucoma. Doyne Memorial Lecture, 1975. Trans Ophthalmol Soc U,K. 95:288-296, 1975.

18. Susanna R, Drance SM: Use of discriminant analysis. I. Prediction of visual field defects from features of the glaucoma disc. Arch Ophthalmol 96:1568-1570, 1978.

19. Drance SM, Schulzer M; Douglas GR, Sweeney VP: Use of discriminant analysis. II. Identification of persons with glaucomatous visual field defects. Arch ophthalmol 96:1571-1573, 1978.

20. Drance SM, Schulzer M, Thomas B, Douglas GR: Multivariate analysis in glaucoma. Use of discriminant analysis in predicting glaucomatous visual field damage. Arch Ophthalmol 99:1019-1022, 1981.

21. Taylor DM: How early is early surgery in the management of strabismus? Arch Ophthalmol 70:752-756, 1963.

22. Taylor DM: Congenital strabismus. The common sense approach. Arch Ophthalmol 77:478-484, 1967.

23. Ing M, Costenbader FD, Parks MM, Albert DG: Early surgery for congenital esotropia. Am J Ophthalmol 61:1419-1427, 1966.

24. Ing M: Surgical treatment and motor results. In: Symposium: infantile esotropia. Am Orthopt J 18:11-14, 1968.

25. von Noorden GK, Isaza A, Parks ME: Surgical treatment of congenital esotropia. Trans Am Acad Ophthalmol Otolaryngol 76:1465-1474, 1972.

26. Ing MR: Early surgical alignment for congenital esotropia. Trans Am Ophthalmol Soc 79:625-663, 1981.

27. Bateman JB, Parks MM, Wheeler N: Discriminant analysis of infantile esotropia: predictor variables for short and long term surgical outcomes. Submitted for publication.

28. Mathewson GH: Convergent strabismus changed to divergent without operative interference. Am J Ophthalmol 9:608, 1926.

29. Moore S: The natural course of esotropia. Am Orthop J 21:80-83, 1971.

30. Burian HM: Hypermetropia and esotropia. J Pediatr Ophthalmol 9:135-143, 1972.

31. Parks MM: Management of acquired esotropia. Br J Ophthalmol 58:240-247, 1974.

32. Folk ER, Whelchel MC: The effect of the correction of refractive errors on nonparalytic esotropia. Am J Ophthalmol 40:232-236, 1955.

33. Fletcher MC, Silverman SJ: Strabismus: a study of 1,110 consecutive cases. Part II. Findings in 472 cases of partially accommodative and non accommodative esotropia. Am J Ophthalmol 61:255-265, 1966.

34. Uemura Y: Surgical correction of infantile esotropia. Jpn J Ophthalmol 17:50-59, 1973.

35. Dankner SR, Mash AJ, Jampolsky A: Intentional surgical overcorrection of acquired esotropia. Arch Ophthalmol 96:1848-1852, 1978.

THE ASSOCIATION FADENOPERATION - ADJUSTABLE SURGERY

A. Spielmann

ABSTRACT

The Cuppers' Fadenoperation and the adjustable procedures are to be associated in adult patients any time the deviation has a dynamic component. The Fadenoperation takes care of the dynamic part of the deviation and the adjustable procedures are used as a complement to conventional surgery to fine tune the correction of the static part of the deviation. Their association is reported in Esotropias, in Palsies (N. III palsy) and in Retraction Syndromes.

INTRODUCTION

Every ocular surgeon will adapt new surgical techniques to his own philosophy of strabismus. Thus, for almost ten years I have added Cuppers's Fadenoperation,(1) for two years Jampolski's adjustable procedures(2) and a personal adjustable tucking technique of the superior oblique muscle(3,4) to the so-called conventional surgery in my adult patients. I have assigned those procedures distinct and well-defined goals.

ESOTROPIAS

The Basic and the Dynamic Deviations

A new interest in the well-known basic and dynamic deviations has developed with Cuppers's work(5) upon the hyperadduction phenomena, the blocking syndromes and their surgical cure by the Fadenoperation.

Without going deeply into etiology, we can consider variable convergent strabismus to be a functional, innervational esotropia similar to a convergence "spasm". This functional "dynamic" deviation is superimposed on a basic primary position of the eyes which may be esotropia, exotropia, hypertropia or even orthophoria if the origin of the functional esotropia is a sensorial defect.

STRABISMUS II
ISBN 0-8089-1424-3

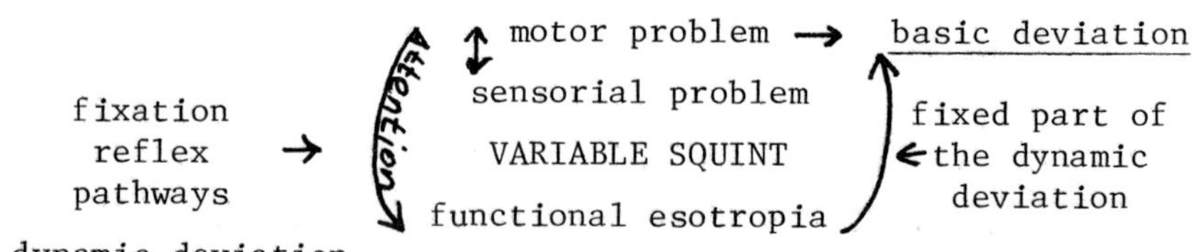

Logically, at the two poles of the deviation in those cases of variable strabismus, we are bound to have a minimal deviation and a maximal one which depend on the effort of attention. The minimal deviation is usually found in far vision. I measure it by means of a rapid cover-uncover test, with the glasses on. Its value suggests the value of the basic deviation. The maximal deviation is usually found in the near fixation while viewing detailed objects. I measure it by means of an alternate cover test, with and without glasses, and evaluate the accommodation factor. The maximal dynamic deviation is the value of the maximal deviation minus the minimal deviation. In this value I include the so-called accommodative deviation. This gives an estimate of the favorable influence of the Fadenoperation upon this factor. I use it as a basis to quantify the Fadenoperation (monolateral or bilateral) without risks for the convergence since I know the maximal contraction of the medial recti. It does not mean that patients do not have to wear their glasses - indeed they must nor that we cannot play games with the AC/A ratio which is favorably influenced by the Fadenoperation.

Surgery

1. The dynamic deviation may be cured by any procedure which introduces a "motor brake" on the medial recti.

Large recessions (especially adjustable ones) may correct (global surgery)(6) the dynamic deviation when the recession happens to coincide with the needed change in the arc of contact or when the paresis created by an excessive contraction of the recessed muscle neutralizes the dynamic factor. Yet we do not know how they act on each component of the deviation. The evolution during the days after surgery is unpredictable in the absence of resection. Recessions can hardly be used in the case of a basic deviation equal to zero.

The Fadenoperation, on the contrary, does not affect the basic position in the cases of relative orthophoria (Scott(7)-Spielmann(8)). It is the only possible procedure in the case of an isolated dynamic deviation for far vision as well as for near vision, in nystagmus for instance. But its action is only predictable with precision in an orthophoric position of the eyes. So it has to be associated with a carefully planned surgery of the basic position in what I call a specific "dissociated" surgery.

I perform a monolateral Fadenoperation if the dynamic deviation is less than 25 prism diopters (case 1). I perform a bilateral Fadenoperation if the dynamic deviation is greater than 25 prism diopters (case 2).

2. The basic deviation is treated by conventional surgery which has to follow the rules of isotony (light, equilibrated recess-resect procedures) if we want to limit its action to the correction of the basic deviation.

I resort to conventional surgery when a Fadenoperation is performed, on the basis of the formula: $\Delta = R(2) + 3S$ where Δ is the basic deviation, R(2) is the square of the recession measured in millimeters, and 3S is three times the resection in millimeters (Spielmann and Laulan(8)). When the retinal correspondence is abnormal, I operate on the basis of the "subjective deviation", i.e., Δ = the prismatic value of the deviation where the Bagolini's striated lenses imaged are crossed or when a crossed diplopia appears. The subjective deviation is treated by a "fixed" surgery and the rest of the deviation by an adjustable one.(9)

In this surgery, a major problem is the clinical approach to the basic deviation and the fear of a postoperative diplopia in adult patients, because an error in its evaluation may be the cause of a consecutive divergence. So, at least in some cases, we have to use an adjustable surgery to make up for the difficulty of its diagnosis.

A lateral rectus muscle resection is the adjustable part of my surgery. Up to 15 prism diopters, I use it without a medial rectus recession (R = 0).

Examples

Esotropia with a NRC and a dynamic deviation $< 25\Delta$ = Monolateral Faden. Case 1. (Fig 1) was a case of residual esotropia in a 17-year-old girl operated on 10 years ago.

The minimal deviation was 12 prism diopters so I performed an adjustable lateral rectus resection. The maximal deviation was 35 prism diopters. The dynamic deviation being 23 prism diopters (35-12), I performed a monolateral medial rectus Fadenopration. (Other deviations: near vision deviation with glasses = 25 prism diopters. Far vision deviation measured by an alternate cover test = 16 prism diopters. Subjective deviation = 12 prism diopters). The result was orthophoria for far and near vision with the glasses, a 6 prism diopters esophoria without glasses.

Esotropia with an ARC and a dynamic deviation >25Δ = Bilateral Faden. Case 2 (Fig 2): in this case of esotropia with abnormal retinal correspondence, I operated for the value of the stable subjective deviation (16 prism diopters) by a 4 millimeter medial rectus recession. For the uncertain value of the minimal deviation (35 prism diopters) and

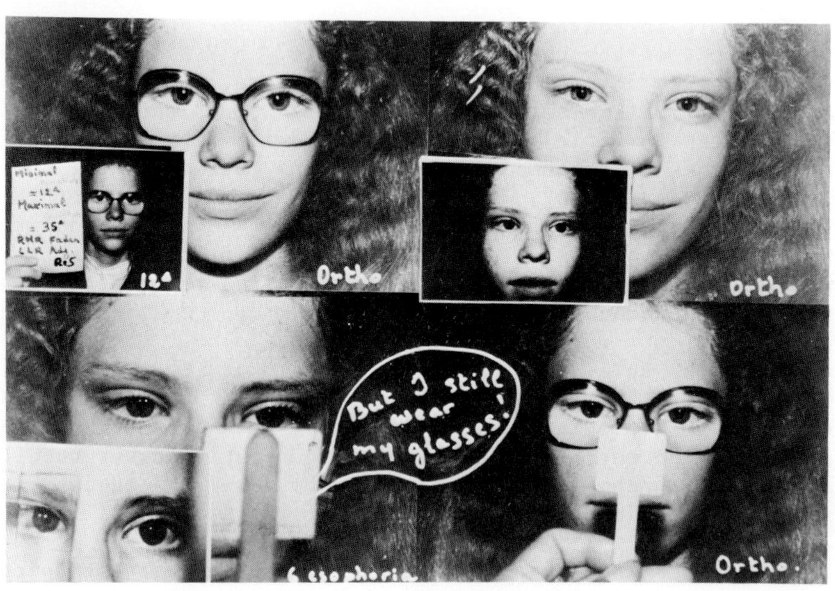

Figure 1. (Case 1): Variable strabismus with NRC and dynamic deviation < 25Δ. Minimal deviation (far vision with spectacles) = 12Δ. Surgery = RLR muscle: adjustable resection. Maximal deviation (near vision without spectacles) = 35Δ. Surgery = RMR m Fadden 14 mm. RESULT = orthophoria with glasses for far and near vision. 6Δ esophoria without glasses. Convergence = good.

because of the risk of a diplopia, I performed a lateral rectus muscle adjustable resection (which in fact was left recessed). The maximal deviation being 70 prism I performed a 14 mm bilateral Fadenoperation (plus an adjustable tucking of the superior oblique muscle). The result was an 8 prism diopters microstrabismus with good motility and no change one year later.

CRANIAL NERVE PALSIES

The Primary and the Secondary Deviations

The choice of the procedure is similar in mechanical or neurogenic palsies. Our conception of a specific surgery allows us to say that, by and large: a) A conventional surgery combined with an adjustable procedure is used for the primary deviation of the eyes. b) A Fadenoperation is used for the secondary deviation and has to equiliberate (paresis against paresis) the motility in the field of the paretic muscle.

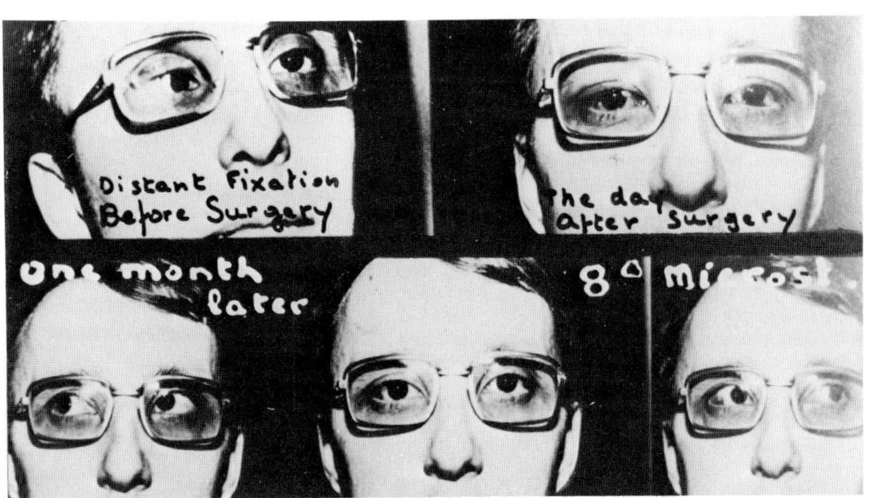

Figure 2. (Case 2): Esotropia ARC dynamic deviation $> 25\Delta$. Subjective deviation = 16 prism diopters (scotoma 16). Minimal deviation = 35 prism diopters. Maximal deviation = 70 prism diopters. Surgery = 4 mm RMR m Recession for the fixed subjective deviation + RLR adjustable resection. Bilateral Faden 14 mm + S.O. muscle adjustable tucking. Result = 8 microstrabismus.

Examples

III Cranial Nerve Palsy (Case 3 - Fig 3): in this case, I performed an adjustable lateral rectus recession plus a medial rectus muscle resection on the dominant paretic eye. Fadenoperations on the lateral and on the superior recti muscles were performed on the non-paretic eye associated with an adjustable left inferior rectus muscle resection. The result was a binocular vision with a large central field of gaze.

Retraction syndrome (Case 4 - Fig 4): in this case of unilateral Duane's Syndrome I applied my usual technique:(10) Fadenoperation on the two horizontal recti of the paretic eye. The lateral rectus muscle recession was an adjustable one. The improvement was noticeable in the retraction and the incomitance. An extended field of binocular vision was transferred into the primary position suppressing the torticollis.

DISCUSSION

We have demonstrated the association "Adjustable procedures Fadenoperation" in esotropias, exotropias with III cranial nerve palsies and unilateral retraction syndromes. I have also used it in many other cases: nystagmus, Brown's syndromes, double elevator palsies, and DVD. That is, the

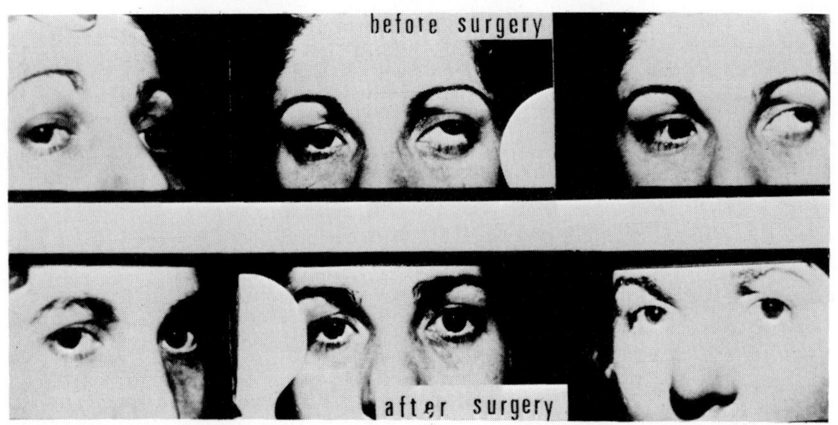

Figure 3. (Case 3): N. III Palsy: Fixation of the paretic eye. Surgery = Paretic eye: RLR m Adjustable recession. RMR m 6 mm resection. Nonparetic eye: LSR m Faden 13 mm and LLR m Faden 18 mm L Inferior R adjustable resection. Result: Binocular vision in the PP.

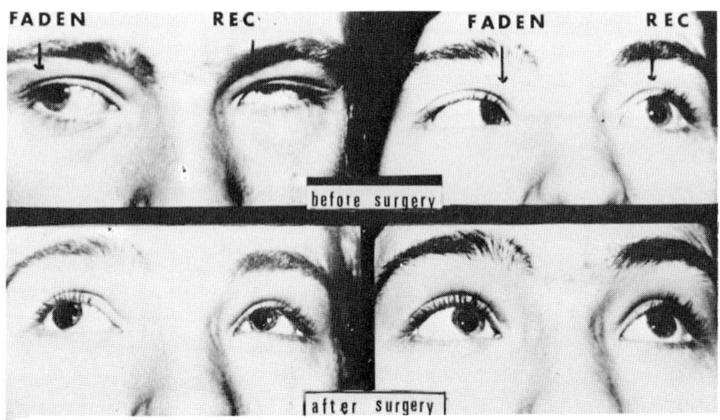

Figure 4. (case 4): Left Unilateral Duane Syndrome. Surgery = Recession of the 2 horizontal recti of the paretic eye. Fadenoperation on the 2 horizontal recti of the non paretic eye. Result: Binocular Vision in the P.P.

combined procedure is used any time I was faced with the problem of a variable deviation in adults. In all those cases the Fadenoperation took care of the variable part of the deviation due to the hyperinnervational factors. The adjustable procedures which compensate for the imprecision of our measures were added to conventional surgery to correct the abnormal position of the eyes. The suppression of the dynamic component of the deviation by the Fadenoperation combined with the use of an isotonic surgery probably account for the consistency of the results as studied previously.(11)

It is clear that the conventional strabismus surgery remains important. But every surgeon has experienced unsatisfactory results, more dramatic in adult patients because of the diplopia. That is why our surgery has to be improved at times by the addition of new procedures such as the Fadenoperation and the adjustable sutures which in my opinion are to be used in a "selective" and "dissociated" surgery.

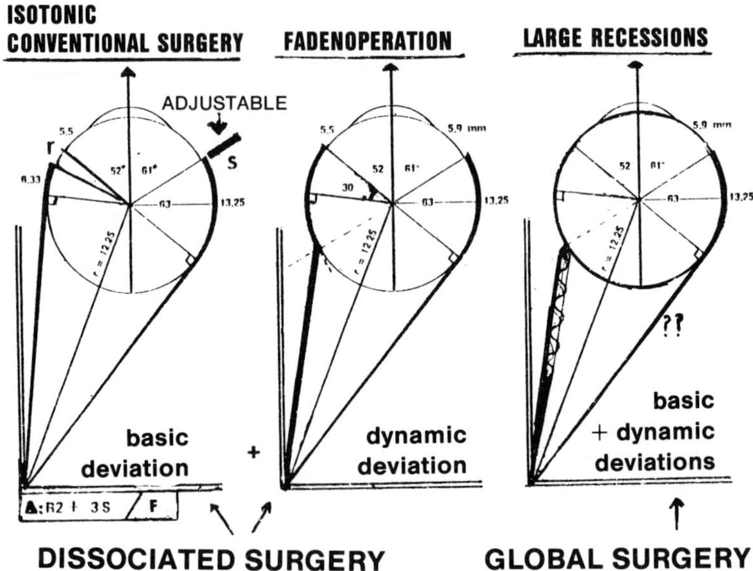

Figure 5

REFERENCES

1. Cuppers C: The so-called Fadenoperation. In Fells P (ed): Second Meeting of the International Strabismological Association, Marseille, Diffusion generale de libraire, 1974, p 395-400.

2. Jampolsky J: Adjustable Strabismus Surgical Procedures. Transactions of the New Orleans Academy of Ophthalmology, St. Louis, CV Mosby, 1978, pp 321-349.

3. Spielmann A: Plicature reglable du grand oblique. Bull Soc Ophthalmol France No 11, 1980, pp 1079-1083.

4. Spielmann A: An adjustable tucking technique for the superior oblique muscle. Monaco 1st International Meeting of Ocular Surgeons, October 1981.

5. Cuppers C, Adelstein F: Zum problem der echten und der Sheinbaren abducenslatmunf (das sog Blockierung-syndrom). In Bucherein das Augenarzts (BE Mbl Augenheik, H 46 271-278, 1966.

6. Spielmann A: Techniques chirurgicales actuelles dans les esotropies fonctionnelles. Mode d'action et indications. Bull Soc Ophthalmol France 81:865-871, 1981.

7. Scott AB: The fadenoperation. Mechanical effects. Am Orthopt Journal 27-44-47, 1977.

8. Spielmann A, Laulan J: Action of recessions and resections when associated with a fadenoperation in esotropia. Statistical Results. (Kyoto-I.S.A.) in Strabismus, Reinecke RD (ed), Grune and Stratton, 1978, pp 355-369.

9. Spielmann A: Indications for Adjustable Symposium on Strabismus CESO. Florence, 1983 (in press).

10. Spielmann A: Le syndrome de retraction de stilling Duane. J Fr d'Orthoptie 11:105-123, 1976.

11. Spielmann A: La chirurgie reglable dans les exotropies. Bull Soc Ophthalmol France 83:259-266, 1982.

MODIFICATION TO THE CLASSIC CONCEPT OF OBLIQUE MUSCLES GLOBAL INSERTION

M. H. Bernasconi, S. Dobsky, E. Rivas,
Y. Palma, and A. Pacheco

ABSTRACT

Strabismus surgical anatomy was studied in respect to global insertions of oblique muscles. The classical concept was: the superior oblique (SO) had linear insertion on the posterior, superior and external quadrant of the sclera, the inferior oblique (IO) had linear insertions on the posterior, inferior and lateral quadrant.

Fifty eyes from fresh corpses were studied. Stress lines were built. The muscles were recognized, photos were taken, and histology was made. Our new anatomical concept is summarized: 1. The superior oblique insertion can have linear insertions but also has area insertions. The insertion can be on the nasal side and its tendon may form a dihedral angle. 2. The inferior oblique insertion is almost all area in type, it is 100% above the classical descriptions of the insertion and is a thick and oval muscle.

INTRODUCTION

We investigated the reason for hypertropias secondary to vertical muscle surgery by studying the ocular global insertions of both oblique muscles. We report the type and magnitude of the various insertional patterns.

The classic anatomic concepts are as follows: The anatomists and ophthalmologists state that the superior oblique muscle (SO) has a linear insertion which is on a scleral quadrant located posteriorly, superiorly, and externally in respect to the whole globe. They further state that the inferior oblique muscle (IO) has a linear insertion on a scleral quadrant which is located posteriorly, inferiorly, and laterally in respect to the whole globe.

MATERIALS AND METHOD

It was impossible to use preserved corpses. The muscles were fragil and the eyes hypotonic. We used fresh corpses and studied 50 eyes. Data were recorded in respect to the insertion characteristics, lines of force, and the relation

STRABISMUS II
ISBN 0-8089-1424-3

of the insertions to each other.

Work was done always with a surgical view, respecting the scleral insertions. All globes were removed. In enucleation, a muscle hook was used only for the 4 rectus muscles, never for an oblique muscle. The oblique muscles were cut from their global insertion by carefully raising them gently with forceps and not breaking their fine structures. Finally the lines of force were determined.

Data included:

1. Drawings of both obliques of each eye on their correspondent part of the scheme.
2. Measuring the distances from muscles to optic nerve and equator.
3. Photography of demonstrative cases.
4. Histologic study of fresh material, preserved material, and representative photos.

Lines of force were determined on the eye in respect to the anterior posterior meridian (APM) the mid-point of the superior rectus to the exterior optic nerve, and in respect to the horizontal meridian (MH), from a point in mid lateral rectus insertion to mid optic nerve, and in respect to the equator (E) and the maximum curvature measure from the limbus, with a compass.

RESULTS

Insertion pattern: both obliques have linear insertions. Ten SO and 36 IO had area insertions. The SO: the width was 1.5 to 6.0 mm and the length of insertion was 9 to 16 mm. The IO: width was 1.5 mm to 10 mm and the length was 5 mm to 20 mm. Linear insertions in both muscles were simply straight or curved, cornered, recurrent, complex and ravine.

The SO tendon is not in the same angle as the muscle, but forms a dihedral angle (forms a tent). In a linear pattern insertion which forms a fan. Both cases have to vertex toward the pulley.

Insertion quadrant: SO with nasal insertion 9 times, naso-temporal 13 cases, and temporal 28 cases. The IO had no cases above the horizontal meridian but was over the horizontal meridian 26 times, down below the horizontal meridian, and "hanging" from it, 24 times.

OTHER CHARACTERISTICS

The SO has insertions variable in surface, place, form, size and position. The IO has less variable insertions; it's not a muscle like a ribbon, but is thick, with an oval section.

HISTOLOGY

We studied 13 IO's from fresh bodies and observed the following: linear insertions were less than 1 mm and area insertions were more than 1 mm, broad and open.

Macroscopy showed area insertions presenting always with the same pattern - similar to a tent, with the external face of the muscle, fibrotic, extended on the sclera; the internal face was only muscle. The width of the tent base was 1.2 mm to 8.8 mm.

Microscopy showed an external face in continuation with the sclera. The external face was made of fibers of the tendon, but internal face was only muscular. The interior of the tent was occupied by muscle fibers, or by muscle fibers and conective tissue. In 8 muscles suspected of area insertion, 7 were area insertions; 5 suspected to be linear but were in area. So, from 13 cases studied, 11 were area insertions.

SURGERY VERIFICATION IN HUMAN BEINGS

IO photos made of surgery showing the same things mentioned above.

DISCUSSION

From over 50 eyes we found that scleral insertions of both obliques had variations from the classical descriptions. The variations were marked in two senses: They showed largely 1) area insertions and 2) inserted on different places on the globe.

We think that with a fine dissection, similar to the one used in the operating room by an ophthalmologist, is possible to see the true insertions of the oblique muscles. Only a fine strabismus surgeon is able to look for the new types of insertions. There seems to be more area insertions than the linear classical ones. The SO varies enormously as to the place of insertion and, the IO is inserted 100% higher than the classical description. SO tendon occupies a dihedral angle. The IO is a thick muscle, with oval section.

In conclusion, neither SO nor IO have linear scleral insertions 100% of the time. Nor are they in the strict scleral place as the classical descriptions describes them.

We document a new anatomical concept verified by dissection, photography (corpses and living patient), and histology (fresh and conserved).

In 50 eyes the scleral insertions are:

Superior Oblique	Inferior Oblique
80% linear	72% area
20% area	28% linear
44% nasal	52% up above the horizontal mer.
	48% "hung" from the horizontal mer.
	(100% higher than the classical concept)
Very variable: form, surface position, size, place.	Not so variable. Thick muscle Oval section
Tendon: dihedral angle	

REFERENCES - Not Included by Author

ACKNOWLEDGEMENTS

Technicians: I. Lopardo
M. Melognio
A. Martin
Histology: Dr. N. Reissenweber
Anatomy: Dr. D. Varela (Bibliography and conserved corpses)

DISCUSSION BY T. NAKAGAWA

We frequently encounter motor anomalies of the oblique muscles. However, their anatomy has not been pursued in recent times. The insertions of the obliques are famous for their variability. These two papers are further verification of their variability. Dr. Bernasconi concluded that the superior oblique has both linear and area insertions. In some cases insertions are on the nasal side of the anteroposterior meridian of the globe and are placed 100% higher than the classical description. The cross section of the inferior oblique was thick and oval. Dr. Fuchs, in his text book of ophthalmology published in 1923, noted that the S.O. has two kind of insertions, one broad and the other linear. Dr. Bernasconi reconfirmed Dr. Fuch´s description and presented beautiful slides demonstrating various kinds of insertions and precise statistical analysis. It is also interesting that some of the insertions of superior obliques are nasal to the anteroposterior meridian, a controversial point in previous papers. These results may come from the meridian proposed in this report which is somewhat more temporally situated than the conventional anteroposterior plane. The insertion of I.O. in this report lies above the horizontal meridian in 52% of cases which has been believed below the meridian. (This is contraversial to Dr. Emmel´s paper.) Finally not only I.O. but also all extraocular muscles are oval in their cross section except in their tendinous portions.

THE HISTOPATHOLOGY OF HUMAN STRABISMIC EXTRAOCULAR MUSCLE

K. W. McNeer

ABSTRACT

Until recently there was no identifiable pathologic alteration in human strabismic extraocular muscle in either light microscopic or electron microscopic sections. Moreover, the normal microscopic anatomy of human extraocular muscle is not well defined since the bulk of material reported in the literature is based on material from sub-human species. There are conflicting reports between the physiological and the anatomic classifications of fiber systems in the extraocular muscle of all mammalian species. It is generally agreed that there are at least fast and slow functions of mammalian extraocular muscle but disagreement remains on defining the fiber types as seen under light microscopy and electron microscopy. The histopathologic findings found by the author are presented. The microscopic alteration occurred in the fast fiber system of the orbital muscle layer and involved primarily the mitochondria.

STRABISMUS II
ISBN 0-8089-1424-3

DISCUSSION BY T. NAKAGAWA

Dr.McNeer has beautifully demonstrated the histopathological findings and concluded that the microscopic alternation in strabismic extraocular muscles occurred primarily in the fast fiber system involving mitochondria. The mammalian extraocular muscles have two layers, orbital and global. Each layer has several fiber types. Dr. Furuno reported fiber types on human I.O. by histochemical methods. In general slow fibers are small in diameter with numerous mitochondria and are located on the orbital side. Fast fibers are large in diameter, located on the global side and their mitochondoria are not numerous. However, these two major fibers are difficult to differentiate when the cross section of the muscle is near its tendinous part, usually losing their characteristics. Slow fibers seem to be losing their mitochondria. Control study of cross section of the same area is indispensable to confirm the conclusion. In 1980 Dr. Martinez reported a minimal but constant morphological difference between strabismic and non-strabismic extraocular muscles. It would be desirable to study a complete cross section area of the muscle at different levels. Dr. McNeer´s excellent presentation has given us further knowledge of the human strabismic muscles.

DEVELOPMENT OF THE NERVES OF THE EXTRAOCULAR MUSCLES

D. Sevel

ABSTRACT

This is the first detailed description of the development of the nerves of the extra-ocular muscles. Based on the examination of serial sections of embryos and fetuses ranging in size from 13.6 mm to term a holistic description is given of the development of the extra-muscular and intra-muscular nerves.

The abducent, oculomotor and trochlear nerves can be differentiated in the 22.0 mm sized embryo. The intramuscular nerves, however, only appear to be noted in the 68.5 mm sized embryo. At this stage of development entwining spirals, incomplete rings, flower sprays, and spindle nerve endings are observed. Sympathetic nerves are first observed in the 165.0 mm sized fetus.

The intra-muscular nerves develop in 3 stages:

1. Stage of "Rete" formation (38.2 mm to 54.0 mm)
2. Stage of differential degeneration (54.0 mm to 61.3mm)
3. Stage of specialization

The clinical significance of nerve development in the extra-ocular muscles is considered with reference to Duane's Retraction Syndrome and congenital absence of the abducent nerve.

INTRODUCTION

To date the development of the nerves of extraocular muscles has not been fully studied. The purpose of this investigation is to re-evaluate the embryological development of the nerves within the extraocular muscles.

MATERIALS AND METHODS

Fifty-four embryos and fetuses, ranging in size from 13.6 mm to term were examined.(1) The normal development of the embryo/fetus was an essential pre-requisite, so the conceptus of known induced abortions was not accepted for investigation. If the mother was exposed to teratogenic drugs

STRABISMUS II
ISBN 0-8089-1424-3

during pregnancy the embryos or fetuses were excluded from the survey. Where salpingectomies were done (for ectopic pregnancies), the Fallopian tubes were dissected with the aid of a dissecting microscope and the embryos retrieved.

The age of the embryo/fetus was determined by the crown-rump length. A micrometer gauge was used for measuring the length of the fetus up to 170 mm, thereafter a centimeter metal ruler was used.

Furthermore, the development of the eye was correlated with the development of other organs of the body. It was then possible to assess this interrelationship, and therefore confirm the age of embryo/fetus.(2)

The specimens were examined macroscopically with a dissecting microscope. Small specimens (smaller than 80.0 mm crown-rump length) were fixed for at least one week and larger specimens (larger than 80.0 mm crown-rump length) for at least two weeks.

The specimens were serially sectioned. Every attempt was made to obtain conventional planes of anatomy viz frontal (coronal) and transverse (horizontal) planes. Sections were stained with hematoxylin-eosin, Masson trichrome, methanimine silver, periodic acid schiff, and luxol fast blue.

RESULTS

The nerves of muscle develop pari passu with the maturation of the extra-ocular muscles. Contemporaneously with intramuscular development of the nerves, the definitive extramuscular component of the oculomotor, trochlear and abducent nerves are seen to form and to enter the muscle. At the 26.0 mms stage of maturation, the nerves enter the muscle at right angles but with muscular growth and elongation this "angle" of entry becomes acute (Fig 1). At the junction of the posterior third and anterior two thirds, where the nerve trunk enters the muscle, the branches of the nerve are large. A "T" shaped division of the nerve occurs, the one limb of the "T" passing posteriorly to the origin, the anterior limb of the "T" passing towards the tendon of insertion. The branches become smaller proximally and distally. The nerves show constant division but evidenced no characteristic pattern to this division. The nerves divide and ramify around the early myoblasts. Towards the tendons (origin and insertion) the nerves are in parallel bundles of two to four and are more attenuated than those nerves which end on the motor endplates. The intramuscular nerves develop in distinct stages (Fig 2).

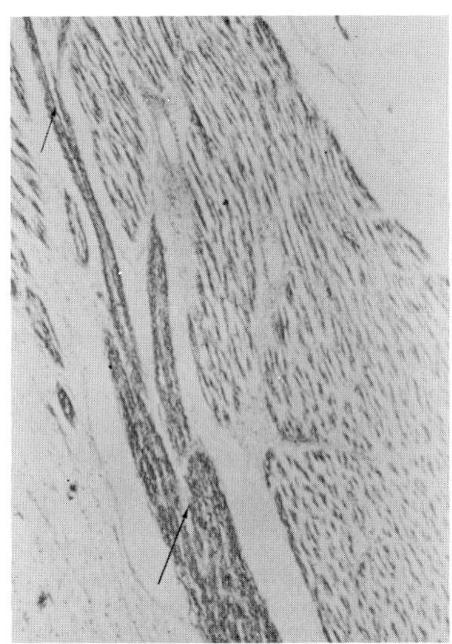

Figure 1. 4/72 22.0 mms Division of abducent nerve (arrowed) occurs on entering lateral rectus muscle. Silver X 40.95

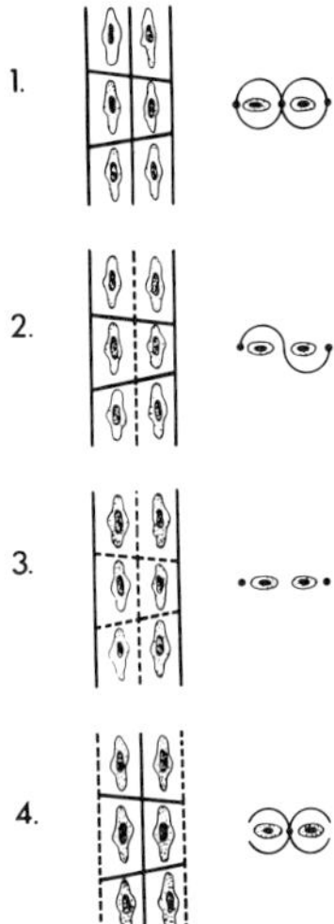

Figure 2. NEUROGENESIS

1. Stage of "rete" formation is present

2, 3 and 4 are stages of differential degeneration indicated by broken lines. Note formation of spiral and annulo-spiral nerves.

The fine nerves are arranged around the myoblasts in a net-like fashion. This enmeshment of the embryonic muscle cells extends the whole length of the muscle, from origin to insertion. The "rete-like nerves" are concentrated at the neuro-vascular hilum.

II. State of differential degeneration (54.0 mms - 61.3 mms) (Figure 3).

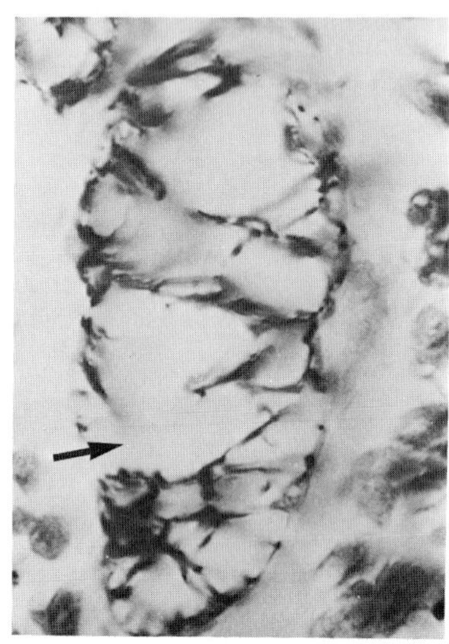

Figure 3. 33/73 59.5 mms
Differential degeneration (arrowed) of nerves has occurred.
Silver x 650

These intramuscular nerves degenerate differentially. The stage of "rete" formation imperceptibly merges with the stage of differential degeneration. The differential degeneration of the developing nerves doe not have a specific pattern. No constant nerve distribution is discernable in any one extraocular muscle.

III. Stage of Specialization (68.5 mms onwards).

Specialized nerve endings (motor, sensory, and their respective specialized nerve endings) are first observed at 68.5 mms stage of development. Characteristic features of the innervation of extraocular muscles are the profusion of the nerves relative to the bulk of its muscle, the frequency with which nerve endings are noted, and the repeated division of the nerves in the muscle (Fig 4).

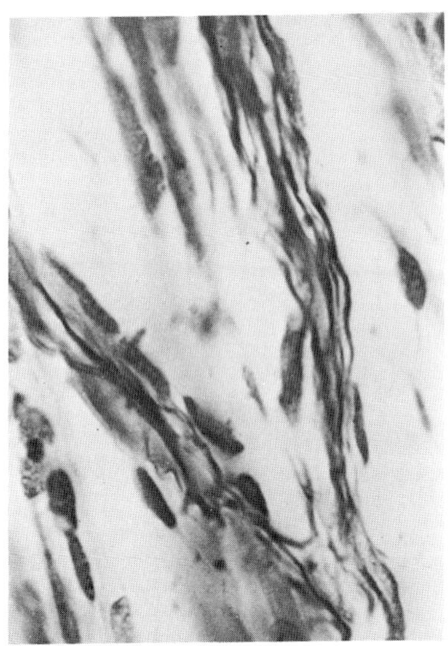

Figure 4. 34/73 80.0 mms
The extraocular muscles have a rich nerve supply. Note the repeated division of the nerves.
Silver x 650

IV. Specific Nerves

A. Motor Fibres

Motor fibers are recognized morphologically by a gradual thickening at their endings. These fibers cross the muscle fibers transversely and then divide. Each division ends on a muscle or on a motor end-plate (Fig 5).

B. Sensory Fibres

These are found both in the muscle and in the tendon. The sensory fibers are abundant, do not end on motor end-plates but do have specific sensory nerve endings. It can be difficult with light microscopy to differentiate motor from sensory nerves if their specific nerve endings are not visualized. This difficulty is compounded if the muscles examined are cut transversely. A sensory fiber may pass distally and then reverse its direction, thus retracing its course and only then end on a sensory end-organ (Fig 6). At varying positions on the musculo-tendinous junction the sensory nerves divide frequently and terminate in the tendon

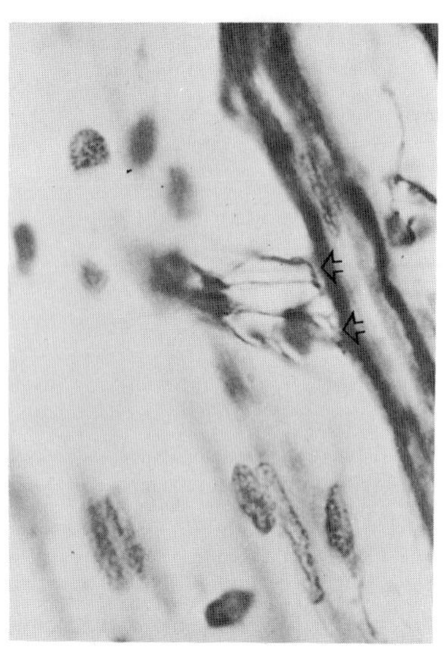

Figure 5. 2/72 88.6 mms
Motor-end plate is on muscle fiber (arrowed)
Silver x 650

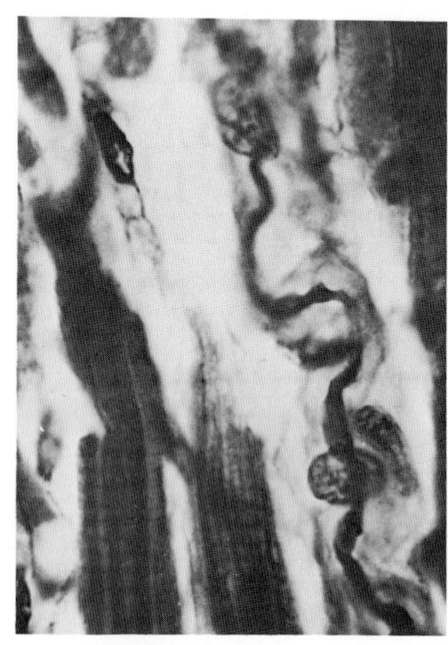

Figure 6. 14/72 115 mms
Tortous spiral nerve ending is adjacent to muscle fibres.
There are varicosities present on the nerves.
Silver x 650

fibers. In this series tendon organs are not seen in the sections examined.

C. Vasomotor nerves

The sympathetic nerves are first noted in the 165.0 mms sized fetus and can only be recognized in this investigation by their location in relation to blood vessels (Fig 7). The sympathetic nerves in spindles can not be distinguished with any certainty. The nerves around the vessels develop much like the nerves in the muscle. Thus up to the 80.0 mms stage of development a "rete"-like arrangement of nerves occurs around the muscle arterioles. From 80.0 mms to 165.0 mms there is differential degeneration of the nerves. After the 165.0 mms stage of development the sympathetic nerves are entwined around the arterioles and are morphologically recognizable as autonomic nerves.

D. Myelinization of Nerves

Myelinization of the extra- and intramuscular components of the oculomotor, trochlear, and abducent nerves is not noted in the embryos and the early fetuses. Only scanty myelinization of these nerves is present in the full term fetus. In the adult specimens, however, myelinization of nerves are distinctly observed.

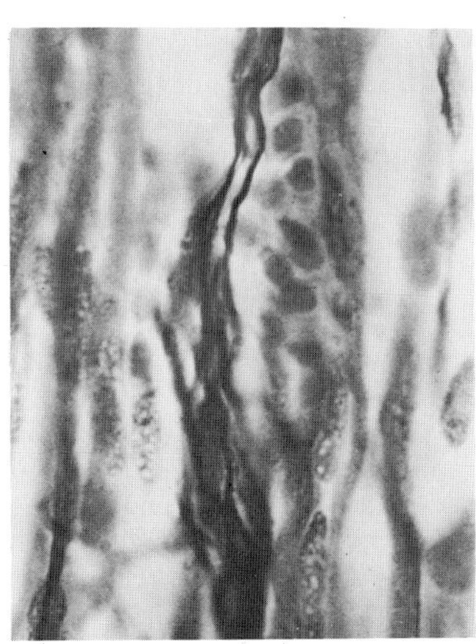

Figure 7. 68/74 210 mms
Autonomic nerves are adjacent to the blood vessel
Silver x 650

DISCUSSION

No consensus of opinion prevails about the development of nerves in skeletal muscle. Boeke(2) first noted nerves in muscle at the myotube stage of muscle development. Iwanaga(3) only recognized nerves in developing human muscle at the 19 mms stage of development. Tello(4,5) observed that nerves developed in voluntary muscles at different stages and that the muscle and the nerve endings of the tongue were the first to develop. The extraocular muscles were among "the latest to differentiate". Sensory nerve endings developed before the motor nerve endings. At the 8 week stage of development myofibrils began to differentiate and bulbous nerve endings were seen. At the 10-12 week stage of development, the amount of connective tissue increased and large numbers of nuclei were present in the muscles. Varicose nerve endings were noted in the myotube stage of development. Between 12-22 weeks, myotubes multiplied, and spindles were noted. From the 22-26 week, the myotubes "disassociate from one another" and their nuclei became peripheral. Between 26-28 weeks, the motor end-plates developed.(6) To determine the age, Tello(4,5) used time of gestation rather than the length of the embryo/fetus. The accuracy of the gestation period (as determined by clinical history) is questionable. Furthermore, the author does not define or describe the terms used, e.g., myoblast, myotubes, muscle cells, spindles and motor end-plates. Straus and Weddell(7) first noted nerves in limb muscle at 65 weeks stage of development. By the 8th week of development discrete nerve bundles were noted and these had the appearance of adult nerve. Rexed(8) investigated the development of peripheral nerves in muscle and concluded that only in the newborn, could motor nerves be differentiated from sensory nerves. Medullation of the nerves commenced at the 4th month of development and was only completed at 3 years of age.(9)

Wolter(10-13) used a silver stain technique to demonstrate the nerves of the extraocular muscles. He distinguished motor nerve endings (endings on the muscle) vegetative nerve endings (endings on vessels) and sensory nerve endings viz:-muscle bud-like endings, aboreal endings, and brush-like endings. The latter were morphological descriptions of the sensory nerve endings and were situated in the interstitial tissue and not in contact with the muscle fibers. The oculomotor or trochlear and abducent nerves in human embryo were first observed at six weeks, seven weeks and eight weeks respectively.(14) Sakamoto(15) noted that the motor nerves of the extraocular muscle all reached their respective muscles by the eighth week of development. Okamoto(16) examined 45 fetuses between 2-9 months of development and commented that nerve fibers were first seen in the extraocular muscles in the third month of development, the motor endplates at eight months and the spiral nerve endings were only observed in the ninth month of development.

In this investigation, it is not possible to differentiate between the motor and sensory fibers except if the fibers were examined in relation to their respective termination to a motor endplate on to sensory nerve endings.

Motor endplates are first noted on the extra and the intrafusal fibers at the 68.5 mms stage of development. It is not possible to distinguish the different plate endings vis. P_1, P_2 and motor endplates within the spindles. Plate-endings can be differentiated from the trail endings and are discrete while the trail endings extend over a long area of intrafusal surface.

Nerve fibers are observed which entwine around the equatorial region of the nuclear bag and the nuclear chain region of spindles. Spiral and incomplete rings are noted as well (Fig 8). It is not possible, however, to distinguish with any certainty between primary and secondary sensory nerves. Spray arrangements of nerve endings are also noted. Nerve endings are not visualized on tendons.

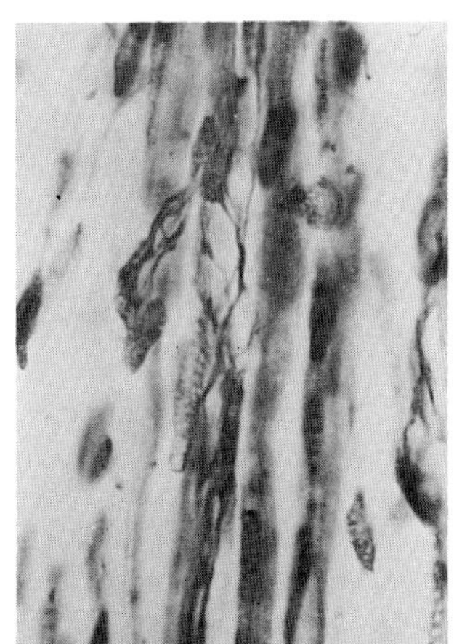

Figure 8. 5/72 70.0 mms
The spiral nerves are in relation to the multinucleated myoblasts
Silver x 650

Entwining spiral incomplete rings and flower-spray nerve endings are observed infrequently at the 68.5 mms stage of development, but are observed with greater frequency in the 80 mms sized fetus. The entwining spiral and incomplete ring nerve endings are more frequently observed than the flower-spray form of nerve endings.

Free nerve endings are profuse and are the most commonly observed nerve fibers. These free nerve fibers are characterized by the presence of varicose filaments along their course and are predominantly related to the muscle spindles, the interstitial tissue of the muscle, the fat and the blood vessels. These nerves are first observed in the 68.5 - 80 mms sized fetuses.

Occasional spindles are distinguished at the 68.5 mms stage of development. As the fetus matures, spindles become more evident. More spindles are present per field of observation in the adult extraocular muscles as compared to a corresponding field in the full-term fetus (Figure 9). Only once the muscle is cut longitudinally is it possible to differentiate the nuclear chain from the nuclear bag region of the spindle. Furthermore, it is only in longitudinal sections that nerve endings on the spindle can be seen with any certainty. In this investigation, it was not possible to distinguish the spindle motor from sensory fibers unless the terminal ends of these fibers were examined in relation to either motor or sensory endings.

The arterioles are first observed in the 165.0 mms sized fetus but are more evident in the larger fetus. The sympathetic nerves develop soon after the development and maturation of the arterioles. Fine nerves are observed to entwine and surround these vessels. Again as the muscle matures more arterioles are observed. Hence more entwining sympathetic nerves are noted in the adult as compared to the number observed in the full-term fetus.

There appears to be no advantage of the solochrome cyanine method for staining myelin over the luxol fast blue stain.(17) The most satisfactory method of demonstrating myelin in the nerves would be with the electron microscope. Cottrell(18) examined the peripheral nerves of the newborn and found that "myelin was exceedingly scanty in the newborn". Furthermore, axis cylinders of peripheral nerves were only observed after birth until the age of four years. At two and one-half years, only one-third to one-half of the nerve fibers were myelinated. Rexed(8), contrary to the above

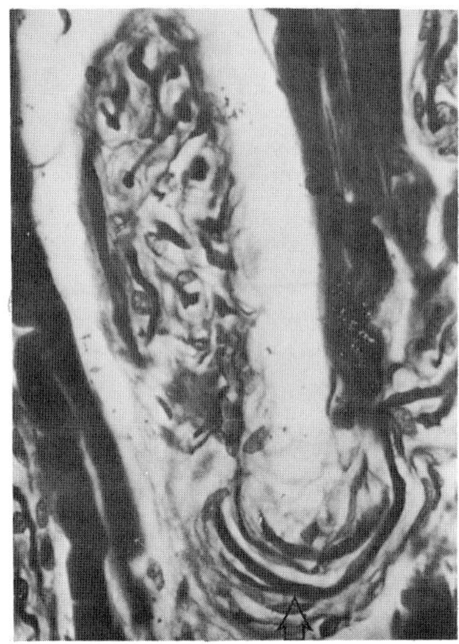

Figure 9. 71/74 Adult
Nerve fibres (arrowed) terminate on spindle which is surrounded by muscle fibres
Silver x 260

investigation, found myelinization of peripheral nerves in 150 mms sized fetuses. Lewis(17) commented that human myelinated nerve fibers increased in size only in the early post-natal period. These nerve fibers then continued to become myelinated for some months after birth.

Myelin sheaths may be missed, because in the preparation of the specimens, the nerves are passed through alcohol, which may dissolve the fat of the myelin sheath.

In this investigation myelinization of the nerves of muscle is only present in the full term fetus and in the adult specimens so no comment can be made prior to this time on the different types of sensory nerves viz. types I-IV sensory nerves.

REFERENCES

1. Sevel D: A reappraisal of the origin of human extraocular muscles. Ophthalmology 88(12):1330-1338, 1981.

2. Boeke J: Anat Anz 35:193-224, 1909. As quoted by Tiegs OW. Physiological Reviews 33:90-144, 1953.

3. Iwanaga I. Mitt Allg Path u Path Anat (Sendai) 2:257-341, 1923-1926. Quoted by Tiegs OW. Physiological Reviews 33:90-144, 1953.

4. Tello JF: Genesis de las terminaciones nerviosas motrices y sensetivas. En el sistema locomotor de lasvertebrodos superiores. Histogenesis-muscular. Trab Lab Invest Biol (Madril) 15:101-199, 1917.

5. Tello JF: Die entstehung der motorischen und sensiblen nervendigungen. 1. Indem loko motorischen systeme der Hoheren Wirbeltiere. Ztschr Anat Entwicklung 64:384-440, 1922.

6. Hewer EE: The development of nerve endings in the human foetus. J Anat 69:369-379, 1935.

7. Straus WL, Weddell G: Nature of the first visible contractions of the forelimb musculature in rat fetuses. J Neurophysiol 3:358-369, 1940.

8. Rexed B: Contributions to the knowledge of the post-natal development of the peripheral nervous system in man. Acta Psychiat Neurol (Suppl) 33:1-206, 1944.

9. Langworthy OR: Development of behavior patterns and myelinization of the nervous system in the human fetus and infant. Contrib to Embryol No. 24:1-57, 1933.

10. Wolter JR: Die nervenendigungen in der ausseren augenmuskalatur. Ber Kongr Deutsche Ophthalmol Gesellsch Heidelberg 57:285-287, 1951.

11. Wolter JR: Uber nervenendigungen in der ausseren augenmuskalatur. Acta Neurovegt 4:343-353, 1952.

12. Wolter JR: Morphology of the sensory nerve apparatus in striated muscle of the human eye. Arch Ophthalmol 53:201-207, 1955.

13. Wolter JR: Moderne neuropathologie am auge angewandt. Klin monatblatter fur augenheilk. 126:670-678, 1955.

14. Cooper ERA: The trochlear nerve in the human embryo and foetus. Brit J Ophthalmol 31:257-275, 1947.

15. Sakamoto M: Embryology of the 3rd, 4th and 6th cranial nerves. Acta Soc Ophthalmol Jap 57:146-148, 1953. Quoted by Mann I. The Development of the Human Eye. New York: Grune and Stratton Inc., 1969.

16. Okamoto T: A study on the genesis of the spiral nerve ending in the extrinsic ocular muscle. Jap J Ophthalmol 4:12-15, 1960. Quoted by Duke-Elder S and Cook C. System of Ophthalmology. Normal and Abnormal Development 1963; Vol III.

17. Lewis PD. Personal communication. 1975.

18. Cottrell L: Histologic variations with age in apparently normal peripheral nerve trunks. Arch Neurol & Psychiat 43:1138-1150, 1940.

DISCUSSION BY T. NAKAGAWA

Dr. Sevel reported his outstanding work on the development of intra-muscular nerve. The first stage of rete formation, the second stage of differential degeneration and the third stage of specialization. I wonder whether or not all kinds of neuro-muscular junctions can be found in human skeletal muscles that can be found in human extraocular muscle in relation to their properties of responses.

THE USE OF A SCAN ULTRASONOGRAPHY TO DESIGN THE STRABISMUS OPERATION

W. E. Gillies and A. McIndoe

ABSTRACT

In this technique, 3 pre-operative measurements are important:

1. The diameter of the eye which allows calculation of the circumference of the eye and the distance from the central cornea to the geometric equator.
2. The length of the oculomotor axis from the front of the eye to the orbital apex.
3. The oculomotor angle between the oculomotor axis and the anterior-posterior axis from which it is about 10 degrees divergent. The position of the oculomotor equator is about 2 mm closer to the limbus on the medial side than the geometric equator and 2 mm further on the lateral side. At operation, the corneal diameter and the position of the rectus muscle insertions are measured and the muscle length calculated.

The operation is designed by estimating the amount of recession from the angle of deviation and the circumference of the eye. This must be accompanied by a corresponding resection to take up the slack in the antagonist or else a similar recession should be performed upon the opposite eye. To maintain full muscle action, it is preferred not to recess a muscle beyond the oculomotor equator and resections are usually 0.20 to 0.30 of the muscle length.

INTRODUCTION

It often seems that the Micawber principle applies in squint surgery, so recession required: 5 mm, recession performed: 5 mm, result, happiness with perfect parallelism. On the other hand recession required: 5 mm; recession performed: 4 mm, or 6 mm, result, misery and we sit around, Micawber-like, waiting for something to turn up --- or in --- or out.

Ultrasonography enables more accurate planning of the strabismus operation although we recognize that many other

STRABISMUS II
ISBN 0-8089-1424-3

factors influence the behavior of the eyes at and following strabismus surgery.(1,2) Although we must remember these other factors, if we ignore the geometry of the strabismus operation we can hardly hope for optimal results. A considerable variation of dimensions occurs in strabismic eyes. The purpose of this paper is to systematically evaluate the data available for the surgeon's consideration.

METHOD

Using A scan ultrasonography, the following measurements are made:

1. The diameter of the eye, this may be done in an A-P direction or along the oculomotor axis. Since the eye is usually spherical, the circumference is easily calculated and then the measurement of a quadrant from the center of the cornea to the equator. (See Fig 1.)

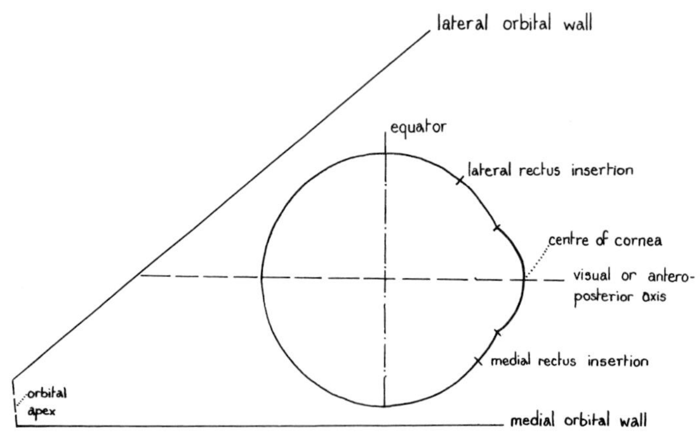

Figure 1. Measurement of the A-P diameter of the eye by A scan which allows calculation of the circumference of the eye and a quadrant from the central cornea to the geometric equator.

2. The length of the oculomotor axis, this is the axis around which the recti muscles are disposed and act. It runs from the front of the eye through the center of the eye to the apex of of the orbit where the recti muscles arise and it is divergent to the antero-posterior axis of the eye. The

oculomotor equator of the eye is at right angles to this axis and it will be about 2 mm nearer the limbus on the nasal side than the transverse equator but 2 mm further on the lateral side so one may easily over-recess a medial but not so easily a lateral rectus. (See Figs 2 and 3).

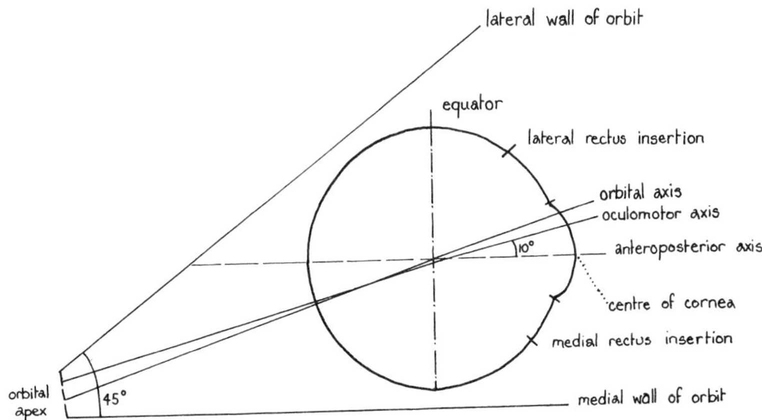

Figure 2. Measurement of the oculomotor axis and the distance from the front of the eye to the orbital apex. The oculomotor axis is about 10 degrees divergent to the antero-posterior axis and the orbital axis further divergent again.

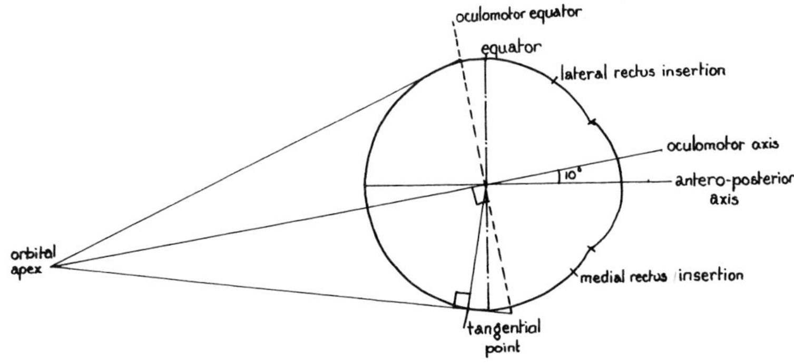

Figure 3. Measurement of the oculomotor equator which lies about 2 mm closer to the limbus on the medial size than the geometric equator and 2 mm further on the lateral side. The tangential point of maximum torque in the primary position is about 5 mm behind the oculomotor equator.

CASE REPORTS

Case 1: Age 10 years: originally an esodeviation.

Previous surgery: Bilateral medial rectus recession with recurrence. The surgery was reported once and produces a gross exotropic secondary deviation.

1979: Right recession of the lateral rectus and resection of the medial rectus muscle.

1982: Preoperatively left exodeviation was greater than 45 prism diopters (p.d.) far and near with some left medial rectus muscle weakness.
Axial lenghts: Right 22.94 mm, left 22.39 mm.
Oculomotor axis: Right 38 mm, left 38 mm.
Oculomotor angle: 10° - correction 2.04 mm.
Circumference (allow 1 mm for chorioretinal thickness) = 73.51 mm.
Quadrant (1/4 circumference) 18.38 mm.
Oculomotor equator 16.34 mm from corneal center medially but 20.42 mm laterally.
At operation: corneal diameter 12 mm.
Lateral rectus: 6 mm; medial rectus insertion 4 mm but previously recessed 5 mm.
So limbus to oculomotor equator
medially: 10.34 mm
laterally: 14.42mm
Safe lateral rectus recession 8.42 mm
Correction needed 30°
= 30/360 x 73.51 = 6.13 mm
∴ 8.5 mm recession of lateral rectus

Medial rectus length = distance from orbital apex to oculomotor equater + distance from insertion to oculomotor equator
= 28.79 + [Quadrant - (½ corneal diameter + distance from limbut)]
= 28.79 + (18.38 - 15)
= 32.17 mm
0.25 of muscle length ≃ 8 mm
Operation performed
Left recession lateral rectus - 8.5 mm
Left resection medial rectus 5 mm and advancement to old insertion. (total shortening ≃ 10 mm)
Post operatively 2 months
Near exo 2Δ - Distance eso 4Δ
Convergence fails at 20 cm

Case 2: Age 13 years

Left exotropic deviation 35Δ left hypertropia/6Δ
V pattern

Left I.O. overation: +++ Right I.O. overation: ++
Axial length: Right 21.4 mm Left 21.6 mm
Orbital apex: Right 36 mm Left 39 mm
Oculomotor angle: 10°
Circumference: 71.03 mm
Quadrant: 17.76 mm
Central cornea to oculomotor equator:
Medially: 15.79 mm
Laterally: 19.73 mm
At operation: corneal diameter: 11.0 mm; Lateral rectus insertion: 6.5 mm; Medial rectus insertion: 5.0 mm
So medial rectus to oculomotor equator
= 15.79 - (5.5 + 5.0)
= 5.49 mm
Lateral rectus to oculomotor equator = 19.73 - (6.5 + 5.5)
Corrections needed ≃ 17.5°
= 17.5/360 x 71.03
= 3.45 mm
Lateral rectus to oculomotor equator
= 29.92
Lateral rectus length = 29.92 + 7.73
= 37.65
0.25 of lateral rectus - 9.4 mm
Operation:
Left eye: recession medial rectus 5 mm, resection lateral rectus 8 mm, and recession inferior oblique 10 mm.
Right eye: recession inferior oblique 7 mm.
Post operatively:
No V pattern,
Distance: 10Δ Esotropia Left Hypertropia 2Δ
Near: 2Δ Exotropia Left Hypertropia 2Δ

At operation two measurements were made:

1. The corneal diameter - 'white to white'.

2. The distance of the rectus muscle insertion from the limbus.

Knowing the circumference of the eye and the oculomotor angle, the position of the oculomotor equator may be calculated and its distance from the limbus estimated. If it is decided not to recess a muscle behind the oculomotor equator then the maximal recession may be estimated at operation when the distance of the muscle insertion from the limbus is measured. The length of a rectus muscle may also be estimated by calculating the length from the orbital apex to the oculomotor equator and adding the distance to its insertion. The maximum resection as a proportion of muscle length may then be calculated. Our regard for the different characteristics of the muscles, caused us to prefer not to exceed a ratio of 0.25 resection for a medial rectus muscle or 0.3 resection for the lateral rectus muscle.

To calculate the amount of surgery, the angle of deviation to be corrected is first estimated. Then the recession necessary to correct this angle of deviation is estimated in mm from the circumference of the globe and an additional 1mm - 2 mm added to allow for loss of effectivity in cutting and suturing the muscle. As residual slack in the antagonist muscle will take up about half of this recession the antagonist muscle will take up about half of this recession the antagonist must be subjected to an appropriate shortening or else an equal recession of similar degree must be performed on the opposite eye in order to fully correct the deviation.

SOURCES OF ERROR

The use of ultrasonography to measure the dimensions of the eye involves some approximation which may lead to small errors which should be recognised.

The antero-posterior diameter is from the front of the cornea to the anterior surface of the retina and if this is to measure the diameter of the globe a correction for the thickness of retina choroid and sclera should be added. We have used a correction of 1 mm.

Measurement of distances on the surface of the eye,

e.g., corneal diameter involves an error, for these are chord measurements and not circumferential measurements. The error is small, e.g., for a cornea of 12 mm in an eye of 24 mm it is less than 0.5 mm.

It should be remembered that although the recti muscles of the eye are arranged about the oculomotor axis, this axis does not necessarily pass through the center of rotation of the eye, the position of which may vary in different positions of gaze and differs between eyes. It is assumed that the center of rotation lies near the geometric center of the eye.

Because of the technical factors we have measured the oculomotor axis in relation to the fixation axis which is somewhat divergent from the antero-posterior axis of the eye, so that we are probably understating a little the divergence of the oculomotor axis from the antero-posterior axis. As the angle (α) involved is up to 5 degrees the understatement will be up to 1 mm, but again this is variable and may be different for myopic eyes.

Measurement of the diameter of the eye is highly reproducible to a level of ± 0.01 mm, the measurement to the orbital apex is only reproducible to ± 2 mm and the orbital apex is not measured as a single point. The oculomotor angle is accurate to ± 2 degrees.

DISCUSSION

Measurement of strabismic eyes with ultrascan shows a considerable variation in ocular dimensions and if surgery is designed taking these dimensions and the angle of deviation into account there is a considerable variation in the amount needed to produce a given result. This is particularly so for recessions but less so for resections, since the muscle length varies proportionately less than the distance of the insertions from the equator, in particular the medial rectus insertion is often fairly close to the oculomotor equator.

If a rectus muscle is recessed behind the oculomotor equator, loss of torque in the primary position will only occur if the muscle is recessed behind the tangential point where the line of action of the muscle is tangential to the globe and which is about 5 mm behind the oculomotor equator.(3,4) On the medial side this represents a movement of about 20 degrees adduction before the oculomotor equator reaches the tangential point and loss of torque starts to occur. Only if a muscle is recessed behind the tangential point will muscle action be weakened in the primary position. If a muscle is recessed to a site behind the oculomotor equator but in front of the tangential point there will be a progressive weakening of the muscle the further it is recessed in its direction of action but this may be acceptable in large deviations where the surgeon is aware of the factors involved. The surgeon may decide that to secure parallel visual axes an acceptable price may be some weakness of adduction.

Another factor which may limit the action of a recessed muscle is excessive shortening of the distance between its origin and its insertion so that the muscle can no longer contract effectively. This is less likely to apply with the medial rectus where the amount of recession possible is limited but it may be significant for the lateral rectus where large recessions are often possible and some shortening of the muscle may already have occurred in a longstanding exotropic deviation. We believe caution should be exercised if a recession approaches 0.25 of the muscle length.

In planning resections, we try to:

a) carry out a shortening appropriate to the amount of the recession performed, and

b) avoid excessive tightening of a muscle which will limit its ability to relax against the action of its antagonist.

We plan a resection of 0.20 to 0.30 of the muscle length and tend to smaller resections of the medial rectus because of its greater stiffness.

These ratios are still somewhat empirical but should be exceeded with caution and an understanding of the likely consequences.

We realize that many other factors affect the outcome of strabismus operations. We may deliberately under or overcorrect a deviation of we may deliberately under or overcorrect one muscle. Many other allowances must be made, e.g., with amblyopic eyes, with accommodative strabismus or with variation of the angle in different directions of gaze. It is unlikely that the correction of strabismus will ever be a purely geometric exercise.

ACKNOWLEDGEMENTS

We thank Kerrie Shegog for secretarial assistance, Miss J. Quilter for assistance with references and the help of the Melbourne University Department of Ophthalmology.

REFERENCES

1. Gilles WE, McIndoe A: Measurement of strabismus eyes with a scan ultrasonography. Aust J Ophthalmol 9:231-232, 1981.

2. Gillies WE, McIndoe A: The use of ultrasonography in determining the amount of extraocular muscle surgery in strabismus. To be published, Aust J Ophthalmol, Aug 1982.

3. Beisner DH: Reduction of ocular torque by medial rectus recession. Arch Ophthalmol 85:13-17, 1971.

4. Boeder P: The cooperation of extraocular muscles. Am J Ophthalmol 51:469-481, 1961.

DISCUSSION BY D. DUNLOP

Dr. Gillies has used ultrasonography to measure the size of the eye and the orbit so that he can calculate the torque potential of the relevant muscles and assess more accurately the optimum muscle displacement. It is obvious that the recession of the lateral rectus muscle can be greater than the recession of the medial rectus muscle before the onset of limitation. What is not so obvious is that he has shown that more that twice as much recession is possible in some eyes on the same horizontal muscle because of differences in the size of the globe and the length of the orbit.

We should pay more attention to such factors and perhaps in the future the use of CT scans will help to establish orbital size, shape and angulation standards. The use of calibrated tension forceps or muscle dynamometers might also help us achieve better precision in surgery.

ANATOMICAL VARIATION OF THE INSERTION OF THE INFERIOR OBLIQUE MUSCLE

D. K. Emmel, L. Apt and R. Foos

ABSTRACT

The existence of multiple ("bifid") insertions of the inferior oblique muscle is questioned by many ophthalmic surgeons. We carefully studied 200 autopsy eyes to delineate the extent of variability of the insertion of this muscle. One hundred muscles had single lines of insertion. The remaining 100 muscles had multiple separate and distinct insertions with a variety of dimensions. This study refutes the notion that bifid insertions are usually iatrogenic. The difference between the surgical and anatomic isolation of the insertion helps explain the discrepancy between the high incidence of multiple insertions and the infrequency of complicaitons of surgery involving the insertion of the inferior oblique muscle.

INTRODUCTION

Knowledge of the anatomy of the insertion of the inferior oblique muscle, particularly with regard to its variations and anomalies, is essential for accurate and reliable surgery on the muscle. Although early anatomic studies of the extraocular muscles(1-4) called attention to anomaliesof their insertions, many modern day surgeons have come to regard the occurrence of these anomalies as rare and their significance is minor. For example, one complication of inferior oblique muscle surgery is the occurrence of a residual overction of the muscle after a weakening procedure. Many ophthalmologists on finding at reoperation a portion of the insertion still intact are likely to regard this finding to result from previous iatrogenic splitting of the muscle rather than from the existence of an unrecognized supernumerary ("bifid") insertion.

In a previous study of the anatomy of the inferior oblique muscle Apt and Call(5) noted the occasional occurrence of supernumerary insertions of the inferior oblique muscle. (Mentioned in presentation of this paper at the annual meeting of the American Association of Pediatric Ophthalmology, April 6, 1977, San Francisco, CA) Recently, Wilson and Landers(6) reported the incidental finding during retinal detachment

STRABISMUS II
ISBN 0-8089-1424-3

surgery of an anomalous duplication of the inferior oblique muscle. The present study was undertaken to document with precision the major variations of the insertion and specifically to assess the prevalence of multiple insertions of the inferior oblique muscle.

MATERIALS AND METHODS

We studies from 100 patients 200 autopsy eyes which were undeformed and without volume change. None of these individuals were documented to have strabismus. Age ranged from 4 to 95 years with a median age of 62 years. Only two individuals were less than 10 years old. The eyes originated from 76 males, 24 females, 66 whites, 25 blacks, 5 Hispanics and 4 Orientals.

The inferior oblique muscle was separated carefully from the globe to its point of insertion by blunt dissection and was examined at a magnification of 10 to 20 times by means of a stereomicroscope. All measurements were made to the nearest tenth of a millimeter with either calipers or a calibrated reticle, and appear in the text as the mean value plus or minus one standard deviation.

RESULTS

All inferior oblique muscles were found to insert on the globe in a linear fashion.

One hundred of 200 inferior oblique muscle insertions were found to be single, having the usual, classically described configuration and position. Single insertions were gently curved, convex upward, and tiled slightly from the horizontal meridian so that te anterior end of the insertion was 1-2 mm (mean 1.8 mm) lower than the posterior end of the insertion. The center of the insertion was, on the average 0.8 mm above the horizontal meridian. The single line of insertion averaged 10.1 ± 1.0 mm in length; the anterior end of the insertion averaged 16.4 ± 0.9 mm posterior to the external limbus and the posterior end 5.7 ± 1.0 mm anterior to the optic nerve sheath.

Only 15 of the 100 inferior oblique muscles with single insertions had a smooth line of insertion. The remaining 85 specimens in this group contained from 1 to 6 small thin reflections which projected diagonally backward from the inferior surface of the anterior end of the insertion. These reflections ranged in length from 0.4 to 3.9 mm (mean 1.7 mm), rarely were longer than 2.0 mm and except in four cases never extended more than 2.5 mm (mean 1.3 mm) below the line of insertion.

One hundred of the 200 inferior oblique muscle specimens had multiple insertions. Multiple insertions were composed of two to six distinct and separate insertions, although double and triple insertions accounted for 89% of the total number of muscles with multiple insertions. A typical pattern or configuration was identified and found to occur in 87 of 100 of the muscles with multiple insertions. This pattern consisted of a larger or primary insertion and a series of one to five smaller secondary insertions 1 to 3 mm in length, which were arrayed in a stack just below and slightly in front of the anterior end of the primary insertion. All components of multiple insertions were linear and roughly parallel to each other. Muscle bodies were found to divide at a point which ranged 1.2 to 18.2 mm proximal to the insertion with a mean distance of 5.6± 1.6 mm between the two most widely separated components.

The primary insertions averaged 8.3± 1.9 mm in length; their anterior end averaged 17.2± 2.1 mm from the external limbus and their posterior ends 5.9± 1.2 mm from the optic nerve sheath. Their centers were located on the average 1.4 mm above the horizontal meridian and they were most often found to be convex upward and tilted slightly in the opposite direction from the single inferior oblique muscle insertions so that the anterior end was approximately a millimeter (mean 1.3 mm) above the posterior end.

The secondary insertions averaged 3.3± 1.2 mm (range 0.6-6.3 mm) in length; their anterior ends averaged 16.8±1.6 mm from the external limbus and their posterior ends 11.5± 2.3 mm anterior to the optic nerve sheath. Secondary insertions nearly always were located below the horiontal meridian. Hence the secondary insertions were somewhat anterior in position compared with the primary insertions, their anterior ends corresponding closely in position to the anterior ends of single insertions.

Thirteen of the inferior oblique muscles with multiple insertions did not closely fit this pattern, having lines of insertion which were not parallel t each other, or having secondary insertions located in unusual positions such as posterior and superior to the primary insertion.

DISCUSSION

This study precisely documents the conformation of the insertions of the inferior oblique muscle and establishes the high frequency of multiple insertions of this extraocular muscle. This finding may be surprising tomany ophthalmic surgeons. The lack of published reports or discussion suggests that the high incidence and variety of multiple insertions is not widely appreciated; and the complications that might be expected to arise from such variations do not appear to occur frequently.

We feel that this discrepancy can be explained by the difference between thesurgical and anatomic isolation of the inferior oblique muscle. The deep anatomic positionof the insertion of the inferior oblique muscle and the reasonable constraints imposed by time and minimally disruptive surgery tend to limit the extent of dissection possible during the operation. These restrictions do not apply to the examination of autopsy specimens where the enucleated specimen can be optimally manipulated and dissected at leisure. Also, the inferior oblique muscle body often is isolated surgically with a muscle hook at a distance from its insertion (in most cases probably proximal to the point at which the muscle divides) and thus all of the insertions are gathered together as the hook is brought up to the actual insertion site. Nevertheless, multiple insertions of the inferior oblique muscle occur in sufficient numbers and are of sufficient dimensions to allow portions of a multiple insertion to be separately isolated, thus accounting for some cases of incomplete recession of the muscle or incomplete success from other operations that require a change in the position of the insertion.

On the basis of this study it apears that variations of the insertion of the inferior oblique muscle is substantial and potentially significant. The complications associated with surgery on the inferior oblique muscle near its insertion, including incomplete recession, may result from the presence of multiple ("bifid") insertions that are undetected by the ophthalmic surgeon, rather than from faulty technique in isolating the muscle.

ACKNOWLEDGEMENTS

Supported in part by Public Health Service Center Grant EY00331 and research grant EY00725, National Eye Institute, National Institutes of Health, Bethesda, MD

REFERENCES

1. Stevens T: A Treatise on the Motor Apparatus of the Eyes, Embracing an Exposition of the Ocular Adjustments and their Treatment with the Anatomy and Physiology of the Muscles and their Accessories, Philadelphia: FA Davis, p. 54, 1906.

2. Howe L: On the primary insertions of the ocular muscles. Trans Am Ophthalmol Soc 9:668-678, 1902.

3. Salzmann M: The Anatomy and Histology of the Human Eyeball in the Normal State. Its Development and Senescence. Chicago: University of Chicago Press, p. 9, 1912.

4. Duke-Elder S, Wybar KC: System of Ophthalmology, Vol 2, the Anatomy of the Visual System. London: Henry Kingston, p. 427, 1961.

5. Apt L, Call NB: Inferior oblique muscle recession. Am J Ophthalmol 85:95-100, 1978.

6. Wilson RS, Landers JH: Anomalous duplication of inferior oblique muscle. Am J Ophthalmol 93:521-522, 1982.

DISCUSSION BY T. NAKAGAWA

Dr. Emmel reported the impressive findings that the half of 200 insertions of I.O.´s were multiple and the secondary insertions were usually arranged in a stack below the anterior end of the primary insertion. We would like to see a statistical analysis as to how far from the insertion the I.O. divided. Since we usually operate the muscle several millimeters from its insertion, most of the cases do not have complications due to variations of the insertions of I.O´s.

THE POSITION OF THE EYES UNDER GENERAL ANESTHESIA IN ESOTROPIA

THE OPTO-MOTOR REFLEX AND THE STRETCH TEST

P. V. Berard, R. Reydy, and D. Jordan

ABSTRACT

Under deep general anesthesia the eye devisation is often not the same under light stimulation and may change after four to five minutes in the dark (light-dark effect). After studying a group of esotropic patients three provisional conclusions may be stated: (1) The variations of convergence under general anesthesia are not connected only with spasm of the contracture, nor the age of the child nor the duration of the strabismus, but vary with the opto-motor reflexes which evidence the degree of suppression. (2) The variations of the opto-motor reflex (with or without light stimulation) seem to demonstrate the dominance of the temporal retinal half in esotropia. (3) From a therapeutic point of view, the eye position under general anesthesia prior to surgery is an unreliable measurement. The muscle stretching test must show large abnormal modifications to be considered clinically reliable. We must rely only on the clinical examination and make a strict rule to eleiminate by surgery all obstacles which prevent fusional reflexes from being re-established.

INTRODUCTION

Many authors have studied the position of the eyes under general anesthesia in the hope of improving surgical technique.(1,7,15,16,18,19,22,25) Their researches resulted in several divergent opinions that can be summarized as follows:

(1) The position of the eyes is not predictable and one cannot draw any practical conclusion. This is the opinion held by Ardouin.(2)

(2) The position of the eyes is a function of muscular spasm and of contracture in connection with the visco-elastic modifications of the muscle. This view is held by Souron et al(23), Quere et al.(19)

STRABISMUS II
ISBN 0-8089-1424-3

(3) The position of the eye is contradictory; therefore, in congenital esotropia with large deviation some have observed a reduction in the strabismic angle under general anesthesia;(3,8,9,12) and others(18,19) have observed the persistance or the exaggeration of the deviation. Some authors even notice that the younger the child the higher the probability of persistance or exaggeration of the deviation under general anesthesia(18,19,25).

We believe that these views represent new interpretations if we take into account the opto-motor reflexes in the course of general anesthesia. One perceives that the esotropic deviation is often different according to whether the subject is in the darkness or under the operating light. These clinical observations have been confirmed by the electromyographic researches of Mitsui and Tamura.(15)

On the other hand, a correlation between muscular elasticity and variation of the esotropic deviation under general anesthesia has been sought. For instance, Quere(18,19) thinks that muscular elasticity should diminish when the convergent deviation persists under general anesthesia. According to us, the modifications of muscular elasticity indicated by the stretching test are purely random.

Because of these contradictions we regrouped 100 cases in which (1) the esotropic deviation under general anesthesia had been studied in relation to the level of brightness; and (2) the stretching test had been studied in relation to the esotropic deviation under general anesthesia.

MATERIALS AND METHODS

We studied 100 cases of operated esotropia with ages ranging from 1.5 to 31 years; only 5 cases were older than 11 years. All these strabismus had normal ductions before surgery and had no previous surgery.

The type of anesthesia

The anesthetic procedure was always the same. Premedication in the young child (2 years of age) consisted of Phenobarbital suppository (3mg/kg) given 45 minutes before surgery; older children are given an intramuscular injection of atropine (1.0mg/kg) plus another injection of Diazepan (1mg/kg). Induction stage is obtained with increasing concentrations of Halothane conveyed with nitrous-oxygen. Intubation stage is carried out up to 6-7 years of age with

Halothane only; after 7 years of age Halothane is associated with Suxamethonium (lmg/kg). After intubation stage we study the eye position; Halothane is then suppressed and Euflurane with Droperidol-Fentanyl (potentialisator) is given to older children. No curarizing drug is contained in the anesthetic adminitered.

Strabismic deviation under general anesthesia in relation to brightness

Once the patient was deeply asleep, we had studied the strabismic deviation after 10 minutes in the darkness and after 2 minutes under the light of the skialytic lamp.

The darknesswas obtained by total elimination of light or by placing on both eyes a cloth drape folded many times. We noted the position of the eyes immediately after turning on the room light of the operating room or after removal of the drape. We then switched on the skialytic lamp and observed the possible variation of the position of the eyes; the brightness of the skialytic lamp was 100.000 lux (hundred thousands). The deviation is measured by the Hirschberg test using the corneal reflection. This method is difference from that used by Quere(19) which only takes into account the variations of the deviation under the lighted skialytic lamp. The passage from the darkness to the light involves a modification of the strabismic deviation most often bilateral, but sometimes unilateral, and especially on the nondominant eye. This variation of the strabismic deviation in relation to the level of brightness is a type of opto-motor reflex.

The stretching test

We performed tests in the following manner: the medial rectus muscle after disinsertion was stretched with two sutures previously placed on its tendon near the insertion, whereas the globe is maintained in primary position by a forceps in taking care not to push it into the orbit. This is te method of Quere(19). In operating on esotropia, we made a systematic recession of both medial rectus muscles without operating on lateral rectus muscles; the stretching test is, therefore, systematic on both medial rectus muscles. The importance of the stretching is codified in relation with the limbus:

Grade 1: we can attain the nasal limbus or just behind it

Grade 2: we can attain the nasal third of the corneal radius

Grade 3: we can attain the middle of the corneal nasal radius or beyond. This test is very problematic.

RESULTS

Variation of the convergent deviation in relation to brightness

We classified the results into four groups:

Group A: No deviation in the darkness and in the light for both eyes: 29 cases (29%)

Group B: No deviation in the darkness and convergence in the light: 37 cases (37%). In this group we can distinguish two subgroups:

1. No deviation in the darkness for both eyes: (a) convergence in the light for both eyes (22 cases); (b) convergence in the light for one eye (8 cases)

2. No deviation in the darkness for one eye (7 cases) but both eyes are convergent in the light

Group C: Convergence in the darkness for both eyes: 25 cases (25%). Convergence in the light:

1. No deviation for both eyes (1 case)

2. Unchanged deviation (12 cases)

3. Increased deviation (11 cases for both eyes; 1 case for one eye)

Group D: Atypical forms:

1. No deviation in the darkness and in the light for one eye, deviation in the darkness and in the light (sometimes increased) for the other; these are mixed forms (3 cases)

2. Divergence in the darkness for both eyes (3 cases): (a) two cases remain divergent in the light; (b) one case is straight in the light

3. No deviation in the darkness and divergence in the light (2 cases); no deviation in the darkness for one eye, divergence for the other; no deviation in the light for both eyes (1 case)

Stretching test (100 cases)

A. Identical stretching for both eyes (85 cases)

Grade 3: 45 cases
Grade 2: 21 cases
Grade 1: 19 cases

B. Different stretching for one eye in comparison with the other (15 cases)

Grades 3/2: 9 cases
Grades 2/1: 6 cases

Correlation with the variation of the convergent deviation in connection with brightness

The histograms show:

1. in Group A (no deviation in the darkness and in the light) in the stretching test, the medial rectus muscle does not exceed the nasal limbus in 7 cases out of 29 (Table I)

2. In Group B (no deviation in the darkness, deviation in the light) in the stretching test, the medial rectus muscle does not exceed the nasal limbus in 6 cases out of 37 (Table II)

3. In Group C (deviation in the darkness and in the light) in the stretching test, the medial rectus muscle does not exceed the nasal limbus in 7 cases out of 25 (Table III)

4. In Group D (atypical forms) in the stretching test, the medial rectus muscle does not exceed the nasal limbus in 2 cases out of 9 which deal with two patients straight in the darkness and divergent in the light (Table IV)

Correlation between the variation of the convergent deviation in connection with brightness, stretching test and the age of the onset of strabismus

We have distinguished the convenital esotrpias appearing before one year and the acquired esotropias appearing after

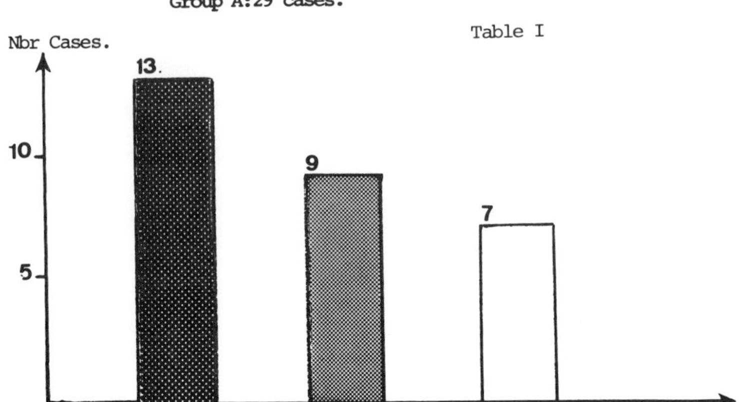
Group A:29 cases.
Table I
Nbr Cases.
13.
10
9
7
5
St3
St2
StI
Stretching Test

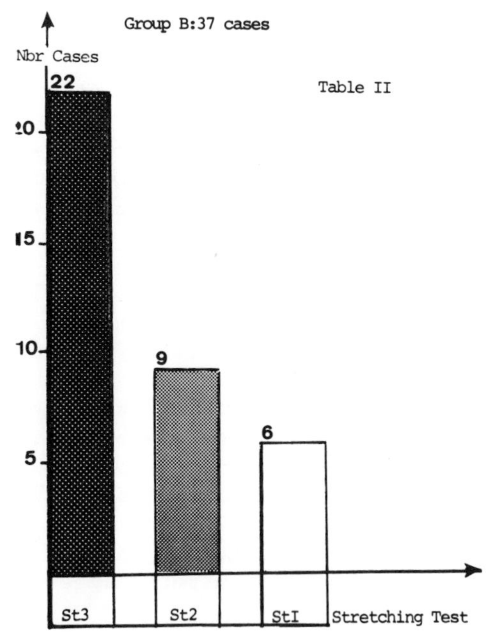
Group B:37 cases
Nbr Cases
22
Table II
20
15
10
9
6
5
St3
St2
StI
Stretching Test

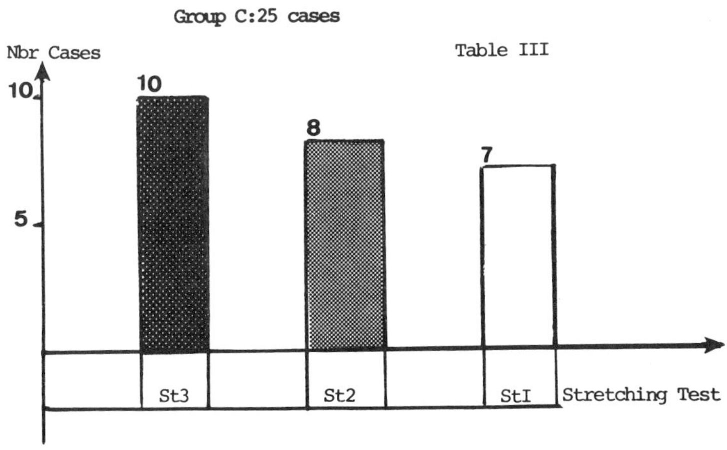
Group C:25 cases
Nbr Cases
Table III
10
5
10
8
7
St3
St2
StI
Stretching Test

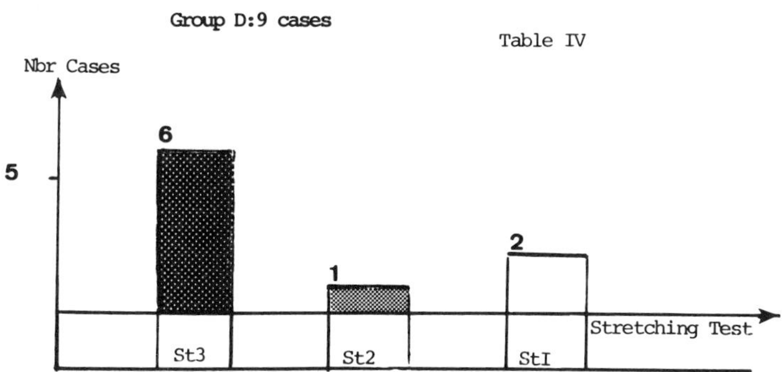
Group D:9 cases
Table IV
Nbr Cases
5
6
1
2
Stretching Test
St3
St2
StI

one.

Group A: out of 29 cases, 6 are congenital esotropias
Group B: out of 37 cases, 20 are congenital esotropias
Group C: out of 25 cases, 9 are congenital esotropias
Group D: out of 9 cases, 6 are congenital esotropias

All the results are summarized in Table V below:

Groups	Congenital	Acquired	Total
A	6	23	29
B	20	17	37
C	9	16	25
D	6	3	9
Total	41	59	100

Moreover, we ahve considered on one hand the cases with a stretching test Grade 3 (1/2 nasal corneal radius or beyond), on the other hand the cases with stretching test Grade 2 (nasal third of corneal radius) and 1 (nasal limbus or below). We notice in Table VI below that out of 35 congenital esotropias (Group A, B and C) 16 have a stretching test Grade 3, 19 have a stretching test Grade 2/1.

	Grades		
Group	3	2 and 1	Total
A	1.5	4.5	6
B	10.0	10.0	20
C	4.5	4.5	9
Total	16.0	19.0	35

DISCUSSION

Variation of the convergent deviation under general anesthesia in connection with brightness

For a long time the authors(1,7,16,18,19,23,25) have stated that under general anesthesia the angle of deviation in esotropia was according to the cases, identical, diminished, cancelled, or even inverted. We have even verified this. In Group A the deviation disappeared under general anesthesia. In Group B and C it persisted. We have been the first authors(4-6) to report the observations of esotropic patients in which the strabismic deviation varied according to brightness under general anesthesia.

In this new work, we state that in 37% of the cases (Group B), the deviation persisted ordiminished under general anesthesia in the light but disappeared in the darkness. In rare cases (atypical forms of Group D) the variation of the deviation was asymmetrical; one eye became straight in the darkness and te light, the other remained convergent.

We are convinced that these variations of the deviation in relation to brightness are not attributable to a weak anesthesia. Each time we ensured that a full surgical anesthesia plane was reached and remained constant during the different phases of examination. These variations could only be attributed to a modification of the innervational tonus which is bound to the brightness at the level of the retina and consequently to an opto-motor reflex.

According the Keiner's conceptions(13) which have been resumed by Govin(10,11), there would be normally a balance between the opto-motor action of adduction of the temporal retinal half and the opto-motor aciton of abduction of the nasal retinal hald. But we know from experience that suppression of the nasal half of the retina is easier to obtain than suppression of the temporal one. Convergent strabismus, resulting fro example of the decompensation of esophoria, suppression is localized in the nasal reinal half which leads to the prevailing action of adduction of the temporal retinal half; it follows that the degree of esodeviation which occurs depends in part on the extent and the depth of the suppression scotoma. According to its importance, the suppression disappears or persists under general anesthesia with correction on noncorrection of the deviation.

When under general anesthesia the deviation disappears in the darkness and in the light, the suppression scotoma would not be very deep and the balance between the opto-motor action of adduction of the temporal retinal half and the opto-motor action of abduction of the nasal retinal half is easily re-established. On the other hand, when the deviation persists in the darkness, as well as in the light, the suppression remains deep and, consequently, the action of adduction of the temporal retinal half remains preponderant. In intermediate cases, however, the suppression persists in the light, but is cancelled in the darkness with more or less complete disappearance of the strabismic deviation. Tamura and Mitsui(24) confirmed by electromyographic methods that the temporal retina is more sensitive than the nasal retina in esotropia.

Mitsui(15) argues that the reflex is passing through the subcortical pathway with a synapse located in the superior colliculus and once the opto-motor reflex hs been elicited, a proprioceptive reflex, starting in the medial rectus muscle,is superimposed; this proprioceptive impulse would have a synapse located in the superior colliculus.

This interpretation is clearly opposed to that which would make the vatiations of the deviation depend on a spasmodic factor, possibly associated with a contracture secondary to visco-elastic and mechanical factors(18,19). In our opinion these factors play a milited role in concomitant esotropia which has never had surgery.

The stretching test and correlation with variations of the deviation in connection with the brightness

In 85% of the cases the stretching is identical in both eyes. We believe that it is difficult to speak in terms of normal or abnormal stretching, for no series of the stretching test have been practiced on normal subjects. Rosenbaum et al(20,21), however, did try to measure exactly the strength of the muscular stretching; they found no significant difference between the normal and pathological patients. For our purpose, we differentiated arbitrarily three goups of stretching.

Moreover, the stretching test is extremely subjective. To make the test more objective, Roth(22), Paliaga(17), Rosenbaum et al(20) have attempted to use a dynamometer in order to apply a uniform and observable traction force.

The histograms show undoubtedly that there is no correlation between strabismic deviation under general anesthesia and the stretching test. Thus in Group A (no esotropic deviation in the darkness and under the light of the skialytic lamp) and in Group C (esotropic deviation persisting in the darkness and under the light of the skialytic lamp) we have the same percentage in the stretching test group 1, where the muscle attains the limbus, that is in 25% of the cases. In other wods, it is possible to observe reduced stretching in child with straight eyes under general anesthesia and conversely stretching surpassing the nasal half of the corneal radius in child with convergent eyes under general anesthesia.

This lack of correlation has also been confirmed by numerous clinical assessments; in particular, it is frequent that active and passive ductions are strictly normal in subjects in which the stretching does not surpass the nasal limbus. Even obvious modifications of muscular elasticity, as can be seen almost automatically on rectus muscle that has had previous surgery on, do not always involve a clinical modification of the duction test.

Our research, therefore, is in contradiction iwth that of Quere(18,19) who discovered a satisfactory correlation between the deviation under general anesthesia and the stretching test. He concluded that if the esodeviation disappears under general anesthesia, there is a spasm without contracture, that is to say without visco-elastic modifications of the muscle. The stretching test is then qualitatively normal. On the other hand, if the esodeviation persists under general anesthesia, there is a contracture secondary to the visco-elastic modifications of the muscle. The stretching is then qualitatively reduced or stopped, the muscle having become more or less inextensible. In fact, it seems to us that the lack of correlation that we have observed logically stems from our pathogenic interpretation of the variations of the convergent deviation under general anesthesia; given that the possibility of persistance of the deviation under general anesthesia is a function, above all, of the depth of suppression and not of the visco-elastic factors, it is to be expected that the stretching test be in direct relation with the deviation under general anesthesia.

Moreover, the importance of the stretching does not permit us to presume the importance of the convergent deviation; in the esotropia of small angle, the stretching cannot surpass the nasal limbus and conversely in the esotropia of large angle, the stretching cn surpass the half of the nasal corneal radius. We will try to confirm this opinion in our future researches.

Correlation between the variation of the convergent deviation in connection with the brightness, the stretching test and the age of the onset of the strabismus

We observed that in 35 cases of congenital esotropia of Groups A, B and C, 26 have no deviation in the darkness, but 29 keep the same deviation under the light of the skialytic lamp. This confirms the opinion of the authors(3,8,9,12) who believe that congenital esotropia becomes straight under general anesthesia.

Among these 35 cases of congenital strabismus of Groups A, B and C, close to half of the subjects (16 cases) has a stretching attaining or surpassing half of the nasal corneal radius. Among the 19 cases which have less stretching, 14.5 cases (Groups A and B) have the eyes straight in the darkness with esodeviation under the operating light in 10 cases (Group B) Therefore, the persistance or the disappearance of the deviation under general anesthesia is not a function of the elasticity of medial rectur muscles. We think that the congenital esotropia does not exhibit more particular characteristics to the stretching test than it exhibits under general anesthesia. Those statements are in agreement with the fact that the congenital esotropia with pseudo-paralysis of both lateral rectus muscles recovers most frequently a normal abduction by a correct preoperative medical treatment.

SUMMARY

Under general anesthesia, the position of the eyes in esotropia is bound to the opto-motor reflexes. One hundred cases of operated esotropia were studied. Once the patient was deeply asleep, the esodeviation was measured after 10 minutes in the darkness and after 2 minutes under the skialytic lamp. During surgery a stretching test was performed on both medial rectus muscles. There was no deviation in the darkness and in the light both eyes in 29% of the cases; no deviation in the darkness and deviation in light, ost often both eyes, in 37% of the cases; persistance of the esodeviation in the darkness in 25% of the cases and atypical results in 9% of the cases. The stretching test was graded in three arbitrary groups and has no correlation with the variation of the esodeviation in connection with brightness nor with the age of onset of the strabismus. The variations of esodeviation under general anesthesia do not depend on a spasmodic factor possibly associated with a contracture secondary to visco elastic and mechanical factors. The variations could be attributed to modifications of the balance between the opto-motor action of abduction of temporal retinal half and the opto-motor action of adduction of nasal retinal half. In esotropia, the temporal retina would be more sensitive than the nasal retina. The stretching test in nonoperated medial rectus muscles is not reliable because most often it is contradictory with the clinical findings. From a therapeutic point of view, the position of the eyes under general anesthesia and the elasticity of medial rectus muscles should not be taken into account in primary surgery of concomitant strabismus.

REFERENCES

1. Apt L, Isenberg S: Eye position of strabismic patients under general anesthesia. III INternational Orthoptic Congress. Boston, 1975, pp 417-422.

2. Ardouin M: Communication aux journees de strabologie. Paris, le 16 et 17 Novembre 1979. Hotel Lutetia.

3. Arruga A: Early operations for strabismus. The first International Strabismological Association. Acapulco, March 1970. h. Kimpton, London 1971, pp. 1-22.

4. Berard PV: Discussion de la communication de MA Quere et coll a la Societe Francaise d"Ophthalmolgie. L´examen electro-oculographique de la convergence. Aspects physiologiques et dereglements specifiques. Seance du 9 Mai 1979, Paris.

5. Berard PV: Discussion de la communication de MA Quere et coll a la Societe Francaise d´Ophthalmologie. Le signe de l´anesthesie dans les etropies fonctionnelles. Etude statistique de 318 cas. Seance du 13 Mai 1980, Paris.

6. Berard PV, Reyde R, Mouillac-Gambarelli N: Le reflexe opto-moteur (eclairement-obscuration) et le test d´elongation sous anesthesie generale dans les esotropies. (Nice, Juin 1981, sous presse).

7. Breinin GM: The position of rest during anesthesia and sleep. Electromyographic observations. Arch Ophthalmol 57:323-326, 1957.

8. Cuppers C: Probleme der operativen therapie des ocularen nystagmus. Klin Monatsbl Augenheilkd, 159:145-157, 1971.

9. Cuppers C: Historique et physiopathologie des blocages. J Franc Orthopt 8:15-26, 1978.

10. Gobin MH: The limitation of suppression to one half of the visual field in the pathogenesis of strabismus. Brit Orthopt J 25:42-49, 1968.

11. Gobin MH: Nouvelles conceptions sur la pathogenie et le traitement du strabisme. First Part: J Fr Ophthalmol 3:541-556, 1980.

12. Gomez de Llano F, Zato MA, Castiella JC: Der

diagnostische wert der anasthesie fur die chirurgie des strabismus. Klin Monatsbl Augenheilkd 175:355-359, 1979.

13. Keiner GBJ: Physiology and pathology of the opto-motor reflexes. Am J Ophthalmol 42:233-251, 1956.

14. Mitsui Y, Hirai K, Akazawa K, Masuda K: The sensoriomotor reflex and strabismus. Jpn J Ophthalmol 23:227-256, 1979.

15. Mitsui Y, Tamura O, Berard PV, Reydy R: An electromyographic study on the opto-motor effect in esotropia under general anesthesia. The IVth Congress International Strabismological Association. Asilomar, October 1982 (to be published).

16. Ohmi E, Oguri K: Eye position of the squint under general anesthesia. Acta Soc Ophthalmol Jpn 79:540-546, 1975.

17. Paliaga GP: Intraoperatory strabometry. International Symposium on Strabismus. XIIth Meeting Consilium Europaeum Strabismi Studio Deditum. Florence, May 1982 (to be published).

18. Quere MA, Perchereau A, Clergeau G, Gouray A, Van Cauter O, Bernardet N: Operation du fil et chirurgie classique dans les esotropies fonctionnelles. La clinique Ophthalmologique 1978, 2. Ed. Laboratoires Martinet, Paris.

19. Quere MA, Pechereau A, Calvez B, Clergeau G: Le signe de l´anesthesie dans les estotropies fonctionnelles: etude statistique de 318 cas. Bull Mem Soc Fr Ophthalmol 92:308-319, 1980.

20. Rosenbaum AL, Myer J: New instrument for the quantitative determination of passive forced traction. Ophthalmol 87(2):158-163, 1980.

21. Rosenbaum AL, Weiss SJ, Bateman JB, Liu PY: Quantitative analysis of spring forces in esotropia and exotropia during surgery. J Pediatr Ophthalmol and Strabismus 19(1):7-11, 1982.

22. Roth A, Montard M: Le test d´elongation musculaire sans desinsertion dans la chirurgie due strabisme. Bull Soc Ophthalmol Fr 8-9, 81, 707-709, 1981.

23. Souron R, Quere MA, Pechereau A: La position des globes oculaires au cours de la chirurgie du strabisme. Influence de

l'anesthesie generale. Anesth Analg (Paris) 37:393-397, 1980.

24. Tamura O, Mitsui Y: Role of the temporal and nasal retina in the light-motor reflex in esotropia. The IVth Congress of the International Strabismological Association. Asilomar, October 1982 (to be published).

25. Uemura Y: Ocular movement during induction of general anesthesia in children. XXII Concilium Ophthlmologicum, Paris 2:215-219, 1974. Masson, Paris 1976.

ELECTROMYOGRAPHIC AND FORCED DUCTION FINDINGS IN MOEBIUS' SYNDROME

I. M. Strachan

ABSTRACT

In the six cases of Moebius' syndrome described, horizontal gaze palsy, 6th nerve palsy and vertical gaze palsy have been investigated by EMG. Irregular bursts of activity from the muscles described by other workers were not found. EMG findings were as expected from clinical examination of eye movements. Frequency analysis was normal. Quantitated forced duction showed contraction of the ipsilateral medial rectus in 6th nerve palsy and normal ductions in horizontal gaze palsy, both in adduction and abduction. Adduction in gaze paresis can be achieved by convergence, however, there seems to be no mechanism to abduct the eye. Lack of movement alone there is inadequate to produce contracture.

INTRODUCTION

Moebius (1) described a case of congenital bilateral facial paresis with horizontal gaze palsy and compared it to a similar case described by Von Graefe and a case of Chisholm's which had a bilateral VI nerve paresis associated with the facial palsy.

Since then the definition of the syndrome has widened. Henderson (2) collected 60 cases of facial diplegia from the literature and added one of his own. Forty-five of these had oculomotor defects, half of which were gaze palsies as they were straight in the primary position and half probably had VI nerve pareses. The limits of the syndrome are poorly defined. Electromyographic (EMG) investigation in these cases have been sporadic as the syndrome is somewhat rare and its occasional association with low intelligence makes some cases difficult or impossible to examine by EMG.

Breinin (3) investigated an infant of 18 months with horizontal gaze palsy and good convergence. Vertical movements were intact. Little activity was found in a

STRABISMUS II
ISBN 0-8089-1424-3

lateral rectus. Van Allen and Blodi (4) reported one case in a 26 year old woman with convergent strabismus and an atrophic tongue. All horizontal recti showed electrical activity but the lateral recti showed less than normal. The medial recti showed no change in firing pattern with attempted versions. Spindle-shaped volleys of activity giving co-contraction of horizontal recti were reported. There was no oculomotor response to caloric stimuli and forced duction testing showed no restriction. Two sisters with affected antecedents were examined by Papst and Esslen. (5) They had poor intelligence and other associated defects. The first had only convergence present and electromyography of the right lateral rectus showed no activity. The second was unusual in having a divergent strabismus and clinically resembled a bilateral internuclear ophthalmoplegia with loss of vertical movements. The right medial rectus and right lateral rectus muscles showed good activity and some convergence impulses were recorded. Merz and Wojtowicz (6) found active medial and lateral rectus muscles in 2 cases and Andreani et al (7) reported a case with 30 degrees esotropia with a constant interference pattern in the right lateral rectus muscle. A further case with loss of horizontal gaze and elevation was reported by Orfila et al. (8) No activity was shown electromyographically from the left lateral rectus muscle but the medial rectus muscle was inhibited in attempted left gaze and gave an enhanced response with convergence and attempted right gaze.

An affected father and son were described by Ricker and Merten. (9) The son who was examined by EMG had absent horizontal and vertical gaze but good convergence. The medial and lateral rectus muscles showed a relatively normal but unvarying EMG from the right medial rectus muscle. The response from the lateral rectus muscle was somewhat diminished but also did not vary with attempted change of gaze. Finally, Schmidt (11) reported one case with horizontal gaze palsy and esotropia. Recordings from the left medial rectus and lateral rectus muscles showed good firing patterns in all gaze positions. Attempted saccades showed synchronous bursts from the horizontal rectus muscles. The vestibulo-ocular reflex was absent.

Huber (12) described the EMG findings in Moebius' syndrome but not as a case report. He stated that there were short bursts of innervation in the lateral rectus muscles and retained convergence impulses of short duration in the medial rectus muscles. The medial rectus muscles failed to show inhibition on attempted abduction.

REPORT OF CASES

Over the last 10 years, I have collected 6 cases of Moebius' syndrome, 5 of which have had electromyographic investigation (Table 1).

Case 1

A male, 17 years old, had bilateral upper facial weakness and a right esotropia. The right eye did not move to midline. Horizontal gaze palsy was present and no horizontal eye movements were elicited on caloric testing. Previous Hummelsheim operation had been performed on the right eye. VA = 6/9 right and 6/9 left.

EMG of the right lateral rectus muscle revealed a normal trace unvarying with gaze position including convergence. The right medial rectus muscle showed a normal interference pattern which did not change with gaze position except for increasing firing on convergence.

Forced duction test disclosed limited movement of right eye on attempted abduction.

Case 2

A female, 13 years old, has lower bilateral VII cranial nerve palsies. The eyes were straight in primary position. A horizontal gaze palsy with good convergence was found. VA = 6/9 right and 6/9 left. No response was found to caloric testing for horizontal movements.

EMG of the right lateral rectus muscle showed normal response in primary position and decreased on convergence. The right medial rectus muscle showed normal response in primary position and increased on convergence.

Force duction test revealed no restriction of movement.

Case 3

A male, 29 years old, had complete bilateral facial palsies and a left esotropia of 40 degrees. The right eye was operated in childhood, details unknown. No horizontal movements including convergence were seen. Caloric testing gave no response. VA = 6/12 right and 6/36 left.

TABLE 1

Case No.	Ocular Movements	Electromyography	Forced duction Test	Calorics	VII
1	RCS + horiz. gaze paresis	RLR ++ RMR ++ - +++ on convergence	R eye limited abduction	- VE	Bilateral upper paresis
2	Str in primary horiz. gaze paresis conv. intact	RLR ++ + convergence RMR ++ +++ convergence	No restriction Rt. eye	- VE	Bilateral lower paresis
3	Large LCS No horiz. movements.*	LLR -	N.D.	- VE	Complete bilateral paresis
4	L VI paresis R gaze paresis upgaze absent.	RMR ++ RLR ++ Both change on conv. LLR -	R restriction on abduction L on restriction	- VE	Bilateral lower paresis
5	Straight in primary. Absent horiz. gaze conv. normal	RMR ++ RLR ++ both change on convergence	No restriction R & L eye	- VE horiz. + VE Vert.	L severe paresis. R mild.
6	RCS + 5° Horiz. gaze palsy conv. poor*	N.D.	Restricted abduction R & L eye	N.D.	R complete paresis. L slight.

N.D. = Not done *Previous operation - See text.

EMG of the right lateral rectus muscle showed no activity.

Forced duction test - not done.

Case 4

A female, 35 years old, (Fig 1) had bilateral lower facial palsies and a large angle left esotropia. No upward gaze except a Bell's phenomenon was found and horizontal versions were absent. The right eye could converge and no caloric responses were found. VA = right eye 6/9 and left eye 6/12.

EMG of the right lateral rectus muscle gave a normal pattern for primary position which was unchanged by gaze but inhibited by convergence. The left lateral rectus muscle showed no activity (Fig 2).

The forced duction test showed no restriction to movements of the right eye. The left eye showed gross restriction on abduction.

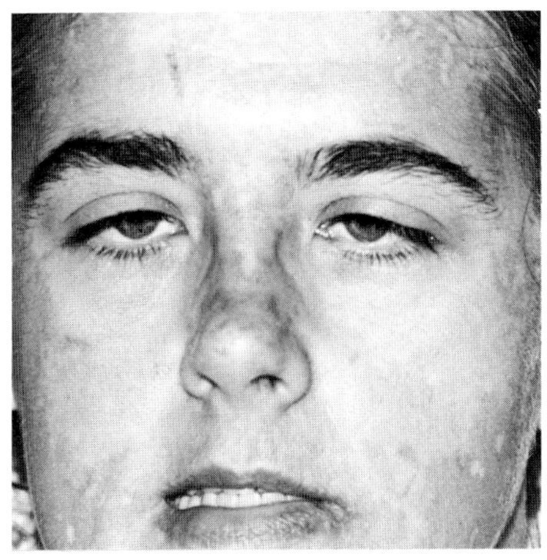

Figure 1.

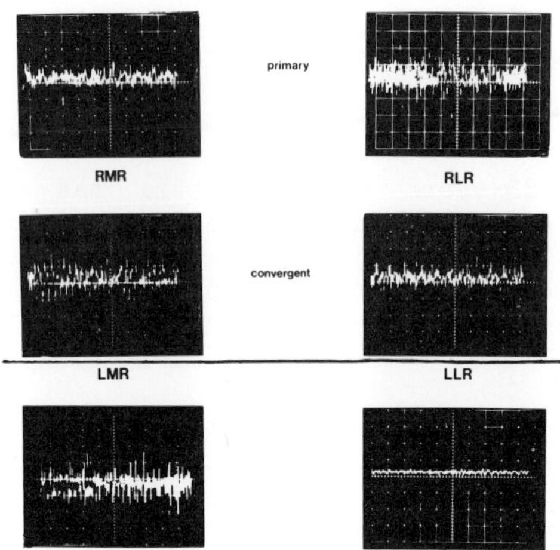

Figure 2.

Case 5

A male, 13 years old, had asymmetric bilateral VII cranial nerve weakness, with the left more severely affected. A horizontal gaze palsy allowed straight eyes in the primary position. Convergence was intact. Calorics were absent for horizontal but present for vertical movements. VA = 6/9 right and 6/9 left.

EMG of the right medial rectus and right lateral rectus muscles gave a normal trace for primary position, but no change was elicited except appropriate excitation of medial rectus and inhibition of lateral rectus on convergence. There was a normal frequency analysis.

Force duction test gave no restriction of movement.

Case 6

A female, 16 years old, had complete right VII cranial nerve paralysis, slight weakness of the cranial nerve, a 5 degrees esotropia and a horizontal gaze palsy. Convergence was intact but weak (bilateral medial rectus recession age 3). Calorics were not investigated.

EMG was refused by the patient.

Forced duction test showed restricted abduction of both eyes, but adduction was normal.

DISCUSSION

All cases in the present study conform to the original definition of the syndrome. (1) The electromyographic findings confirm, as Moebius originally described, either a gaze or lower motor neuron VI cranial nerve palsy. No abnormal motor units were detected. Vertical gaze was normal except in Case 4 in which upward gaze was absent. Interestingly, Bell's phenomenon was preserved in this case.

Forced duction testing showed no restriction in the pure gaze palsy cases even though those eyes have presumably never abducted past the midline. Case 1 was anomalous in showing restricted forced abduction in the presence of apparently normal lateral rectus electromyography. Previous surgery here makes this difficult to interpret. Could the surgery itself have reduced adhesions or caused neurotisation of a defective lateral rectus? It was also difficult to know exactly what was being recorded electromyographically after the Hummelsheim operation.

Of the previously reported cases electromyographically investigated, all would accord with Moebius's original description except Papst and Esslen's (5) second case which had excellent abduction in both eyes.

Vestibular testing when recorded has shown absent responses at least horizontally. (13,14) This is presumably a common phenomenon in all cases as head thrusts to produce horizontal movements have not been reported in Moebius' syndrome which is a differential feature from Cogan's oculomotor apraxia which also has a defect of voluntary horizontal gaze.

REFERENCES

1. Moebius PJ: Ueber angeborene doppelseitige Abducens-Facialis-Lahmung. Munchener Medicinische Wochenschrift 35:91-94, 1888.

2. Henderson JL: The congenital facial diplegia syndrome: Clinical features, pathology and aetiology. A review of 61 cases. Brain 62:381-403, 1939.

3. Breinin GM: New aspects of ophthalmoneurologic

diagnosis. Arch Ophthalmol 58:375-388, 1957.

4. Van Allen MW, Blodi FC: Neurologic aspects of the Mobius' syndrome. A case study with electromyography of the extraocular and facial muscles. Neurology 10:249-259, 1960.

5. Papst W, Esslen E: Elektromyographischer Beitrag zum Moebius -Syndrom. Klin Monatsbl Augenheilkd 137:401-410, 1960.

6. Merz M, Wojtowicz E: The Moebius' syndrome. Report of electromyographic examinations in two cases. Am J Ophthalmol 63:837-840, 1967.

7. Andreani D, Gandini S, Gandini-Collodel E: Osservatione su un cas di sindrome di Moebius con registrazione elettromiografica del muscolo retto esterno. Rivista Oto-neuro-oftalmologia 43:315-322, 1968.

8. Orfilla E, Montagna P, Massanisso JE, Vina R: Sindrome de Moebius. Archivos Oftalmologia (Buenos Aires) 45:165-168, 1970.

9. Ricker K, Mertens HG: Storungen der innervation beim Moebius Syndrom. Klin Monatsb Augenheild 156:551-557, 1970.

10. Goldsztajn M, Reichowa J: Badanie electromiograficzne w zespole Moebiusa. Neurol Neurochir Pol 6(1):123-126, 1972.

11. Schmidt D: Congenitale augenmuskelm-paresen. Albrecht von Graefes Arch Klin Exp Ophthalmol 192:285-312, 1974.

12. Huber A: Topographische und aetiologische analyse von augenmuskellahungen in elektromyogramm. Ophthalmologica 149:359-374, 1965.

13. Wollensak J, Fleischer-Peters A, Hovels O: Uber die angeborenen okulo-fazialen Lahmungen. Klin Monatsbl Augenheild 140:383-396, 1962.

14. Danis P, Brihaye-Van Geertruyden M: Nouvelle observation de paralysie oculo-faciale congenitale. Bull Soc Belge Ophthalmol 102:624-634, 1952.

ROLE OF TEMPORAL AND NASAL RETINA IN OPTOMOTOR REFLEX OF ESOTROPIA UNDER GENERAL ANESTHESIA

O. Tamura and Y. Mitsui

ABSTRACT

The role of the temporal and nasal retina in the optomotor reflex of esotropia under general anesthesia was studied by electromyography. Visual input caused ipsilateral esodeviation under all conditions, and the temporal retina was more sensitive than the nasal retina. In contrast to Keiner's observation, version was not excited even when the nasal retina was illuminated. However, the present findings do not conflict with Keiner's observation, because they are related to a reflex through a subcortical transmission pathway while his phenomenon is related to a reflex through the cortex.

INTRODUCTION

There is much evidence that an optomotor reflex is important in manifestation of esotropia.(1-4) Keiner(1) first reported that visual input from the temporal retina causes esodeviation of the ipsilateral eye, while that from the nasal retina causes version in the direction of the light. Different roles of the temporal and nasal retina in the pathogenesis of strabismus were also suggested by Gobin. (2) The optomotor reflex in esotropia occurs even under general anesthesia, as first observed clinically by Berard and his associates (4) and later confirmed by Mitsui and his associates with electromyography. (5) In the present study, the roles of the temporal and nasal retina in esotropic cases under general anesthesia were examined by electromyography.

MATERIALS AND METHODS

The materials and methods used were essentially as reported previously by Mitsui and his associates. (5) Electromyograms (EMGs) of the four horizontal rectus muscles were examined in 7 cases of constant esotropia under general anesthesia, in 5 of which active discharges from the medial rectus muscles were demonstrated. These 5 cases, 2 boys and

STRABISMUS II
ISBN 0-8089-1424-3

3 girls, ranging from 3 to 18 years old, were selected as subjects for continuous recordings.

The subjects were divided into two groups and treated as follows: First, the presence of active discharges from the medial rectus muscles under general anesthesia was confirmed under illumination with skialytic light, and then the room was made completely dark for 10 minutes. Then, in group I (3 cases), both eyes were spot-lighted from the left side as shown in Fig 1. The spot-light used was a round disk of opaque glass 43 mm in diameter illuminated from the back. It was placed 1 m from the patient's face at an angle to the left of 45 degrees of the center. Leakage of light to surrounding areas was prevented by a hood. The intensity of illumination was about 1 lux on the patient's cornea. In this way, lighting of about half the diameter of the optic nerve disk was focused on the nasal retina of the left eye and the temporal retina of the right eye. Spot-lighting was continued for 5 minutes, during which time the EMG was recorded continuously.

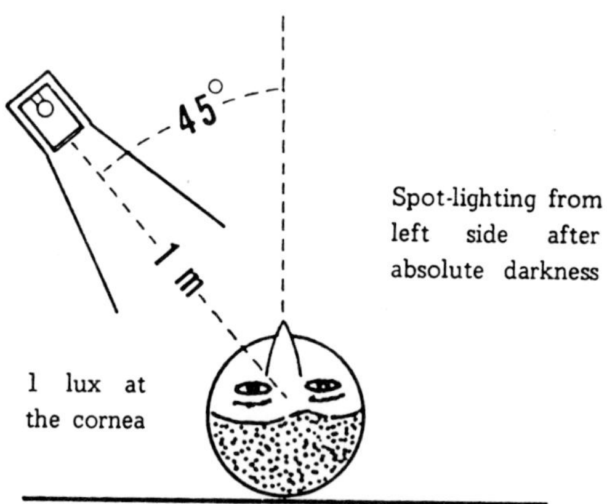

Figure 1. Diagram of method of spot-lighting from the left side after absolute darkness. Illumination on the cornea was about 1 lux.

Group II (2 cases) was treated as group I, except that a screen was placed in the center of the face and a black contact lens was used to cover the right eye during spotlighting so that only the nasal retina of the left eye was illuminated (Fig 2). Recordings were made continuously for 10 minutes during spot-lighting.

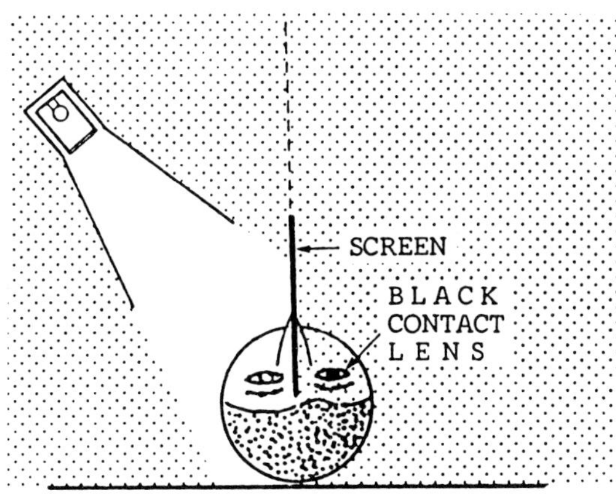

Figure 2. Diagram of spot-lighting of the nasal retina of the left eye after absolute darkness. Illumination of the right eye was prevented by a screen at the corner and a black contact lens on the right eye.

The general anesthesia used and the method of EMG recording were the same with those reported previously. (3)

RESULTS

In group I, when the nasal and temporal retina were spot-lighted after 10 minutes in complete darkness, all 3 esotropic patients under general anesthesia gave similar EMG patterns. An example of the pattern is shown in Fig 3. The four horizontal rectus muscles became essentially silent after the period of darkness (Fig 3a). Discharge from the right medial rectus began to increase about 57 seconds after the beginning of spot-lighting (Fig 3b), whereas that from the left medial rectus began to increase after about 108 seconds of spot-lighting (Fig 3c).

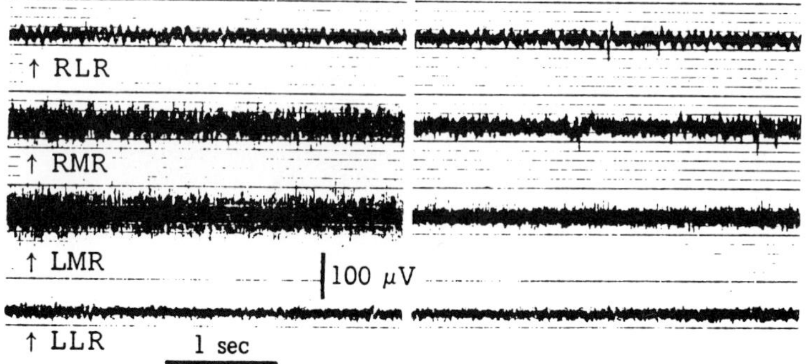

Figure 3: (a) EMGs of the four horizontal rectus muscles of an esotropic case under general anesthesia. Left: under skialytic light. Right: after 10 minutes of absolute darkness.

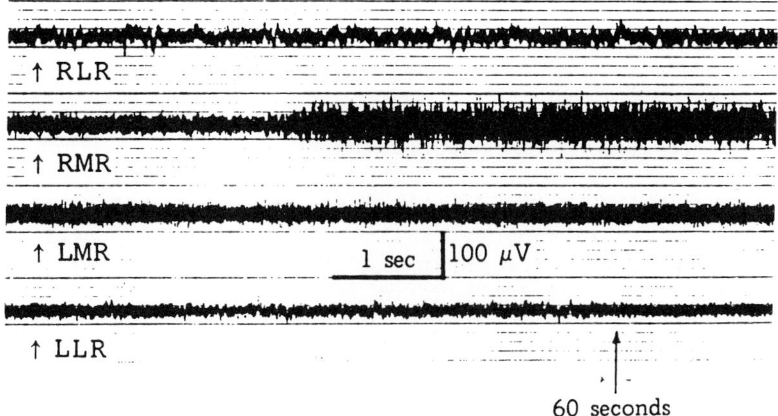

(b) The same as above when both eyes were spot-lighted from the left side after 10 minutes of darkness. The recording around 1 minute after the beginning of spot-lighting is shown.

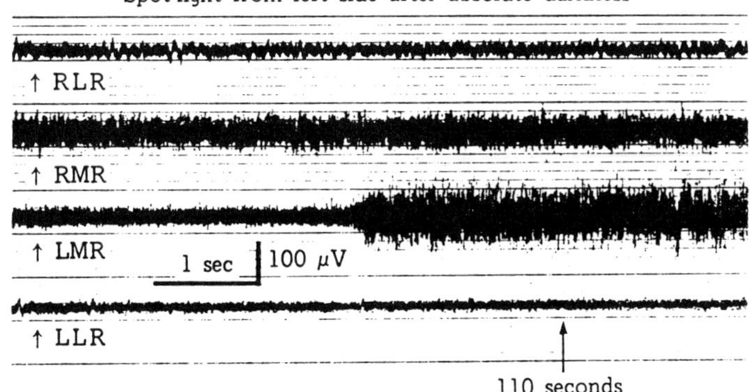

(c) The same as b, showing the recording around 110 seconds after the beginning of spot-lighting.

Fig 4 shows the same EMG recorded at a slow paper speed to show the difference in lag times for re-appearance of discharges in the right and left medial rectus clearly in one continuous section of the EMG. The lag time after spot-lighting in the right and left medial rectus in the 3 cases are tabulated in Table 1. The lag time is consistently shorter in the right medial rectus than in the left.

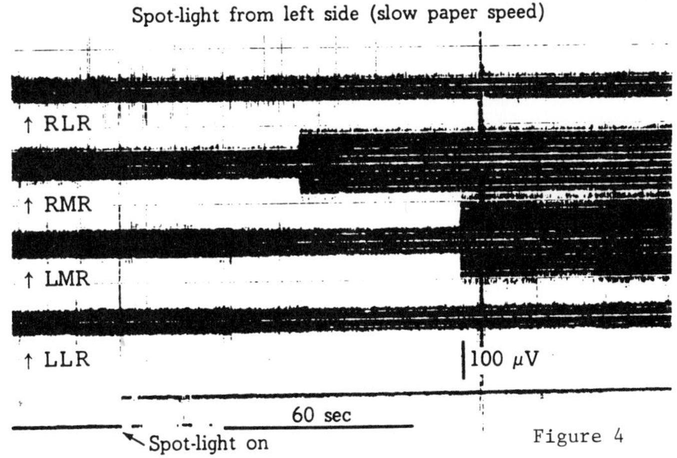

Figure 4

TABLE 1

Lag Time Until Refiring from the Medial Rectus Muscles on Spot-lighting fromt he Left Side after Absolute Darkness

Case No.	Lag Time: Right Medial Rectus	Lag Time: Left Medial Rectus	Difference (sec)
1	116	135	19
2	105	139	34
3	57	108	51

In the 2 cases of group II refiring in the left medial rectus muscle occurred after a much longer lag time of 2 minutes or more. There were no obvious changes in the EMGs of the other three muscles, even after spot-lighting for 10 minutes (Fig 5).

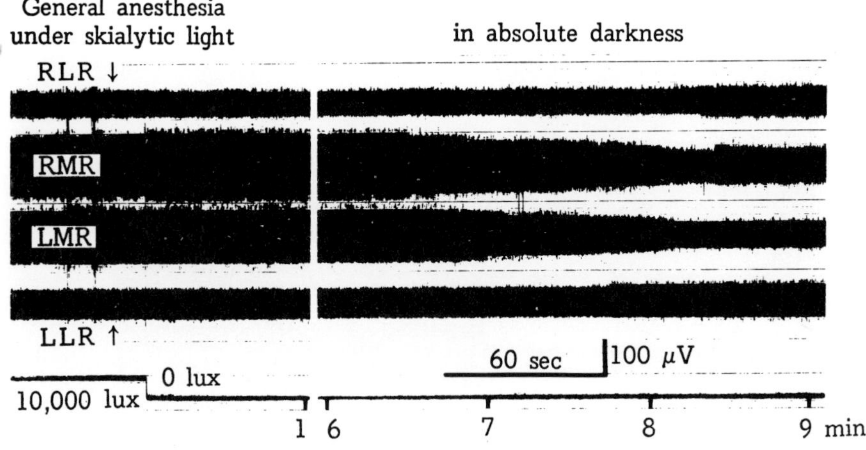

Figure 5. (a) EMGs of the four horizontal recti of an esotropic case under general anesthesia recorded at very low paper speed. Left: Record from 1 minute before to 1 minute after darkening the room. Right: Record from 6 to 9 minutes after darkening the room.

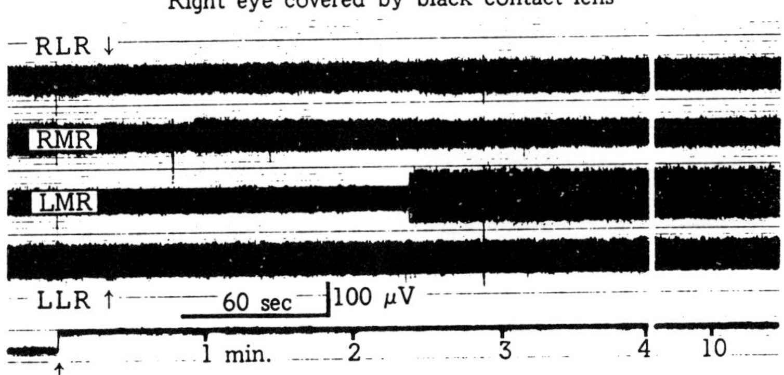

(b) The same as above showing the record when the nasal retina of the left eye was spot-lighted after the period of darkness. Left: Record for 4 minutes after beginning of spot-lighting. Right: Record after about 10 minutes of spot-lighting.

DISCUSSION

The lag time, until re-firing of the medial rectus muscle on re-exposure to light after darkness, is known to decrease with the intensity of illumination. (5) In the present study the intensity of light on the cornea in group 1 was about 8% more on the left eye than on the right, because the spot-lighting was from the left (Fig 1). Nevertheless, the lag time of the left medial rectus was consistently longer than that of the right medial rectus (Table 1). Thus the findings must be attributed to lower sensitivities of the nasal retina than of the temporal retina in this optomotor reflex.

This reflex was strictly restricted to the ipsilateral medial rectus, regardless of whether the nasal or the temporal retina was illuminated (Fig 5). Keiner's observation (1) that illumination of the nasal retinal causes version in the direction of the light was not demonstrated. However, Keiner's observations were made on conscious patients where the pathway through the cortex may predominate. Therefore, the present results are by no means giving a denial to Keiner's observation. On the contrary, Keiner's observation that the nasal and temporal retina have different behaviours in the optomotor reflex in esotropia must be highly evaluated.

It should be noted that this kind of optomotor reflex is applicable to esotropic cases only. It has been suggested that the optomotor reflex in exodeviations is contralateral, (3) and we plan to study this problem next.

ACKNOWLEDGEMENTS

Authors wish to thank Dr. Takao Saito, Professor of Anesthesiology, Tokushima University, who undertook the general anesthesia in absolute darkness throughout the study.

REFERENCES

1. Keiner GBJ: New Viewpoints on the Origin of Squint. A clinical and statistical study on its nature, cause and therapy. The Hague, Martinus Nijhoff, 1951.

2. Gobin MH: Limitation of suppression to one half of the visual field in the pathogenesis of horizontal deviation of squint. Ophthalmologica 155:297-298, 1968.

3. Mitsui Y, Hirai K, Akazawa K, Masuda K: The sensorimotor reflex and strabismus. Jpn J Ophthalmol 23:227-256, 1979.

4. Berard PV, Reydy R, Mouillac-Gambarelli N: Le reflexe opto-moteur (eclairement-obscuration) et le test d'elongation sours anesthesie generale dans les esotropies. Bull Soc Ophthalmol Fr 82(8-9):1037-1042, 1982.

5. Mitsui Y, Tamura O, Hirai K, Akazawa K, Ohga M, Masuda K: An electromyographic study on the optomotor effect in estropia. Br J Ophthalmol 65:161-166, 1981.

HISTOPATHOLOGICAL STUDY ON THE MONKEY EXTRAOCULAR MUSCLES UNDER BOTULINUM TOXIN INJECTION

K. Mukuno, A. B. Scott, and S. Ishikawa

ABSTRACT

Histopathological study of botulinum toxin A injected medial rectus of 3 rhesus monkeys was made. One monkey (the dosage of 3 X 10-4 micrograms) demonstrated almost no change when examined at 6 days after the injection. One monkey examined at 45 days after the injection with the moderate dosage of 2 X 10-2 micrograms produced the change at the nerve terminals of injected medial and lateral rectus muscles. Mild degree of demyelinative change close to the nerve terminal and complete regeneration were the major findings. Since the dosage is rather high in this animal, the use of lesser dosages would be used to treat a patient.

The third monkey was treated 3 times in the medial rectus muscle. Light microscopy disclosed almost normal muscle fibers and myelinated nerve bundles. A few regenerated neuromuscular junctions were noted indicating complete morphological regernation which could be expected even after triple injections.

INTRODUCTION

An injection of botulinum toxin into extraocular muscle as an alternative to strabismus surgery has been proposed by one of the authors. Histopathological evaluation of extraocular muscle after the injection of botulinum toxin has been considered to be important for application of this technique to the human being.

In the present report, histopathological study was carried out on the botulinum A toxin injected medial rectus muscle of three rhesus monkeys under different dosages of injection with varied durations after the injection. The animals were sacrificed and their muscles were examined. Histopathological findings obtained from the animals will be mentioned.

STRABISMUS II
ISBN 0-8089-1424-3

METHODS

Three adult rhesus monkeys (A, B, and C) were used. Botulinum A toxin was injected only in the right medial rectus muscle in each monkey, except monkey C, by microsyringe via transconjunctival route under surface anesthesia. The dosages used were; A: 3 X 10-4 micrograms only one time, B: 2 X 10-2 only one time, and C: 4 X 10-4 (Dec 18, 1975), 1 X 10-2 (June 28, 1976), and 1 X 10-2 (Sep 13, 1976) three times in the right eye and 1 X 10-2 in the left eye, respectively. Histopathological studies were made in A: 6 days, B: 45 days, and C: 3 days after the last injection of the right eye and 64 days after in the left eye, respectively, followed by sacrifice under pentobarbital anesthesia. Histopathological study was made by haematoxylin and eosin staining, Masson trichrome staining and toluidine blue staining for light microscopy. Standard technique for electron microscopic observation has been used. Only medial and lateral recti of the injected side were examined and other eye's muscles were used for control. All extraocular muscles were examined only in animal A.

RESULTS

General Observation:

No systemic toxic effect caused by injection was seen in any of the animals. After the injection, no local irritation of the eye was seen in all animals. The lid opening as well as eye movement was more or less involved.

Lid Opening and Eye Movements:

Animal A demonstrated a moderate degree of exotropia and moderate underaction of the medial rectus muscle as well as a slow adduction of the eyeball during version movement. These changes were seen at least one day after the injection and lasted until 6 days later at the time of the histopathological examination.

Animal B demonstrated moderate ptosis with inability to adduct the eyeball. In addition, the eye movements toward all directions were moderately affected at the time of histopathological examination.

Animal C: Ocular signs following the previous two injections were gone about 2 months after the injections. No residual involvement of the left eye was noted 2 months after injections. Right complete ptosis with inability of the adduction and moderate limitation of eye movement toward all directions was present at 3 days after the last 3rd injection.

Histopathological Findings:

Animal A: All extraocular muscles, except injected medial rectus, demonstrated normal histopathological findings by light microscopy. The injected medial rectus muscle revealed the following change. The point of injection was located at 5 mm to 6 mm from the insertion. The thinning of muscle suggesting local atrophy of the injected area was seen at 5mm to 10 mm from the insertion by macroscopic observation. By light microscopic observation of this atrophic area, mild degree of round cell infiltration was seen at a small lesion of disorganized muscle fibers and connective tissues. Very mild perivascular infiltration adjacent to the sclera was noted. These changes were not observed in the other muscles nor in the other animals, therefore, this could be due to transient cell infiltration after the injection. No change was seen among myelinated nerve bundles in the medial rectus muscle. In general, the change due to the injection was mild. No change was noted in other extraocular muscles including the neighboring superior oblique muscle.

Animal B: Needle point and local atrophy of the muscle could not be noted in the injected medial rectus muscle by macroscopic observation, 45 days after injection. Cellular infiltration was not seen. The main change was located at the nerve terminal. Thinly myelinated nerve fibers were seen close to the neuro-muscular junction of the injected site. Typical onion bulb formation was observed. Nerve terminal without junctional folds at twitch fibers were frequently seen. Sprouting neuromuscular junction of slow fibers was also seen. No change was seen in the nerve axons. Therefore, the changes were considered to be due to regeneration of the nerve terminals followed by demyelination. Vacuole formations, as well as disarrayed myofibrils, were scarcely seen within the muscle fibers. The variation in size of muscle fibers in a small area suggested residuals of incomplete denervation. Similar slight regenerative changes were seen at the lateral rectus muscle. The changes were seen in both slow and fast fibers' group. The changes produced by injection were, in general, located mainly at the nerve terminals with regeneration.

Animal C. There was no thinning of the muscle or needle scars in the medial rectus muscle in spite of triple injections during 10 months. Cellular infiltration was not found. No apparent change was seen in the nerve bundles as well as no formation of the vacuoles within the muscle fibers. Increased connective tissues among muscle fibers in a small restricted area were seen in the lateral rectus muscle. Neuromuscular junctions showed regeneration. This muscle seemed to be almost normal in appearance. Left medial rectus, 2 months after injection, appeared similar to that of animal B.

By histopathological observation, botulinum toxin A injection produced mild changes mainly localized at the nerve terminal with regeneration. These were characterized by onion bulb formation and newly formed sprouting neuromuscular junctions at the medial rectus as well as in other muscles to a lesser grade.

SURGICAL MANAGEMENT OF DETERIORATED ACCOMMODATIVE ESOTROPIA

E. R. Crouch

ABSTRACT

A prospective study was designed to determine the amount of surgery to perform on deteriorated accommodative esotropia and to evaluate the possibility of removing the hyperopic correction postoperatively. Patients excluded from the study were all patients with associated ocular pathology, patients with infantile esotropia who had developed accommodative esotro- pia, patients with a hyeropia greater than +5.00, and patients who had had previous strabismus surgery. The forty-three patients included manifested greater than 20 prism diopters of esotropia while wearing full hyperopic correction. Patients were followed for a postoperative period of at least twelve months with a maximum of six years. Over 70 percent have been followed for a period of four years or more. The amount of surgery was determined by measurements based on the amount of Fresnel prisms required to make the patient orthophoric prior to surgery with the full hyperopic correction in place. Postoperatively, of the forty patients studied, 19 of the patients (47.5%) had an esotropia greater than 10 prism diopters which required glasses. No patient developed an exotropia of greater than 6 prism diopters post- operatively. Twenty-one of forty patients (52.5%) did not require glasses postoperatively.

INTRODUCTION

The majority of patients with accommodative esotropia do not develop a nonaccommodative element. However, a portion deteriorated to a constant esotropia with full hyperopic correction in place. The presence of both accommodative and nonaccommodative components are attributed to a deterioration of the initial purely accommodative element.(1,2) The term deteriorated accommo- dative esotropia or partially accommodative esotropia has been used to identify this condition. Unlike the large angle esotropia found in congenital esotropia, the nonaccommodative esotropic angle is usually moderate. The mechanism causing the nonaccom- modative component is most likely an acquired anatomic change

STRABISMUS II
ISBN 0-8089-1424-3

that requires surgical correction if the deviation is significant and is not controlled by fusion.(3-7)

Important determining factors in surgery include the amount and comitancy of the esotropia, the relationship between the distance and near deviation, and the fusional capacity of the patient. A bilateral medial rectus recession is the preferred surgical procedure.(5,8) The quantity of the bilateral medial rectus recession is generally based on measurements of the esotropia at distance wearing the full hyperopic correction. The full hyperopic correction is applied postoperatively.

A prospective study was designed to determine the amount of surgery to perform on deteriorated accommodative esotropia and to evaluate the possibility of removing or reducing the full hyperopic correction postoperatively.

METHODS

All consecutive patients with deteriorated accommodative esotropia with a prismatic deviation greater than 20 prism diopters while wearing the full cycloplegic refraction were included in the study. The hyperopic correction range varied between +2.00 and +5.00 diopters. Both patients with a normal AC/A ratio (same distance and near measurements) and patients with an abnormal AC/A ratio (distance-near disparity of greater than 10 prism diopters) were included in the study. Specifically excluded from the study were:

1. Patients with greater than +5.00 diopters of hyperopia.
2. Congenital esotropia patients who had developed an accommodative esotropia.
3. Patients with any organic ocular disease such as toxoplasmosis, cataracts, or glaucoma.
4. Patients with neurological disease or paralytic strabismus.
5. Patients who had undergone previous strabismus surgery.

Data on each patient included sex, age of onset of accommo- dative esotropia, age of onset of deteriorated accommodative component, amblyopia therapy, visual acuity, cycloplegic refractive error, age and date of surgery, millimeters of surgery, and preoperative and postoperative diopters of esotropia with and without glasses. Worth-4-dot (at 6 meters and 0.33 meters), Titmus stereotest, and prism adaptation results were recorded. Preoperative visual acuity was 20/30 or better in both eyes or good, central and maintained fixation bilaterally prior to any surgery. Cycloplegic refractions were performed thirty minutes after instillation of two drops of 1% cyclopentolate hydrochloride and two drops of 1% tropicamide with a five minute interval between drops. Refractive errors were expressed as the spherical equivalent. Esotropias were measured by cover-uncover test and by alternative cover test and were expressed in prism diopters. All distance measurements were made at 6 meters with accommodative targets and all near measurements were made with an accommodative target at 0.33 meters.

After the basic deviation was determined, base out Fresnel prisms were placed on the glasses in increments of 5 prism diopters until the patient was orthophoric. For instance, if a patient measured 20 prism diopters of deviation initially, 20 prism diopters of base out prisms were placed on the glasses. The patient then returned 30 minutes later and had remeasurements. If there was still a greater deviation, additional Fresnel prisms were added until the patient's angle of deviation was stable. Frequently, the total deviation with Fresnel prisms and the measurements without glasses were similar. Therefore, the decision was made to base the millimeters of medial rectus recession on the distant (6 meters) esotropic angle as measured without glasses. Preoperative prismatic deviations were measured on three separate visits. All surgery was performed by the same surgeon utilizing a fornix-based approach and bilateral medial rectus recession.(9) Postoperative examinations were performed on the first postoperative day, at one week, two weeks, one month, three months, and then every three months thereafter. Patients were followed for a minimum period of twelve months and a maximum period of six years. The mean followup time was 37 months. Sixty-two percent of the patients were followed for a period of four years or more. Postoperatively, if the patient manifested greater than 10 prism diopters of esotropia, glasses were prescribed. The amount of the hyperopic correction was determined by starting initially at 1/2 of his normal hyperopic correction. The glasses were increased in 1/2 diopter steps until the patient was orthophoric in the primary position. Surgical results were evaluated and determined as follows:

1. An undercorrection was considered a prismatic deviation of greater than 10 prism diopters of esotropia without glasses.

2. An overcorrection was considered a prismatic deviation of greater than 6 prism diopters of exotropia without glasses.

RESULTS

Forty-three patients were included in the study. Twenty-three were male, twenty were females. Four patients in the study had an identical twin who did not have or develop accommodative esotropia in spite of greater than two diopters of hyperopia in each twin. The age of onset of deteriorated accommodative esotropia component was 3.6 years. Amblyopia treatment was required in eight of 43 patients.

The initial preoperative prismatic deviation with glasses varied between 20 and 35 prism diopters. The median amount of increased deviation with prism adaptation was 15 prism diopters with a range of 0 to 25 prism diopters. The median amount of increased deviation without glasses was 17 prism diopters with the range of 0 to 30 prism diopters. Surgical decisions were based on measurements of the deviation without the hyperopic correction. The median amount of increased surgery was 1.5 mm per muscle. For example, if the basic deviation was 20 prism diopters with glasses and 35 prism diopters without glasses, surgery was performed for the 35 prism diopter deviation, a bilateral medial rectus recession of 5 mm. The amount of surgery required varied between 3.5 mm bilateral medial rectus recessions and 6 mm bilateral medial rectus recessions. Table 1 summarizes preoperative and postoperative deviations during the first three months of followup. Twenty-four of the 43 patients were less than 10 prism diopters esotropic after surgery and have been maintained out of glasses. No patients have developed an exotropia postoperatively.

TABLE 1

Summary of Preoperative and Postoperative Measurements

Preoperative Deviation Total = 43	Postoperative Deviation Total = 43	Postop Deviation Requiring Glasses Total = 19
20-25 sc = 20	0-4 ET sc = 15	0-10 cc = 16
26-35 sc = 14	5-10 ET sc = 9	11-25 cc = 3
36-50 sc = 7	11-20 ET sc = 16	
51-65 sc = 2	20 ET sc = 3	
	0-6 XT = 0	

Long-term surgical results are listed in Table 2. Forty of 43 patients (93%) were corrected with glasses and/or surgery. Twenty-four of the 43 patients (56%) were able to remove their glasses after surgery and to maintain a prismatic deviation of less than 10 prism diopters esotropia. The 95% confidence limits interval for this result are between 40 and 71 percent. Sixteen of 43 patients (37%) were straight with glasses plus surgery. At 8 to 14 months postoperative, three patients (7%) developed a residual esodeviation of greater than 20 prism diopters while wearing full hyperopic correction. These patients required a second procedure of a bilateral lateral rectus resection. They have had a residual deviation of less than 0-10 prism diopters while wearing full hyperopic correction.

Table 2. Surgical Results

	%
Corrected with glasses and/or one surgery 40/43	93
Eyes straight out of glasses 24/43	56
Eyes straight with glasses plus surgery 16/43	37
Eyes straight with glasses plus two surgeries 3/43	7

Table 3 illustrates the hyperopic correction preoperatively and the hyperopic correction in the 19 patients requiring glasses postoperatively. The mean preoperative hyperopic correction was +3.00 diopters. Fifteen of the 19 patients required a hyperopic correction as early as the second day postoperative and as late as four weeks postoperative. Four patients required hyperopic correction as late as four to six months after surgery. In nine of the 19 patients, a reduced hyperopic correction enabled them to maintain straight eyes.

Table 3

Hyperopic Correction	Preoperative	Postoperative*
+2.00 to +3.00	21/43 (49%)	11/19 (58%)
+3.25 to +4.00	16/43 (37%)	4/19 (21%)
+4.25 to +5.00	6/43 (14%)	4/19 (21%)

*19 of 43 patients required hyperopic correction postoperatively

+5.00	6/43 (14%)	4/19 (21%)

* 19 of 43 patients required hyperopic correction postoperatively

Additional observations were noted. Twenty-nine of the 43 patients demonstrated a normal distance-near relationship. Twenty of these 28 patients did not require glasses postoperatively (71%). However, the results were not as successful for those patients with an abnormal distance-near relationship (high AC/A ratio). Of the fifteen patients with an abnormal distance-near disparity, only four (27%) were able to remove their glasses postoperatively.

Postoperative fusion was also evaluated by Worth-4-dot and Titmus stereotest (Table 4). Of the 43 patients studied,16 were too young to fully evaluate. Results on the remaining twenty-seven: Gross fusion as determined by the Worth-4-dot test at distance and near was present in 16 of 27 patients (59%); fifteen of these patients had better than 100 seconds of stereopsis on the Titmus stereotest; eleven of 27 patients (41%) demonstrated a definite monofixation syndrome as described by Parks.(10)

TABLE 4

Postoperative Fusion*

	Worth 4 Dot D + N	Titmus Steropsis 100 Sec or Better	Monofixation
Out of Glasses	9/14	8/14	5/14
With Glasses	7/13	7/13	6/13

*27 patients tested; 16 too young to evaluate

These patients were subdivided into those requiring glasses and those out of glasses postoperative. In patients requiring glasses, 7 of 13 (53%) had fusion on Worth-4-dot at distance and near and better than 100 seconds of stereopsis. In patients out of glasses, 9 of 14 (64%) had fusion at distance and near on Worth-4-dot and 8 of 14 (57%) had better than 100 seconds on Titmus stereotest.

DISCUSSION

Treatments to alter accommodative esotropia have included full hyperopic correction as determined by cycloplegic refraction, pharmacologic alteration of the AC/A ratio, and surgery. Surgery is usually recommended for the nonaccommodative component of deteriorated accommodative esotropia when the deviation is greater than 20 prism diopters and fusion is not controlled.(3-7) Previous studies have indicated that recession of both medial rectus muscles is an effective surgical procedure in patients with high AC/A esotropia.(5,8,11) Rosenbaum et al excluded patients of greater than +3.75 diopters from their series because of the concern of possibly developing exotropia. The present series excluded patients with greater than +5.00 diopters of hyperopia because of the same concern. In the present series, 6 patients had greater than +4.00 diopters. Only two of the six were able to remove their glasses postoperatively while the remaining four required a full hyperopic correction postoperatively. No patients in the present series have developed an exotropia with a mean followup time of 37 months. Sixty-two percent have been followed for four years or longer. The results of the present study do not apply to patients with anisometropia, untreated amblyopia, or patients with cerebral palsy. These patients have been shown to develop secondary exotropia postoperatively.

It has been recommended that patients with high accommodative convergence to accommodation ratio (high AC/A ratio) require 1 mm additional surgery per muscle to correct the nonaccommodative esotropic angle.(2) The present series mean increase in surgery was 1.5 mm per muscle for both patients with a normal AC/A ratio and with a high AC/A ratio.

Comparison of postoperative fusional ability were essentially equal between those patients requiring glasses and those patients out of glasses postoperatively.

Additional studies with prism adaptation may provide information regarding the management of deteriorated accommodative esotropia and prove helpful in predicting the postoperative result.(12) In the present series, the median increased deviation with prism adaptation was 15 prism diopters as compared to a median increased deviation without glasses of 17 prism diopters was not significant.

Recession of both medial rectus muscles is a highly effective surgical procedure in deteriorated accommodative esotropia. The amount of surgery is based on the prismatic deviation without glasses. The median amount of additional surgery required in patients with deteriorated accommodative esotropia was 1.5 mm per muscle. When this additional surgery was performed, twenty-four of 43 patients (56%) were able to remove their glasses postoperatively.

ACKNOWLEDGEMENTS

Friendly D (reviewed the manuscript), Moser D., Ph.D. provided statistical assistance.

REFERENCES

1. Burian HM, von Noorden GK: Binocular Vision and Ocular Motility. St. Louis, CV Mosby Co., 1974, pp 282-292.

2. Parks MM: Ocular Motility and Strabismus. Hagerstown, MD, Harper & Row, 1975, pp 102-108.

3. Breinin GM, Swann KC, Costenbader FD: Symposium: Accommodative esotropia. Trans Am Acad Ophthalmol Otolaryngol 61:375-396, 1957.

4. Breinin GM: Accommodative strabismus in the AC/A ratio. Am J Ophthalmol 71:303-311, 1971.

5. Parks MM: Abnormal accommodative convergence in squint. Arch Ophthalmol 59:364-380, 1958.

6. Swann KC: Classification and diagnosis. Trans Am Acad Ophthalmol Otolaryngol 61:383-389, 1957.

7. Knapp P: The clinical management of accommodative esotropia. Am Orthopt J 17:8-13, 1967.

8. Rosenbaum AL, Jampolsky A, Scott AB: Bimedial recession in high AC/A esotropia: A long term followup. Arch Ophthalmol 91:251-253, 1974.

9. Parks MM: Fornix incision for horizontal rectus muscle surgery. Am J Ophthalmol 65:907-915, 1968.

10. Parks MM: The monofixation syndrome. Trans Am Ophthalmol Soc 67:609-657, 1969.

11. Bateman JB, Parks MM: Clinical and computer-assisted analyses of preoperative and postoperative accommodative convergence and accommodation relationships. Ophthalmol 88:1024-1030, 1981.

12. Jampolsky A: A simplified approach to strabismus diagnosis, in Burien HM (ed): Symposium on strabismus. Transactions of the New Orleans Academy of Ophthalmology, St. Louis, CV Mosby Co, 1971, p. 66.

REVERSED FIXATION TEST (RFT)
A NEW TOOL FOR THE DIAGNOSIS OF
DISSOCIATED VERTICAL DEVIATION (DVD)

G. Kommerell and S. Mattheus

ABSTRACT

Dissociated vertical divergence (DVD) depends on the balance of visual inputs coming through the right and left eyes. In the classical Bielschowsky test, the balance of visual inputs is altered by darkening the retinal image of one eye with a filter. We found out that shifting the fixation to the other eye while darkening the previously fixing eye reveals additional amounts of DVD and discloses cases of DVD which have been concealed with classical filter testing. The main clinical value of the new test is a sensitive differential diagnosis between DVD and esotropia with elevation in adduction (overaction of the inferior oblique muscle).

Reversed Fixation Test (RFT). On the synoptophore, the objective angle of squint is determined with right eye fixation. The illumination is then switched to the left eye which now fixes in an elevated position. A few seconds are allowed for possible upward drift of the right eye. The amount of upward movement represents the "DVD component" of the strabismus, and is determined by aligning the right tube of the synoptophore with the visual axis of the right eye.

Results. Of 30 strabismic patients who showed a DVD component with the RFT, only 15 were positive with Bielschowsky's test. In the 15 patients positive with both tests, the average amount of DVD was 11.1 degrees using our test, and only 5.4 degrees with the Bielschowsky test.

INTRODUCTION

Distinguishing between (DVD) and elevation in adduction (also called strabismus sursoadductorius or primary overaction of the inferior oblique muscles) can be difficult as demonstrated in Fig 1. The picture shows a patient with congenital esotropia. When the right eye (RE) fixes in the

STRABISMUS II
ISBN 0-8089-1424-3

primary position, the left eye (LE) is adducted and elevated, and when the LE fixes in the primary position, the RE is adducted and elevated. In such cases we are faced with the differential diagnosis of the patient having either bilateral elevation in adduction, or DVD, or a combination of both. Bilateral elevation in adduction can easily be corrected by surgery, but DVD cannot if we are dealing with a patient who habitually alternates fixation. Thus, distinguishing between these is important for planning surgery.

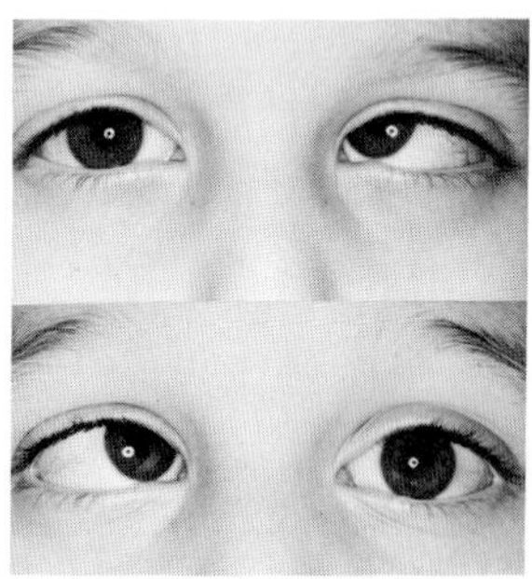

Fig 1. Patient with congenital esotropia. The aspect is compatible with both DVD and bilateral elevation in adduction.

Although the typical DVD is present in abduction as well as in adduction, this criterion does not always clarify the differential diagnosis, because, in some cases with DVD, one eye deviates upward if its visual axis is interrupted by the nose, i.e., in adduction. Moreover, bilateral elevation in adduction often occurs in combination with DVD.

In this paper, we suggest a new test which isolates and accentuates the characteristic of DVD, namely, the dependence of the deviation on the balance of visual inputs entering the right and the left eyes. This test was termed the "Reverse Fixation Test" (RFT) and preliminary reported by Mattheus et al (1978).

METHODS

Reversed Fixation Test (RFT)

The patient is seated at the synoptophore, and the angle is determined with the RE fixing in the primary position.

The light is repeatedly switched from the right to the left tube, and the left tube is adjusted until the refixation saccade of the LE is nullified (Fig 2, upper part). Then, the LE is induced to fix, not in the primary position, but with the left tube remaining in the non-primary position (Fig 2, lower part). In the case of elevation in adduction, or any kind of paretic strabismus, the RE will stay in the primary position, even though fixation has been changed to the LE. But in the case of DVD, the RE will slowly drift up (with a time course determined by Helveston, 1980). The degree of this upward movement represents the "DVD component" which can be determined by aligning the right tube with the visual axis of the RE. It is essential that the left tube remains in its previously determined upward position during this procedure.

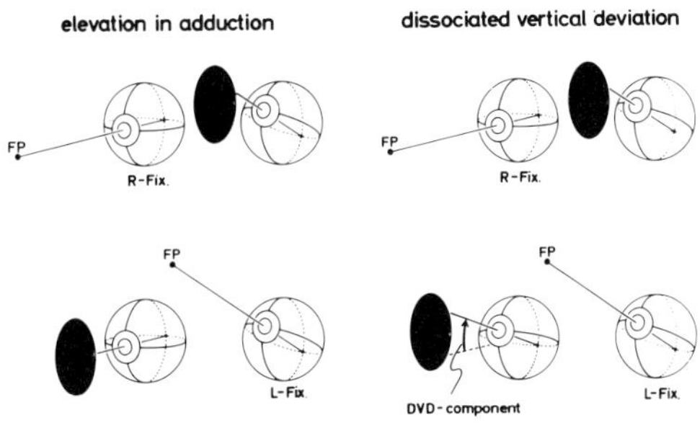

Fig 2. The Reversed Fixation Test reveals unchanged position of the right eye in patients with elevation in adduction, and updrift of the right eye in patients with dissociated vertical deviation.

In order to investigate whether the RFT really brings out a greater alteration of the deviation than does the classical Bielschowsky test, we compared the two in a series of 30 patients. The selection criterion was a DVD component of at least five degrees on the RFT. Only one of the 30 patients had bifoveal fusion ("alternating hyperphoria"), the others had permanent deviations.

Bielschowsky Test

To keep all other parameters unchanged, the Bielschowsky test was also performed at the synoptophore and the angle determined with the LE fixing using the same bright picture as the one employed with the RFT. (The LE was made to fix in the non-primary position which had previously been found as the angle of strabismus with RE fixation.) Then, the bright picture in the left tube was replaced by a dark slide which provided only a dim fixation point at the same location as the fixation target on the bright picture. The downward movement of the RE after darkening the LE was taken as the measurement of the Bielschowsky test. We consider this procedure to be equivalent to darkening the fixing eye with a filter.

RESULTS

The correlation of the RFT with this Bielschowsky test is shown in Fig 3. If the correlation had been perfect, all points would lie on the 45 degree line. It can be seen, however, that the Bielschowsky test resulted in lower values in all cases. In 15 patients, the Bielschowsky test deviation was even zero, although a considerable DVD component was found with the RFT.

Repeating the two tests in the same patient after some weeks, we have found the values to be quite variable; but the DVD component was consistently higher with the RFT than with the Bielschowsky test.

A variant of the Bielschowsky test was performed in only five of the 30 patients. One eye was covered for a few seconds. When uncovered, this eye moved down in all five cases. The amount of downward movement was smaller than the RFT valune in four cases and equal in one case.

Using the RFT, we have occasionally encountered a dissociated horizontal deviation (DHD). This ocular motor abnormality has already been reported by Urist (1976, his patient No. 4). DHD can be mimicked by uncorrected anisometropia. Therefore, the diagnosis of DHD requires full spectacle correction of both eyes.

DISCUSSION

The characteristic of DVD and of the more rare DHD is the dependence of the angle of strabismus on the balance of visual inputs coming through the right and the left eyes. This balance is shown schematically in Fig 4. If the RE is fixing a target on a bright picture, and the LE is presented with a dark, contourless field, the balance of visual inputs is shifted strongly to the RE. In the case of DVD, this imbalance of the visual inputs drives the LE up (Fig 4A).

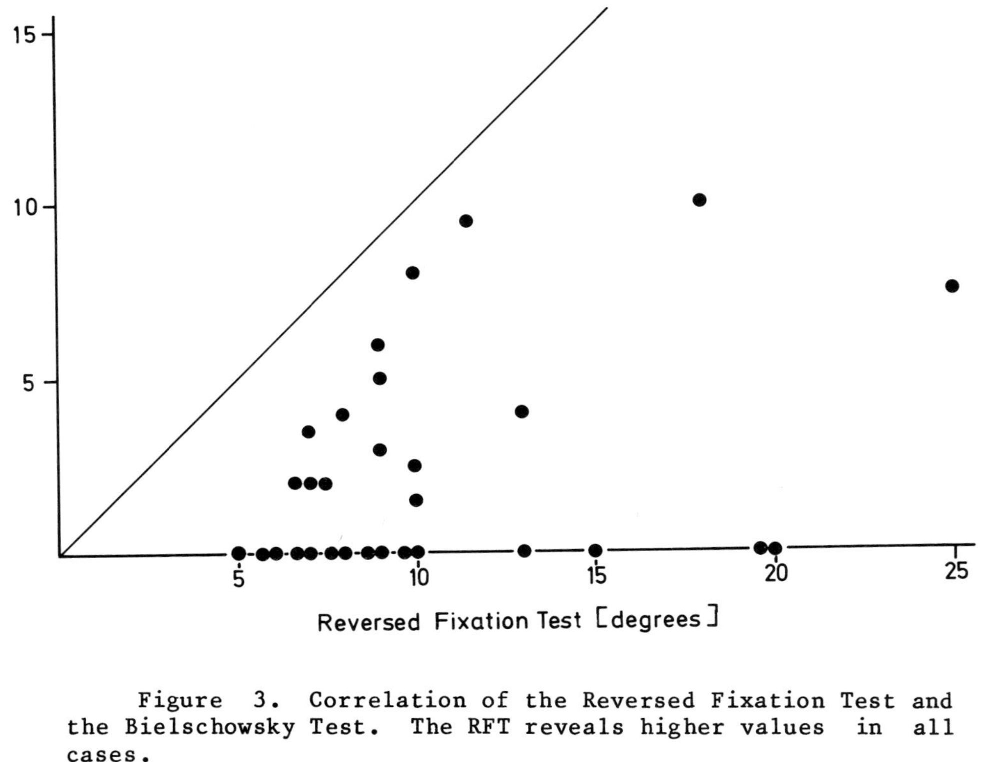

Figure 3. Correlation of the Reversed Fixation Test and the Bielschowsky Test. The RFT reveals higher values in all cases.

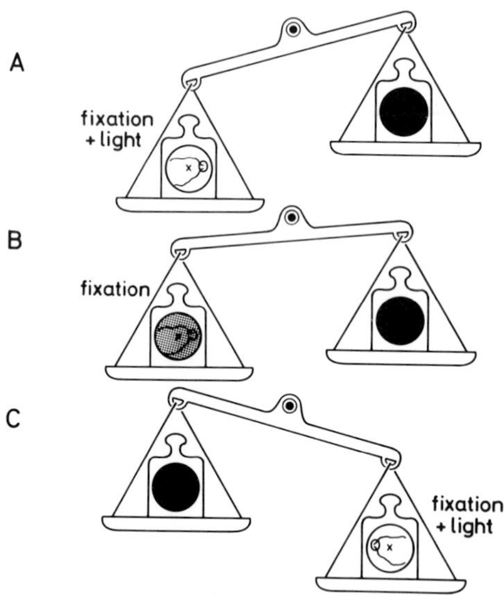

Figure 4. Balance of visual inputs coming through the right and the left eyes. Switching light and fixation to the opposite eye (C) is more effective than darkening the fixing eye with a filter (B).

In the classical Bielschowsky test, this imbalance of visual inputs is decreased by placing a dark filter before the fixing RE, thus reducing the dominance of the RE and allowing the LE to come down (Bielschowsky 1930, p 504). (Fig 4B).

Using the Reversed Fixation Test (RFT), we proceed two steps further. Not only is the RE darkened but the LE is brightened and, in addition, the LE is induced to take over fixation (Fig 4C). Thus, the imbalance is actually reversed to a dominance of the LE.

Our results show that there are indeed many cases in which darkening the fixing eye has little or no effect on the ocular motor system whereas switching fixation from one eye to the other has a marked influence.

Although the balance of visual inputs coming from the right and the left eyes is the pathognomonic determinant of DVD, the variability of the results obtained with both the RFT and the Bielschowsky test indicates that DVD also depends on non-visual, as yet unknown factors, such as attention or vigilance.

The simple alternate cover test also reverses the imbalnce of visual inputs, but it does not allow one to make a clear distinction between DVD and esotropia with elevation in adduction, or with a co-existing paresis. The crucial point is that the simple alternate cover test compares the angles with the right or the left eye each fixing in the primary position, whereas in the RFT, the LE fixes in the non-primary position which previously determined as the angle of squint. In this way, we avoid confusion with the "secondary" angle of paretic strabismus.

Theoretically, our test could be performed with the alternate cover test and prisms. Practically, however, this is difficult. For instance, in the case of an esotropia with elevation in adduction, accompanied by DVD, one would need a prism base out and a prism base down in front of the LE to neutralize the angle with the RE fixing in the primary position. Then, a third prism base down in front of the RE would be necessary to determine the upward movement of the RE when the LE takes over fixation. A single examiner can hardly handle all of these prisms, and at the same time do the cover testing. Thus, it is obviously more practical to perform the RFT at the synoptophore than with prisms.

If a synoptophore is not available, the DVD component can be estimated using a fixation light and an occluder. With these simple instruments, the RFT is performed in the following three steps. First, the RE is induced to fix in the primary position while the LE is occluded. Second, the position of the LE under cover must be remembered. Third, the LE is induced to fix in the remembered, non-primary position holding the fixation light in the appropriate oblique direction, while the RE is covered. Any deviation of the right eye from the primary position represents a DVD component.

In conclusion, we do not claim that our investigators have elucidated the mechanisms underlying the DVD, but we propose the Reversed Fixation Text (RFT) as a diagnostic tool which isolates and accentuates the DVD in patients with other, co-existing ocular motor abnormalities. A positive

RFT in patient with spontaneously alternating fixation should warn us that the vertical deviation includes a DVD component which cannot be completely eliminated by any type of surgery. Corresponding to DVD, a dissociated horizontal deviation (DHD) also defies complete surgical elimination, if the patient habitually alternates fixation.

REFERENCES

1. Bielschowsky A: Die einseitigen und gegensinnigen ("dissoziierten") Vertikalbewegungen der Augen. Albrecht von Graefes Arch Ophthalmol 125:493-553, 1930.

2. Helveston EM: Dissociated vertical deviation, a clinical and laboratory study. Trans Amer Ophthalmol Soc 78:734-779, 1980.

3. Mattheus S, Deberitz I, Kommerell G: Differentialdiagnose zwischen inkomitierendem und dissoziiertem Schielen. Arbeitskreis Schielbehandlung , Berufsverband der Augenartte Deutschlands 10:135-137, 1978.

4. Urist MJ: The fusional balancing innervation in heterophoria for control of antipodal deviations at a null point: A previously undescribed type of binocular innervation. J Pediatr Ophthalmol 13:65-71, 1976.

SURGICAL TREATMENT OF TORSION: AN OBJECTIVE ASSESSMENT

W. E. Scott and G. Gitschlag

ABSTRACT

Correction of cyclotorsional deviation has heretofore been measured by subjective methods, primarily the double Maddox rod. As has been recently pointed out, cyclotorsion can be objectively diagnosed by fundus photography, noting the relationship of macula and disc. We report a series of 10 patients with cyclotorsion, due either to superior oblique palsy or thyroid myopathy, in whom the correction of cyclotorsional deviation is objectively quantified by comparing the relationship of macula to disc on pre- and post-operative fundus photos.

INTRODUCTION

Correction of cyclotorsional deviation has heretofore been measured by subjective methods. As has been recently pointed out, cyclotorsion can be objectively diagnosed by fundus photography, noting the relationship of macula and disc. We report a preliminary series of thirteen patients with superior oblique palsy or thyroid myopathy in whom the correction of cyclotorsional deviation was objectively quantified by comparing the relationship of macula to disc on pre- and post-operative fundus photographs.

BACKGROUND DISCUSSION

Cyclodeviation is a misalignment of the eyes around the Y axis of Fick, the sagittal axis, resulting in a torsional rotation of the globe, either clockwise or counter-clockwise. It is most frequently produced by paresis of one of the cyclovertically acting extraocular muscles, i.e., the vertical recti and the obliques. The torsional action of the obliques is relatively greater than the vertical action, in contradistinction to the vertical recti. Consequently, cyclodeviations are more likely to occur and to be of greater magnitude from paresis of the obliques than of the vertical recti. However, as Caygill has pointed out in 1972, cyclotropias are not infrequent in thyroid myopathy with inferior rectus involvement. Cyclodeviation may also occur

STRABISMUS II
ISBN 0-8089-1424-3

in association with dissociated vertical deviation and A and V patterns in the absence of any apparent paretic component.

Since the cyclovertically acting muscles have both a torsional and vertical component, purely torsional complaints are not the rule in cases of paresis of these muscles. However, in a significant number of patients the torsional component will be of such magnitude as compared to the vertical that it will be the main cause for the patient's distress. This may result, for example, in partially recovered superior oblique palsy or post-operatively in patients with superior oblique palsy or thyroid myopathy in whom the vertical deviation has been corrected but in whom a bothersome residual cyclodeviation persists.

Several clinical methods are available for assessing cyclodeviation. These can be divided into subjective and objective techniques. Subjective methods may include the double Maddox rod, the major amblyoscope, the Lancaster or Hess red/green tests, and perimetry. Our personal preference is the double Maddox rod, primarily because it is convenient and expeditious in the clinic. However, all of these tests are dependent upon the patient's subjective responses to different stimuli and require normal retinal correspondence and the absence of suppression to be valid. (They are based either on the diplopia principle or the haploscopic principle.)

The presence of cyclodeviation can also be detected by ophthalmoscopy in an objective fashion. In 1856, von Graefe described apparent vertical displacement of the macula in incyclotropia. Since then, other investigators, Weiss in 1966 and Zahoruk and Levine in 1972, have also reported an altered relationship of macula and disc in patients with cyclodeviation. As von Noorden pointed out in 1979, under normal circumstances, a horizontal line drawn through the fovea crosses the optic disc between the lower and central third (Fig 1). In incylcotropia, the fovea is apparently displaced upward and in excyclotropia downward (Fig 2). This is most easily observed using the indirect (vs. the direct) ophthalmoscope, allowing simultaneous visualization of both macula and disc. Fundus photography is excellent for diagnostic and recording purposes. It is important that the patient's head be held erect and that the eye not being examined be fixing steadily.

MATERIALS AND METHODS

We would like to present a preliminary report on a series of thirteen patients with torsional complaints and with subjective evidence, by double Maddox rod, and objective evidence, by fundus photography, of cyclodeviation pre-operatively (Table 1). These tests were repeated post-operatively for comparison. Eleven of these patients had superior oblique palsy, either unilateral or bilateral, one had thyroid myopathy, and one had a third nerve paresis. The amount of subjective torsion as measured by the double Maddox rod is indicated, as is the surgical procedure performed. Pre- and post-operative fundus photographs demonstrating the relative position of macula and disc were obtained on all patients. Representative fundus photographs of the objective cyclodeviation will be presented with the results. In all cases in which the Harada-Ito procedure was performed, the tendon of the anterior half of the superior oblique was lateralized on an adjustable suture. This allowed the torsional correction to be more easily titrated.

RESULTS

Following operation, all patients reported improvement or resolution of their torsional symptoms. Furthermore, as Table 1 demonstrates, cyclodeviation was also reduced as measured subjectively by the double Maddox rod test. This could be corroborated in each case by post-operative fundus photographs, providing objective evidence of alteration in the cyclodeviation, even in the patients with thyroid myopathy, in whom no oblique muscle was operated. Figs 3-5 are composites of pre- and post-operative fundus photographs of representative patients. Figure 6 is that of a patient with thyroid myopathy with inferior rectus involvement. An inferior rectus recession with an adjustable suture was performed to relieve the restriction. The photographs demonstrate objective evidence that torsional correction can be effected even when the surgical procedure does not involve an oblique muscle.

Initial results appeared to indicate that in patients with superior oblique palsy who underwent the Harada-Ito procedure, the amount of esotropia in downgaze could be affected by the anterior-posterior placement of the anterior segment of superior oblique tendon at the time of lateralization: the more posterior the insertion site was placed, the greater the esotropia in downgaze corrected.

Several patients reported an initial post-operative incyclotorsion which quickly reverted to an excyclotorsion smaller than that present pre-operatively. This corresponds, as described by Guyton, to the period of sensory adaptation to the new cycloposition of the globe, during which a reordering of the retinal meridians occurs (Fig 7). In this immediate post-operative period, the patient may transiently report tilting of a vertical line.

As more data are gathered, we hope to determine if an accurate correlation can be made between the millimeters of displacement of macula and disc and the degrees of torsion. Fundoscopy or fundus photography could then be used as a quantitative as well as qualitative means of diagnosing cyclodeviation. This would be especially helpful in the pre-verbal patient. Fundus evaluation intraoperatively could then be used as a guide in correcting torsional problems.

In summary, fundus photography offers an objective method of measuring cyclodeviation. This may serve to document subjective measurements of torsion or may be used to help diagnose cyclodeviations (e.g., superior oblique palsy) in patients too young or uncooperative for subjective measurement. It also serves to demonstrate that under certain circumstances cyclodeviations can be effectively treated by surgical procedures involving other than the obliques.

REFERENCES

1. Caygill WM: Excyclotropia in dysthryoid ophthalmopathy. Am J Ophthalmol 73:437-441, 1972.

2. von Noorden GK: Clinical observations in cyclodeviations. Ophthalmology 86:1451-1461, 1979.

3. Weiss JB: Ectopies et psuedoectopies par rotation. Bull Mem Soc Fr Ophthalmol 79:329-349, 1966.

4. Levine MH, Zahoruk RM: Disk-macula relationship in diagnosis of vertical muscle paresis. Am J Ophthalmol 73:262-265, 1972.

5. Locke JC: Heterotopia of the blind spot in ocular vertical muscle imbalance. Am J Ophthalmol 65:362-374, 1968.

FUNDUS HAPLOSCOPE AND THE MEASUREMENT OF CYCLODEVIATION

A. Inatomi, F. Takahashi, and K. Kani

ABSTRACT

We have developed a new type of haploscope, named "Fundus Haploscope," utilizing infrared TV cameras, by which fundus pictures of both eyes of subjects are taken and shown on a TV screen simultaneously with target slides. By using the Fundus Haploscope, the relationship between the fundus and the target in respect to their location can be precisely defined. Therefore, the instrument is useful for investigations of binocular conditions.

In this method, using the projected negatives of fundus pictures and a digitizing tablet connected to a computer, the angle is measured between the horizontal and the line linking the center of gravity of the optic disc to the fixation point (P-F angle). By using the relative angle, which is measured in both right and left eyes, the tilt of the head can almost be ignored. Additionally, the subjective angle of cyclodeviation is measured with a horizontal or a vertical line target. In 55 normal subjects, the mean relative P-F angle was 11.9 degrees and the standard deviation was 4.0 degrees. The relative angle provides the basis for measured cyclodeviations.

INTRODUCTION

The binocular visual function test with the major amblyoscope is a prevailing method for strabismus examination and is based on subjective responses and observations of eye positions and of eye movements. However, the judgement as to the relationship of the fundus to the subjective state is principally conjectural.

To solve this problem we have used an infrared TV fundus camera to make a trial model haploscope. With the TV camera, fundus pictures of both eyes of the subject are taken and shown on the TV screen simultaneously with the target slides. That is why this instrument is named "Fundus Haploscope" (Fig. 1).(1)

STRABISMUS II
ISBN 0-8089-1424-3

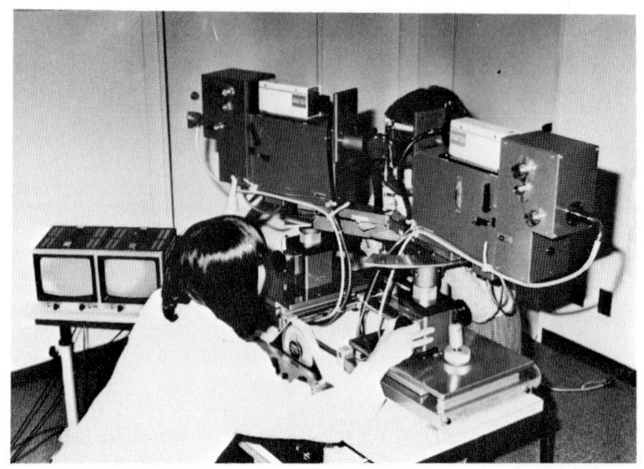

Figure 1. Fundus Haploscope in use

By using the Fundus Haploscope, the relationship between fundus and target in respect to the subjective location can be precisely defined. Therefore, the instrument is useful for investigating the state of binocular conditions, such as determination of retinal correspondence, observation of fine ocular movements under binocular fixation, analysis of motor and sensory components in fusional movements and the measurements of cyclodeviations.

METHOD

Fundus pictures are taken under binocular conditions through the Fundus Haploscope. Then by using the projected negative and digitizing tablet connected to a computer, the center of the optic disc is located (Fig. 2).

The angle is measured between the horizontal and the line linking the center of the optic disc to the fixation point. We call it the P-F angle.

The relative P-F angle (< a + < b) which is measured in both right and left eyes simultaneously give an accurate measurement of the torsional position of the fundus (Fig. 3).

RESULTS

In 55 normal subjects, the mean relative P-F angle was 11.9 degrees and the standard deviation was 4.0 degrees (Table 1). The relative P-F angle provides the basis for measured cyclodeviations. A 12 degrees relative angle is

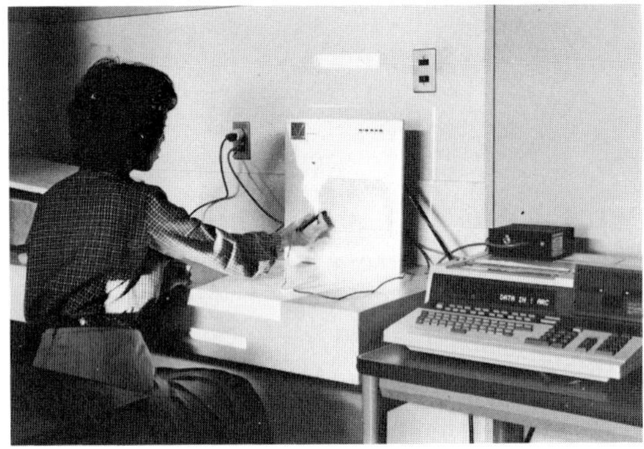

Figure 2. Actual measurement of cyclodeviation. The projected negative and digitizing tablet connected to a computer are used.

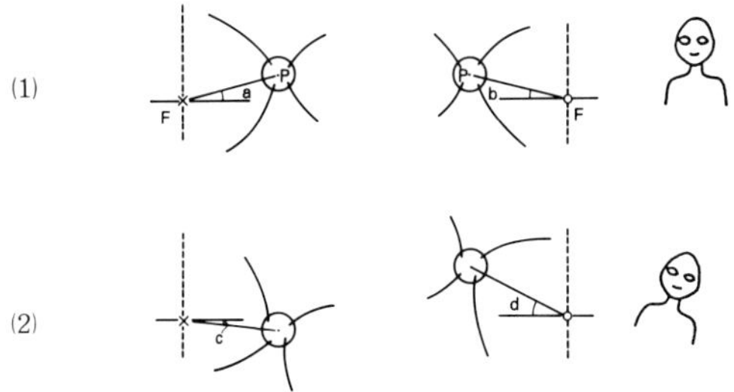

Figure 3.

(1) P : The center of gravity of the optic disc (Papilla)
F : Fixation point (foveola)
a : P-F angle of the right eye
b : P-F angle of the left eye

(2) When the head or body tilts, the P-F angles change but the relative P-F angles do not change.

$$\angle c + \angle d = \angle a + \angle b$$

normal. Under 12 degrees is incyclodeviation and over 12 degrees is excyclodeviation (Fig. 4). Using this method, the quantitative measurement of cyclodeviation was performed on 68 cases with various types of strabismus. There was no significant difference between the average P-F angle of subjects with horizontal strabismus and those with normal eyes. However, the standard deviation was larger in cases of strabismus.

	Mean	S.D.	Max	Min
R-eye	6.4	2.7	12.2	0.3
L-eye	5.5	3.2	12.2	0.1
R-L	3.4	2.6	11.9	0
R+L	11.9	4.0	20.3	4.6

(Relative angle)

Table 1: P-F angle (degree) in 55 normal subjects

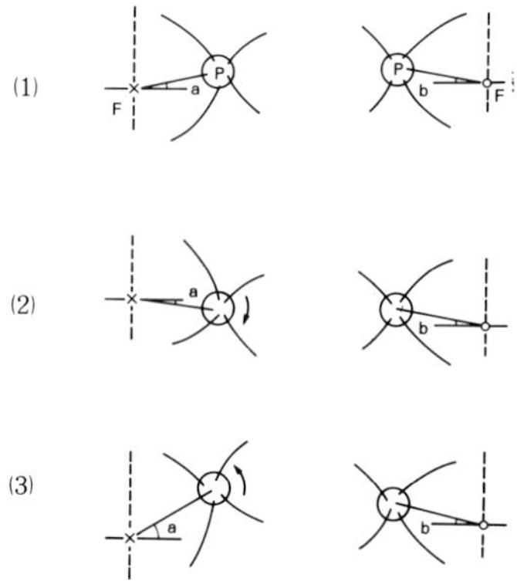

Figure 4.
(1) Normal subject. Mean relative P-F angle is 12°. The standard deviation is 4°.
(2) $\angle a + \angle b < 12° \pm 4°$: incyclodeviation
(3) $\angle a + \angle b > 12° \pm 4°$: excyclodeviation

Excyclodeviations usually were present in cases with paresis, underaction of either intorter, or with overaction of either extorter. Incyclodeviations were usually present in cases with paresis, underaction of either extorter, or with overaction of either intorter. However, in some cases, cyclodeviations contrary to the above rules were observed.

Large cyclodeviations usually were present in disturbances of the vertical rectus muscles (Fig. 5).

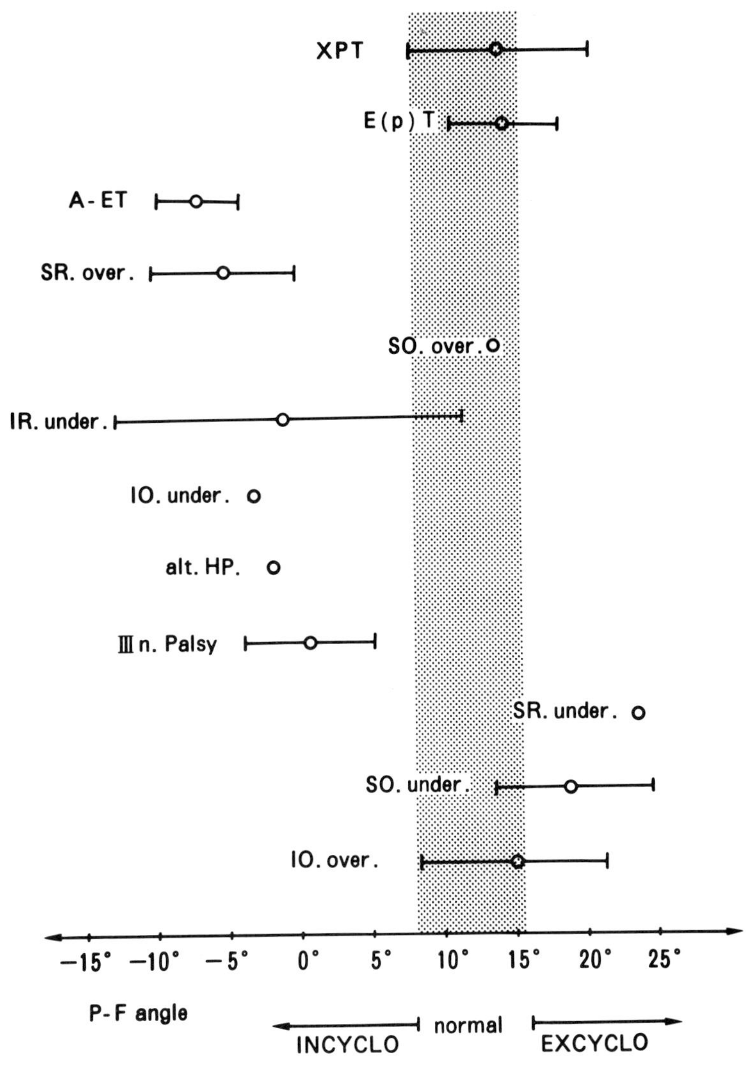

Figure 5. : Cyclodeviation in strabismus

XPT : Exophoria-tropia ET : Esotropia
A-ET : A pattern esotropia
SR. over. : Overaction of superior rectus
SO. over. : Overaction of superior obliquus
IR. under. : Underaction of inferior rectus
IO. under. : Underaction of inferior obliquus
alt. HP. : Alternative hyperphoria
IIIn. Palsy : Oculomotor palsy
SR. under. : Underaction of superior rectus
SO. under. : Underaction of superior obliquus
IO. over. : Overaction of inferior obliquus

DISCUSSION

The subjective measurement of cyclodeviation is more commonly done than the objective measurement, as it is clinically more practical. But in cyclotropia, which is congenital or of early onset, sensory adaptation usually has occurred. Guyton and von Noorden have reported different results between usual subjective tests and objective measurements by the fundus photographic method.(2) Thus, the subjective method of measuring torsion has become more important. However, it presents many difficulties, such as no horizontal or vertical marks on the cornea or in the fundus. Recently Bixenman and von Noorden has provided us with an improved basis for measuring tortion.(3)

Our method is similar to theirs concerning the use of apparent disk displacement. In our test the center of the disk is used, because it is an unchangeable point even if the form of the disc is irregular and tilted. The center of the disk can be easily located by the fundus photograph and digitizing tablet connected to a computer. When the head tilts, the amount of compensatory cycloduction is so small that the eyes tilt in the same direction and the P-F angle changes proportionately. However, by using the relative angle, which is measured in both eyes simultaneously, the tilt of the head can be almost ignored (Fig. 3). The relative angle (< a + < b) can give a more accurate measurement of the torsional position of the fundus.

The average of the relative angle is 12 degrees in normal subjects, and provides the baseline for measuring the torsional position of the fundus by this method.

REFERENCES

1. Inatomi A, Terao N, Kani K, Abe K, Ohno T: A new Fundus Haploscope. Rinsho Coanka 34:815-819, 1980.

2. Guyton DL, von Noorden GK: Sensory adaptation to cyclodeviation. In: Reinecke RD (ed) Strabismus. New York, Grune and Stratton, 399-403, 1978.

3. Bixenman WW, von Noorden GK: Apparent foveal displacement in normal subjects and in cyclotropia. Ophthalmology 89:58-62, 1982.

FURTHER STUDIES ON THE BIELSCHOWSKY HEAD TILT TEST

Y. Watanabe, R. Mori, H. Ohtsuki, R. Ichikawa,
K. Egi, M. Hitomi

ABSTRACT

1. We reconfirmed the existence of counter-rolling of the eyes by an objective method when the head was tilted toward the shoulder. 2. The elevation of the affected eye is mainly caused by the function of the superior rectus muscle in the Bielschowsky Head Tilt Test (BHTT). 3. The BHTT has been shown to be a valuable test for the diagnosis of superior oblique palsy as well as for the evaluation of postoperative improvements of the abnormal head posture. 4. Surgical treatment of superior oblique palsy should be designed with consideration of the BHTT findings and in respect to the ocular dominance.

INTRODUCTION

The physiological basis of the Bielschowski Head Tilt Test (BHTT) is the existence of counter-rolling of the eyes when the head is tilted toward the shoulder.(2)

The authors proved the value of the BHTT for the diagnosis of vertical strabismus using a photographic method in cases with positive BHTT.(23-26)

Recently, however, some investigators such as Levine and Jampel deny the occurrence of the counter-rolling of the eyes induced by head tilt, and consequently, declare that the BHTT is to be labelled as an unreliable test for diagnosing the superior oblique palsy.(11,12,14,15) They favor the theory that it is the inferior oblique muscle that causes the elevation of the eye when the head is tilted toward an affected side in the presence of the superior oblique palsy.

Goodier also supports Levine's opinion and states that BHTT often can produce misleading results in the diagnosis of vertical strabismus.(3,14,15)

The purposes of this paper are: first, to reconfirm the existence of the counter-rolling by Mori's method;(16) secondly to show the BHTT to be a valuable test for the diagnosis of the superior oblique palsy; and thirdly to demonstrate that through the clinical observations in the

STRABISMUS II
ISBN 0-8089-1424-3

surgical treatment of the superior oblique palsy the elevation of the affected eye in the BHTT was mainly caused by the superior rectus muscle.

MATERIALS AND METHODS

The material consisted of 45 cases of unilateral superior oblique palsy with positive BHTT. None of them had either neuro-otologic or orthopedic disorders. The details are shown in Table 1. The total number of cases were divided into two groups in respect to ocular dominance.

The methods used in this paper are given in Table 2. The side of ocular dominance was determined by the "hole in card test." To assess the BHTT, photographic documents were taken in all cases. Mori's procedure, however, was performed in some of the cases who had a close relation to the test and who cooperated in the procedure.

Final assessments of grade of cures of all cases treated in this study were based on the standards of the Japanese Association of Strabismus and Amblyopia (JASA).(22) The cases were reexamined after an average of three and a half years (from one year to seven years) from the last operation.

Mori's methods uses an instrument with a periscope-like function and a camera with motor drive unit, and the head tilt is caused by an electrical apparatus to obtain a continuous tilt up to 30 degrees in five seconds.(16) Figure 1 shows a close-up of fitting the subject to the apparatus. (The subject is Dr. D.A. Robinson, who visited us several years ago.)

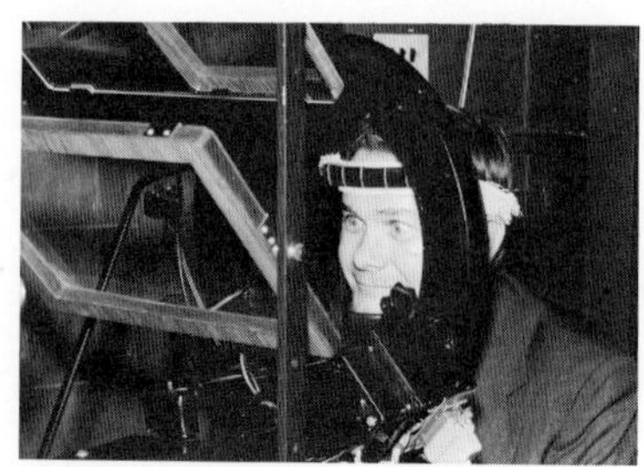

FIGURE 1. Moris Apparatus

Table 1.

MATERIALS

Unilateral Superior Oblique Palsy	45 cases
congenital	43 cases
acquired	2
dominant eye paretic group (DEP)	19
non-dominant eye paretic g.(NDEP)	26
years of age: 2 yrs -- 21 yrs (5.5 yrs in average)	

Table 2.

METHODS

Abnormal Head Posture

Side of Ocular Dominance (Hole in Card Test)

Motility (duction and version)

Bielschowsky Head Tilt Test (BHTT)
(Mori's Method, Photographic Method, quantitative analysis ...)

Deviation

Binocularity

Neuro-otological, Orthopedical Examinations.

RESULTS

The postoperative findings of the head postures and the results of the BHTT in superior oblique palsy with reference to the method of surgery and to the side of ocular dominance are shown in Table 3. Cases who underwent weakening operations on the inferior oblique muscle of the affected eye as the first procedure showed a negative response to the BHTT postoperatively in 40% of the Dominant Eye Paretic group (DEP-group), and in 73% of the NonDominant Eye Paretic group (NDEP-group).

A negative response to the BHTT was found in all cases who underwent recession of the superior rectus muscle of the affected eye.

Cases where weakening operations of the inferior oblique muscle of the affected eye had sufficiently corrected the vertical deviations in the primary position, showed a negative response to the BHTT both in the DEP-group and in the NDEP-group (Table 4).

Table 3. Comparison of postoperative change in the head postures and the results in the BHTT in superior oblique palsies with references to the method of surgery and to the side of ocular dominance.

	Dominant Eye Paretic Group				Non-Dominant Eye Paretic Group			
No. of Cases	19				26			
Postoperative Vertical Deviation in Primary Position (p.d.)	5.1 ± 5.0				2.8 ± 3.6			
Operated Muscles	IO#	SO*	IO+IR	SR	IO#	SO*	IO+IR	SR
No. of Cases	10	2	3	4	15	1	4	7
Abnormal Head Postures								
corrected	4	0	1	3	10	0	4	7
improved	5	1	2	0	4	1	0	0
not improved	1	1	0	1	1	0	0	0
BHTT: negative	4	0	0	4	11	1	4	7
positive	6	2	3	0	4	0	0	0

IO#: weakening operation of Inferior Oblique M., only
SO*: tucking of the affected superior oblique M.

Table 4. The results of the BHTT after the weakening operation of the inferior oblique muscle in the affected eye.

	Cases with negative response to the BHTT		Cases with positive response to the BHTT	
	Dominant Eye Paretic G.	Non-Dominant Eye Paretic G.	Dominant Eye Paretic G.	Non-Dominant Eye Paretic G.
No. of cases	4	11	9	7
Age at operation (years)	6.5 ± 2.7	5.0 ± 2.0	8.1 ± 6.6	3.7 ± 2.2
Vertical deviation in primary position (preoperative) (pd)	13.5 ± 8.5	10.3 ± 4.5	9.7 ± 8.8	8.4 ± 3.7
Amount of correction of vertical deviation in primary p.	9.0 ± 4.9	9.6 ± 5.9	4.1 ± 8.5	3.7 ± 3.2
Preoperative grade of overaction of inferior oblique m.*	1.8 ± 0.5	1.3 ± 0.5	1.8 ± 0.8	1.9 ± 0.7

* Quantitative analysis of the grade of overaction of inferior oblique muscle was performed after Ghi (1969), and the marked degree of overaction corresponds to +++ (3 positive points), the moderate one to ++ (2 positive points) and the mild one to + (1 point).

The relationship between postoperative response to the BHTT and changes in the head posture with reference to the side of ocular dominance is shown in Table 5. A well correlated relationship was noticed between the negative response to the BHTT and a post-surgical improvement of abnormal head posture.

The final results were distributed according to the grade of cures which were recommended by JASA. Cases of the

Table 5. Correlation between the postoperative results in the BHTT and the improvement of abnormal head posture.

Improvement of abnormal head posture,	Positive cases in the BHTT postoperatively	Negative cases in the BHTT postoperatively	TOTAL
not improved	[2], (0)	[1], (1)	[3],(1)
improved	[7], (4)	[2], (1)	[8],(5)
corrected	[2], (0)	[6], (20)	[8],(20)
TOTAL	[11], (4)	[8], (22)	[19],(26)

[ ]: Non-dominant eye paretic group,

( ): Dominant eye paretic group.

Table 6.

GRADE OF CURES

Grade of Cures	DEP-group	NDEP-group
Excellent (IV)	3 (16%)	6 (23%)
Good (III)	1 (5%)	7 (27%)
Fair (II)	2 (11%)	6 (23%)
Poor (I)	12 (63%)	6 (23%)
Not improved (0)	1 (5%)	1 (4%)
Total	19	26
		X^2 : 8.62

NDEP-group showed better improvement than that of the DEP-group. Attention should be paid to the side of ocular dominance in the surgical treatment of the superior oblique palsy (Table 6). EXAMPLES

Case 1 is an 8-year-old boy with a right congenital superior oblique palsy with the right eye dominant. In the upper part of Fig. 2 an overaction of the right inferior oblique muscle is seen in gaze up and left. In the lower part of Fig. 2, with head tilt to the right, the right eye moved upward. When the fixation was changed to the right eye during the head tilting, the left eye went down.

Fig. 3 shows the postoperative conditions following myectomy of the right inferior oblique muscle. No overaction

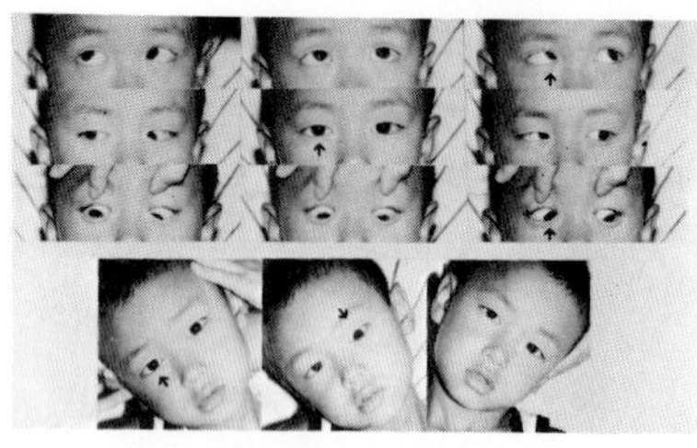

FIGURE 2. Congenital Superior Oblique Palsy, O.D., with the right eye dominant, preoperative

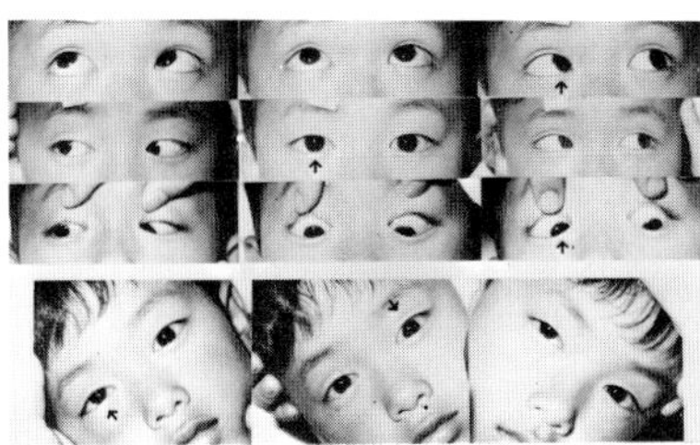

FIGURE 3. Postoperative findings, after myectomy of the inferior oblique muscle of the Right eye. (Aug. 8, 1980)

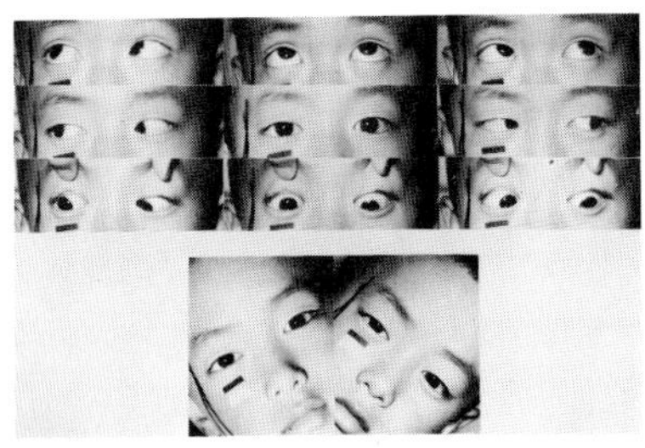

FIGURE 4. Postoperative findings, after recession of RSR (3 mm) (aug. 12, 1981)

of the operated muscle is seen. A positive response to the BHTT, however, is noticed in the lower part of this figure.

The same case underwent a recession of the right superior rectus (3 mm). No elevation of the right eye is found in the BHTT (Fig. 4). Fig. 5 shows a course of improvement of abnormal head posture of the case.

FINDINGS ON THE CURVES OF THE DYNAMIC COUNTER-ROLLING (DCR)

Fig. 6 represents the curves of the DCR of both eyes as well as the amount of vertical deviation of the eyes of the same case corresponding to the degree of head tilt when using Mori's apparatus. The degree of the head tilt is plotted along the abscissa, and the size of the vertical deviation and of the counter-rolling is plotted along the ordinate. The curves of the DCR clearly show that the counter-rolling of the eyes was induced by the head tilt even with paresis of the superior oblique muscle. Regarding the coordination of the DCR curves of both eyes, the figures are to coordinate well during the clockwise tilt but coordinate less with head tilt to the right.

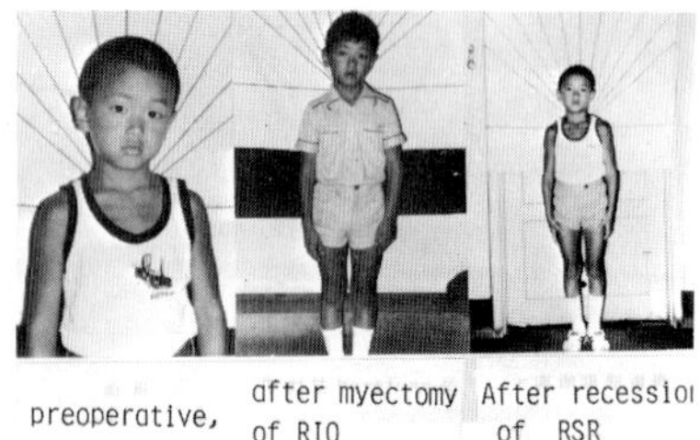

FIGURE 5. Course of abnormal head posture

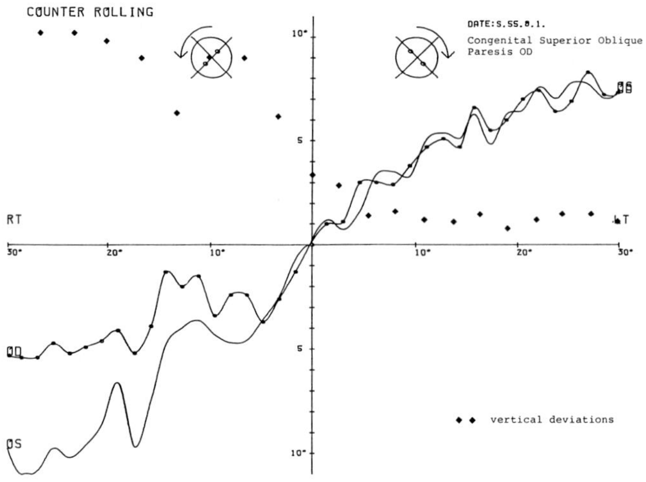

FIGURE 6. Dynamic Counter-Rolling of both eyes and vertical deviation of the right eye, Case KD, postoperative findings of myectomy of the inferior oblique, OD (Watanabe, et al)

The diamond-shaped dots show the vertical deviation of the right eye. The deviation increases with the degree of head tilt. No vertical deviation is found in the oblique position of the head about five and a half degrees clockwise where this case can be suspected to take an abnormal head posture to maintain single binocular vision.

The regression coefficient of the DCR curves of this case show the regression coefficient of the right eye in the second phase (from 10 degrees to 20 degrees of head tilt) to be lower than normal.

Fig. 7 shows the curves of the DCR of the same case after a recession of the superior rectus muscle of the affected eye as the second procedure. The less coordinated DCR curves are seen when the head is tilted to the right shoulder. No elevation of the right eye, however, is noticed in the right tilt.

COMMENTS

It is well known that the counter-rolling was first reported by Hunter in 1786 after he looked in a mirror and noticed that his eyes rotated as he tilted his head.(6) In the counter-rolling studies, however, disparate results have long puzzled numerous investigators of this phenomenon. Those who have studied the counter-rolling are divided into two schools, the one denying any cycloduction with tilting of

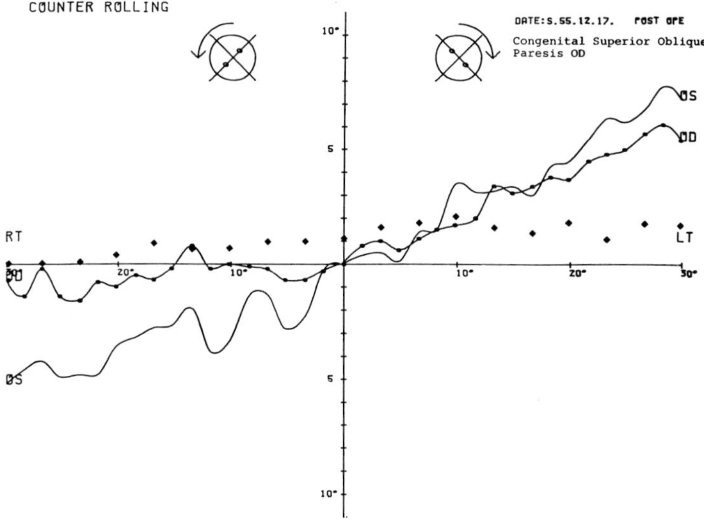

FIGURE 7. Dynamic Counter- Rolling of both eyes and vertical deviation of the right eye, Case KD, postoperative findings, after a recession of the superior rectus mucle of the right eye (Watanabe et al).

the head,(4,5) the other confirming the counter-rolling of the eye as the head is tilted.(1,13) All investigators agree that the greatest error probably arises during the measurement of the ocular torsion. The photographic method is regarded as the best method for detecting the counter-rolling objectively.

Jampel points out that if fixation and head position are not rigorously controlled in photographic experiments, a pseudotorsion may be measured, which is a major artifact in such measurements.(12) In Mori's method, however, details on the consideration of the secondary and the tertiary position of gaze have already been discussed by the authors.(23)

The occurrence of the counter-rolling is also confirmed on normal subjects using infrared television pictures obtained with the Fundus Haploscope which was invented by Inatomi and is regarded as one of the best and the most precise methods for detecting the counter-rolling.(10,21)

The counter-rolling is divided into two categories, Static Counter-rolling (SCR) and Dynamic Counter-rolling (DCR). The former is noticed when the head is maintained at a tilted position in a certain period, the latter occurs during the head tilt. The reasons why the DCR is adopted in a series of our studies are as follows: 1. The DCR has a larger amplitude than the SCR. 2. It is easily measured and clinically applied by using Mori's method.(27) 3. A method of analyzing the curves of the DCRs was established by Ichikawa.(9) The main points in analyzing the curves are coordination of the DCR curves of both eyes and regression coefficient of the curves. 4. It has been proven that the DCR curves provide useful information in the fields of both oculo-motor physiology and neuro-otology.(9)

In normal subjects, according to Mori, both eyes move conjugately during head tilting;(16,17) well coordinated DCR curves are, therefore, found in most instances. Consequently, the amount of regression coefficient of the DCR of both eyes shows almost the same value for a certain degree of head tilt.

In cases with palsy of the superior oblique muscle of the right eye, as shown in Fig. 6, the DCR curves of clockwise tilt are well coordinated. In counterclockwise tilt, the DCR curve of the right eye has a lower amount of regression coefficient than that of the left eye. As a result, coordination of the DCR curves on counterclockwise tilt becomes worse. These findings are noted in the second phase of head tilt in particular. In order to explain the reasons why the two curves are less coordinated with the right tilt, it is clearly pointed out that the amplitude of the DCR of the right eye is smaller than that of the left eye due to underaction of the right superior oblique which intorts the right eye with counter-clockwise tilt.

After reconfirming the existence of the counter-rolling with head tilt, it is easily accepted, as stated by Bielschowsky, that the BHTT has a physiological basis.(2)

In a case presented in this paper where the patient showed a positive response to the BHTT preoperatively, the response to the BHTT did not change even when the inferior oblique overaction was reduced to nil by surgery, but a negative BHTT result was obtained by a recession of the superior rectus muscle of the paretic eye. The clinical course of this case produced counter-evidence to those who deny the diagnostic value of the BHTT and favor the theory that it is the inferior oblique that causes the elevation of the paretic eye with head tilt to the affected side in the presence of a unilateral superior oblique palsy. The results of this paper certainly confirm that the elevation of the affected eye in the BHTT is caused mainly by the superior rectus muscle.

Using Hess charts, Goodier demonstrated the cases who showed a negative response to the BHTT after normalizing an overaction of the inferior oblique by its weakening operation.(3) These findings prompted her to favor Levine's opinion, and to state that a positive BHTT for differentiation between a superior oblique palsy and a contralateral superior rectus palsy is often misleading.

The results of the BHTT, as reported by the authors previously,(23-26) are much influenced by the testing conditions, such as a tilted position of head, the size and contour of fixating targets, the testing distance, correction of refractive errors, the criteria of a positive BHTT, the ocular dominance, and so on. Goodier's survey(3) would have more persuasive power if she could have stated clear criteria for making decisions as to a positive BHTT, and added at least the findings of Hess charts when the head was tilted toward the shoulder.

It is well known that a negative response to the BHTT was found after weakening operations on the inferior oblique muscle of the paretic eye as the first procedure. In our series this tendency was noted in 40% of the Dominant Eye Paretic group, and in 73% of the Non-Dominant Eye Paretic group. The larger the size of vertical deviation of the primary position which was corrected by weakening surgery of the inferior oblique muscle of the affected eye postoperatively, the higher was the percentage of cases which showed a negative response to the BHTT (Table 4).

Regardless of the side of ocular dominance, however, a negative response to the BHTT was noted in all cases which underwent recession of the superior rectus muscle of the paretic eye (Table 3). The weakening surgery of the superior rectus muscle is closely related to changing the BHTT to negative.

According to a series of studies by the authors, it is well known that the results of the BHTT are much influenced by the side of ocular dominance in the presence of unilateral superior oblique palsy.(23-26) Recently some sensorimotorial disorders have been reported on nonparetic eye when the paretic eye is fixating in cases with unilateral superior oblique palsy.(19)

Classification of unilateral superior oblique palsy according to the side of ocular dominance has been reported by White(28) and others.(20) Unfortunately there are few papers concerning surgical treatment of a unilateral superior oblique palsy with notation as to the side of ocular dominance.

SURGICAL MANAGEMENT OF UNILATERAL SUPERIOR OBLIQUE PALSY(7,8)

The following general principles should serve as a useful guide for treating unilateral superior oblique palsy with reference to the side of ocular dominance. 1. First, the side of ocular dominance may be determined by means of the "hole in card" test. 2. Regardless of the side of ocular dominance, a weakening procedure of the inferior oblique muscle is performed as the first procedure in the presence of overaction of that muscle. 3. Without overaction of the inferior oblique muscle of the affected eye, a weakening operation of the inferior rectus muscle of the non-paretic eye is performed in cases of Dominant Eye Paretic group for releasing an overaction of the yoke muscle of paretic muscle. 4. A weakening surgery of the superior rectus muscle of the affected eye is scheduled in the presence of its secondary contracture in cases of Non-Dominant Eye Paretic group. 5. With some exceptions, strengthening procedure on paretic muscle cannot be adopted because of the ineffectiveness in most instances.

Improvement of abnormal head posture is adopted as one of the important points of standard of cures of the Japanese Association of Strabismus and Amblyopia.(22) A well correlated relationship between the negative response to the BHTT and a postsurgical improvement of abnormal head posture suggests that the BHTT gives useful information of assessing postoperative head postures in cases with unilateral superior oblique palsy.

ACKNOWLEDGEMENTS

The authors are grateful to Dr. Nobuhiko Matsuo, Professor and Chairman, Department of Ophthalmology, Okayama University Medical School, for his constant interest and guidance in this investigation, and wish to thank the following specialists who contributed to this investigation by taking pictures and analyzing data: Dr. Reiji Hashimoto, Professor, Department of Electronic Science, Okayama University of Science, Mr. Akira Hosoda, Ms. Hiroka Takasaki and Miss Yumiko Oyama, Department of Ophthalmology, Okayama University medical School. We are also grateful to dr. Shinobu Awaya, Associate Professor, Department of Ophthalmology, Nagoya University School of Medicine, for his valuable suggestions as well as his sincere help in preparing this manuscript, and wish to thank Dr. Akio Ohshima, Department of Oto-laryngology, Okayama University Medical School, for his helpful criticism of the manuscript.

REFERENCES

1. Adler FH: Physiologic factors in differential diagnosis of paralysis of superior rectus and superior oblique muscles. Arch Ophthalmol 36:661-673, 1946.

2. Bielschowsky A: Lectures on motor anomalies, VIII. Paralysis of individual eye muscles: Abducens-Nerve paralysis Am J Ophthalmol 22:357-367, 1939.

3. Goodier HM: The evaluation of the Bielschowsky's head Tilting Test, Orthoptics, Research and Practice, Transactions of the Fourth International Orthoptic Congress, 189, Kimpton, London, 1981.

4. Helmholz H: cited by Duke Elder: Textbook of Ophthalmology, Vol 1., 624. St. Louis: CV Mosby, 1938.

5. Hewitt RS: Torsional eye movements. Am J Ophthalmol 34:253-260, 1951.

6. Nelson JR, Cope D: The otoliths and the ocular countertorsion reflex. Arch Otolaryngol 94:40-50, 1971.

7. Ichikawa R: Surgical treatment of superior oblique palsy. Part 1. Longterm surgical effects with reference to ocular dominance and the Bielschowsky Head Tilt Test. Rinsho Ganka 35:611-620, 1981.

8. Ichikawa R: Surgical treatment of superior oblique palsy. Part 2. Longterm effect of superior rectus recession of the paretic eye. Rinsho Ganka 36:925-932, 1982.

9. Ichikawa R et al: Dynamic counter-rolling and unilateral labyrinthine disorders. Jpn Rev Clin Ophthalmol 76:1933, 1982.

10. Inatomi A et al: A new "fundus haploscope." Rinsho Ganka 34:815-819, 1980.

11. Jampel RS: Ocular torsion and the function of the vertical extraocular muscles. Am J Ophthalmol 79:292-304, 1975.

12. Jampel RS: Ocular torsion and the primary retinal meridians, Am J Ophthalmol 91:14-24, 1981.

13. Javal E: In Traite des Maladies de Yeux by L. Wecker, Paris, Delahaye, 2:815, 1866.

14. Levine MH: Evaluation of the Bielschowsky Head Tilt Test. Arch Ophthalmol 82:433-439, 1969.

15. Levine MH: Pendulum-like eye movement, compensatory cycloversion challenged. Am J Ophthalmol 75:979-987, 1973.

16. Mori R: Studies on the binocular counter-rolling induced by head tilt in man. Part 1. The coordination of the counter-rolling of both eyes in normal subjects. Acta Soc Ophthalmol Jpn 77:753-760, 1973.

17. Mori R: Studies on the binocular counter-rolling

induced by head tilt in man. Part 2. Analysis of the dynamic counter-rolling and the static counter-rolling of both eyes in normal subjects. Folia Ophthalmol Jpn 27:76-83, 1976.

18. Mori R: Studies on the binocular counter-rolling induced by head tilt in man. Part 3. Experimental and clinical studies in normal and pathological subjects. Jpn J Clin Ophthalmol 32:607-613, 1978.

19. Olivier P, von Noorden GK: Excyclotropia of the nonparetic eye in unilateral superior oblique muscle paralysis. Am J Ophthalmol 93:30-33, 1982.

20. Scott WE: Differential diagnosis of vertical muscle palsies. Symposium on strabismus, 118. St. Louis: CV Mosby, 1978.

21. Takahashi K: Eye movement with body tilt. Nippon Ganka Gakka 85:952, 1981.

22. Uemura K: Standard of cures of strabismus, authorized by The Japanese Association of Strabismus and Amblyopia (JASA). Jpn Rev Clin Ophthalmol 72:1408, 1978.

23. Watanabe Y, et al: Studies on the Bielschowsky Head Tilt Test. Part 1. An argument against Dr. Levine's opinion. Folia Ophthalmol Jpn 28:23-33, 1977.

24. Watanabe Y, et al: Studies on the Bielschowsky Head Tilt Test. Part 2. On the vertical deviation patterns of both eyes during head tilt in patients with positive response to the Bielschowsky Head Tilt Test. Folia Ophthalmol Jpn 28:34-42, 1977.

25. Watanabe Y, et al: Studies on the Bielschowsky Head Tilt Test. Part 3. On the vertical deviation pattern of both eyes in head tilting positions in patients with positive response to the Bielschowsky Head Tilt Test. Folia Ophthalmol Jpn 28:43-65, 1977.

26. Watanabe Y, et al: Studies on the Bielschowsky Head Tilt Test. In Reinecke RD (ed) Strabismus, Proceedings of the Third Meeting of the International Strabismological Association, 387-389. New York: Grune & Stratton, 1978.

27. Watanabe Y, Ichikawa R: Dynamic counter-rolling and its clinical application. Jpn Rev Clin Ophthalmol 76:1856, 1982.

28. White JW: The choice of the fixation eye in paralytic and nonparalytic strabismus. Am J Ophthalmol 27:817-819, 1944.

QUANTITATIVE FORCED TRACTION MEASUREMENTS IN STRABISMUS

H. S. Metz and G. Cohen

ABSTRACT

In the evaluation and management of human strabismic disorders, both innervational and mechanical factors play an important role. The innervational component has been investigated by the use of such techniques as ocular electromyography, active force generation testing and ocular saccadic velocity determinations. The mechanical components, both from the extraocular muscles and the orbital tissues, have been mainly determined by qualitative forced duction testing. This clinical technique has some inaccuracies and is often not repeatable among different observers.

We have developed and tested instrumentation which will quantitatively measure the amount of force necessary to move the globe a known distance. Quantitative forced traction testing was performed prior to and during surgery in a group of "non-strabismic" patients as well as in patients with esotropia, exotropia, vertical strabismus, thyroid ophthalmopathy, orbital floor fracture and one patient with muscular dystrophy. The findings were compared among different groups of patients as well as before, during and after muscle surgery in patients with strabismus.

INTRODUCTION

For proper strabismus management, there is a need to differentiate between neurogenic versus mechanical restriction of eye movement. Unequivocally differentiation of neurogenic from mechanical causes of strabismus requires more than can be learned from a usual clinical examination of the patient's dynamic ductions, versions and static deviation. The management of strabismus requires knowledge of the mechanical and innervational properties of the extraocular muscles, as well as the mechanical and viscous properties of the passive, restraining tissues. In most clinical situations, the passive elements are determined by the "calibration" of the educated hand of a skilled physician as he moves a forceps applied to the limbus of the eye. Without question, the diagnosis would be more accurate if the

STRABISMUS II
ISBN 0-8089-1424-3

results of quantitative measurements of the mechanical properties of the muscles and orbital tissues were available, such as static force-duction data, as well as dynamic measurements including saccadic velocity and acceleration.

The usefulness of passive force duction testing has been reiterated in the literature for more than 15 years. At present, the test is either performed qualitatively, and is dependent upon the examiners experience to be of value or is available quantitatively only as a laboratory tool. We have developed instrumentation and techniques to quantitatively measure and make the diagnostic procedure simple enough to be used by the general ophthalmologist caring for strabismus patients.

PROCEDURE

Our strain gauge force transducer can be used in the operating room. A forceps is mounted in a thick plastic holder with a stainless steel hook clamped at the flexible tipped end (Fig 1). The hook engages a small loop of suture (6-0 silk) sewn through partial thickness sclera at the limbus (at the 9 and 3 o'clock mericians for horizontal movement and at the 12 and 6 o'clock meridians for vertical movements). The horizontal or vertical projection of the angular rotation is measured by a millimeter scale with the limbus as the index of movement. An ink mark on the lid and brow is used as a point of reference. Grams of force necessary to achieve the movement is read directly from a digital readout. The strain gauge force transducer is gas sterilized for use in the operating theater.

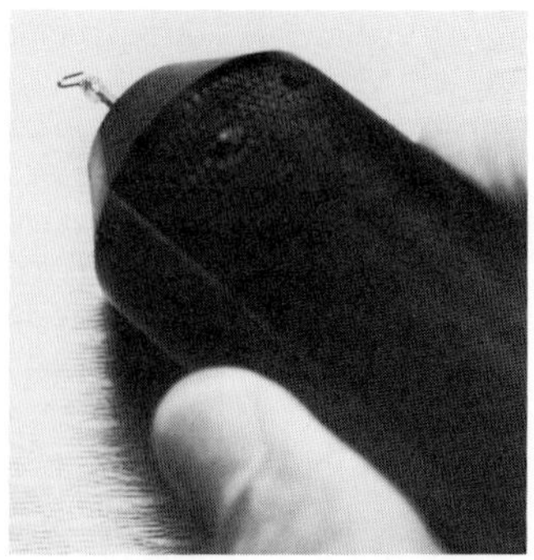

Figure 1. Strain gauge force transducer.

A plastic holder minimizes the effect of temperature change on the sensitive semiconductor strain gauge mounted on the tines. It has proven to be a reliable force transducer. The strain gauge is connected to a bridge circuit amplified by an integrated circuit operational amplifier so that the range 0-100 grams appears as a 0-100 mv signal which is in turn fed to an LED readout (Fig 2).

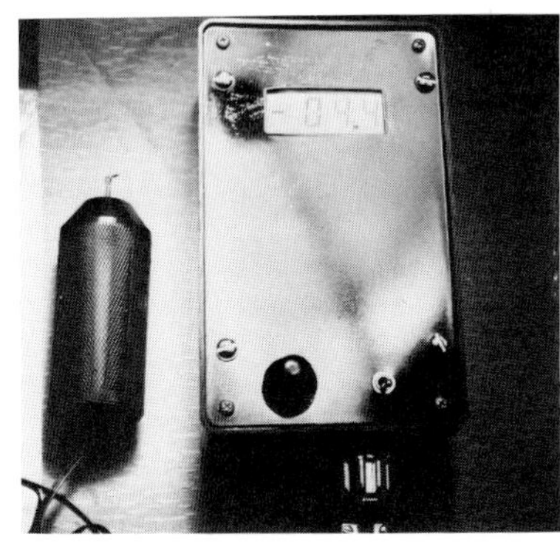

Figure 2. LED readout of strain gauge force transducer.

We have studied patients at surgery, determining the passive duction results quantitatively. Tension was measured as the globe was rotated horizontally (or vertically) 3 mm, 5 mm, 8 mm, and 10 mm from the resting position. Distance was measured visually by aligning the limbus with a ruler and three separate trials were made. The results in normal patients and strabismus patients are described.

RESULTS

Sixty patients have been studied by quantitative forced duction testing under general anesthesia at the time of surgery.

Controls

Thirteen non-strabismic patients (seven adults and six children) composed a "normal" group. The patients all had eye surgery (cataract, glaucoma, nystagmus surgery), other than strabismus repair. There was good correlation. The length-tension curves correlated well with the measurements comparing adults and children (Fig 3). An even tighter fit was seen between two eyes of the same patient in two cases. Several "normal" individuals had increased tension required to move the globe upwards from the starting position (Fig 4). It is possible that the depth of anesthesia was not as great in these patients so that the starting eye position was higher than normal. Therefore, more force might be required for upward rotation since the globe started at a high level.

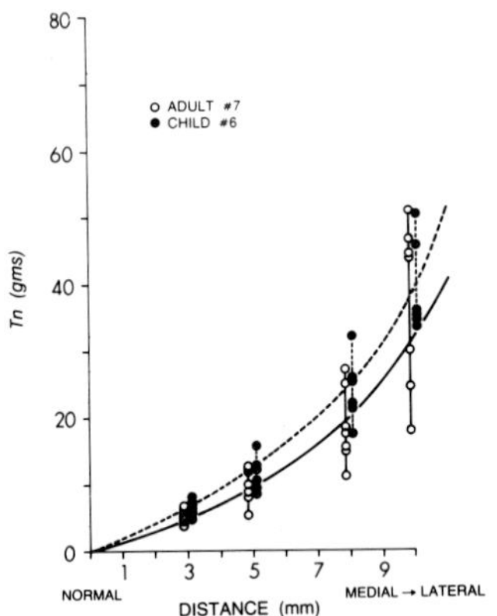

Figure 3. Length-tension curve of ocular rotation in non-strabismic adults and children.

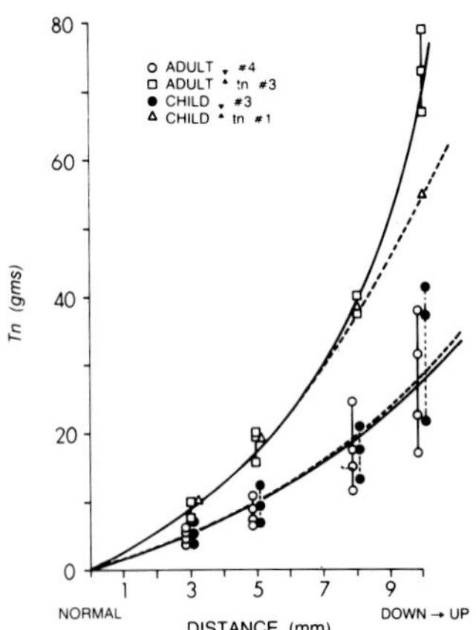

Figure 4. Length-tension curve of ocular rotation upward showing increased tension required in some patients.

Strabismic Patients

The strabismus patients included 21 cases of esotropia, 16 cases of exotropia, 4 with hypertropia, 3 with thyroid ophthalmopathy, 1 with dissociated vertical divergence (DVD), 1 early re-operation following undercorrected esotropia in a child with muscular dystrophy and 1 patient with an orbital floor fracture. In these patients undergoing strabismus surgery, quantitative forced traction measurements were made prior to surgery, after rectus muscle disinsertion and then after rectus muscle recession, resection or advancement. The zero position for all measurements was the starting position of the globe prior to muscle surgery.

Exotropia

In 16 patients with exotropia, 12 had recession-resection surgery and 4 had bilateral lateral rectus recessions. After the rectus muscle was disinserted, starting eye position was displaced in a direction opposite that of the action of the muscle. The length-tension curve was also displaced, but the shape of the curve was essentially unchanged. If the muscle was resected (or advanced), the globe was displaced towards the operated muscle beyond the starting point, and the length-tension curve displaced in a similar manner. The first portion of the curve had a similar shape but often was noticeably steeper as rotation extended beyond 5 mm (Fig 5). When the muscle was recessed, ocular position occasionally remained the same as in the disinserted state but, more often, was displaced towards, but short of the starting position. The length-tension curve was similarly displaced between the curve drawn prior to surgery and that when the muscle was disinserted (Fig 6). The shape remained the same. When a large recession was performed (or a smaller recession in a re-operation when the muscle had been previously recessed), the curve recorded following disinsertion and recession essentially overlapped, suggesting that this amount of recession left the muscle in a slack state.

Esotropia

In 21 esotropic patients, 14 had recession-resection surgery while 7 had bilateral medial recti recessions. The effect upon eye position and the length-tension curve was similar to those found in exotropic patients. In some cases

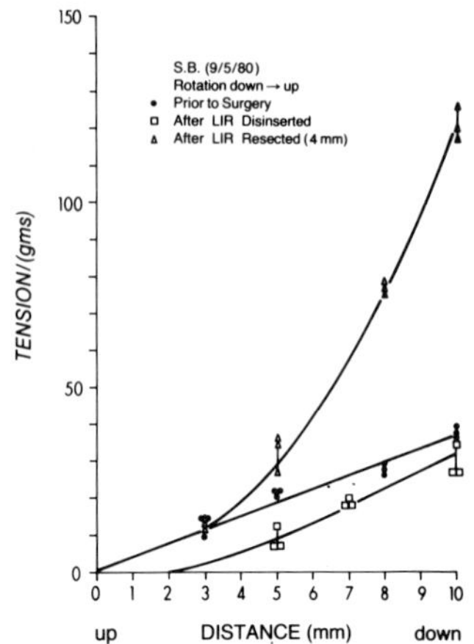

Figure 5. Length-tension curve of ocular rotation showing effect of rectus muscle disinsertion and recession.

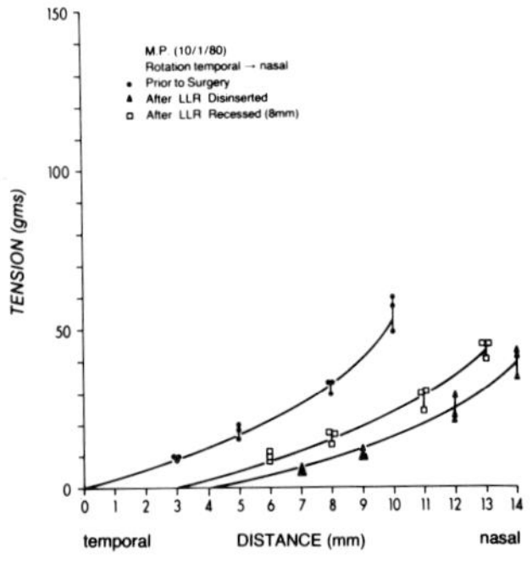

Figure 6. Length-tension curve of ocular rotation showing effect of rectus muscle disinsertion and recession.

with a large angle esotropia, disinsertion of the lateral rectus had little effect on the position or shape of the length-tension curve. This might be due to the lateral rectus being "stretched out" by the large esotropia, producing little effect when this thin, "stretched" muscle was disinserted.

In general, the force necessary to rotate the globe from the starting position a given distance (length-tension curve) did not differ when esotropic or exotropic patients were compared with normals (up to 10 mm of rotation). This suggests that in most cases, the esotropes and exotropes studied did not demonstrate mechanical difficulties with ocular rotation in the range studied.

Verticals

All 4 patients with vertical deviations had recession-resection procedures of the vertical recti. The effect of disinsertion, recession or resection was similar to that found with the horizontal recti. Length-tension measurements prior to surgery rotating the globe downward showed that increased force was required (compared to "controls") in 3 hypertropic eyes while in 1 hypotropic eye, increased force was needed to rotate the globe upwards. This suggests that more of a mechanical component was present in these patients with vertical strabismus than in the horizontal strabismus group.

Thyroid

The 3 patients with thyroid disease were all somewhat different. One had only a vertical deviation and required considerably more force to elevate the hypotropic eye than "controls" (Fig 7). Another case had only a horizontal deviation with significant limitation of abduction monocularly. Force to rotate the eye laterally in the other eye was unremarkable while a noticeable increase in force was needed in the esotropic eye with limited abduction. The third patient had both a horizontal and vertical strabismus with limitation upwards and nasally. Both upward rotation of the hypotropic eye and nasal rotation of the exotropic eye required increased force for eye movement. Mechanical factors in all 3 cases were obvious and significant. Recession of these tight muscles provided an increased range of rotation and large displacement and flattening of the length-tension curve (Fig 7).

DVD

The patient with DVD had a large superior recti muscle recession bilaterally. The length-tension findings prior to surgery were normal. Muscle recessions had only a modest effect on the position of the curve while the shape of the curve was unchanged.

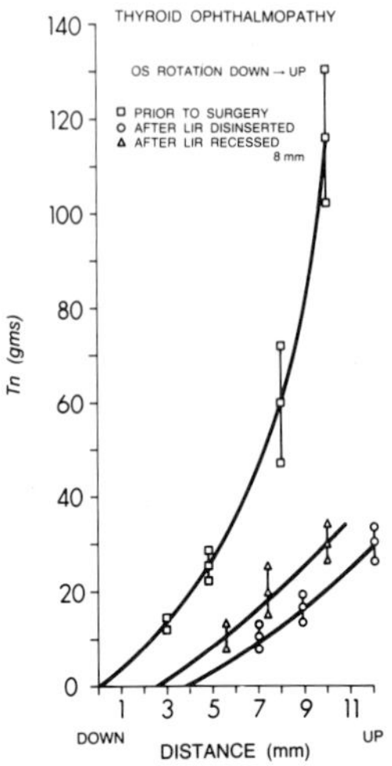

Figure 7. Length-tension curve of ocular rotation in a patient with thyroid ophthalmopathy, hypotropia and limited upgaze, before and after inferior rectus recession.

Muscular Dystrophy

One patient had congenital esotropia and an undetermined type of generalized muscular dystrophy. Prior to the start of surgery, measurements indicated that a large amount of force was needed to move the globe laterally in each eye (Fig 8). Medial rectus muscle recession displaced the curve and flattened the shape minimally. Although the result one day after surgery was excellent, a large esotropia recurred in 3 weeks. The length-tension curve of one eye prior to re-operation 7 weeks later showed an increased slope when compared with the curve at the end of the first surgery. This may account for the early recurrence of significant esotropia following what initially appeared to be a satisfactory outcome. Re-recession of the medial rectus displaced the curve but did not change its shape.

Orbital Floor Fracture

A patient with orbital floor fracture with entrapment demonstrated an increase in force required for upward rotation of the involved eye. After the tissue had been

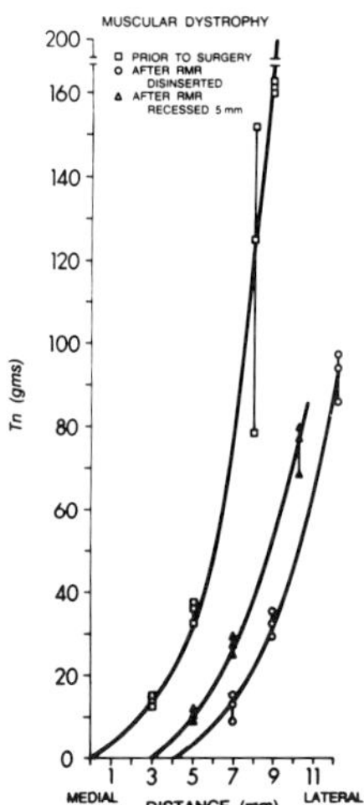

Figure 8. Length-tension curve of ocular rotation in a patient with muscular dystrophy, before and after medial rectus muscle recession for a large angle esotropia.

surgically extricated from the fracture site, the force needed for elevation was diminished markedly (Fig 9). The increased slope of the length-tension and the change following surgery confirmed the restrictive nature of this problem. Quantitative forced traction results may assist the surgeon in determining whether the tissue has been removed from the entrapped position.

DISCUSSION

Strabismus surgery is performed for functional and cosmetic purposes. It produces a mechanical change of the position of the globe in the orbit. The amount of surgical correction (prism diopters per mm of surgery) is dependent upon several variables (e.g., pre-operative deviation, which muscles are operated upon, whether previous surgery has been done, muscle and conjunctiva-tenons contracture, etc.). Each surgeon must necessarily try to establish a standardized technical routine to attempt to produce similar results with similar findings. However, each surgical procedure must be tailored to the individual patient rather than use one procedure for all patients. Quantified test procedures go a long way toward achieving this goal. Each surgeon must be

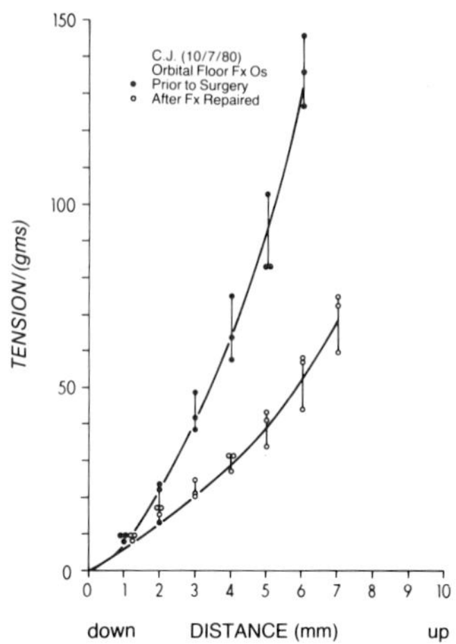

Figure 9. Length-tension curve of ocular rotation in a patient with an orbital floor fracture, before and after the release of tissue entrapped in the floor fracture.

able to use the quantitative data, adapted to his own purposes. The strain gauge transducer with an electronic digital readout can accurately measure the force needed to produce the observed rotation.

Qualitative techniques used in the past involved the use of surgical forcepts with the examiner using experience to estimate the force needed to produce rotation. Various types of calibrated forceps have also been developed(1) but most have proven to be inaccurate because of significant variability in the readings and design problems. A spring forceps or oculomyodynameter method also proved inaccurate and difficult to use.(2) Quantitative measuring devices and techniques have also been described by Strachan,(3) Rosenbaum,(4) Stephens and Reinecke(5) and Madroszkiewicz.(6)

Kaneko et al(7) carefully analyzed the length-tension relationships in normal individuals and compared this curve with measurements taken in patients with mechanical restrictions. As expected, a steep curve was found as a result of these restrictions.

Modern, integrated circuit techniques employing strain gauges, carrier amplifiers and analog-digital convertors for digital readout are now inexpensive and small enough to make a clinical electronic strain gauge recording transducer quite feasible. This device should be useable even by an inexperienced clincian, as long as the measurement of tangential force is made over a predetermined arc.

Quantitative data can help the surgeon in his decision to determine the amount of recession and/or resection required to produce the desired balance of forces to allow the eye to come to a desired, central position postoperatively.

The types of strabismus cases which would be particularly amenable to this method of analysis would be those with limitations of ocular rotations. This would include extra-ocular muscle palsies (sixth and third nerve palsies), long-standing large deviations, thyroid ophthalmopathy, cases with multiple re-operations and various neuro-ophthalmic eye movements abnormalities with strabismus.

These studies indicate that passive force measurements can be performed quantitatively with repeatable results. Improved accuracy and consistency are likely to be achieved if the distance of rotation is measured accurately. These measurements can also be improved by the use of automatic zeroing and computer control for rapid display and calculation of results in the operating room during surgery.

REFERENCES

1. Scott AB, Collins CC, O'Meara DM: A forceps to measure strabismus forces. Arch Ophthalmol 88:330-332, 1972.

2. Schillinger RJ: The prevention of over-correction and under-correction in horizontal strabismus surgery. J of Ped Ophthalmol 3:38-41, 1966.

3. Strachan IM et al: An apparatus for measuring forces in strabismus. In Moore S, Mein J, Stockbridge L: Orthoptics - Past, Present, Future, New York, Stratton Intercontinental Med Book Corp, 1976, pp 123-128.

4. Rosenbaum AL, Meyer JH: New instrument for the quantitative determination of passive forced traction. Ophthalmology 87:158-163, 1980.

5. Stephens KF, Reinecke RD: Quantitative forced duction. Tr Am Acad Ophthalmol & Otolaryng 71:324-328, 1967.

6. Madroszkiewicz M: Oculomyodynamometry. The strength and work of extra-ocular muscles in squint. Ophthalmologica 161:491-498, 1970.

7. Kaneko H, Koga A, Adachi K: Quantitative designation of the forced duction test. 1. Difference between normal and pathological extra-ocular muscles. Acta Soc Ophthalmol Jpn 75:1515-1523, 1971.

MUSCLE INJECTION TO CORRECT STRABISMUS

A. B. Scott

ABSTRACT

We have injected 79 patients with Oculinum (botulinum toxin A) for correction of strabismus or eyelid disorders. Horizontal strabismus has been benefited in nearly every instance. Vertical strabismus is more difficult to treat, since a sufficiently paralyzing dose tends to have an effect on adjacent extraocular muscles or the levator. Nevertheless, significant effects can be obtained. There is a moderate variability in the response of individual patients to injection, the effect being a much greater one in smaller individuals and in women, and much less effect occurring in males. There is no substantial difference in dose response for individuals from ten to adulthood, when corrected for weight. The treatment has been helpful in preventing medial rectus contracture during the healing phase of lateral rectus palsy. When total lateral rectus palsy persists requiring surgery, the uncontracted medial rectus requires no surgical recession, allowing confining of surgery to the lateral rectus and to transposition of vertical muscles with large amplitudes of movement resulting. Long-term corrections are seen especially in cases where fusion is gained or regained, with corrections in several patients for over two years.

STRABISMUS II
ISBN 0-8089-1424-3

THE 1982 COSTENBADER LECTURE

We are honored to have Joseph Lang as our ninth Costenbader Lecturer. Professor Lang studied medicine in Zurich under the guidance of Marc Amsler who interested him in the field of ocular motility. He is Professor and in charge of the Orthoptic Department of the University Eye Clinic in Zurich, and for the past 8 years, Secretary of the European Strabological Society.

His book, Strabismus, has two editions in German, one in Spanish and French. His book on Microtropia recently had its second edition. He was awarded the Vogt-Award of the Swiss Ophthalmological Society in 1974 for work on microtropia. His papers are benchmarks of original observations and thought, especially in our understanding of sensory adaptations to strabismus.

The Costenbader Lecture is presented annually at the AAPO&S meetings in memory of Frank D. Costenbader (1905-1978) of Washington, D.C., the father of pediatric ophthalmology in the USA. Beyond recognizing his many contributions to knowledge of strabismus, we memorialize also his kindness to patients, his helpfulness to colleagues, and his inspiration to a generation of ophthalmologists. The lecture was initiated in 1974 by the Costenbader Alumni Society and adopted by the American Association of Pediatric Ophthalmology and Strabismus at its first meeting in 1975.

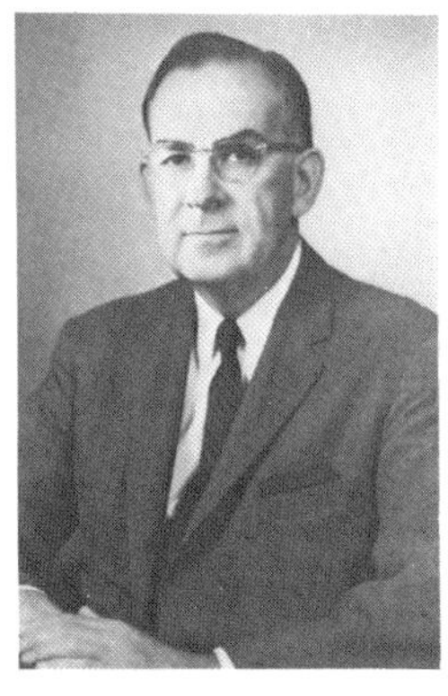

Costenbader Lectures

1974 Marshall M. Parks
1975 Robert N. Shaffer
1976 Lorenz E. Zimmerman
1977 T. Keith Lyle
1978 Jules Francois
1979 D. Robison Harley
1980 David G. Cogan
1981 Philip Knapp

STRABISMUS II
ISBN 0-8089-1424-3

SPECIAL FORMS OF COMITANT STRABISMUS

J. Lang

ABSTRACT

This lecture is concerned with some special forms of comitant strabismus. The congenital strabismus syndrome is characterized by early onset, latent nystagmus, dissociated vertical divergence, excyclorotation of the nonfixating eye and anomalous head posture. Microtropia is an inconspicuous strabismus of less than 5 degrees, showing no motor but only sensorial defect with harmonious anomalous correspondence. Normosensorial late convergent strabismus is a motor form of strabismus with acute, intermittent onset and normal retinal correspondence showing excellent surgical prognosis. Theoretical and practical importance and frequency of these forms are discussed.

Three new diagnostic methods are also discussed: the two pencil-test, the fourth image of Purkinje and the new Lang-Stereotest.

INTRODUCTION

First I would like to thank the officers of the American Association for Pediatric Ophthalmology and Strabismus for the kind inviation to give the Costenbader Lecture. If is, of course, a great honor and pleasure for me to speak in front of such a famous audience. It is also a pleasure for me to discuss with you some of my views on strabismus problems, which to you may have some European flavor.

I had the great privilege to meet Frank Costenbader personally twice, for the first time at the First International Strabismus Symposium in Giessen in 1966, and for the second time at the First Congress of the International Strabismological Association in 1970 in Acapulo. I had the good fortune to have a long discussion on strabismus with him on our pleasant two-day bus trip from Mexico City to Acapulo. I was deeply impressed by the wisdom, the modesty and the honesty of this great man. He confessed that he regarded himself not as a scientist, but as an ophthalmological practitioner devoted to the welfare of his patients. Knowing him personally made me glady accept the honor and the task of speaking to you. I know that Dr. Costenbarder would have appreciated that I prefer to speak to you more on clinical experience than on scientific aspects of strabismus.

I would like to discuss with you three clinical entities, namely the congenital strabismus syndrome, microtropia and normosensorial late strabismus. Together with accommodative strabismus they represent four model forms which can give a better survey on the vast field of convergent strabismus.

I would also like to offer you three small diagnostic pearls, namely the two-pencil test, the forth image of Purkinje and the new Lang-Stereotest.

CONGENITAL STRABISMUS SYNDROME

In 1961, Costenbader(1) published his thesis on infantile esotropia which means an esotropia known to be present before the age of one year. Prior to that(2) he had defined congenital esotropia as "strabismus present by 6 months of age, characterized by a large deviation unresponsive to spectacle treatment of the existing hyperopia" But do congenital cases always show a large deviation? Are there other signs which characterize congenital convergent concomitant strabismus?

At the first International Congress of orthoptists in London in 1967, I(3) discussed a very simple question: Do children who squint from birth or from the first few months of life show a characteristic form of strabismus which may be differentiated from other forms?

At that time, in 82 such cases, I found 92% with dissociated vertical divergence, 57% with latent nystagmus, 65% with excyclorotation of the nonfixing eye and 70% with abnormal head posture. Twenty percent showed A-pattern, 17% showed V-pattern and 15% had, in addition to the strabismus, cerebral damage. The percentage of these characteristics may vary, but I have found the picture as a whole, to have been confirmed ever since that time.

The different characteristics could best be seen in a short film. In this film a girl with congenital strabismus syndrome was shown at the age of 8 months and at the age of 10 years. She was operated on when she was 6 years and 7 months (No. 106 in Malcolm Ing's thesis).(4) At the age of

10, the two pencil test was positive when both eyes were open, but negative when the deviating eye was covered.

Dissociated vertical deviation was first described by Bielschowsky(5) and may also be called occlusion hypertropia. The eyes may seem to be vertically aligned, but the occluded eye slowly drifts upward and after uncovering may drift down again. The darkening phenomenon of Bielschowsky shows the same movements. This phenomenon is of innervational origin and must not be confused with elevation in adduction as seen in V-patterns which sometimes is also called alternating sursumduction. Dissociated vertical divergence is not usually present in the first year of life, but appears in congenital strabismus only at the age of two years.

The second sign of the congenital strabismus syndrome is latent nystagmus. If one eye is occluded jerking nystagmus with a rapid phase to the side of the fixating eye is observed. This jerking nystagmus sometimes is present when both eyes are open, and from it the fixating eye can be recognized in small angles: the rapid phase of the nystagmus is always directed to the fixating eye. In addition, there may be a rotatory component of the nystagmus. Latent nystagmus must be carefully differentiated from congenital pendular nystagmus. Its correlation with strabismus is very high. I once found that in patients with latent nystagmus almost 99% have strabismus, whereas with congenital pendular nystagmus only 30% have a strabismus and between them mainly cases with albinoti fundi. This differentiation has never been made by the advocators of the nystagmus-blockage syndrome - an entity which anyway seems to lose its importance.

Cyclorotational movements are often seen in the congenital strabismus syndrome: the eye that takes up fixation makes an incyclorotation and the eye that relinquishes fixation makes an excyclorotation. Sometimes spontaneous rotational movements are seen.

Abnormal head posture is often seen in the congenital strabismus syndrome. Usually the head is tilted towards the shoulder of the fixating eye and the face is also turned to this side. All these signs must be carefully looked for, be it by slit lamp, by carefully watching rotation movements on the iris, and by funduscopy. Recently, I had the opportunity to examine these cases on the television monitor of an infrared fundus camera. It is impressive how the whole picture of the congenital strabismus syndrome is even more apparent with this device.

We call this picture a syndrome because it fulfills the conditions of a syndrome. A syndrome should be a group of apparently unrelated symptoms and signs which have the tendency to appear together and to characterize a clinical entity. This congenital squint syndrome largely corresponds to the entity described in 1954 by Crone(6) as alternating hyperphoria, in 1959 by Anderson(7) as latent nystagmus and alternating hyperphoria and in 1962 by Ciancia(8) as esotropia in infants with limitation of abduction.

What is the pathogenesis of the congenital squint syndrome? Nobody knows for sure. We once thought it had its seat in the brain stem and was due to an imbalance between vestibular and visual influence upon the oculomotor mechanisms. Now we believe that it may be due to an imbalance between the geniculo-striate and the extra-geniculo-striate system and that latent nystagmus is the dominating feature of this syndrome. Clinical observations and neuroanatomical facts support this hypothesis.

Clinical observations show that in almost 99% of cases with latent nystagmus, a strabismus is present. Cases with orthotropia and latent nystagmus are extremely rare. In infants with the congenital strabismus syndrome both eyes are in a convergent position at first. On ophthalmoscopical examination of fixation, the fixation object does not lie in the fovea but on the nasal side of the fovea. Only gradually does fixation move into the foveola. We got the clinical impression that only when fixation has moved to the foveola, latent nystagmus can manifest itself. The fixation object in the nonoccluded eye slowly moves from the foveola to the nasal side and by a saccade returns to the foveola. Imbalance of optokinetic nystagmus may result from this. In some adult cases, one can see that in binocular vision the leading eye does not fixate exactly with the foveola, since when the squint eye is occluded, an adjustment movement of the fixating eye can be observed.

Concerning the neuroanatomical facts, one must bear in mind that beside the retino-geniculo-striate system other pathways exist, the most important being the extra-geniculo-striate pathway to the colliculus superior and to the pulvinar and from there to the cortex, as shown in the diagram by Trevarthen and Sperry.(9) This second visual pathway is claimed to be responsible for ambient vision.

Furthermore Bernheimer(10) in 1899 demonstrated that 20 to 30% of the fibers of the optic nerve do not reach the corpus geniculatum laterale, but pass to the pretectal and tectal area. According to Minkowsky(11) these are probably only uncrossed fibres which stem from the nasal parts of the retina. In addition, it is known that, in the early stages of human fetal development, the primitive phylogenetic arrangement of a complete decussation of the nerve fibers occurs in the chiasm. It is not until the 11th week that uncrossed fibers begin to appear.

Keeping in mind that congenital strabismus is often seen in cases of prematurity or of cerebral damage, we may expect that in these cases the phylogenetic older extra-geniculo-striate system, based on the nasal halves of the retina and on the crossed optical fibers subserving ambient vision, is dominant. This accounts for the convergent position of the eyes and for the tendency to fixate in the nasal part of the retina. As visual development goes on in the first months of life, fixation moves into the fovea to fulfil the task of discriminating forms.

When both eyes are open, no nystagmus is seen since opposite movements of the eyes are counterbalanced. When one eye is occluded counterbalance does not exist any more. Fixation then slowly glides from the foveola to the nasal part of the retina due to the tendency of ambient vision, and then quickly returns to the foveola again (Fig 3), bringing back the object in the area of discrimination.

I am fully aware that this is a hypothesis based only on clinical impressions and on possibly insufficient neuroanatomic facts.(12) But since nowadays everybody is speaking mostly of the work by Hubel and Wiesel on the geniculo-striate system, I find it worthwhile to mention other works and pathways. Maybe this view also explains why patients with congenital esotropia cannot be cured just by aligning them even by the most sophisticated surgical techniques.

MICROTROPIA

But now let us go to another clinical entity which may seem less important, but which is interesting for the whole pathogenesis of strabismus, namely microtropia.(13)

Microtropia or microstrabismus may be defined briefly as

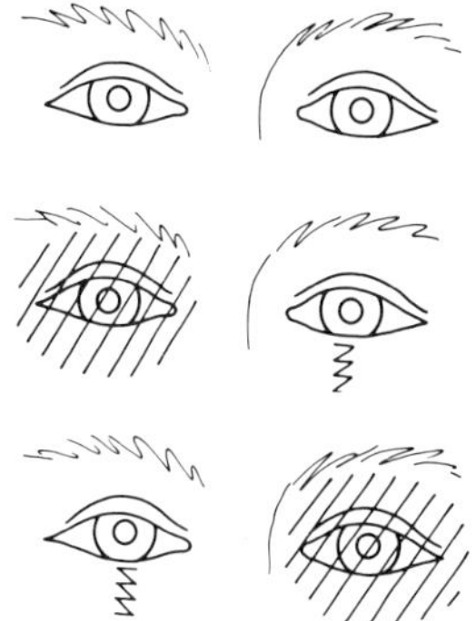

fig. 1: Latent nystagmus. a. both eyes open - no nystagmus. b. right eye covered - nystagmus to the left. c. left eye covered - nystagmus to the right.

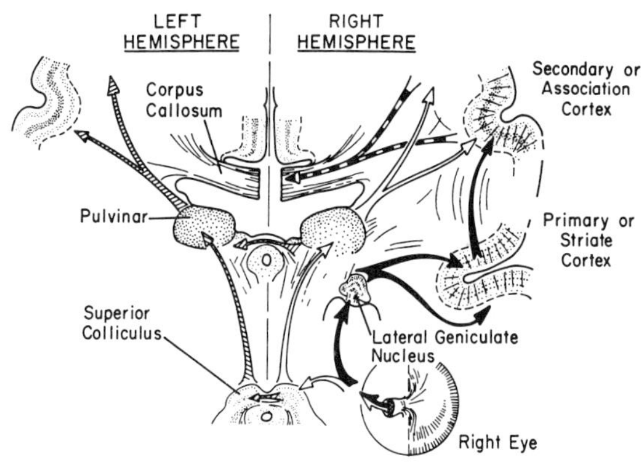

fig. 2: From Trevarthen and Sperry: extra-geniculo-striate pathway.

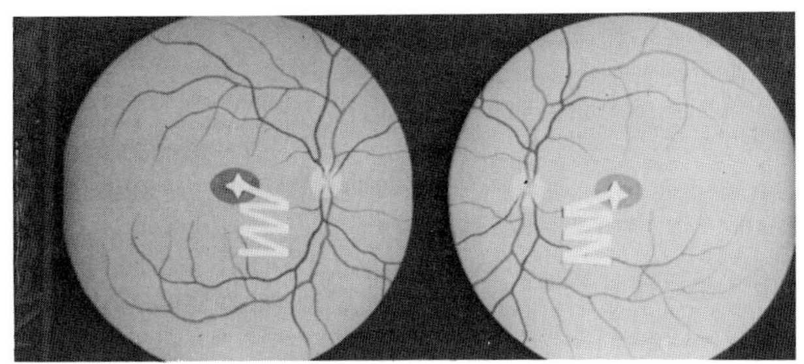

fig. 3: Latent nystagmus as seen in the fundi.

an inconspicuous strabismus of less than 5 degrees, usually with harmonious anomalous correspondence. Three forms can be distinguished: primary constant, primary decompensating and consecutive microtropia, which has also been called secondary microtropia.

There are three situations in which the ophthalmologist may be confronted with microtropia:

a. in amblyopia apparently without strabismus (In the past this has usually been diagnosed as congenital amblyopia);

b. in hereditary or familial problems of strabismus;

c. in residual strabismus after treatment, which each of us sees more often than he would like to.

Microtropia does not seem to have been familiar to well-known early strabismologists as Javal, Worth, Duane and Bielschwosky. Let us quote Maddox(14) who in 1898 wrote that "minute squints were exceedinly rare, the natural desire for single vision being too strong to allow minute squints to exist".

Observations of small angles have been made only in the last few decades. There were plenty of theories on the causes of this condition and on the ways of avoiding it, be it by orthoptics, by prisms, by surgery and/or by other sophisticated treatment. Here once again strabismologists have fallen into the same old trap. Before knowing the nature of a condition one already knows where it comes from and how to treat it.

But before dealing with consecutive microtropia, where treatment can produce almost every sensorial perturbance, except, of course, a real cure, one should try to study and to learn as much as possible from primary microtropias. In primary microtropia no treatment has changed the original sensory conditions and more insight may be gained into a fascinating experiment of primary binocular pathology made by nature itself.

As far as I know, cases of primary microtropia were described for the first time by Jampolsky(15) in 1951 under the name of fixation disparity. I will not go further in details about terminology of microtropia, be it retinal slip, cortical slip, fusion disparity, ultrasmall angle, eso flick or other terms. But since this condition is, in the US, mostly called Monofixation Syndrome, I will say a few words later on about that.

For many years I have carefully looked for primary microtropias in my practice. Out of a total of 41,678 there were 7,751 motility patients who were listed on special punch cards. In 3,338 cases of convergent strabismus there were 1,176 total microtropias and 626 cases of primary constant microtropia, which means 18.7%. Whereas in convergent strabismus, I found 35.2% microtropia, in divergent strabismus there were only 3.3% of microtropias. In order to understand these figures I should add that I worked as a general ophthalmologist at that time and only later became a full-time strabismologist. From these numbers I estimate that 1% of the general population in Switzerland has a microtropia.

The most important characteristic of microtropia is amblyopia. What are the clinical findings in microtropic amblylopia? In 113 children with untreated primary microtropia we found 69% with isometropia whereas 31% had an anisometropia. Again we found 51% with central fixation whereas 49% had eccentric fixation. In isometropia central fixation prevailed with 58%, whereas in anisometropia central fixation was found in only 37%. Vision was best in cases with isometropia and central fixation, the mean value being 0.58. Vision was worst, as can be expected in anisometropia with eccentric fixation, the mean value being 0.08. Isometropia with eccentric fixation and anisometropia with central fixation range in between.

We have done a lot of interesting studies in adult microtropias on the nature of fixation behaviour, on the nature of the scotomas and on reading capacity, but time does not allow us to go into details. More details can be found in the second edition of my monograph on microtropia.

Let us come to hereditary problems of microtropia. Since the times of Hippocrates one knows that squinters stem from squinters and it has recently become apparent, that microtropia here plays a role. Oggel and Rochels(16) recently published a pedigree of a family with three generations and 23 members, where 10 members had a primary microtropia and 4 a large angle strabismus. I would also like to report on three sisters (Fig 4). The youngest and the eldest sister started to squint at the age of 3 years. Both had a hyperopia of about 3.5 diopters and an amblyopia of one eye. After correction of hyperopia and treatment of amblyopia a consecutive microtopia resulted. The second girl never squinted, but at the age of seven years a microtropia of the left eye was found with amblyopia of 0.2.

I am sure that all of you have seen similar situations and agree with me that microtropia plays an important role in hereditary factors in strabismus, although we do not yet know the exact hereditary mode.

This example also shows the importance of microtropia in the pathogenesis of large angle strabismus.

We all assume that there are some factors which cause an aligned patient to develop strabismus. When this is true for parallel cases, this must even more be probable in cases with microtropia, since there exists a primary disturbance of binocularity. Factors which predispose to decompensation may be a hyperopia, a convergent position of rest, convergence excess and an amblyopia. Such factors may also be combined. From there results a large convergent deviation. Cases with this mechanism may be suspected when shortly after the onset of strabismus a deep amblyopia already exists, or when in intermittent cases in the apparent parallel position, there is microtropia or eccentric fixation. Since anomalous correspondence exists already, it can easily adapt to the large angle. After successful treatment, be it by glasses, orthoptics or surgery, not orthotropia, but the preexisting microtropia shows up again. This supplies a simple answer to the question, why even after careful treatment not an orthotropia but a consecutive microtropia usually results.

Now I may be allowed to explain differences which exist between microtropia and the monofixation syndrome of Marshall Parks. I have, of course, studied carefully Marshall Parks fine thesis on the monofixating syndrome.(17) In analysing the 100 cases in his thesis I interpreted 12 cases as primary microtropias, 59 cases as consecutive microtropias, 5 cases as amblyopia ex anisometropia, 6 as stereoamblyopias, 6 as fully accommodative cases, 8 as cases of normosenorial late strabismus, 3 as cured intermittent divergence and 1 as a macular lesion. All these different conditions have one symptom in common, namely subnormal stereopsis with supression of one eye. By definition microtropia describes only cases with manifest deviation, discovered by the cover-test or by eccentric fixation, whereas the monofixation syndrome includes also cases with orthotropia.

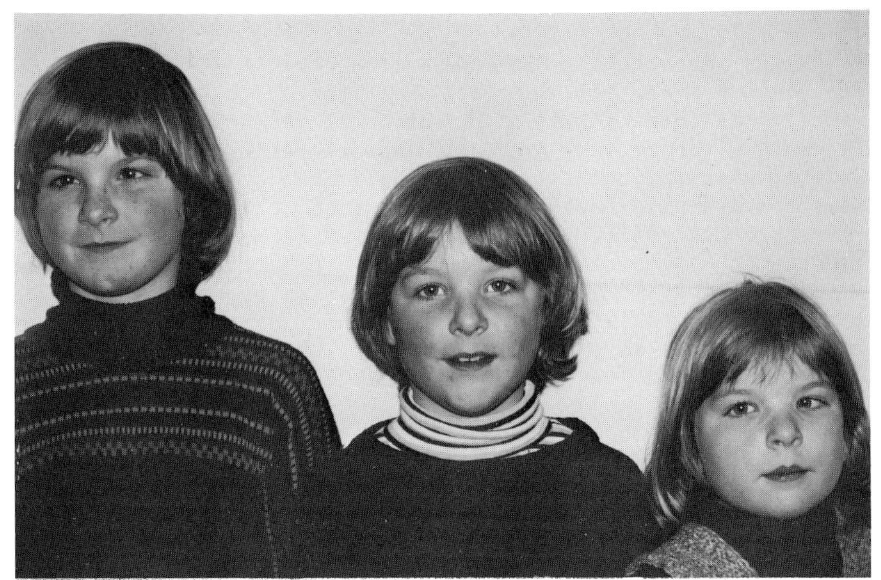

fig. 4: Three sisters, two with large angle strabismus, one with primary microtropia.

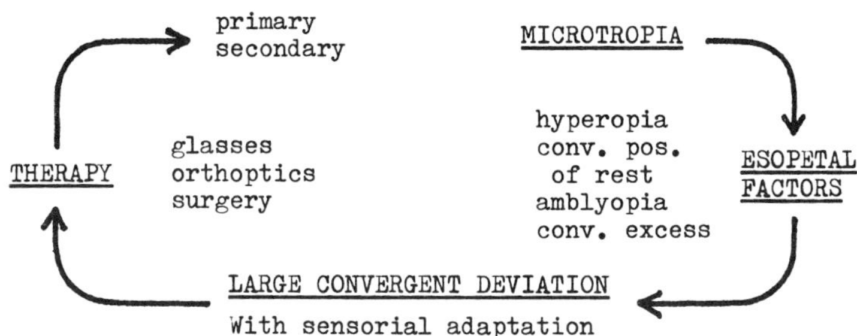

fig. 5: Decompensation of primary microtropia into a large angle and return to microtropia after treatment.

This may be explained by the example of anisometropic amblyopia, where there is no deviation, whereas in microtropia there exists a deviation of less than 5 degrees. In anisometropic amblyopia a normal retinal correspondence exists, whereas in microtropia usually there is a anomalous correspondence. Amblyopia ex anisometropia is essentially a refractional condition and must be treated mainly by optical correction whereas microtropia is primarily a sensorial defect and its amblyopia should be treated by occlusion. Of course, both conditions may be combined, as a cataract can be combined with a maculopathy - but they should all the same be differentiated as carefully as possible.

I know the opinion that in microtropia the presence of an anomalous correspondence is not shared by all strabismologists. This difference is most probably due to different examinations. I, myself, have relied mostly on ophthalmoscopical examination of correspondence and I can not just neglect my findings. I have also developed a photographic method to show anomalous correspondence.(18) I admit that this is, of course, easier done in adults than in children. But I think that results from these studies are also valid for children. Curiously enough nowadays results from animals, such as cats and monkeys, who naturally do not squint - are readily accepted for humans, whereas results from strabismic adults are not regarded as valid for strabismic children.

THE FOURTH IMAGE OF PURKINJE

Now I would like to speak about two diagnostic methods which I have developed in the last years(19) and which to me are real pearls and which may help to further clarify some points of discussion. Hirschberg's method of assessing strabismus by using the first image of Purkinje is well known, but so is the limitation of this test for small angles. By chance I discovered that by using the fourth image of Purkinje, the one resulting from the posterior surface of the lens, our discrimination threshold for small angles can be sharpened. The fourth image of Purkinje is very weak but can be seen in photographs when these are centered exactly on the plane of the iris. The patient should fixate in the objective and the electronic flash must be positioned exactly vertical above the objective. The fourth Purkinje image can then be seen below and temporal from the first reflex. In cases of microtropia the fourth image is less temporal, as can be seen in a case of microtropia. Once you are familiar with this method, you automatically check every photograph for the fourth image of Purkinje.

LANG STEREOTEST

The other test I would like to acquaint you with is the new Lang-Stereotest(19) which is a combination of the random-dots of Julesz(20) with cylinder screens. Most of you know cylindrical screens or panography from postcards where the attraction does not exactly correspond to their ethical value. But nobody knows that these cylindrical gratings were invented by the same Walter Robert Hess(21) who had described coordimetry for examination of eye muscles. Beneath each fine cylindre there are two fine strips of pictures (Fig 7).

I have combined these two methods which has the advantage that no glasses are necessary for the examination. Children do not always easily accept glasses or time must be spent to make them accept them. Since my test works without glasses, examination in young children is made easier and quicker. Three objects are seen binocularily: a cat, a star and a car. Children may name these objects, or they may point to them or by observation of fixating movements of the eyes a positive results may be found. Interestingly enough, children recognize the figures usually quicker than adults (Fig 8).

In examining about 1000 cases, I have found that patients with anisometropic amblyopia may pass this test whereas children with microtropia usually fail this test. This is, of course, no hard and fast rule.

This leads us to the question if the patients with constant strabismus have binocular stereopsis. The answer again depends on the methods we use.

TWO PENCIL TEST

When using the two pencil test(22) (Fig 9), which is based on large disparity of gross objects (Fig 10), we can even find in the congenital strabismus syndrome a binocularity. The examiner holds a pencil vertically in front of the patient. The patient is asked to hold a second pencil, bottom down, vertically above the examiner's pencil and to bring his pencil slowly down in an attempt to touch the examiners pencil. This test should be done first with both eyes open, then with the weaker of deviating eye occluded. The binocular and monocular performance are then

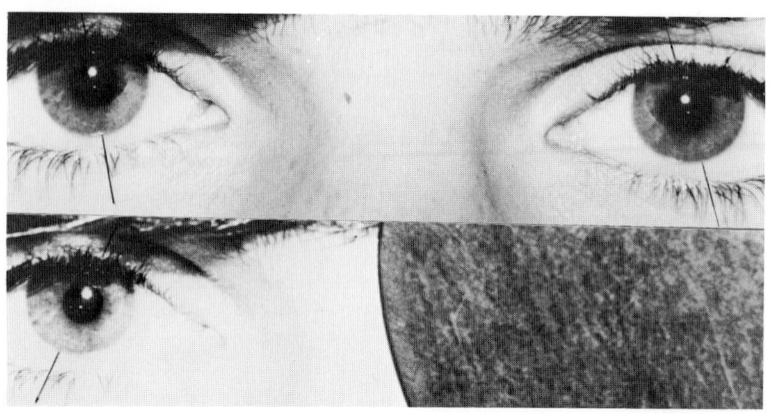

fig. 6: The fourth image of Purkinje in a case of microtropia. a: both eyes open - microtropia of the right eye. The fourth image of Purkinje is on the nasal side of the first in the right eye and on the temporal side in the left eye. b: Left eye covered - adjustment movement of the right eye. The fourth image is now temporal below the first image.

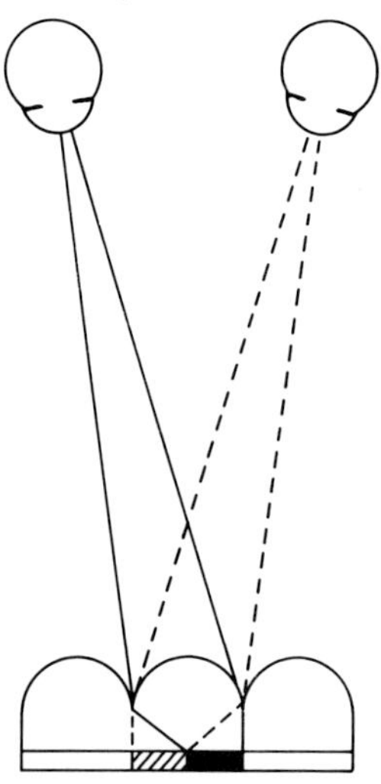

fig. 7: Principle of cylinder screens.

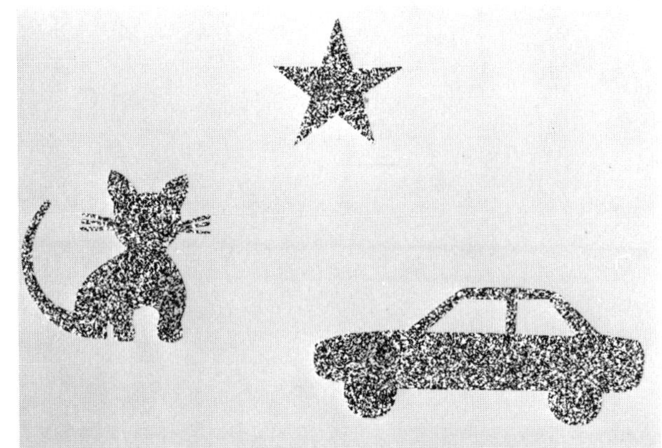

fig. 8: The three pictures of the Lang Stereotest.

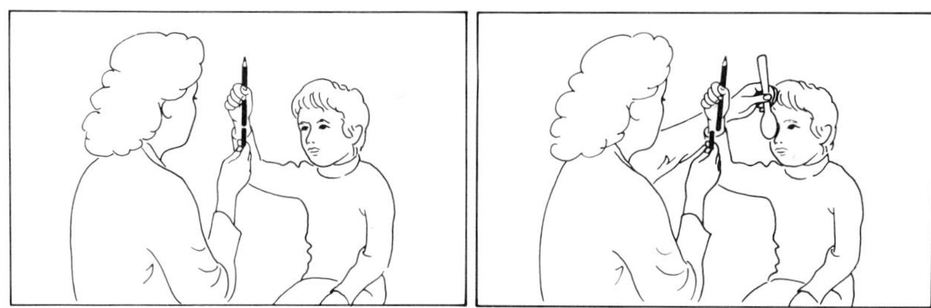

fig. 9: The two pencil test. a: with both eyes open, b: with one eye covered.

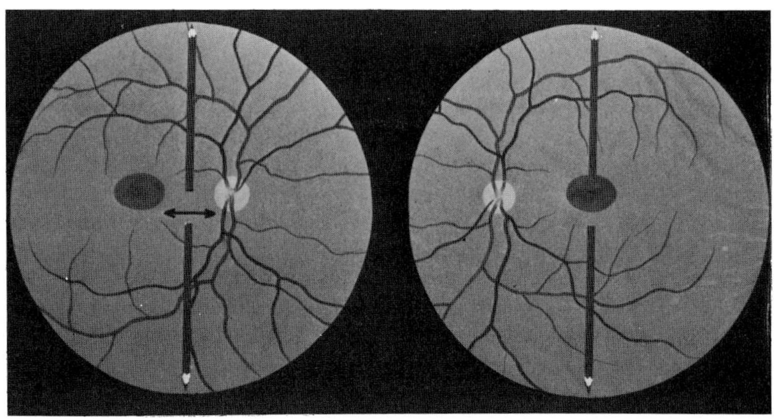

fig. 10: The two pencil test represented in the fundi. Adjustment of large vertical lines is possible with ARC.

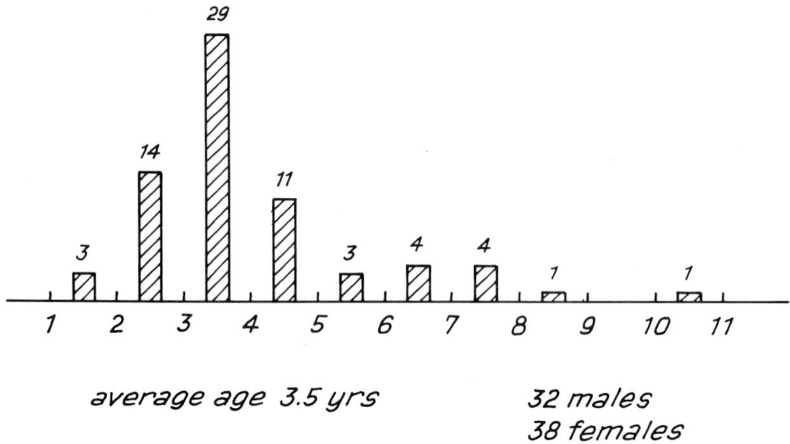

fig. 11: Onset of squint in 70 cured patients with normosensorial late convergen squint (average age 3.5 years).

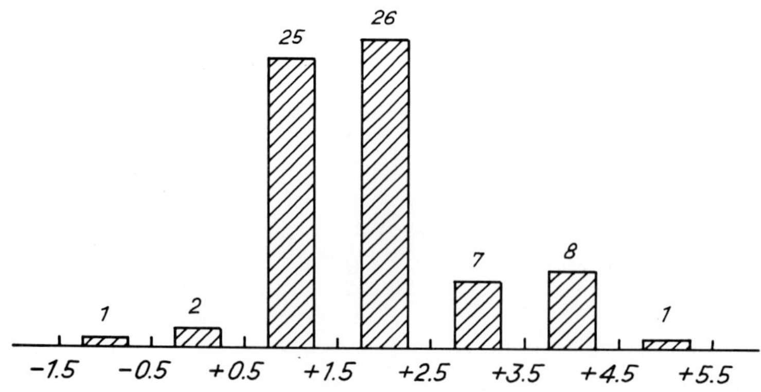

fig. 12: Refraction in 70 cases of normosensorial late convergent squint.

compared.

When we use random dots, then we find a much worse stereoacuity in microtropia than by using tests with lines and contours, such as the Titmus test. There seems to be a fundamental difference between using small random-dots and tests with lines and contours.

NORMOSENORIAL LATE CONVERGENT STRABISMUS

I would like to close my discussion with another strabismus form, the so-called normosensorial late convergent strabismus. Here in the manifest stage, there is no stereopsis at all, even by the two pencil test. But after surgery full stereopsis usually is reached, even with random dots.

For many years, I have been interested by the simple question, what cases of strabismus could really be cured by surgery. Let us look at 70 cases which I reported on some years ago. In studying this strabismus form the importance of case history is revealed and the old saying that in medicine the case history already means half of the findings proves to be true again.

The most striking feature in our 70 patients is the late onset of strabismus: on an average at the age of 3 years and 5 months. In almost all of these cases the onset was not gradual but acute or sudden. At the beginning the strabismus was usually intermittent and then became constant. Often the strabismus did not start in the evening or with fatigue but appeared immediately on waking in the morning, or after a nap. Those children seem to wake up as squinters, but after one or two hours the eyes may return to parallelism.

Recently, the daughter of one of our residents, at the age of 3-1/2 years, suddenly showed a constant convergent strabismus one morning. But the parents had noticed some months before that when woken up at nights the eyes were convergent. Of course, Barbara work up in the morning much earlier than her parents so that an intermittent phase could easily have escaped observation. She was unhappy. Before the onset she loved to draw and to walk on low narrow walls. She stopped doing this immediately. She complained of double vision. She grossly missed the two pencil test. After operation she switched to orthothropia, was happy again and passed the two pencil tests and other more sophisticated stereotests gloriously.

Not all children, of course, complain about diplopia, but closing one eye in a convergent strabismus may be regarded as an objective sign of diplopia. Seventeen out of our seventy children closed one eye. But again it must be taken into account that not all children can close one eye, but rubbing one eye or closing one eye with a hand has the same significance.

You must always ask specifically for this information because it tends to get forgotten quickly by the parents.

With this fresh anamnesis one would believe that the parents could give exact information about trigger factors. In two cases, a short occlusion of one eye was indicated as cause, in a few cases minor chldren's illnesses were connected with the onset, but even the parents doubted if that was really the cause.

Refraction shows almost normal distribution for this age. In all cases full correction was given and in most cases prismatic correction was tried. But not in all cases a prismatic orthotropia was reached. Surgery was the treatment of choice. In most cases, I performed a standard operation with 4 mm recession and 7 mm resection of the nondominant eye.

Besides those 70 successful cases, I had, of course, failures. Time does not allow me to go into details about them and most differential diagnoses.

I hope you agree with me that there is a clinical entity of normosensorial late convergent strabismus, which can be cured by simple surgery, if surgery is not delayed too long after the onset of strabismus. All of the 70 cases reached orthotropia, some of them even orthophoria. Those cases usually are not described as a separate entity, but are reported to show the usefulness of some sophisticated treatment methods and greatly help to improve statistical results on those methods.

With these three clinical entities and with accommodative convergent strabismus now let us come back to our model forms of strabismus and let us try to localise their seat.

Accommodative strabismus without high AC/A is the result of hypermetropia and has its seat in the refraction of the eyes.

The congenital strabismus syndrome may be due to an imbalance in development between the extra-geniculo-striate and the geniculo-striate visual system and has its seat in the midbrain.

Microtropia may be due to a statistical variation in the interplay between the feedback mechanisms of monocular fixation and binocular fusion, and may have its seat in the visual cortex.

Normosensorial late convergent strabismus may simply be due to convergent position of rest with its seat in the orbit.

Be that as it may. I would like to end with a quotation from the great physiologist Hering, whom you know from his law of equal innervation of yoke muscles and from his law on identical visual direction. In 1899, Hering wrote that, concerning strabismus, it is not the judgement of the physiologist that is crucial, but that of the experienced ophthalmologist. I think this quotation would have pleased Frank Costenbader.

REFERENCES

1. Costenbader FD: Infantile esotropia. Trans Am Ophthal Soc 59:397-429, 1961.

2. Costenbader FD: Factors in the cure of squint. In Allen JH (ed): Strabismus Ophthalmology Symposium, St. Louis, CV Mosby, 1950, p. 367-376.

3. Lang J: Squint dating from birth or with early onset. First International Congress of Orthoptists. Kimpton, London, 1968, pp. 231-237.

4. Ing MR: Early surgical alignment for congenital esotropia. Tr Am Ophthalmol Soc 79:625-663, 1981.

5. Bielschowsky A: Die einseitigen und gegensinnigen (dissoziierten) Vertikalbewegungen der Augen. Graefes Arch Ophthalmol 125:493-553, 1930.

6. Crone RA: Alternating hyperphoria. Brit J Ophthalmol 38:591-604, 1954.

7. Anderson JR: Ocular Vertical Deviations and Nystagmus. London, British Medical Association, 1959.

8. Ciancia A: La esotropia con limitacion bilateral de la abeduccion en el lactante. Archivos de Oftalmologia de Buenos Aires, 37:207-211, 1962.

9. Trevarthen CB, Sperry RW: Perceptual unity of the ambient visual field in human commisurotomy patients. Brain 96:547-570, 1973.

10. Bernheimer S: Die Wurzelgebiete der Augennerven, ihre verbindungen und ihr Anschluss an die Gehirnrinde, Handbuch der Gesamten Augenheilkunde, Graefe A, Saemisch ET (eds), 2nd ed vol 1, part 2, chapter VI.

11. Minkowsky M: Uber den Verlauf, die Endigung und die zentrale Reprasentation von gekreuzten und ungekreuzten Sehnervenfasern dei einigen Saugetierenund beim Menschen, Schweizer Archiv fur neurologie und psychiatrie, 6:201-252; 7:268-303, 1920.

12. Lang J: A new hypothesis on latent nystagmus and on the congenital squint syndrome. Docum Ophthalmol Proc Series, Vol 32, 1982, Dr. W. Junk Publishers, The Hague.

13. Lang J: Evaluation in Small Angle Strabismus or Microtropia. Strabismus Symposium Giessen 1966, Karger Basel, 1968, 219-222.

14. Maddox EE: Tests and studies of the ocular muscles. Bristol (1898).

15. Jampolsky A: Retinal correspondence in patients with small degree strabismus. Arch Ophthalmol 45:18-25, 1951.

16. Oggel K, Rochels R: Ueber die Hereditat des Mikrostrabismus und die Pradisposition zum groben Schielwinkel. Klin Mbl Augenheilk 175:697-703, 1979.

17. Parks MM: The monofixation syndrome. Tran Am Ophthalmol Soc 67:609-657, 1969.

18. Lang J, Wurth A: Photographic representation of anomalous retinal correspondence. Ophthal Res 1:88-93, 1970.

19. Lang J: Mikrostrabismus, Heft 62, Bucherei des Augenarztes, 2. Auflage, Enke Verlag Stuttgart, 1982.

20. Julesz B: Foundations of Cyclopean Perception. Chicago, The University of Chicago Press, 1971.

21. Hess WR: Direkt wirkende Stereokopbilder. Zeitscher. fur wissenschaftliche Photographie. XIV Band, 34-38, 1914, Leipzig.

22. Lang J: Der Treffversuch zur Prufung des Stereoskopischen Sehens, Klin Monatsbl fur Augenhk 165:895-897, 1974.

23. Lang J: Normosensorial late convergent squint. In: Orthoptics, Proceedings of the Fourth International Orthoptic Congress, Kimpton, pp 230-233, 1981.

24. Hering E: Ueber die anomale Localisation der Netzhautbilder bei Strabismus alternans. Deutsches Archiv fur klinische Medicin, 64:15-32, 1899.

MEASURED GRADUATED RECESSION OF THE SUPERIOR OBLIQUE MUSCLE

P. Romano and P. Roholt

ABSTRACT

1. Superior oblique recession can be performed through a single superior nasal fornix incision. The keys to performing this procedure this way include marked infraduction of the eye with a superior rectus bridle suture, a narrow malleable retractor of good exposure, and Katzin corneal scissors to sever the muscle from the globe.

2. There is a good correlation between the amount of reduction in an A-pattern from this procedure and the amount of surgery performed when the amount of recession is measured directly from the original anterior point of the superior oblique insertion. The first 4 mm of surgery on each superior oblique has 2o effect, but thereafter one obtains 2 diopters of reduction in the A-pattern for each mm of superior oblique surgery. Measuring the recession indirectly from the nasal corner of the superior rectus insertion does not seem to work in this regard.

3. There was a good correlation between the amount of superior oblique overaction prior to surgery and the effect obtained, but a poor correlation between the amount of recession performed and the effect obtained in reducing superior oblique overaction. This is probably due, at least in part, to inaccurate measurement techniques. As a result of this study, we have dispensed with the old +1 to +5 system and now measure superior oblique overaction directly relate to millimeters of misalignment of the corneal light reflexes in the field of action of the obliques.

INTRODUCTION

Six patients underwent bilateral superior oblique recession for A-pattern strabismus with overacting superior obliques. The established technique was modified to permit the entire procedure to be carried out through a single nasal fornix incision. The amount of recession was graduated and measured both directly from the point of the original

STRABISMUS II
ISBN 0-8089-1424-3

incision anteriorly and indirectly from the nasal of the corner of the superior rectus insertion based on anatomical measurements.

A good correlation was found between the amount (measured directly) of recession performed and reduction in the A-pattern. The relationship was linear. By extrapolataion the first 8 mm total of superior oblique surgery had no effect but thereafter the effect obtained was 2 diopters reduction in A-pattern for every mm of superior oblique surgery. No similar correlation was found for the amount of recession performed measured indirectly.

There was no correlation between reduction in superior oblique overaction and the amount of recession performed. This was believed to be due, at least in part, to an inaccurate system of measurement of superior oblique overaction. We now, therefore, measure superior oblique overaction in mm using the corneal light reflexes.

There was, however, a good correlation between the amount of preoperative superior oblique overaction in mm using the corneal light reflexes.

Attempts at weakening the superior oblique muscles have lagged behind advances in surgery of other extraocular muscles. Special problems in dealing with the superior oblique arise because 1) access to muscle is difficult resulting in postoperative adherences, 2) attempts at weakening can change the direction of action, and 3) the fragility of the superior oblique tendon demands special care in manipulation.

Previous procedures which have been used (tenotomy, tenectomy, trochlear recession) are nongraduated and irreversible. Therefore, in 1970 Ciancia(1) and Diaz(2) proposed a method of recession of the superior oblique. Later, Caldeira(3) used a similar method of recession which he graduated but only in general terms.

The purpose of this report is to relate our efforts in the realm of bilateral superior oblique recession for A-pattern strabismus with superior oblique overaction. Previous techniques have been modified to facilitate performing the procedure through a single incision. This modification is demonstrated. Six cases in which graduated surgery were performed were reviewed to determine if the amount of surgery can be correlated with effect and to determine whether one can indirectly measure the amount of superior oblique recession to advantage in determining how much surgery to perform in these cases, as has been done for inferior oblique surgery by Apt and Call.(4)

MATERIALS AND METHODS

All six patients studied were patients of and operated upon by the senior author. They have been followed for a period of at least 6 months following surgery. The date on these patients in presented in Table 1. All had A-pattern strabismus with superior oblique overactions.

TABLE 1: Case Data

CASE NO.	PREOP DEV. A Pattern	PREOP DEV. SO OA	AMOUNT SO RECESSION*	POSTOP DEV. A Pattern	POSTOP DEV. SO OA	CHANGE A Pattern	CHANGE SO OA
1 RE		+4	12		+2		-2
LE	46	+5	14	10	+1	-36	-4
2 RE		+5	10		+1		-4
LE	23	+4	10	- 5V	+2	-28	-2
3 RE		+5	14		+1.5		-3.5
LE	40	+3.5	12	6	+2	-34	-1.5
4 RE		+4	13		0		-4
LE	30	+3	11	3	0	-27	-3
5 RE		+4	10		+2		-2
LE	43	+4	12.5	12	+1	-31	-1
6 RE		+3	12		+1		-2
LE	15	+3	12	-13V	+1.5	-28	-1.5

*direct measurement (mm)

A pattern: in prism diopters--the difference between upgaze and downgaze at distance.

SO OA: graded on a scale from 0 to +5, with +5 including a "rollout" of the eye.

The surgery was performed as follows: A single superior nasal fornix incision was made through the conjunctiva, parallel to the fornix and about 2 mm anterior to the fornix, between the medial rectus and superior rectus insertions. Tenon's capsule was opened at right angles to the conjunctival incision. A muscle hook was then placed beneath the superior rectus and a bridle suture passed beneath this which was then fixed with a hemostat to the drapes inferiorly. Maximal infraduction of the eye with this bridle suture is a key point to obtaining the exposure desirable for reaching the superior oblique insertion through this nasal approach. At times it is best that this bridle suture be directed toward the foot of the patient. At other times it seems best to angle this bridle suture slightly medially or temporally to obtain best exposure. The lid speculum is removed and a Desmarres retractor is placed in this incision and the superior oblique tendon is visualized directly. It is isolated on a muscle hook and dissected out of Tenon's capsule to its insertion. A thin malleable orbital retractor is useful at this point to obtain the desired exposure. We have a malleable retractor which has been narrowed to the width of approximately 1/4 inch for this purpose. Then, under direct visualization the superior oblique tendon is severed from the globe using Katzin curved corneal scissors (Fig 6). These are recommended because they have a significant curve to them permitting the easy severance of the tendon from the globe without endangering surrounding tissues, leaving a small stump. The tendon is brought forward in the wound and the end of the tendon is imbricated with a 6-0 Vicryl suture with knots at each corner. The superior oblique tendon is recessed and re-sewn to the globe at a point along the line of action of the tendon. This line of action (see Fig 4) passes about 2 mm behind the nasal corner of the superior rectus muscle at an angle of about 30 degrees to the corneal limbus. It crosses a line parallel to the corneal limbus, 3 mm nasal to the nasal corner of the superior rectus insertion. These are good reference points to determine the proper angulation of the new insertion site.

Two methods were used to measure the amount of surgery to be performed. Prior to the disinsertion of the tendon, a narrow ruler with a slight curve to it was passed beneath the superior rectus to the anterior corner of the superior oblique insertion. The point to which the tendon was to be recessed was then measured and marked directly on the sclera along the line of action of the superior oblique tendon. A measurement was also indirectly taken of the amount of recession based on the anatomical location of the new point of insertion as in Fig 4. The wound was closed with one or two 8-0 Vicryl sutures. Postoperatively, no patches, drops or ointments were used. The patient was examined the morning following surgery, again 4 days later, and 6 weeks and 6 months after surgery, at which time measurements were taken.

RESULTS

The specific result data may be seen in the Case Data in Table 1. The amount of superior oblique directly measured varied from 10 to 14 mm and the amount of change in the A-pattern from such surgery varied from 27 to 36 prism diopters. The results of the 6 cases are represented in Fig 1.

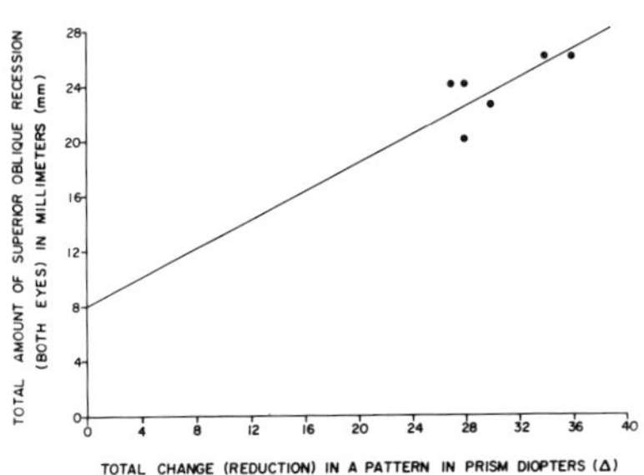

Figure 1. Correlation between amount of surgery and reduction in A-pattern.

There is a linear correlation between the total amount of superior oblique recession performed and the total change in the A-pattern obtained. This is a linear relationship. There was 2 prism diopters of effect for each mm of surgery performed on the superior obliques after the first 8 mm. That it is say, you can recess each superior oblique 4 mm and expect essentially no effect on an A-pattern from that, but thereafter one may expect approximately 2 prism diopters for each mm of surgery performed on the superior obliques. For example, a measured 12 mm recession O.U. should provide 32 mm of correction of an A-pattern. The first 4 mm in each eye do not count. In each eye, therefore, effectively 8 mm of surgery was performed. For a total of 16 mm of surgery, one would expect 32 prism diopters of effect.

With regard to the amount of superior oblique recession and its correlation with the amount of reduction in superior oblique overaction, there was no correlation (Fig 2).

When, however, we took a look at the change in the superior oblique overaction, compared to the amount of superior oblique overaction prior to surgery, there seemed to be a fair correlation here: the greater the superior oblique

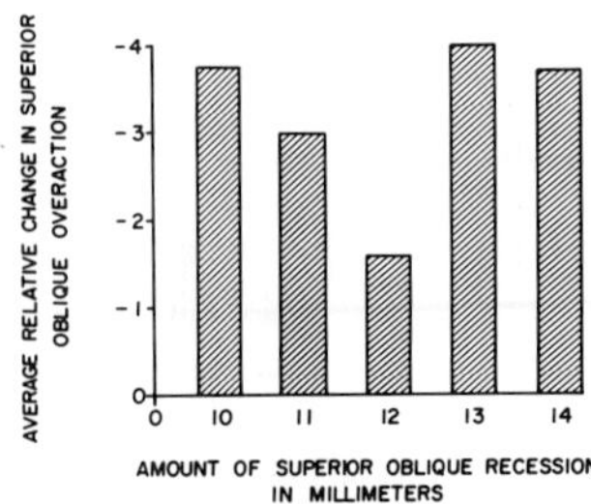

Figure 2. Correlation between amount of surgery and reduction in superior oblique overaction.

overaction prior to surgery, the greater the change in superior oblique action noted regardless of the amount of surgery performed (Fig 3).

We also tried to correlate the amount of recession measured by the indirect method with the amount of effect on A-pattern. This is represented in Fig 5. Again, there is no correlation. The actual difference in the 5 cases in which both measurements were performed is shown in Table 2. As noted, the indirect measurement always seemed to be less in magnitude than the direct measurement. Even so, there was no correlation with indirect measurement.

DISCUSSION

The amount of effect that we obtained by performing this procedure is of the same order of magnitude of that obtained using other methods such as tenotomy or tenectomy. It is also of the same order of magnitude as that previously reported for the technique of recession of the superior oblique.

We found a specific linear relationship between the amount of surgery performed and its effect on A-pattern. This relationship can be described simply by saying that the first 4 mm on each superior oblique do not count and thereafter one may expect 2 prism diopters for each mm of surgery performed on the superior obliques in terms of closing an A-pattern.

Caldeira(3) graduated his recessions but made only general recommendations. We charted out his data and found it supported our findings. His data suggest a zero extrapolation at about 12 mm of total superior oblique

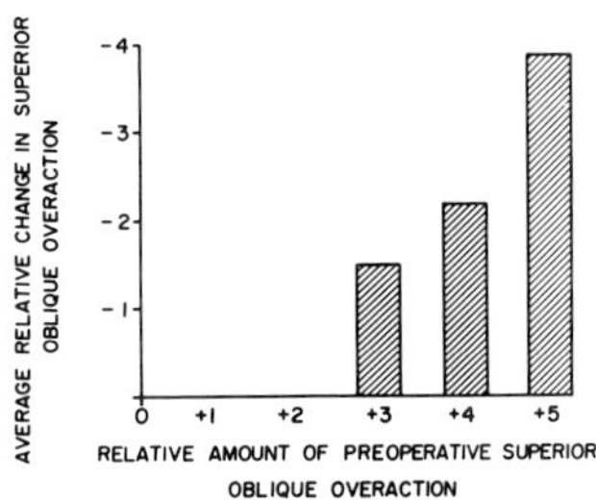

Figure 3. Correlation between preoperative amount of superior oblique overaction and reduction of overaction by surgery, without regard to amount of surgery.

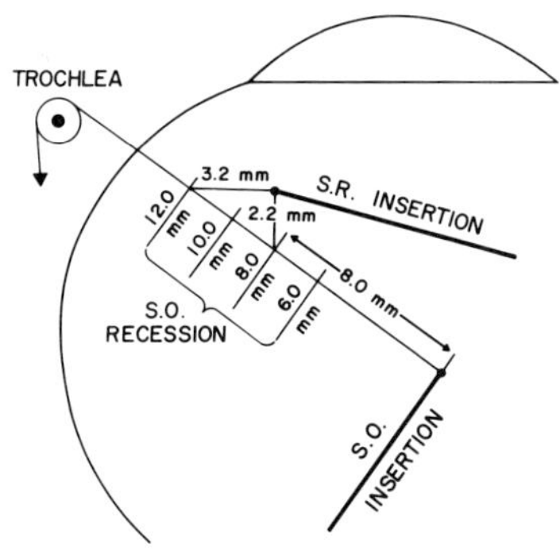

Figure 4. Diagrammatic representation of method of indirect measurement of graduated superior oblique recession.

TABLE 2: Difference (in Millimeters) Between Direct and Indirect Measurement of S.O. Recession Site

Case No.	2	3	4	5	6
Right eye	$-3\frac{1}{2}$	-3	-1	-3	-2
Left eye	$-3\frac{1}{2}$	-2	-2	-4	-1

*indirect measurement was always less in magnitude than the direct measurement.

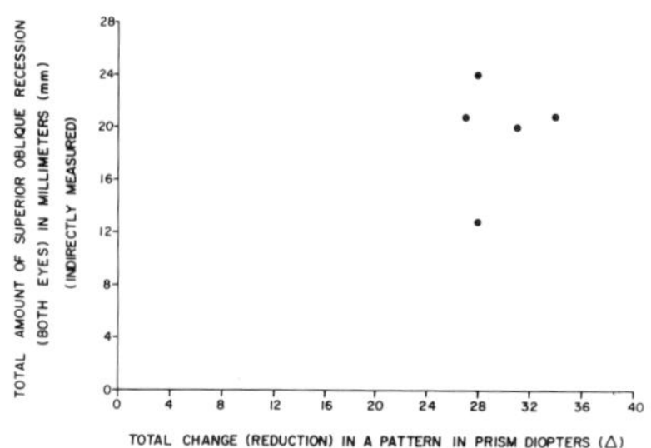

Figure 5. Correlation between amount of surgery (indirectly measured) and reduction in A-pattern.

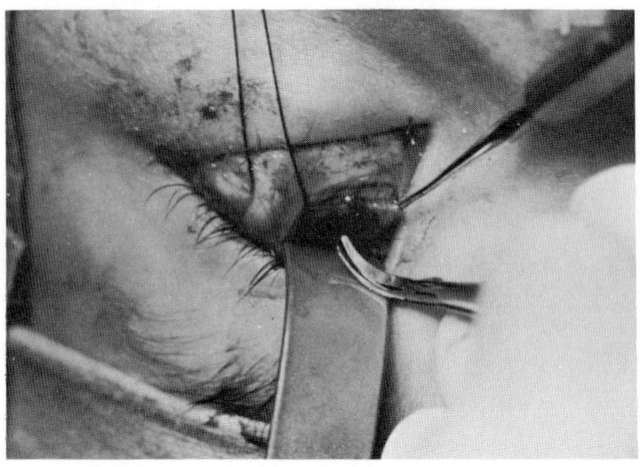

Figure 6. Recession of superior oblique muscle of left eye (surgeon's view) demonstrating (a) single superior nasal fornix incision (b) bridle suture holding eye in marked infraduction (c) superior oblique tendon on Steven's muscle hook (d) malleable orbital retractor exposing superior oblique tendon (e) Katzin curved scissors poised prior to disinsertion of superior oblique.

surgery with a slope of 3 prism diopters of change of the A-pattern for each total millimeter of superior oblique recession.

His data, interestingly, also demonstrate, as ours did, a poor correlation between the amount of superior oblique surgery performed and the amount of reduction in superior oblique overaction. He also confirmed our positive correlation between the amount of preoperative superior oblique overaction and the effect obtained from recession in reducing that overaction.

Such results have been described elsewhere, not only for oblique surgery but for horizontal surgery. Namely, a given amount of surgery always seems to have more effect on a larger deviation than it does on a smaller deviation.

On the other hand, it was certainly apparent (even with 3 people obtaining measurments at each sitting: the surgeon, the resident on the case, and one of our orthoptists), that the number of disagreements over the degree of oblique overaction demonstrated that a rating system such as used here (+1, +2, +3, +4, and +5) simply is not very good, especially for scientific purposes. Therefore, we have changed our method of measuring oblique overactions at our clinic. We use the corneal light reflexes and measure the amount of difference in mm of difference of corneal light reflex in the 4 oblique positions. When there seems to be distinct exo deviation at the end of excursion, a so-called "rollout" movement, we still denote this as a +5 as we did with the old system in addition to whatever mm of vertical misalignment is present. It has been surprising to find, using this system of measurement, that there are some cases which have a small amount of vertical misalignment, perhaps only 1 or 2 mm, but who may also have a "+5" rollout. Nor do all the 4 mm or greater vertical misalignments have a "5+" rollout. This warrants perhaps further study.

We were disappointed to find that indirect measurement of the superior oblique was not an accurate method or certainly one which did not seem to correlate well with the effect obtained as did direct measurement. Because of the distortions inherent in obtaining direct measurement, we though that indirect measurement might be more accurate but the converse, in fact, turned out to be true.

ADDENDUM

Following presentation at the combined Fourth Meeting of the International Strabismological Association and Sixth Annual Meeting of the American Association for Pediatric Ophthalmology and Strabismus, Monterey, California, October 24-30, 1982, three of four previous authors on this subject, Drs. A. Ciancia, G. Velez, and J. Caldeira warned of a complication of this procedure they have observed, namely, limitation of depression in abduction.

To avoid this, they recommended respectively:

1. (Ciancia) The anterior corner of the new insertion should be placed 13 mm posterior to the limbus.

2. (Velez) The anterior corner of the new insertion should be placed 5 mm posterior to the nasal corner of the superior rectus recession (about the same point recommended by Ciancia).

3. (Caldeira) Be sure the width of the new superior oblique insertion is at least 6 mm.

Because of their combined extensive experience, we recommend that their advice be followed.

REFERENCES

1. Ciancia AO, Diaz JP: Retroceso del oblicuo superior. Primeros resultados. Arch Oftal (B Aires) 45:193-200, 1970.

2. Diaz JP: Mesa redonda: "Tratamiento de sindromes A, V, X" Resultados Y complicaciones del retroceso del oblicuo superior. Memorias del IV Congreso del Consejo Latinoamericano de Estrabismo (CLADE) Litografia Bybsa, Mexico, D.F., 1976, pp. 186-192.

3. Caldeira JAF: Graduated recession of the superior oblique muscle. Brit J Ophthalmol 59:553-559, 1975.

4. Apt L, Call NB: Inferior oblique muscle recession. Am J Ophthalmol 85:95-100, 1978.

DISCUSSION BY S. VERONNEAU-TROUTMAN

Dr. Romano and Roholt have analyzed in depth the effect of bilateral recession of the superior oblique in six patients with "A" patterns. They came to the conclusion that when the recession was measured from the anterior point of the insertion of the superior oblique each mm of recession will correct 2 prism diopters, taking into account that the first 4 mm of recession will have no effect. Therefore, the amount of recession to be done will be found following this simple formula:

$$\text{Total Recession} = \frac{A}{2} + 8$$

Applying this formula to the six cases presented, only small overcorrections or undercorrections should have resulted. (Table I)

One may question, however, the indication for this bilateral procedure in case No. 6, with 15 prism diopters of A pattern, to correct 11 prism diopters of the pattern, especially if horizontal muscle surgery had to be done. The authors have made also the observation that the amount of superior oblique overaction does not parallel the A pattern. Indeed in two of their six cases (case No. 2 and csse No. 6) a superior oblique overaction persisted while a V pattern

Case No	Preop A Pattern (in)	SO Recession Done (in mm)	Postop A Pattern (in)	Recession Advocated (in mm)	Anticipated Results
1	46	26	10	31	+
2	23	20	-5 V	19.5	-4 V
3	40	26	6	28	2
4	30	24	3	23	5
5	43	22.5	12	29.5	-2 V
6	15	24	-13 V	15.5	4

Table S. Veronneau-Troutman - After Romano and Roholt, results of measured graduated bilateral recession of superior oblique on six cases.

developed, not an X pattern. Although a weakening procedure of the superior oblique affects the A pattern, it would seem that the superior oblique per se is not responsible for the pattern.

Done under direct visualization, recession of the superior oblique as described by the authors is a safe procedure. In my hands, it is even safer if the surgeon uses the microscope. The measured recessions are preferable to Tenectomy or Tenotomy.

BROWN´S SYNDROME FOLLOWING SUPERIOR OBLIQUE TUCK

R. A. Saunders and J. L. Grady

ASTRACT

Nineteen eyes of 16 patients underwent tuck of the superior oblique tendon in the surgical management of unilateral or bilateral superior oblique palsy. In each case, the amount of tuck was determined intraoperatively by performing forced ductions after the superior oblique tendon had been isolated temporal to the superior rectus muscle and provisionally tied. Optimal surgical results were obtained when resistance to elevation in the adducted eye was first detected as the inferior limbus reached the horizontal meridian. Moderate limitations of elevation in adduction were usually present in the immediate postoperative period and corresponded to intraoperative findings. However, ductions tended to improve with time and only one tuck was removed for postoperative Brown´s syndrome. All patients could eventually fuse in primary position and reading position without prismatic assistance.

TECHNIQUES USED FOR WEAKENING THE INFERIOR OBLIQUE

D. Romero-Apis and S. Martinez-Oropeza

ABSTRACT

Landolt was the first surgeon to operate on the inferior oblique. He made a tenotomy at the muscle´s origin through skin. Myectomy on nasal side is made by Duane(2), Dunnington (7), White(6) and Berke(3). Tenotomy at the insertion was popularized by Brown(8). Recession was recommended by Fink (9), and variations were made by Dyer(5), Parks(11), Prieto-Diaz and Souza-Dias(18). Myectomy at the middle third was introduced by McNeer, Scott and Jamplolsky(14). Surgical dennervation was recommended by Gonzalez(16). Chemical dennervation with botulinum toxin was reported by Scott(17). Romero-Apis and Martinez recommended Fadens on the middle third(19). Since 1980 the authors are doing triple myectomies on the middle third. Seventy-five cases are here analyzed: 30 esotropias and 45 exotropias. The results are compared to a series of 179 cases in which a middle third myectomy was performed. Results are: 1. Inferior oblique residual overaction: 2.6% in triple myotomy cases; 13.4% in myectomy cases. 2. Adhesion syndrome: 2.6% in triple myotomy cases (mild all of them); 9% in myectomy cases (severe two of them). 3. Superior oblique consecutive overaction: 7.8% in triple myotomy cases; 4.5% in myectomy cases. Results are discussed.

INTRODUCTION

Landolt(1), in 1885, was probably the first surgeon operating on the inferior oblique and made the tenotomy at the orbital origin through the skin. This procedure was used with enthusiasm by Duane(2) and later Berke(3). White and Brown(4) advocated a disinsertion, and later Dyer(5) awakened further interest in this procedure. Recession was popularized by White(6), Dunnington(7), Brown(8), Fink(9), and Berens(10), and later variations were reported by Dyer(5), Parks(11, 12), and Prieto-Diaz and Souza-Dias(13). Myectomy in the middle third of the muscle was introduced by McNeer, Scott and Jampolsky(14) in 1965. Wertz, Romano and Writhe(15) reported their results in rhesus monkeys as unpredictable and resulted in frequent reattachments of the proximal half of the muscle to the sclera following myectomy. Surgical denervation was advocated by Gonzalez(16) in 1974 and chemical denervation with small concentrations of botulinum toxin (Oculinum) was proposed and tried by Scott et al(17) and has given promising

STRABISMUS II
ISBN 0-8089-1424-3

results(18) seven years later. Romero-Apis and Martinez-Oropeza(19)performed Fadens on the middle third of the muscle in six patients with null results. Triple marginal myotomy in the middle third of the muscle has been advocated by Martinez-Oropeza(20) and Ramirez-Barreto and Murillo-Murillo(21).

Since 1979 the authors have been operating the inferior oblique by means of triple marginal myotomy, and herein report their results.

MATERIALS AND METODS.

Seventy-five cases (30 esotropias and 45 exotropias) were studied. Sixty-four cases had bilateral overaction, and 11 unilateral, giving a total of 139 surgical procedures.

Follow-up observations were made weekly during the first post-operative month, and monthly during the next eleven months. Final evaluation was made one year after surgery.

The results are analysed in three main aspects: a) Residual inferior oblique overaction. b) Consecutive homolateral superior oblique overaction. c) Adhesion syndrome.

A comparison was made with the results of a series of ours in which 197 cases were operated by means of middle third myectomy (101 esotropias and 78 exotropias) of which 161 had bilateral overation and 18 unilateral, giving a total of 340 muscles operated.

TECHNIQUE

The muscle is exposed by an approach in the inferotemporal quadrant near the fornix; when lateral rectus is operated an inferior extension is made of the limbal approach. The middle third of the muscle is disected in 15 mms and a Martinez clamp (special device for this purpose) bent at the right angle holds the muscle (Fig 1). Three incisions are made with an electrocautery (8 to 10 volts), one from the inferior edge in the middle of the two branches, and the other two from the superior edge at the sides of both branches (Fig 2). Each incision cross 2/3 (70%) of the width of the muscle. The Martinez clamp is removed leaving the muscle lengthened (Fig 3), and the conjunctivia is closed.

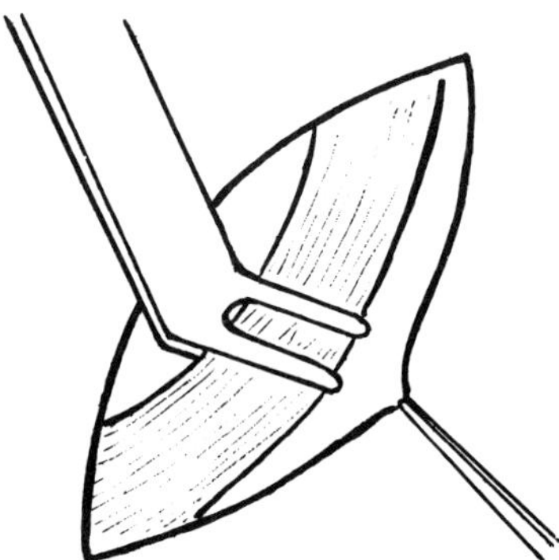

Figure 1. Martinez clamp holding the muscle.

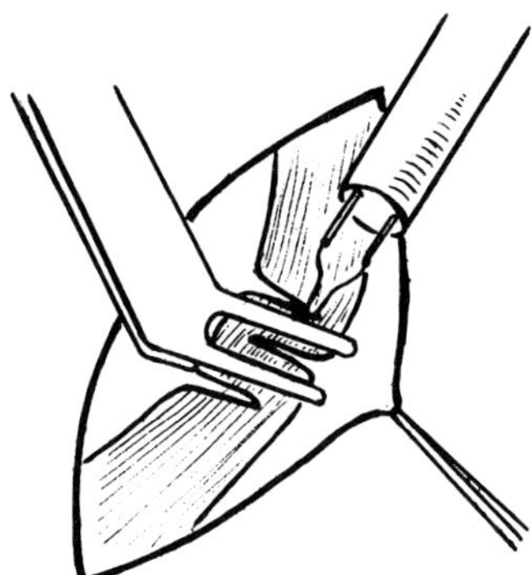

Figure 2. Three opposite incisions made with an electrocautery.

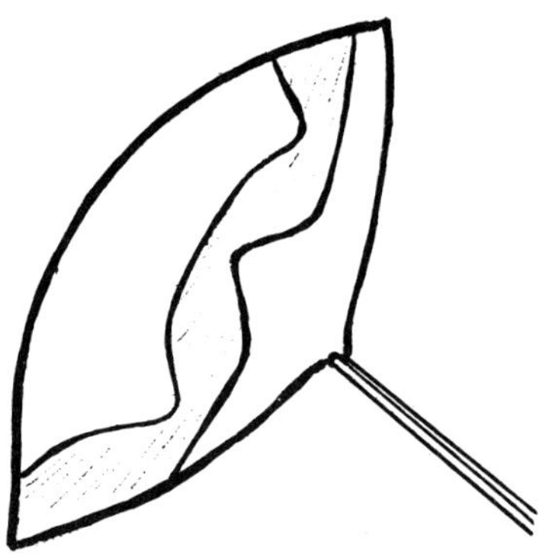

Figure 3. The muscle lengthened.

RESULTS

One year after surgery the following observations were made:

a. With triple marginal myotomy residual overaction was present in 2.6% of the cases. This is compared with our previous series of myectomy in which it was observed in 13.5%.

b. With triple marginal myotomy consecutive homolateral superior oblique overaction was present in 7.8% of the cases. This is compared with our previous series of myectomy in which it was observed in 4.5%.

c. With triple marginal myotomy the adhesion syndrome was present in 2.6%; all these cases had only mild degrees of adhesion with partial limitation of elevation in aduction. This is also compared with the previous series of myectomy in which it was observed in 9%; but two of these cases had a severe degree of adhesion with total limitation of elevation in aduction as well as in abduction, and had hypotropia in the primary position.

DISCUSSION

Surgery of the inferior oblique in the middle third is definitively easier and faster than disinsertion and recession procedures. For several years we used the myectomy procedure. Nevertheless we have found some disadvantages with this technique: residual overaction in 7.8% of the cases, finding in the reoperations the muscle reattached somewhere on the sclera; also adhesion syndrome was present with some frequency: 9% of the cases, some of them severe with limitation of elevation in all directions and hypotropia in the primary position.

With the triple marginal myotomy procedure, made in the third of the muscle, the same fast and easy way of operating is preserved, but with more predictable results than with myectomy. Residual overaction was observed in just 2.6% of the cases, and adhesion syndrome was present less frequently: 2.6% of the cases, all of them of only mild degree.

The possibility of consecutive homolateral superior oblique overaction is greater with the triple marginal myotomy (7.8%) than with myectomy (4.5%), and this might be interpreted as a more vigorous weakening procedure. Naturally cases with small degree of inferior oblique overaction, with normal homolateral superior oblique, should be avoided.

SUMMARY

The history of the inferior oblique muscle weakening procedures are reviewed. A series of 75 cases (30 esotropias and 45 exotropias) operated by means of triple marginal myotomy are presented. Results are compared with previous results by the same authors using the middle third myectomy procedure.

REFERENCES

1. Landolt E: La tenotomie de l´oblique inferieur. Arch Ophthalmol (Paris) 5:402-405, 1885.

2. Duane A: Tenotomy of the inferior obliqueand consideration of the conditions that may call for the operation. Read before the 74th Annual Meeting of the British Medical Association, Section on Ophthalmology, Toronto August 21-25, 1906. Abstract in Brit Med J pp. 1867-1868, 1906.

3. Berke RN: Surgery of oblique muscles. Highlights Ophthalmol 2:264-274, 1958.

4. White JW, Brown HW: Occurrence of vertical anomalies associated with convergent and divergent anomalies. Arch Ophthalmol 21:999-1009, 1939.

5. Dyer JA: Tenotomy of the inferior oblique muscle at its scleral insertion. Arch Ophthal 68:176-181, 1962.

6. White JW: Recession of the inferior oblique muscle. Arch Ophthalmol 29:1033-1034, 1943.

7. Dunnington, JH: A discussion in White JW: Recession of the inferior oblique muscle. Arch Ophthalmol 29:1034, 1943.

8. Brown HW: Surgery of the oblique muscles. In JH Allen Strabismus Ophthalmic Symposium (ed). C V Mosby, St. Louis p. 401-422, 1950.

9. Fink WH: Oblique muscle surgery from the anatomic viewpoint. Am J Ophthalmol 34:261-281, 1951.

10. Berens C, Cole HG, Chamichian S, Enos MV: Retroplacement of the inferior oblique at its scleral insertion. Am J Ophthalmog 35:217-227, 1952.

11. Parks MM: The weakening surgical procedures for

eliminating overaction of the inferior oblique muscle. Am J Ophthalmol 73:107-122, 1972.

12. Parks MM: The overacting inferior oblique muscle. Am J Ophthalmol 77:787-797, 1974.

13. Prieto-Diaz J, Souza-Dias C: Estrabismo. C V Mosby, St. Louis, p. 210, 1980.

14. McNeer KW, Scott AB, Jampolsky A: A technique for surgically weakening the inferior oblique muscle. Arch Ophthalmol 73:87-88, 1965.

15. Wertz RD, Romano PE, Wright P: Inferior oblique myectomy, disinsertion, and recession in rhesus monkeys. Arch Ophthalmol 95:857-860, 1977.

16. Gonzalez C: Denervation of inferior oblique as a weakening surgical procedure. Tr Am Acad Ophthalmol 78:816-823, 1974.

17. Scott AB, Rosenbaum AL, Collins CC: Pharmacologic weakening of extraocular muscles. Invest Ophthalmol 12:924-927, 1973.

18. Scott AB: Botulinum toxin injection into extraocular muscles as an alternative to strabismus surgery. J Ped Ophthalmol Strab 17:21-25, 1980.

19. Romero-Apis D, Martinez-Orpeza S: Personal experience.

20. Martinez-Oropeza S: Miotomias marginales como metodo de debilitamiento del oblicuo inferior. Anal Soc Mex Oftal 54:317, 1980.

21. Ramirez-Barreto MA,Murillo-Murillo L: Debilitamiento del oblicuo inferior. Anal Soc Mex Oftal 55:61, 1981.

DISCUSSION BY S. VERONNEAU-TROUTMAN

Drs. Romero-Apis and Martinez have given us an historic review of the inferior oblique muscle weakening procedures and compared in two different large groups of patients the effect of triple marginal myotomy and myectomy procedures. Double myotomies of the inferior oblique have had their popularity and are still used by some authors. Hugonnier´s text book (Hugonnier R, Clayette-Hugonnier S: Strabismus, heterophoria, ocular motor paralysis. Clinical ocular muscle imbalance. Translated and edited by S. Veronneau-Troutman. St. Louis, 1969, the C. V. Mosby Co, p. 610. Fig 43-17 and 43-18) shows the classical technique of double myotomies which can be compared with the triple myotomies of the authors. Its effect is similar to that described by the Hugonniers´. Many ophthalmologists have abandoned the double myotomy procedure, finding it unpredictable. One may question how the present authors have achieved a greater effect by elongating a muscle rather than cutting it, unless no part of the muscle was removed and reinervation took place. On the other hand, they were successful in 73% of their myectomy cases. If the authors had compared the two procedures in the same patient having bilateral overaction, would their conclusions be different? Perhaps they intend to give us such a study in the future.

SUPERIOR OBLIQUE PLICATION
ITS APPLICATION AND INDICATIONS
IN EARLY ONSET CONVERGENT STRABISMUS

J. L. Van Selm

Superior Oblique plication is a well documented but unpopular operation for correcting the vertical and the cyclorotatory deficit in cases of infantile onset convergent strabismus, weakening procedures on the inferior oblique muscles being preferred.

The results of bilateral inferior oblique recession in 50 cases are compared with a parallel series of 50 cases in which primary plication of both superior oblique muscles was undertaken. Complications of both procedures are discussed and suggestions are made regarding the indications for shortening procedures on the superior oblique muscles.

(No paper was submitted.)

DISCUSSION BY S. VERONNEAU-TROUTMAN

The interest of Dr. Van Selm in the aggressive management of early onset esotropia with bilateral superior oblique palsy goes back many years. In 1973 I had the privilege to be the moderator of the Strabismus session of the 2nd South African International Symposium and to comment on a paper he presented on "Infantial Squint, Its Etiology and Management". In a series of 230 esotropia cases with onset before age one, he found an associated bilateral S.O. palsy in 75% of the cases. Not only did he recommend early surgery but also a four muscle procedure. At that time a bimedial recession with I.O. weakening. (South African Archives of Ophthalmology. Proceedings of the 2nd South Africa International Ophthalmological Symposium: Strabismus. pp 37-41 and 43-53. Vol. 2, No. 1)

To relate early onset esotropia to bilateral superior oblique palsy is tempting. The IV nerves are the only ones with dorsal emergence, they completely decussate and are especially vulnerable. This is well illustrated by the high incidence of bilateral fourth nerve palsy after head trauma. That his cases, operated on early, responded as well to inferior oblique weakening procedures as to superior oblique strenghtening procedures is a little puzzling. One would assume that, although the cases were not selected, in the first group the palsies would have resolved rapidly leaving only a contractured antagonist and in the second group no contracture was present.

DIFFERENCES BETWEEN CONGENITAL AND ACQUIRED SUPERIOR OBLIQUE PALSIES

J. B. Dickson and J. H. Calhoun

ABSTRACT

The records of all patients at Wills Eye Hospital from 1978 through 1981 with the diagnosis of isolated, unilateral superior oblique palsy were retrospectively reviewed. Fifty-eight had sufficient data in records to be included in this study. The patients were divided into two groups. Those with a long history and a vague onset were classified as congenital. Those with a recent, well-defined onset were classified as acquired. Several characteristics other than history distinguished the two groups. Those patients with superior oblique palsies classified as congenital had, in comparison to the acquired group: 1) few complaints of diplopia 2) larger hyperdeviation in primary position 3) hyperdeviation greater in the field of the antagonist (inferior oblique); whereas, greatest hyperdeviation in the field of the palsied superior oblique 4) smaller torsional deviations relative to the amount of vertical deviations

It appears that congenital verses acquired superior oblique palsies can be differentiated on the basis of the clinical findings.

INTRODUCTION

The superior oblique muscle is innervated exclusively by the fourth cranial nerve. Superior oblique palsies can be broadly classified as congenital or acquired. Congenital fourth nerve paralysis may be more common than previously expected, but, diagnosis is less obvious.[1] Etiologies of congenital fourth nerve palsies include birth trauma, developmental anomalies (aplasia or hypoplasis) of the cranial nerve nucleus or fibers, and perinatal infection syndromes.[2,3] The reported causes of acquired fourth nerve palsies are numerous (Table 1). Diabetes- vascular is the presumed etiology in most cases of acquired superior oblique palsy in the over fifty age group. Trauma, which is the number one overall cause in most series, account for most

STRABISMUS II
ISBN 0-8089-1424-3

acquired palsies in the under fifty age group.[4-6] The intent of this paper is to analyze and compare certain characteristics of the congenital versus acquired fourth nerve palsies.

TABLE 1

1)	Diabetes - Vascular	9)	Botulism
2)	Pagets Disease	10)	Orbital Apex Syndrome
3)	Meningitis	11)	Intracranial and Nasopharyngeal Neoplasms
4)	Polyneuritis	12)	Multiple Sclerosis
5)	Cavernous Sinus Disease	13)	Myasthenia Gravis
6)	Superior Orbital Fissure Syndrome	14)	Syphilis
7)	Herpes Zoster	15)	Trauma
8)	Diphtheria	16)	Idopathic

The records of all patients at Wills Eye Hospital from 1978 through 1981 with the diagnosis of isolated, unilateral superior oblique palsy were retrospectively reviewed. Fifty-eight had sufficient data in records to be included in this study. The patients were divided into two groups. Those with a long history and a vague onset were classified as congenital. Those with a recent, well-defined onset were classified as acquired.

Of the fifty-eight patients, thirty-eight were male and twenty were female (Table 2). A higher incidence of trauma was noted in the male population, accounting for the slight male predominance. The youngest patient was twenty-one months and the oldest was eighty-four years of age. Based on the history, twenty-six were classified as congenital and thirty-two as acquired.

TABLE 2

58 Patients	
38 Males	20 Females

The congenital group had a wide range of ages at presentation. The average age was 21.3 years when diagnosed (Table 3). Most patients had long histories of head posturing and/or vague onsets of intermittent vertical diplopia. Of the thirty-two classified as acquired, the average age was 48.1 years (Table 4). All of this group had a rather sudden onset of diplopia. The principle causes were trauma in the young group and diabetes - arteriosclerotic vascular disease in the older group.

TABLE 3

26 Congenital Superior Oblique Palsies
21 Months - 68 Years (Range)
21.26 Years (Average)

TABLE 4

32 Acquired Superior Oblique Palsies
10 Years - 84 Years (Range)
48.1 Years (Average)

On initial examination, thirty-nine of the fifty-eight had diplopia as the chief complaint. Seventeen of the nineteen without diplopia had a head tilt. The remaining two without diplopia or a head tilt, ages thirteen and four, were classifed in the congenital group.

Of the acquired group, thirty-one of thirty-two complained of significant diplopia. The single exception was a ten-year old patient. Eight of the twenty-six congenital superior oblique palsies complained of diplopia, but were not particularly troubled by this in direct contradistinction to the acquired group (Table 5.)

TABLE 5

Diplopia
8/26 Congenital
31/32 Acquired

In the congenital group, the hyperdeviations in primary gaze had a range of 3 prism diopters to 35 prism diopters with a mean of 17.3 prism diopters. The hyperdeviations were greatest in the field of action of the antagonist. Overall this group had large vertical fusional amplitudes. In the acquired group, the hyperdeviations in primary gaze had a range of 2 prism diopters to 18 prism diopters with a mean of 6.5 prism diopters (Table 6). The hyperdeviations were greatest in the field of adtion of the palsied superior oblique.

TABLE 6

Hyperdeviation in Primary Gaze

	Congenital	Acquired
Range	3 - 35	2 - 18
Average	17.3	6.5

The torsional deviation was accurately measured in twelve patients using the double maddox rod. Six were classified as congenital and six were classified as acquired. Per diopter of hyperdeviation in primary gaze, the congenital group had significantly less excyclotorsion. Two patients with congenital fourth nerve palsies demonstrated no excyclotorsion using the double maddox rod (Graph 1).

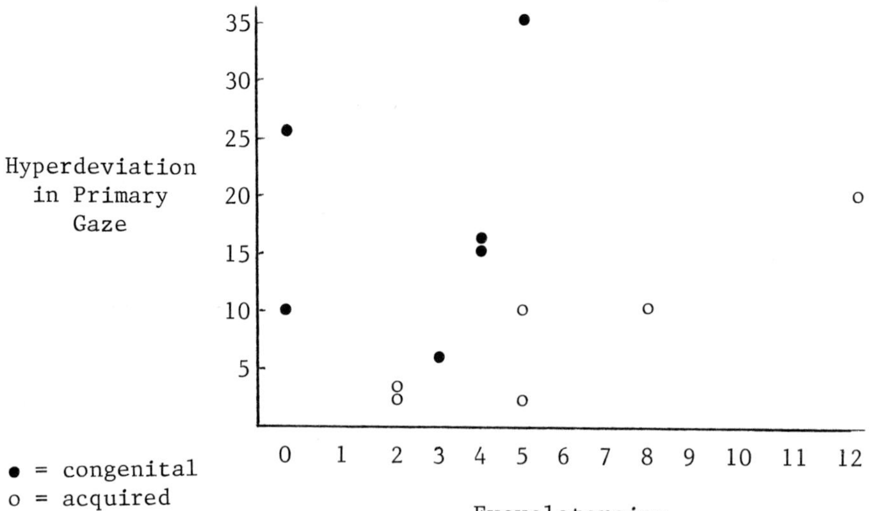

Based on these characteristics, it appears that congenital and acquired superior oblique palsies can be differentiated on the basis of the clinical findings. Using these findings, one can arrive at certain guidelines for surgical treatment. Since congenital superior oblique palsies have the greatest deviations in the field of the ipsilateral inferior oblique, an inferior oblique recession is usually the appropriate surgical choice. A contralateral inferior rectus recession may be indicated when the hyperdeviation in primary gaze is unusually large. In acquired superior oblique palsies, the hyperdeviation is greatest in the field of action of the palsied superior oblique. Here the surgeon may choose between a superior oblique tuck of the palsied muscle or an inferior rectus recession in the opposite eye. Finally, distinguishing a fourth nerve palsy as congenital or acquired may prove helpful in supporting an etiology. This may be helpful in case of trauma when litigation is present.

REFERENCES

1. Coppeto JM, Lessell S: Cryptogenic unilateral paralysis of the superior oblique muscle. Arch Ophthalmol 96:275-277, 1978.

2. Norman MG: Unilateral encepthalomalacia in cranial nerve nuclei in neonates: Report of two cases. Neurology 24:424-427, 1974.

3. Gilles FH: Hypotensive brain stem necrosis. Selective symmetrical necrosis of tegmental neuronal aggregates following arrest. Arch Pathol 88:32-41, 1969.

4. Khawam E, Scott AB, Jampolsky A: Acquired superior oblique palsy. Diagnosis and management. Arch Ophthalmol 77:761-768, 1967.

5. Burger LJ, Kalvin NH, Smith JL: Acquired lesions of the fourth cranial nerve. Brain 93:567-574, 1970.

6. Younge BR, Sutula F: Analysis of trochlear nerve palsies. Diagnosis, etiology, and treatment. Mayo Clin Proc 52:11-18, 1977.

DENERVATION AND EXTIRPATION OF THE INFERIOR OBLIQUE MUSCLE AS THE PRIMARY SURGICAL PROCEDURE IN THE TREATMENT OF SUPERIOR OBLIQUE PALSY

N. N. K. Katz

ABSTRACT

The surgical technique and results of surgery are reviewed in this paper based on 23 consecutive cases where denervation and extirpation of the ipsilateral inferior oblique was performed as the primary surgical procedure of choice. All patients had overaction of the inferior oblique (2 to 4 plus on a 1-4 scale). The rationale for this approach was based on the fact that even "maximal" (14 mm) recession of the inferior oblique may be inadeaute in the face of a nonfunctioning superior oblique. More over geometrically the recommended repositioning of the inferior oblique muscle with 14 mm recessions does not appear more advantageous as a better weakening procedure that the 10 mm recession. Clinically this is borne out. Other weakening procedures such as myotomy and myectomy of the inferior oblique appear even less predictable and more liable to complications of hemorrhage and adherence syndrome.

In our series of cases of denervation and extirpation of the inferior oblique a vertical correction range of 5-15 prism diopters was obtained. The correction seemed to self-adjust with a greater amount obtained for greater hyperdeviations with more contracture of the inferior oblique. Correction of excylcotropia from 0-5o was also obtained, depending on the amount of pre-existing excyclodeviation.

INTRODUCTION

Superior oblique muscle palsy has attracted much attention and controvery with regards to surgical management of the condition. Weakening of its antagonist, the ipsilateral inferior oblique muscle, is generally the recommended surgical procedure in the presence of contracture and overaction of the latter muscle. Various procedures have been described to weaken the inferior oblique muscle.

STRABISMUS II
ISBN 0-8089-1424-3

Results obtained from treating thirteen (13) consecutive patients with unilateral superior oblique muscle palsy with contracture and overaction of the inferior oblique muscle are discussed in this report. The primary surgical procedure employed in all patients was denervation and extirpation of the inferior oblique muscle.

METHODOLOGY

Denervation and extirpation of the ipsilateral inferior oblique muscle was performed as the primary surgical procedure in thirteen (13) consecutive patients on the Ophthalmology Service, Walter Reed Amry Medical Center, with unilateral superior oblique palsy. All the surgery was performed under the supervision of the same surgeon (NNKK). Table 1 details the age, sex, etiology of superior oblique muscle palsy, and pre-operativee hyperdeviation in primary gaze (distance), as well as the presence, if any, of face turn and head tilt. The technique of surgery paralleled that described by Parks.1 The main surgical complication encountered was the formation of an inferior conjunctival and lower lid hematoma which occurred despite cauterizing the cut nerve and vascular stumps and suture ligature and cautery of the proximal cut end of the muscle. However, the hematoma resolved spontaneously in all patients within a period of two weeks. One patient (E.B.) sustained palsy of the pupillomotor fibers of the oculomotor nerve which has resolved partially at this time. Due to his age and retarded mental status, it was not possible to test the accommodation of the affected eye. The overall results are summarized in Table 2. Excluded from this review were patients who had additional muscle surgery done concomiitantly. These were patients with hyperdeviations larger than fifteen (15) prism diopters in primary gaze. These patients generally underwent recession of the contralateral inferior rectus muscle in addition to the inferior oblique muscle.

Paresis of the superior oblique muscle is the most common, isolated cylovertical muscle palsy. Most cases seen in the pediatric and young adult age group are either the congenital type (where the exact mechanism is often unclear), post trauma, or febrile illness. In the older age group, cerebral vascular disease constitutes an important cause of superior oblique muscle palsy. The clinical features of superior oblique muscle palsy include hypertropia, face turn, and head tilt. Diplopia while occurring in adults is often absent in the pediatric age group and anomalous retinal correspondence may be noted. However, in the congenital

Case	Age	Sex	Etiology	Pre-op Hyperdeviation in Prism Diopters	Face Turn	Head Tilt
1	8	M	Congenital	8	+	+
2	18	M	Trauma	8	+	+
3	9	F	Meningitis	6	±	+
4	6	F	Congenital	10	+	+
5	24	M	Trauma	4	+	−
6	1&1/2	F	Congenital	10 ±	−	+
7	29	F	Trauma	8	+	−
8	18	F	Congenital	10	+	+
9	2	M	Congenital (Cerebral Palsy)	10	−	+
10	7	M	Febrile Episode	6	−	+
11	21	M	Trauma	6	+	+
12	25	M	(Unknown)	14	+	+
13	20	F	Trauma	8	+	+

TABLE I

Case	Age	Sex	Period of Follow-Up	Post-Op Hyperdeviation in Prism Diopters	Face Turn	Head Tilt
1	8	M	2&1/2 yrs	0	0	I
2	18	M	2 yrs	0	0	0
3	9	F	2 yrs	Flick	0	I
4	6	F	1&1/2 yrs	2	0	0
5	24	M	1&1/2 yrs	0	0	0
6	1&1/2	F	1&1/2 yrs	6 ±	I	+
7	29	F	1 yr	0	I	0
8	18	F	1 yr	4 ±	+	+
9	2	M	8 mos	8	+	+
10	7	M	8 mos	2	I	0
11	21	M	4 mos	0	0	0
12	25	M	4 mos	2	I	I
13	20	F	2 mos	0	0	I

TABLE II

(I = Improved)

variety apparently the desire for fusion is great enough to elicit a head tilt even in infancy. Often this is noted in the second six months of infancy when the child can raise his head and can sit up and raise himself. However, even with this mechanism, bifoveal or other fusion is not always obtained and anomalous retinal correspondence or total absence of fusion may be seen.

The classification of the various "stages" of superior oblique muscle palsies has been well delineated by Knapp.[2] He notes that in class 1, 2, and 3 there is obvious overaction of the inferior oblique muscle on the same side due to contracture and overaction as a direct antagonist of the superior oblique muscle. A weakening procedure of the inferior oblique muscle is recommended for class 1 and class 3, and tuck of the superior oblique muscle for class 2 (and class 3, if necessary).

The inferior oblique muscle can be weakened by a variety of surgical techniques: myotomy, myectomy, disinsertion at the insertion, disinsertion at the origin, and graded recessions. Traditionally inferior oblique myotomies and myectomies appear to have been the procedures of choice. Parks[3,4] in reviewing and comparing these procedures feels that recession of the inferior oblique muscle is a more controlled, predictable and safe procedure. In the presence of a paretic agonist, however, recession alone may not offer adequate resolution of the problem due to continued contracture of the antagonist and thus result in a recurrence of symptoms. Thus, one hypothetically needs a more predictable as well as a permanent solution to the problem of the overacting antagonist.

Denervation and extirpation of the inferior oblique muscle is predictable so far as eliminating its overaction. We have not encountered a single case of recurrence of overaction of the inferior oblique following this procedure both in this series as well as when the surgery was performed in other types of strabismus associated with its overaction. We have not found underaction of the inferior oblique muscle to be a problem after this procedure. In almost all instances an adequate amount of elevation in adduction persisted even after surgery of the inferior oblique muscle. This is perhaps due to the superior rectus muscle acting as an elevator even in adduction. Boeder[5,6] by mathematic analysis concluded that the superior rectus may be the primary elevator in all fields of gaze. This appears to be borne out clinically.[7]

The only complication met with in the present series was one case of pupillary palsy which is resolving at present. This complication has been noted previously[8] and it must be cautioned that while this problem appears to be usually transient, it could occasionally result in permanent pupillary and accommodative paresis. Although this complication may be due to "surgical, anatomical confusion" at the time of denervation, it is more likely that there may be individual variation in the sites of exit of the autonomic fibers from the branch to the inferior oblique muscle from the oculomotor nerve. It must be emphasized that extreme care must be exercised in this as well as any other inferior oblique surgical procedure to avoid violation of the inferotemporal vortex vein as well as the orbital fat pad to prevent serious hemorrhage and adhesive syndromes. Careful isolation and identification of the entire muscle is mandatory to prevent unexpected recurrences of overaction after surgery due to missed fibres of the inferior oblique muscle. This fact may have been instrumental in the failures following myectomy and myotomy performed without direct visualization of the inferior oblique muscle by the surgical technique well described by Parks.[1]

It is noted from the results that the least benefit appeared in those patients who are younger and had congenital superior oblique palsy with a large head tilt. This has been previously noted and superior oblique muscle tuck has been recommended as the primary surgical procedure of choice in this group of patients.[8] In older patients with sudden onset of superior oblique muscle palsy from cerebral vascular disease, small hyper deviations usually are noted and these patients may do well with prism spectacles and rarely need surgery.

While this represents a small series of consecutive patients and does not make any attempt at a controlled or comparative study with other techniques currently available, it does offer a promising alternative with predictable results and few complications. Other potential indications for employment of this surgery may be in the surgical management of Brown's syndrome where extirpation and denervation of the inferior oblique muscle may be combined with superior oblique tenotomy to prevent superior oblique muscle palsy that may sometimes result from the tenotomy being performed exclusively.

SUMMARY

Thirteen consecutive patients with unilateral superior oblique muscle palsy with less than fifteen (15) prism diopters hyperdeviation and ipsilateral inferior oblique contracture and overaction, were treated by denervating and extirpating the ipsilateral inferior oblique muscle. The results compare favorably with other currently available surgical methods of inferior oblique weakening. This approach appears to hold promise and offers several hypothetical advantages.

REFERENCES

1. Parks MM: Atlas of Strabismus Surgery. Phila., PA, Harper & Row, 1982.

2. Knapp P: Classification and treatment of superior oblique palsy. Am Orthopt J 24:18-22, 1974.

3. Parks MM: The weakening surgical procedures for eliminating overaction of the inferior oblique muscle. Am J Ophthalmol 73:107-122, 1972.

4. Parks MM: The overacting inferior oblique muscle. Am J Ophthalmol 77:787-797, 1974.

5. Boeder P: An analysis of the general type of ocular rotations. Arch Ophthalmol 57:200-206 1957.

6. Boeder P: Cooperative action of extraocular muscles. Br J Ophthalmol 46:397-463 1962.

7. von Noorden GK: Burian-von Noorden's binocular vision and ocular motility. Edition 2, St Louis, 1980, The CV Mosby Co., p 60.

8. Parks MM: Personal communication.

The opinions and assertions herein are the private views of the author and are not to be construed as official or as reflecting the opinions of the Department of the Army or the Department of Defense.

BROWN'S SYNDROME IN THE LIGHT OF FRAGMENTED AND OVERDEVELOPED SUPERIOR OBLIQUE TENDON

W. de Decker and H. G. Conrad

ABSTRACT

While operating on palsied congenital superior oblique tendons, the authors have found seven patients with a fragmented tendon. The defects were located near the insertion, which was missing in 4 and fragmentary in three cases. There is evidence from the zoological literature that the superior oblique tendon develops from 7 to 9 separate "Anlagen" (nuclei). It seems likely that a missing insertion, with some fibers ending in the fascia bulbi, is caused by the lack of two distal "Anlagen", while fragmentation may have its base in only one defective "nucleus".

After this series of defective cases the authors have recently found one patient with a click-syndrome, and one with a Brown's syndrome, both of whom had an overdeveloped terminal tendon. This was partially removed surgically, with good clinical success. The procedure is documented in a film. As such cases are rare and far from being the only explanation for congenital pareses or Brown-like syndromes, the authors would like to hear the opinion of others.

In a patient with an intermittent Brown's syndrome, the tendon of the superior oblique was found to be too thick (overdeveloped?) but of normal length. It could be split, half the cord being resected, and the so-called click-syndrome was cured.

During the last 10 years we have seen seven patients with defective insertions of the tendon of the superior oblique and have reported on the first four cases(2). The subsequently investigated three patients showed the same anatomical findings, which can be divided into two types:

Defective Insertion

Apparently Missing Insertions (5 cases)

The tendons were found in front of the trochlea but did not go to their natural insertions. The distal tendon

STRABISMUS II
ISBN 0-8089-1424-3

"disappeared" within the posterior parts of the fascia bulbi, a structure which is not well defined. The tendon, in other words, of such a patient is not sufficiently attached to the globe (Fig 1). The clinical diagnosis in all five patients revealed a congenital IV nerve palsy with limited convergent microtropia in one child and with moderate compensatory head posture. The anatomical diagnosis was never suspected unless surgery was performed. The surgical correction consisted in hooking the tendon in front of the trochlea (Fig 2) and forming a loop. The vertex of the loop was pulled underneath the superior rectus and attached to the middle of the line where the superior oblique normally inserts (Fig 3). Surprisingly this was successfully done in three patients in a first attempt. The other two patients required a second adjustment, respecting the sagittal position and the degree of tension of the loop.

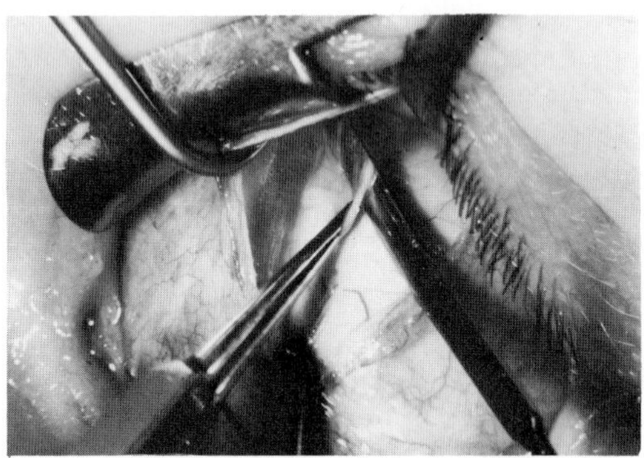

Figure 1. Fragmented insertion of the left superior oblique muscle. The spatula tips from a temporal approach to a thin tendon cord which is not connected to the main tendon (in Fig 2).

Subnormal Development of the Terminal Tendon

This was seen in two patients from whom one presented with the same type of motility disorder. One bilaterally affected patient displayed a V - esophoria with asthenopic complaints. These two patients were corrected by conventional tucking operations temporal to the superior rectus muscle.2

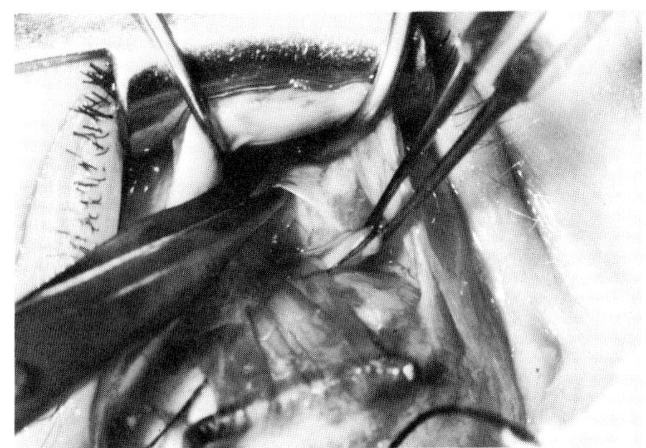

Figure 2. The main pretrochlear part of the tendon is armed with strong silk suture for pulling it underneath the transparent superior rectus. The posterior check ligament is cut to ease the pulling manuever.

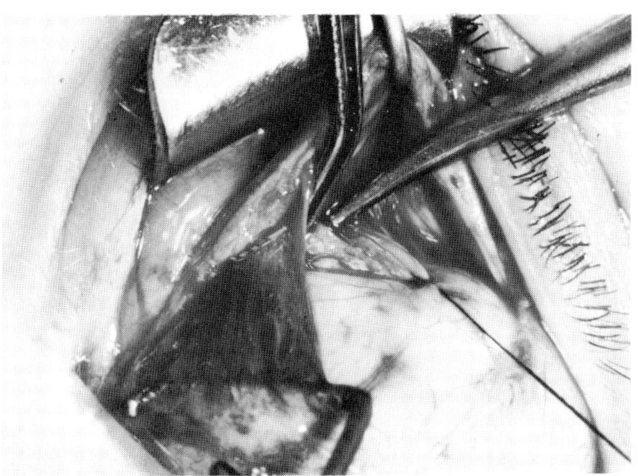

Figure 3. The main part of the fragmented tendon of the superior oblique is pulled to the site of physiological insertion. The tendon forms a loop, the posterior branch "fading" away backwards in the fascia bulbi.

Hyperplasia of the Distal Tendon of the Superior Oblique

Clinically one patient presented a Click-Syndrome, the other a Brown's syndrome. The surgical exposure of the tendon to the trochlea showed in both cases a thick distal

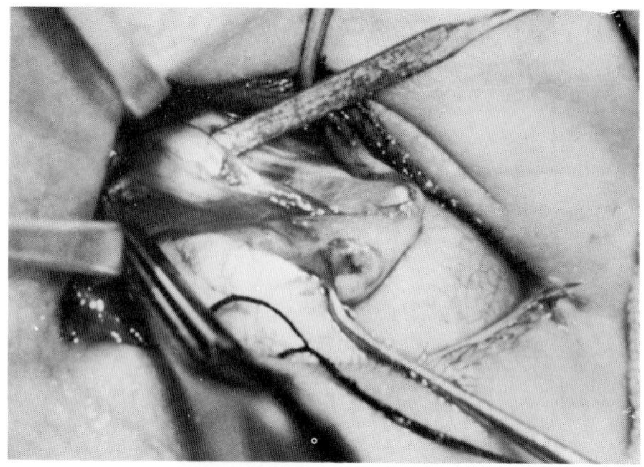

Figure 4. Thick pretrochlear part of the tendon of the superior oblique muscle, indicated by underlying spatula.

portion forming an obstacle to sliding of the tendon (Fig 4). In neither case we could find any signs of former inflammation, nor scars. After pulling all the thick portion vigorously forward the distal tendon could be enfeebled by a longitudinal splitting (Fig 5, 6). This treatment led to unrestricted active and passive vertical rotations in both cases.

DISCUSSION

Gilbert reported that the superior oblique in cats develops from 7-9 "Anlagen" which grow together during ontogenesis.3 We suppose that our findings of underdeveloped terminal tendons in humans may also be based on a weak or lacking formation of the most distal "Anlage". We also speculate that the hyperplastic variation could be caused by an excessive growth of the distal one or two "Anlagen". Two cases cannot prove that all patients with a Brown's syndrome depend on this etiology. But they contribute to the increasingly accepted opinion that the Brown's syndrome and the Click-syndrome are not consistent features.(1,2,5)

We, therefore, suggest that even those colleagues who follow a strictly conservative treatment should surgically inspect the situs. The mentioned anatomical cause seems not to be extremely rare as Dr. Folk could demonstrate a patient with a Click-syndrome in reference who showed an overdeveloped superior oblique including the terminal tendon by a quite readable Computer tomography.

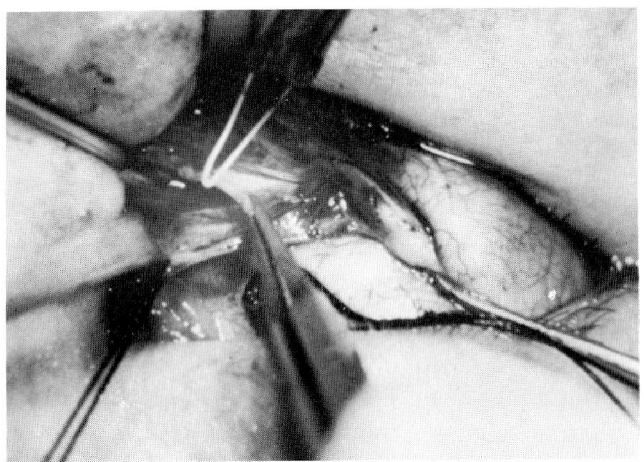

Figure 5. Cutting half the volume of the thick tendon by whiteglowing cauter.

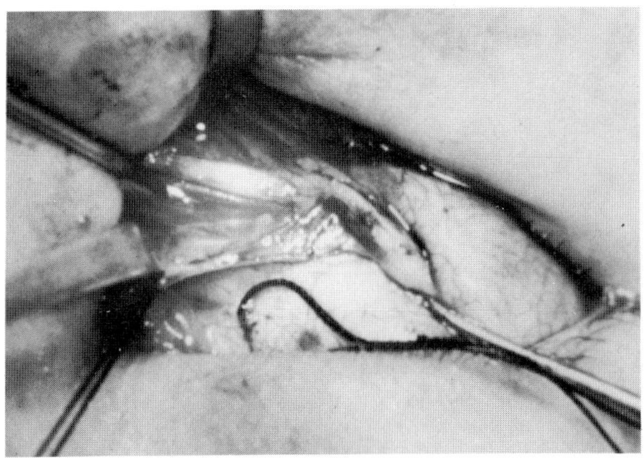

Figure 6. Tendon reduced to normal measures. The underlying tendon sheath remained untouched.

REFERENCES

1. Brown HW: True and simulated superior olbique tendon sheath syndromes. Doc Ophthalmol 34:123-136, 1973.

2. de Decker W, Conrad HG: Surgical transposition of the insertion of the superior oblique in cases of psuedoaplasia and traumatic disturbances. Symp ODG 1977 (Freiburg) Disorders of Ocular Motility, (ed) Kommerell G; Bergmann, Munchen 1978, p. 111.

3. Gilbert PW: Origin and development of extrinsic ocular muscles in domestic cat. J Morphol 8:151-193, 1947.

4. Raab EL: Superior oblique tendon sheath syndrome: An unusual case. Ann Ophthalmol 8:345-347 1976.

5. Roper-Hall MJ, Roper-Hall G: The superior oblique "click" syndrome. Orthoptics; Proc 2nd Int Orthopt Congress Amsterdam 1971, (ed) Mein J et al, Excerpta Medica, Amsterdam 1972, p 360-366.

DESAGITTALIZATION OF THE OBLIQUE MUSCLES AS A SURGICAL TREATMENT OF STRABISMUS

M. H. Gobin

ABSTRACT

Since 1962, we have anteropositioned the inferior oblique muscle for reduction of the elevation in adduction of a V-esotropia. The inferior oblique is detached from the sclera and reattached at the equator of the globe, half way between the lateral and inferior rectus muscles. This anteropositioning was carried out bilaterally and accompanied with recessions of both medial rectus muscles. The results were surprising. Binocular vision appeared spontaneously. The accommodative element of the strabismus disappeared even in cases with a bad prognosis such as a strabimus with an early onset and in adult patients. The good results implied that our surgery removed an obstacle to fusion. It seemed to us that this obstacle was a faculty sagittalization of the oblique muscles. With sagittalization we mean that one oblique muscle has a more anteroposterior course than its antagonist producing a cyclovertical muscle imbalance.

INTRODUCTION

Our anteropositioning of the inferior oblique actually desagittalizes the muscle by enlarging the angle it forms with the visual axis so that the vertical action of the muscle is selectively reduced in favor of the torsional action.

The good results encouraged us to perform a desagitallizing surgery on the superior oblique in order to reduce the depression in adduction of an A-syndrome. When both an elevation and a depression in adduction are present all four oblique muscles are desagittalized. We think that a sagittalization of the oblique muscles plays an important role in the pathogenesis of strabismus (Fig 1).

The surgical techniques of the desagittalization and the indications are presented.

STRABISMUS II
ISBN 0-8089-1424-3

PROCEDURE

An oblique muscle is sagittalized when the angle it forms with the visual axis is smaller than that of its antagonist, the scleral insertion being more posteriorly, or the origin more anteriorly or both. This sagittalization causes a torsional, a vertical and a horizontal imbalance between both antagonists, which can, with or without imposing factors, disrupt binocular vision and cause suppression and strabismus.

We try to reduce the sagittalization of an oblique muscle by a surgical desagittalization; we displace the line of pull of the muscle forwards. A desagittalization of both inferior obliques is performed when an upshoot is present and of both superior obliques when a downshoot is seen.

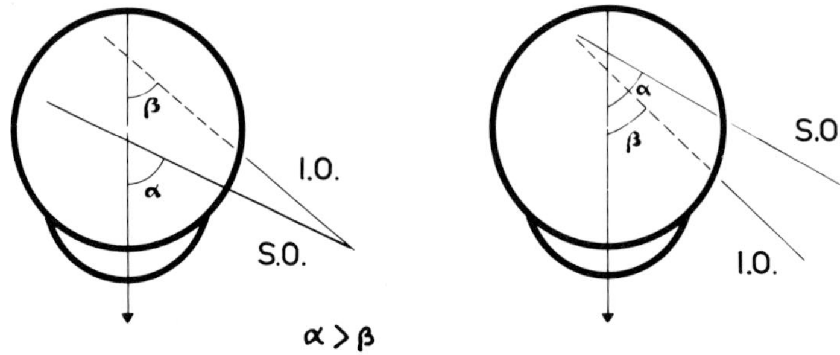

Figure 1. Sagittalization of the inferior oblique muscle. An oblique muscle is sagittalized when the angle it forms with the visual axis is smaller than that of its antagonist, the scleral insertion being more posterioly, the origin more anteriorly or both.

Figure 2 gives a schematical view of the desagittalization of the inferior oblique muscles. From left to right are shown the three types of desagittalization we use: a posterior myectomy, an anteropositioning and a disinsertion. The posterior myectomy consists of cutting the posterior part of the insertion. This insertion is cut over eight-tenth of its width leaving the muscle attached to the sclera with a small strand. To achieve an anteropositioning of the inferior oblique, the muscle's insertion is cut and the anterior tip is reinserted at the sclera, level with the equator of the eye and halfway between the inferior and the lateral rectus. The posterior tip of the muscle is left to retract freely. A disinsertion is carried out by cutting the scleral insertion without reattaching it, the inferior oblique remaining suspended at the height of the crossing with the inferior rectus by means of the connections between both muscles.

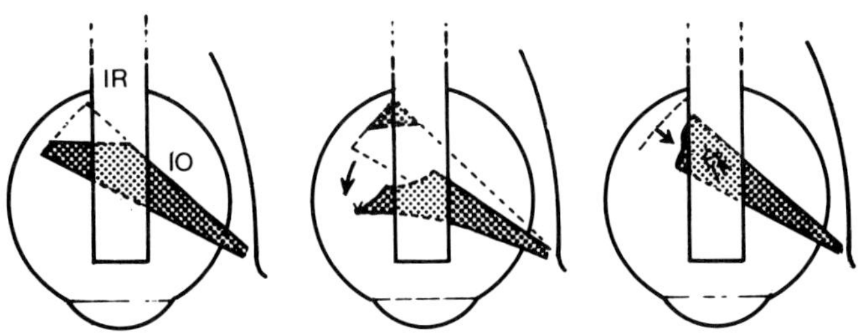

Figure 2. Desagittalization of the inferior oblique muscle. From left to right: posterior myectomy, anteropositioning and disinsertion.

Figure 3 shows the three types of desagittalization of the superior oblique. On the left the posterior tenectomy can be seen: the posterior part of the tendon is cut near the sclera and removed. Next comes the anteropositioning with a loop. The tendon is cut along the sclera and the anterior tip is hung in a loop which is attached to the anterior point of the scleral insertion; the posterior tip is cut away. Finally, on the right, we have the disinsertion of the superior oblique: the tendon is cut and not reinserted so that it will reattach to the sclera somewhere underneath the superior rectus. However, there is a danger for a paralysis of the muscle when the tendon slips back too far and for a reversal of its actions when the tendon attaches to the sclera in front of the equator of the globe.

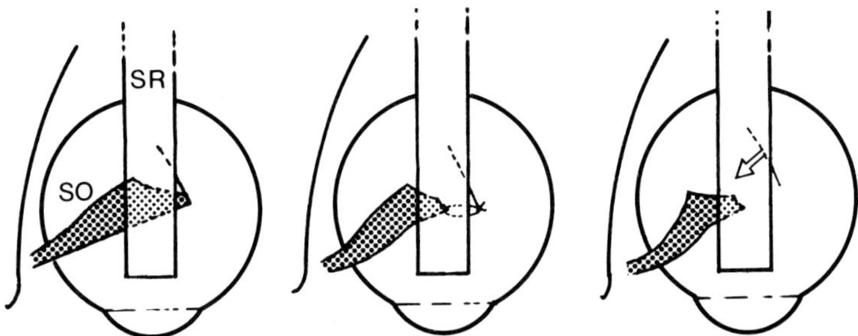

Figure 3. Desagittalization of the superior oblique muscle. From left to right: posterior tenectomy, anteropositioning with a loop and disinsertion.

In our opinion a desagittalizing surgery reduces an important obstacle to fusion, but there is another obstacle which needs to be removed namely the horizontal deviation. To relieve this deviation, we systematically add a bilateral 5 mm recession of the medial rectus in case of an esotropia and of the lateral rectus in case of an exotropia. In large angles we add a loop to the recession (Fig 4). In order to realize a loop recession of a rectus muscle the sutures are placed at 5 mm behind the original insertion and knotted over a probe. The point of attachment of the tendon thus remains in front of the equator of the globe while the muscle can retract further back.

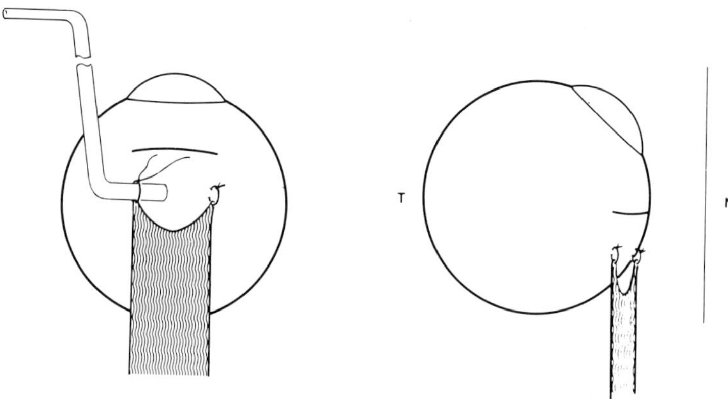

Figure 4. Recession with a loop. The suture is placed at 5 mm behind the original insertion and knotted over a probe, thus resulting in a loop which allows the muscle to retract further backwards without limiting the arc of contact. In order to obtain a large loop we use a probe with a diameter of 2 mm and for a small loop we use a probe of 1.5 mm.

Surgical measurements are impossible with this technique. There are too many parameters which we do not know, such as, the size of the globe so that an exact correlation between the amount of muscle displacement and the angle of strabismus is illusive. Fortunately, in strabismus, suppression is limited to one half of the retina: to the nasal half in convergent strabismus and to the temporal half in divergent strabismus. If we try to correct the deviation exactly there are, of course, a number of cases where we do not know enough; in those cases the image of the dominant eye falls on the suppressed retina half so that the fusion reflexes cannot straighten the eyes. A recurrence of the strabismus will result. If, however, we aim for an overcorrection the image of the dominated eye falls on the nonsuppressed half of the retina so that the motor fusion reflexes can act and reduce the overcorrection.

The motor fusion reflexes are always potentially present even if no sensory fusion is demonstrable. For them to become effective two conditions must be fulfilled: first all obstacles against the fusion reflexes must be eliminated and secondly no new obstacles should be created. The existing obstacles are, as we already said, a sagittalization of the oblique muscles and a horizontal deviation. The most common new obstacles are a vertical deviation and a duction limitation.

A description of the desagittalization technique of the superior oblique follows. The posterior tenectomy is done through an incision in the conjunctive and Tenon's capsule in the temporal upper quadrant. A strabismus hook is placed under the superior rectus muscle and the eye is pulled downwards.

A special spatule, 15 mm long and 5 mm wide, is introduced into the wound in order to lift the capsule of Tenon so that the operation area is clearly exposed.

The anterior tip of the superior oblique inserts about 5 mm behind the insertion of the superior rectus and along the temporal border of this muscle. With a pair of forceps we can pick up the tendon by grasping backwards over the sclera.

A small strabismus hook is introduced underneath the superior rectus and pushed nasalwards until it passes to medial side of the superior rectus. Normally the point of the strabismus hook is directed backwards but if we fail to pick up the anterior tip of the superior oblique the strabismus hook may be introduced underneath the superior rectus with the point directed forwards. Once the hook is in position the point of the strabismus hook is turned backwards.

Now the strabismus hook is swept backwards and the superior oblique pulled temporalwards whilst the assistant releases the superior rectus. During this maneuver the strabismus hook must be directed slightly downwards in order not to catch the superior rectus.

At the moment we pass the temporal border of the superior rectus the point of the strabismus hook is turned up making sure not to catch a vorticose vein.

The anterior border of the tendon is gripped with a pair of forceps and a hole is made in the tendon at 2 mm behind the anterior tip of the insertion. One point of the scissors is introduced into the hole and the posterior part of the tendon is cut along the sclera.

The posterior part of the tendon is resected in order to avoid reattachment to the posterior pole of the globe.

A final control is made in order to make sure that no posterior fibres remain attached to the sclera. The strabismus hook is glided backwards along the sclera insertion and if it bumps against uncut fibres the eye will make an abduction and an intorsion movement.

If we want to perform an anteropositioning with a loop, a Vicryl 6/0 suture is passed through the anterior border of the tendon before the tendon is cut near the sclera. The posterior part of the tendon is again removed in order to avoid reattachment to the posterior pole of the globe. One may not forget gliding a strabismus hook backwards along the scleral insertion in order to make sure that no posterior fibers remain uncut.

The suture is passed through the anterior tip of the scleral insertion and the loop is formed by knotting the thread over the strabismus hook which is in place under the superior rectus. The knot is pushed to the scleral insertion of the superior oblique so that it will not adhere to the superior rectus muscle.

It is important to push the tendon backwards in order to avoid a reattachment to the sclera in front of the equator of the eye. This would inverse the actions of the muscle.

REFERENCES

1. Fink WH: The role of developmental anomalies in vertical muscle defects. Am J Ophthalmol 40:529-552, 1955.

2. Gobin MH: Sagittalization of the oblique muscles as a possible cause for the "A", "V" and "X"phenomena. Br J Ophthalmol 52:13-18 , 1968.

3. Gobin MH: The limitation of suppression to one half of the visual field in the pathogenesis of strabismus. Br Orthoptic J 25:42-49, 1968.

4. Gobin MH: Nouvelles conceptions sur la pathogenie et le traitement du strabisme. L Pathogenie du strabisme, J Fr Ophthalmol 310:541-556, 1980.

5. Gobin MH: Surgical treatment of the A and V phenomena. Trans Ophthalmol Soc UK, 101(2)258-263, 1981.

6. Gobin MH: Surgical management of esotropia. In Evens L (ed): Convergent strabismus. Monographs in Ophthalmology 6. Boston, Dr. W. Junh Publishers, 1982 p. 301-358 and Bull Soc Beige Ophthalmol 195:301-358, 1981.

7. Keiner GBJ: New views points on the origin on squint. Thesis, The Hague, 1952.

SUPERIOR OBLIQUE DYSFUNCTION OF TRAUMATIC ORIGIN

B. Harcourt and F. Spencer

ABSTRACT

Fifty consecutive cases of acquired isolated superior oblique (S.O.) dysfunction have been reviewed. Thirty were found to be post-traumatic; fifteen of these were of central origin (Group A) with no evidence of injury in the trochlear area. Two patients in Group A had a bilateral palsy, representing only 25% of the patients who had suffered a severe head injury. Only 6 Group A patients eventually required ocular muscle surgery in order to regain an extensive field of comfortable binocular single vision; these included 5 with severe head injury and both bilateral cases. In two Group A patients, the affected eye showed a temporary pattern of progressive limitation of elevation in adduction during the recovery period, in the absence of any peripheral injury or evidence of mechanical restriction.

Fifteen patients with injuries in the trochlear area (Group B) all had unilateral S.O. dysfunction. The etiology were varied, but seven out of the 15 had facial lacerations due to windshield injuries. Only two cases in Group B were characteristic of the classical "pseudo" Brown's syndrome. Four patients showed a mixture of S.O. underaction and limited elevation in adduction, and 9 could have been mistaken for IVth nerve palsies of central origin were it not for the fact that they had suffered no significant associated head injury. Seven Group B patients required ocular muscle surgery. Inferior oblique (I.O.) overaction was sometimes masked by mechanical restriction and such patients benefitted from I.O. weakening operations.

INTRODUCTION

We have reviewed 50 consecutive cases of acquired isolated S.O. dysfunction, and found that 29 of these were post-traumatic. We have divided these into a Group A comprising 14 cases of fourth cranial nerve palsy with no injury in the trochlear area or elsewhere in the orbit, and a Group B of 15 cases in which there was evidence of trochlear or orbital injury.

STRABISMUS II
ISBN 0-8089-1424-3

Group A Patients (Traumatic IV Cranial Nerve Palsies)

Seven of these 14 patients had suffered only a trivial head injury, with no loss of consciousness, amnesia or skull fracture. In all those patients the S.O. weakness was unilateral, as it was in all but 2 of the 7 patients who had suffered a serious head injury. Criteria for diagnosing a strictly unilateral compared with a markedly asymmetrical bilateral palsy were principally a lack of any evidence of reversal of vertical diplopia in the right and left lateral depression positions, plus the absence of any evidence of contralateral palsy after surgery in those unilateral cases requiring operation. Only 6 of those 14 patients required surgery in order to regain a good field of binocular single vision (BSV) without a significant compensatory head posture. These included both bilateral cases and 5 of those with serious head injury. That is, only 1 of the 7 with trivial head injury and unilateral palsy required surgery. Two of the unoperated patients during the recovey period exhibited a transient and curious apparent underaction of the ipsilateral inferior oblique, with reversal of vertical diplopia on elevation-in-adduction, in the complete absence of any evidence of trauma in the trochlear region, or of mechanical restriction (Fig 1). The explanation of this is uncertain, but it could have led to misinterpretation as a pseudo-Brown's syndrome if it had been associated with peripheral injury.

Of the 8 patients, all with unilateral palsies, who did not have surgery, only 2 had completely full recovery of ocular movements and binocular muscle balance. Both of these recovered within 4 months, despite one having suffered a serious head injury with a skull fracture, several hours unconsciousness, 2 days retrograde amnesia and diabetes insipidus. Of the other 6, one 68-year-old surprisingly developed a vertical fusion range of 10 prism diopters within 9 months of a parieto-frontal skull fracture, allowing her to maintain, without vertical prisms, comfortable binocular vision in all directions of gaze despite a residual vertical muscle imbalance of 6 prism diopters. One patient had a slight persistent head tilt, avoiding any diplopia, and continued to show marked improvement in ocular movements and muscle balance between 6 and 18 months after injury. Of the other 3, one was rendered completely comfortable in practice although a manifest strabismus could be demonstrated in one case in greater than 30o elevation, and in the other in more than 30o depression of the eyes. In the former case, marked further improvement in muscle balance and the BSV field occurred between 6 and 9 months after injury.

Group B Patients (Peripheral Superior Oblique Injuries)

Every one of these 15 patients had a unilateral SO dysfunction. Although they were all considered to have a local peripheral cause for this, with evidence of soft tissue injury of the eyelids and orbits, and a significant associated head injury in only 3 cases, by no means all showed solely a classical pseudo-Brown's syndrome type of

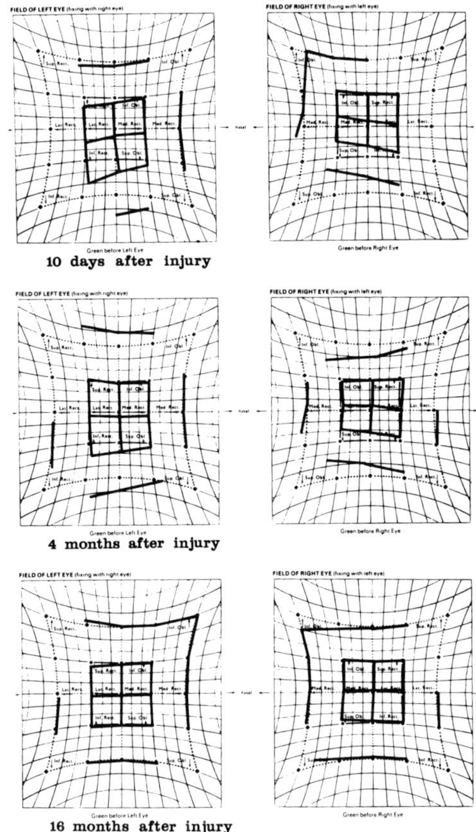

Figure 1. Transient limitation of elevation of right eye in adduction during spontaneous recovery from a traumatic right trochlear nerve palsy. There was marked reversal of diplopia on elevation between 3 and 9 months after injury.

restriction of ocular movement with mechanical limitation of elevation-in-adduction. Indeed, 3 patterns of restricted movements could be differentiated:

Type 1, Pseudo-Brown's Syndrome

Only 2 patients remained in this group 6 months after injury, although initially 2 others appeared to fall into this category.

Type 2, Pseudo-Brown's Syndrome Plus SO Underaction

A mixture of mechanical restriction of elevation-in-adduction and defective depression-in-adduction was found in 5 patients. The limitation of elevation was usually more marked, the main evidence of associated SO weakness being the reversal of vertical diplopia noted on a careful cover-testing in far downgaze.

Type 3, Limitation Only of Depression-In-Adduction; "SO Underaction"

These 8 patients could easily have been mistaken for neurogenic unilateral SO palsies if it had not been for the absence of any significant head injury in all but one instance, and the universal presence either of lacerations in the trochlear region or soft tissue injuries of the orbit. Although there was no obvious clinical sign of mechanical restriction, another indication of a peripheral origin was the incomplete development of muscle sequelae: ipsilateral inferior oblique overaction was either absent or much less than expected, even when SO underaction had persisted for many months, and despite the lack of any mechanical limitation of elevation-in-adduction (Fig 2).

Surgery was required in only 7 of these 15 patients in order for them to recover a comfortable field of BSV during a mean followup period of 16.5 months, although none of the patients showed an absolutely full spontaneous recovery of ocular movements during that period. One Type 1 patient showed little or no recovery of elevation-in-adduction, with diplopia on more than 15o movement into that field of gaze. However, he was a tall man without muscle imbalance in any other direction of gaze, and was in practice symptom-free without having to adopt an abnormal head posture, and did not have surgery.

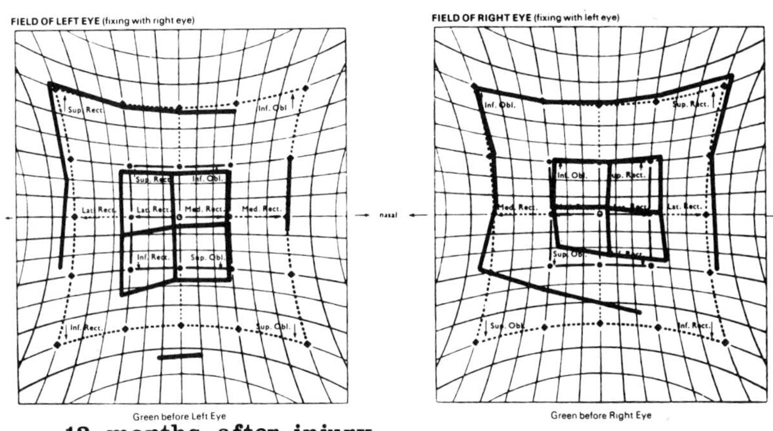

13 months after injury

Figure 2. Incomplete muscle sequelae in a patient with limited right depression in adduction (SO underaction) following orbital trauma. There is evidence of contralateral inferior rectus synergistic overaction, but none of ipsilateral antagonistic inferior oblique overaction.

One Type 2 patient has needed repeated surgery in order to expand his BSV field, and it is especially interesting that his pseudo-Brown's syndrome masked an overaction of the ipsilateral inferior oblique muscle, weakening of which led to marked improvement in his BSV field and compensatory head posture after 2 contralateral inferior rectus recessions had failed to sdo so. One other type 2 patient is now, more than 2 years after injury, exhibiting a late further decompensation with BSV field now restricted to only 10o of elevation and depression from the primary position, a further evidence of the mechanical, and potentially progressive nature of the defect (Fig 3). The patient has previously refused surgery, but contralateral superior and inferior rectus recessions on adjustable sutures have now been strongly advised. Five of the Type 3 patients required surgery, and only one muscle needed adjusting in each case; an inferior rectus recession in two instances, inferior oblique myectomy in two and superior oblique anterior and lateral advancement in one case.

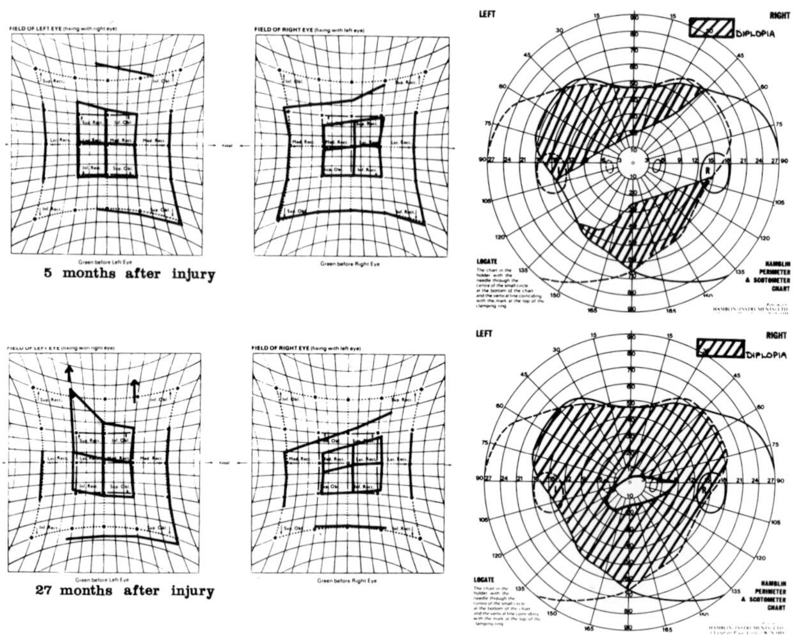

Figure 3. Increasing problems of diplopia in a patient who suffered deep lacerations in the upper inner angle of her right orbit. The field of binocular single vision has continued to shrink in the 2 years after injury due to reversing diplopia from a combination of pseudo-Brown's syndrome and superior oblique underaction of mechanical peripheral origin.

DISCUSSION AND CONCLUSIONS

Retrospective analysis of these cases with a long followup period reveals a number of features which are not entirely consistent with commonly held views. First, the incidence of bilateral SO palsies even after severe head injury was low. Second, despite the rare full recovery of ocular movements and normal muscle balance, less than half the patients required surgery in order to achieve sufficient permanent improvement to allow them comfortable single vision in all the circumstances of their normal life at work and at home. This inferred the absence of any uncomfortable or cosmetically obvious compensatory head posture, and of double vision within the confines of the normally used range of ocular movements. This common comfortable spontaneous recovery may be related to the high incidence of unilateral SO dysfunctions in this particular series. These have none of the problems of constantly reversing vertical and torsional diplopia in the opposite lateral depression positions which afflict those with bilateral palsies, and so may be that much easier for patients to compensate. Incidentally, the conventional 6 months delay for stabilization before surgery would not always have been appropriate in this series, as further spontaneous recovery, and also further deterioration after that period were both noted. Thirdly, many of the peripheral SO injuries were much more similar in pattern to trochlear nerve palsies than to Brown's syndrome, indicating how important it is to seek subtle indications of mechanical limitation of depression-in-adduction in such cases. This altogether varied pattern of post-traumatic SO dysfunction and the complex natural history during the recovery period exemplify the need to assess and treat each patient on individual criteria, and not according to any preconceived set of standard techniques.

COMPARED MEASUREMENT OF A AND V ANISOTROPIA AT THE PERIMETER AND IN FREE SPACE

H. C. de Almeida

ABSTRACT

The measurement of A and V anisotropia is of fundamental importance for the correct treatment of many cases of strabismus. We compared in 30 patients, the measurements of A and V anisotropia obtained by two different techniques: in a perimeter and in free space. The measurements were always made at the same angle of 40 degrees.

This paper allows us the following conclusions:

1-If there is a change of accommodation looking up and down, it should be small and unable to alter the value of A and V anisotropia.

2-The difference between the measurements of the anisotropia in the perimeter (33 cm) and in free space (1.25 m) was minimal and might be forgotten in everyday practice.

3-Therefore either one of the two techniques might be used routinely for the measurement of the A and V anisotropia.

INTRODUCTION

Duane(1), in 1897, described for the first time the variation of the horizontal deviation in the vertical meridian. However, the subject was entirely forgotten for many years, due mainly to Scobee's writings.(4) Friedenwald(2) suggested the term anisophoria to describe the variation of heterophoria in horizontal and vertical gaze when compared with the primary position. Magee(6) suggested the terms anisophoria and anisotropia of the vertical middle meridian to specifically describe the change of the horizontal deviation in looking up, ahead and down.

In 1946, Berke(3) stated that 50% of cases with overaction of the superior obliques showed increased exotropia or decreased esotropia looking down. The opposite

STRABISMUS II
ISBN 0-8089-1424-3

occured looking up. In cases with overaction of the inferior obliques the exotropia increased and the esotropia decreased looking up. The opposite occurred looking down.

Ripple(5) found that the amplitude of accommodation increased looking down and in and decreased looking up and out.

Almeida(7) used a perimeter for the measurement of the anisotropia at 40 degrees up and down. The main criticism to this technqiue is that the aniso-accommodation might interfere with the measurements.

MATERIAL AND METHODS

We compared, in 30 patients, the values of A and V anisotropia measured at 40 degrees, up and down, by 2 techniques: in a perimeter and in free space.

The perimeter used was described in a previous paper(7) and for the measurement in free space we had 3 spots on a wall, at 1.05 m intervals. At this site we placed figures of projected optotypes to control accommodation.

In Fig 1, we apply the following mathematical formula: TGA = a/x or 0.839 = 1/05/x or x = 1.05/0.839 = 1.25 m. In order to maintain the same angle of 40 degrees up and down, the measurements in space should be made at 1.25 m from the central spot. With both techniques a support for the chin and the forehead was used. Glasses were always used, when they decreased the deviation in the primary position. Thirty patients with normal morphoscopic vision OU were examined. Their age varied from 6 to 32 years, with an average of 14.5 years. There were 21 females and 9 males.

There were 15 cases of esotropia, being 6 of small angle, 7 of middle angle and 2 of large angle and 15 cases of exotropia, being 9 of small angle, 5 of middle angle and 1 of large angle. Nineteen patients had V- and 11 showed A-anisotropia.

RESULTS

The V anisotropia varied from 6.0 to 42.0 P.D. with an average of 20.5 P.D., when measured at the perimeter and from 4.0 to 49.0 P.D., average 22.0 P.D. in space. The A anisotropia varied from 8.0 to 32.0 P.D. with an average of 16.5 P.D. at the perimeter and from 6.0 to 36.0 P.D., average

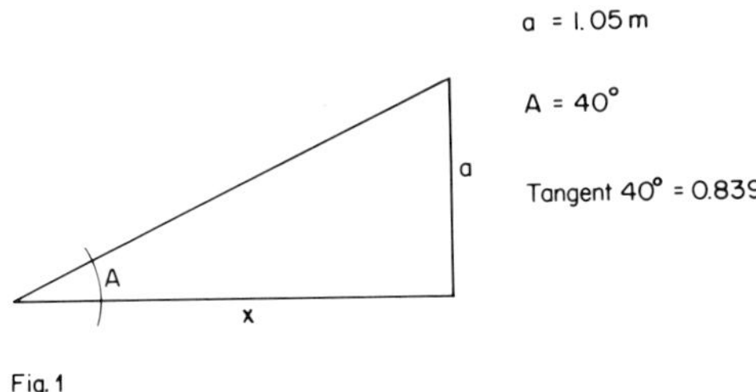

Fig. 1

17.5 P.D. in space. Of the 19 cases of V anisotropia the largest difference between the 2 techniques was 7.0 P.D. and in 3 patients the measurement was exactly the same. The average difference was 3.5 P.D. (Fig 2). Among the V anisotropias the value in space was larger 11 times, but in 5 cases it was smaller. Among the A anisotropias the value in space was larger 8 times, but in 2 cases it was smaller (Fig 3).

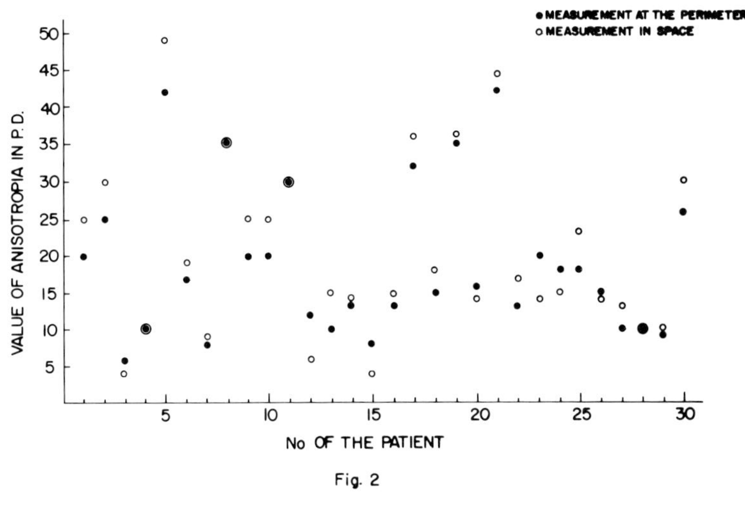

Fig. 2

COMMENTS

The correct measurement of A and V anisotropia is of fundamental importance for the exact treatment of many cases of strabismus. It is astonishing that at present many ophthalmologists still measure the A and V anisotropia by

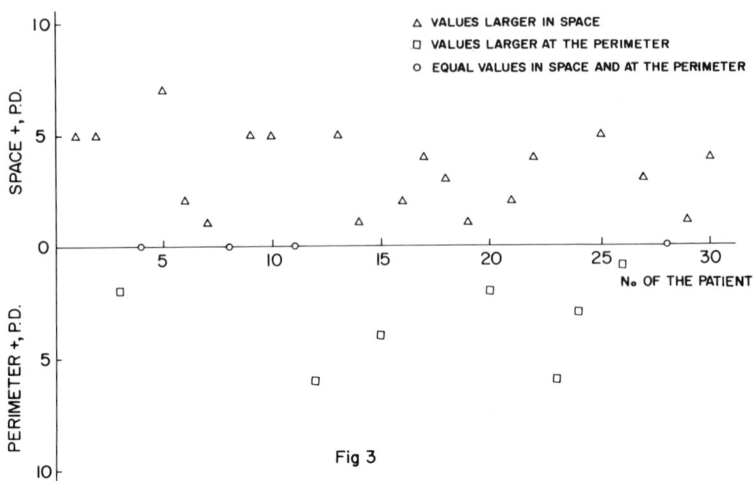

Fig 3

extending and flexing the patient's head, while looking straight ahead.

The incidence of A and V anisotropia found in this work may be considered in agreement with that in world literature.

SUMMARY

The author has examined 30 patients with the A or V anisotropia in a modified perimeter (33 cm) and in free space (1.25 m), keeping always the same angle of 40 degrees between gaze up or down with gaze straight ahead.

If there is a change of accommodation with the eyes looking up or down it should be very small and doesn't alter the value of the A or V anisotropia measured at the perimeter or in space, since the difference between those 2 measurements was minimal and might be discarded in everyday practice.

Therefore either one of the 2 techniques might be used routinely for the measurement of the A and V anisotropia.

REFERENCES

1. Duane A: Isolated paralyses of the ocular muscles. Arch Ophthalmol 26:317-334, 1897.

2. Friedenwald JS: Diagnosis and treatment of anisophoria. Arch Ophthalmol 15:283-307, 1936.

3. Berke RN: Tenotomy of the superior oblique for hypertropia. Trans Am Ophthalmol Soc 44:304-342, 1946.

4. Scobee RG: The Oculorotary Muscles. St. Louis, CV Mosby Co, 1947, p. 40.

5. Ripple PH: Variation of accommodation in vertical directions of gaze. Am J Ophthalmol 35:1630-1634, 1952.

6. Magee AJ: Minimal values for the A and V syndromes. Am J Ophthalmol 50:753-756, 1960.

7. Almeida HC: Correcao cirurgica das anisotropias em A e V pelos deslocamentos verticais monocular e binocular de retos horizontais. Thesis of "Livre Docencia" presented at the Department of Ophthalmol-Otorrinolaryngology of the Medical School of UFMG, Belo Horizonte, MG, Brazil, 1978, p 7-8.

A REMOTE COVER TEST USING CONCAVE MIRRORS

David L. Guyton

A large concave mirror, subtending 6 degrees, is positioned 3 m in front of the patient and forms an aerial image of the patient's eyes in the vicinity of the patient, but laterally displaced. A second concave mirror, located at the image of the patient's eyes, reflects light from a distance cartoon movies onto the first mirror so that the patient sees the image of the cartoon on the surface of the first mirror. Because the patient views the movie by way of the aerial images of his eyes, cover tests may be performed by occluding the aerial image of an eye rather than the eye itself. A small light on the occluder is imaged on the patient's forehead by the first mirror, thus indicating the position of the phantom occluder before the patient's eye. Patient movement is allowed anywhere within a 30 cm circular area, for the occluder is easily moved about to keep one eye covered.

The primary advantage of the remote cover test is the ability to perform a distraction-free cover test, under the conditions of natural seeing, while regarding both of the patient's eyes. Only central vision (6 degrees), however, is occluded by the phantom cover. Patients with strong fixation preference for one eye may not switch fixation to the nonpreferred eye until peripheral vision of the preferred eye is blocked as well. A conventional occluder may be used for this, directly over the patient's eye. Alternately, by decreasing the background illumination during performance of the remote cover test, a measure of the strength of fixation preference may be obtained.

INTRODUCTION

A new type of cover test is described for the detection of strabismus. The test is actually performed without an occluder of any kind in front of the patient's face; in fact, it is all done with mirrors.

Every strabismologist is familiar with the child who is distracted by the occluder during the cover test, and with

STRABISMUS II
ISBN 0-8089-1424-3

small children who are even threatened by the occluder. It would appear desirable, with such children, to be able to perform the cover test without the cover.

In early 1982, I designed and built a system for doing this, using two concave mirrors provided through the courtesy of Humphrey Instruments. Fig 1 shows an optical diagram of the mirror arrangement. The far wall is approximately 3 meters from the patient, and each mirror has a radius of curvature of 3 meters (focal length 1.5 meters). The concave mirror above the patient forms a real inverted image of the cartoon movie on the surface of the second mirror at the end of the room (Fig 2). Note that the movie itself has to be upside down to provide an upright image for the patient to see.

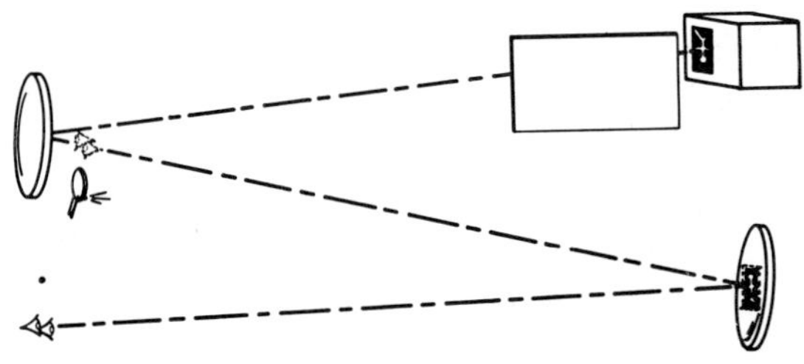

Figure 1. Optical diagram of the remote cover test. A cartoon movie box is mounted high on the far wall with a baffle to prevent the patient from viewing it directly. The patient views the movie via two mirrors, one mounted on the far wall below the movie box, and the other mounted on the refracting stand high over the patient's left shoulder.

The primary function of the concave mirror at the end of the room is to form an image of the patient's eyes back in the vicinity of the examiner (Fig 1), so that the examiner can occlude the image of one eye or the other, and thus block that eye from seeing the movie. All the rays of light that pass from the movie eventually into the patient's eye must pass through the image of the eye's pupil hanging up in space. Occluding the image of the pupil therefore blocks all the rays from the movie which would eventually enter the eye. If one stands up in front of the movie, and looks along the optical path, the view in Fig 3 is obtained. An inverted aerial image of the patient is seen. This is formed just anterior to, and reflected in, the mirror attached to the refracting stand.

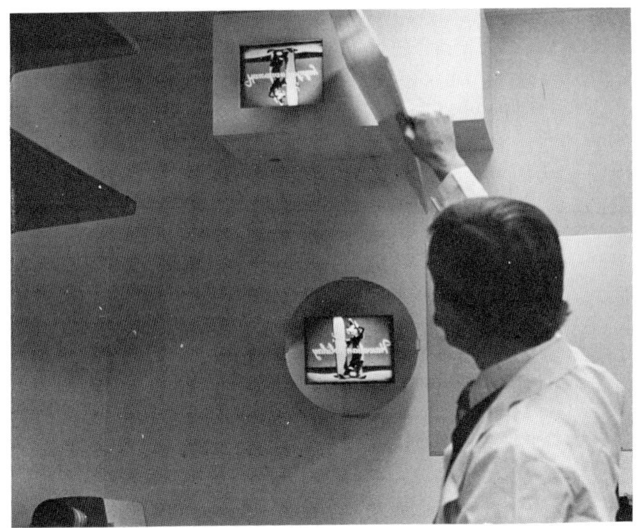

Figure 2. Patient's view of the cartoon movie box mounted high on the far wall with a real inverted image of the movie formed on the surface of the concave mirror below. The baffle is held aside for demonstration purposes. Ordinarily the patient can only see the image of the movie in the mirror below.

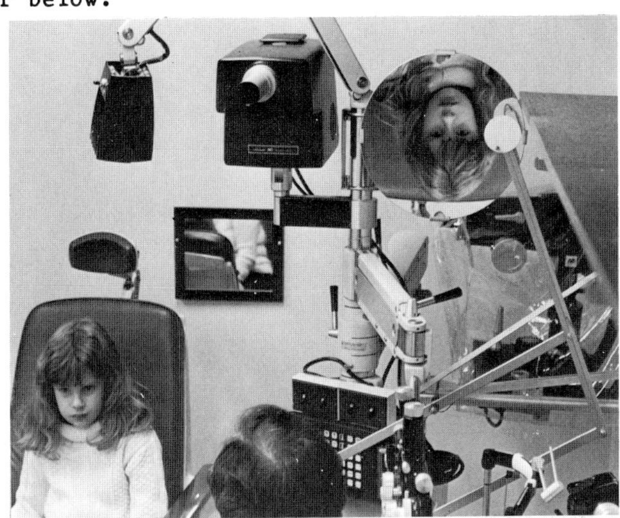

Figure 3. Looking backward along the optical path, with one's head directly in front of the cartoon movie. The inverted image of the patient is seen reflected in the concave mirror attached to the refracting stand.

The actual occluder is placed on the end of an arm reaching up to the image of the patient. Because the image of the patient is upside-down and reversed right-to-left, the occluder must move in the direction opposite to the direction in which the examiner intends to move it. This is accomplished by a pantograph arrangement bolted to the wall, out of the way of the other equipment (Figs 3 and 4). When the examiner's knob moves down, the occluder moves up, and when it moves to the right, the occluder moves to the left, and so forth. A leash is placed on the examiner's knob in such a way as to always keep the occluder within the confines of the mirror.

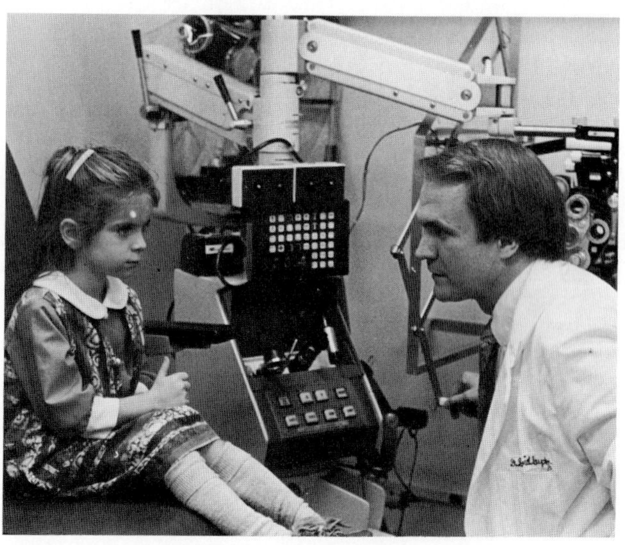

Figure 4. The ordinary testing situation. The patient looks with both eyes open at the image of the movie at the end of the room. The examiner places the spot of light over each eye in turn to perform the familiar cover test.

How does the examiner know the location of the occluder? A small light is mounted on the occluder and is activated when the examiner grasps the knob down below. An image of this light will be formed by the mirror at the end of the room, with the image falling on the patient's forehead, showing the examiner exactly where the phantom occluder is located.

The ordinary testing situation is illustrated in Fig 4, with the examiner watching both the patient's eyes while performing the remote cover test.

Figure 5 illustrates occlusion of the movie for one eye of the patient. Notice that only central vision is occluded by this technique. The mirror subtends an angle of 5.6 degrees, with the movie subtending 3.6 degrees horizontally and 2.7 degrees vertically. 3.6 degrees of horizontal subtends corresponds approximately 6 prism diopters.

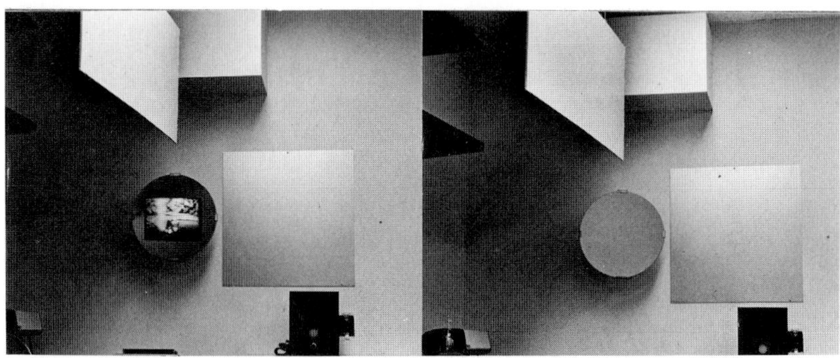

Figure 5. Left: An unoccluded eye's view of the cartoon movie. Right: An "occluded" eye's view of the movie. The occluded eye sees only the light which is diffusely reflected from the front of the occluder, giving the mirror a uniform gray, silver, or white appearance, depending on the reflectivity of the occluder.

Figure 6 illustrates an esotropic child being tested with the remote cover test. Patient movement is allowed anywhere within a 30 cm circular area, for the occluder is easily moved about to keep one eye covered. Because the occluder is constrained to stay within the confines of the upper mirror, placing the light over each eye in turn confirms that the patient is indeed within the 30 cm circular viewing area. Keeping the patient within this area has not presented any problems.

How is this remote cover test useful in the clinical situation? First, it is useful with children, for there is no occluder to distract the child. It should be pointed out, though, that children with strong fixation preference for one eye may not initially switch fixation when the central vision

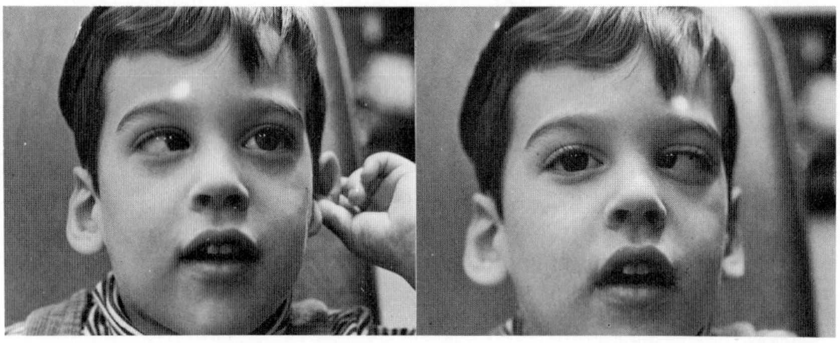

Figure 6. Esotropic child with the phantom occluder over the right eye. Left: Occluder switched to the left eye, causing the right eye to assume fixation.

of that eye is blocked. They may prefer to continue looking at the blank mirror. If they are encouraged, though, to "find the movie; did you see it jump?", they usually quickly learn to switch fixation. The remote cover test is therefore not as reliable as the conventional cover test in detecting the presence of strabismus in these individuals.

Secondly, the remote cover test is useful for demonstration purposes. The parents of the child being examined, or a whole group of medical students, can easily watch the movement of both eyes during performance of the cover test.

Finally, the test is useful whenever a central cover test in free space is desired, leaving peripheral vision intact, and leaving peripheral fusion, if present, intact. It is interesting that the fusion of most intermittent exotropes is not broken up by this test, for peripheral fusion in these patients appears strong enough to maintain alighment even though the central vision of one eye is blocked. If we slowly dim the room lights under these conditions, until fusion is broken, the strength of the peripheral fusion can readily be judged.

Patients with dissociated vertical deviation show an interesting response to the remote cover test. One might think that patients with DVD would use peripheral vision mechanisms to maintain their eyes relatively straight under binocular conditions. The remote cover test suggest otherwise, though, as if central vision is more important in holding the eyes straight. Occluding the central vision in the eye of a patient with dissociated vertical deviation will usually cause that eye to drift up. Occluding the peripheral vision as well, with an ordinary occluder, will sometimes increase the hyperdeviation obtained.

It is not simply the loss of light which causes the occluded eye to drift upward in patients with dissociated vertical deviations. We have experimentally corrected for this light loss to the occluded eye by illuminating the front surface of the occluder. Even with ten times more light to the occluded eye than to the fixing eye, the "occluded" eye still drifts up.

In conclusion, this new cover test not only provides an almost magic test for examination of children, but also promises to provide new information regarding some of the unexplained sensory phenomena in the field of strabismus.

EXPERIMENTAL OBSERVATIONS ABOUT EYE TORSION

C. Souza-Dias, J. C. Bottos and J. Filho

ABSTRACT

By means of an Asahi Pentax camera with a Macro lens and close up ring we took short distance photographs of both eyes of 16 volunteers in order to study eye torsion around the visual axis induced by head tilt. Seven photographs were taken of each eye with the head held vertical and inclined 10 degrees, 20 degrees and 30 degrees toward each shoulder. The inclination of the head was controlled by a device based on a spirit level adapted to the head. The eye torsion was measured by the changes of the angle that was formed by two straight lines. One of these lines was made from two marks made on the conjunctiva, near the limbus, with a hypodermical needle and methilene blue (or 2 natural marks, as blood vessels, when well visible). The other one from 2 marks made on the skin of the eye lids with a thin hydrographic pen (or natural marks). The volunteers were asked to look at the center of the camera lens, in order that the visual axis coincided with the optical center of the camera to avoid parallx. The photographs unequivocally showed that head tilt induced an eye torsion to the opposite side. The statistical study of the results showed the following: 1. intorsion - head tilt of 10 degrees, 20 degrees and 30 degrees induced an intorsion of the ipsilateral eye of 1.98 degrees ± 1.04 degrees, 3.43 degrees ± 1.25 degrees and 4.64 degrees ± 2.21 degrees respectively; 2. extorsion - head tilt of 10 degrees, 20 degrees and 30 degrees induced an extorsion of the contralateral eye of 2.30 degrees ± 1.44 degrees, 3.93 degrees ± 1.94 degrees and 5.19 degrees ± 2.0 degrees respectively. The differences between extorsion and intorsion were statistically insignificant (Student's test). The increase of the eye torsion induced by head tilt from 10 degrees up to 30 degrees was rectilineal.

INTRODUCTION

General agreement exists that the extraocular muscles, in some directions of gaze, have a torsional action upon the eye, when considered isolatedly in their function. However, controversy remains about the torsional movement of the eye in a normal person.

STRABISMUS II
ISBN 0-8089-1424-3

The first author to observe the existence of a torsional movement of the eyes induced by lateral head tilt was John Hunter(5), in the 18th century. Since then, many authors have agreed as to its existence while others have denied it. (8,9,10,11,12,13) Barany stated that for each 15 degrees of head tilt, there is an eye torsion around the sagital axis and in the inverse direction of 2 degrees. He added that the maximum reflex occurs when the head is inclined 60 degrees, when eye torsion varies from 4 degrees to 16 degrees, with a mean value of 8 degrees. Linwong and Herman (5) stated that for a head tilt of 30 degrees, there is a mean incycloduction of the eye in the side of the inclination of 5.13 degrees ± 2.18 degrees and a mean excyloduction of the other eye of 6.5 degrees ± 2.66 degrees. A. Scott (7) demonstrated that for a head tilt of 30 degrees, there is an eye torsion between 5 degrees and 6 degrees.

Hewitt (10), based on studies made with after images, denied the existence of such eye movement. Levine (13) came to the same conclusion, based on retinal photographs, questioning the value of the Bielschowsky's test for the diagnosis of the superior oblique palsy. Jampal, in recent papers (10,11,12), emphasized that the inclination of the head does not induce torsional movements of the eye. He categorically says that one of the functions of the vertical muscles of the eye is to keep the vertical meridian of the cornea parallel to the sagital plane of the skull when the head is inclined to the side. He also says that the mechanic and neurologic mechanism for wheel rotation of the eyes around the pupillary axis apparently do not exist, opposing himself to the conclusions of Woellner & Graibel (14) who affirm that those mechanisms are controlled by the otholith organs.

The impairment of the visual acuity of patients presenting high degrees of astigmatism, already corrected with cylindrical lenses, when their head is tilted to one side and its improvement when the lens is turned some degrees to the opposite side, as well as some thoughts derived from the Bielschowsky's phenomenon observed in patients with superior oblique palsy, strongly suggests the possibility of that movement does exist.

In order to obtain new data about cyclotorsion, we decided to study it with a new method.

MATERIAL AND METHODS

Two groups of volunteers, all ophthalmologists of the Ophthalmological Clinic of the "Faculdade de Ciencias Medicas da Santa Casa de Misericordia de Sao Paulo" and students of medicine from that school were studied. Each group was composed by 16 volunteers, none of whom showed any anomaly of the ocular motility or amblyopia of any nature. By means of an Asahi Pentax photo camera with a close-up device, we took short distance photographs of each one of the volunteers' eyes, with their head erect and inclined to one side and then to the other. They were asked to fixate the center of the camera lens with the eye to be photographed (Fig 1). The degrees of head tilt were different in the two groups. The volunteers of group I were photographed with their head inclined 10 degrees, 20 degrees, and 30 degrees to each side. The inclinations for group II were 30 degrees, 40 degrees, and 50 degrees. The inclinations were controlled by a device specially made for that purpose, based on a spirit level and a protractor (Fig 2).

In the members of the group I, we made two marks on the conjunctiva with methylene blue by means of a hypodermic needle, near the antipodes of the horizontal meridian of the cornea. In view of the resistance of the members of this group to this procedure, we used in the Group II, for the same purpose, the instillation of some drops of an anesthetic collyrium. In this way, a congestion of the conjunctival vessels was provoked allowing an easy visualization of their position. After developing the films, 9 x 12 cm prints were made. Two straight lines were drawn on the prints. One of them, which we call "movable line", passed through the conjunctival marks (those made with methylene blue in the group I and natural landmarks of the conjunctival vessels in the group II, near the limbus, where the conjunctiva is less movable upon the sclera). The other line, the "basic line", passed through two natural landmarks on the peri-ocular skin, near the medial and lateral canti (Fig 3).

The basic line represents the head position with regard to the horizon and the movable line represents the position of a corneal meridian with regard to the basic line. The angle formed by these two lines was called "angle a " and its variation indicates eye rotation around its visual axis. When the vertex of the angle was out of the photo, we used an artifice for its measurement: we traced a peripendicular line to the basic line and measured the angle that it formed with the movable line, which we we call " angle b " and that is the complement of angle a. (90 - b = a). (Fig 2).

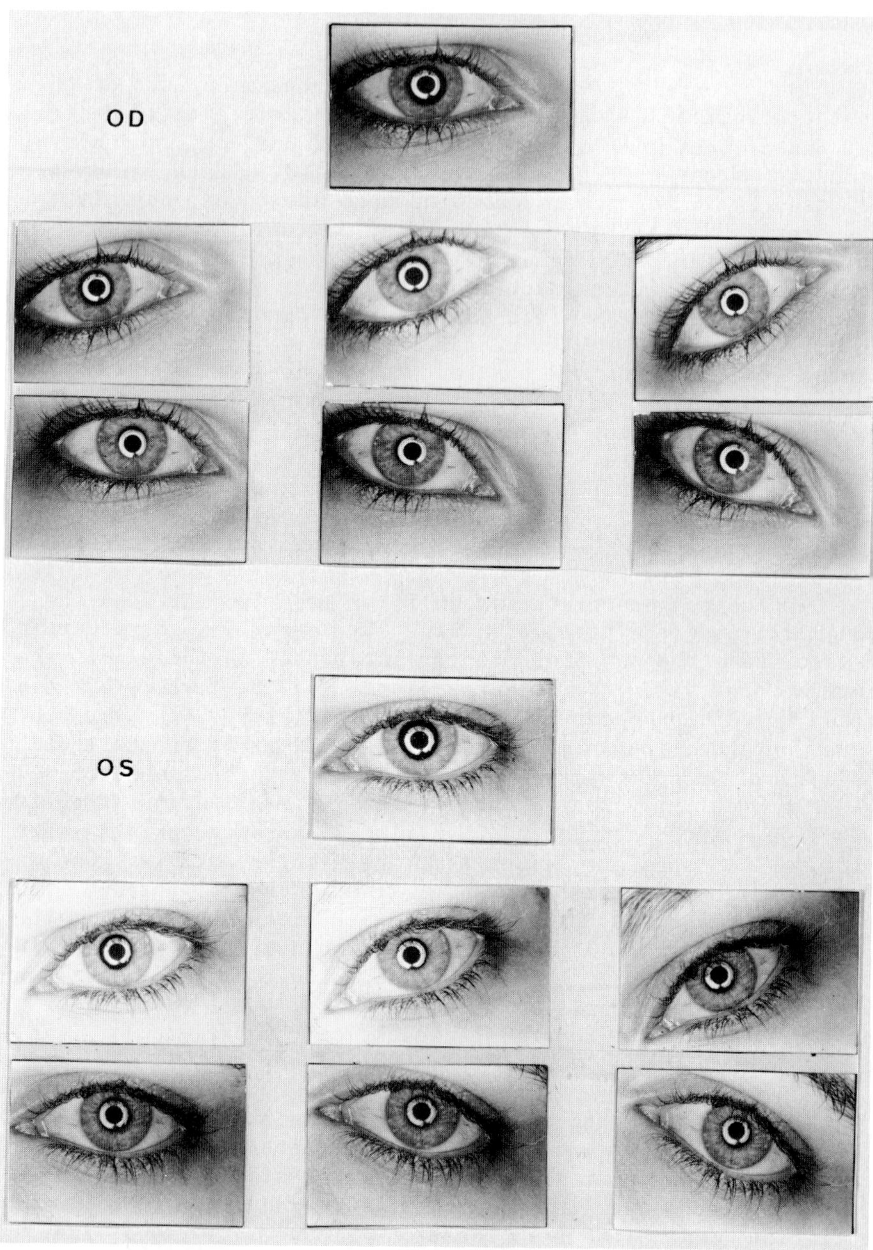

Fig. 1. Photographs of the right (OD) and the left (OS) eyes. At the center and above, the eye with the head erect; below, the eyes with the head inclined 10°, 20° and 30° to the right and to the left sides.

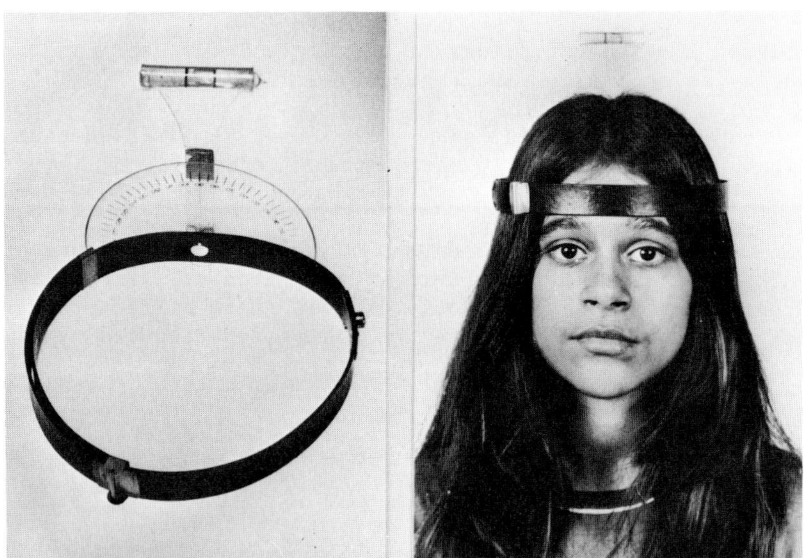

Fig. 2. Special device for controlling the inclination of the head, based on a spirit level and a protractor.

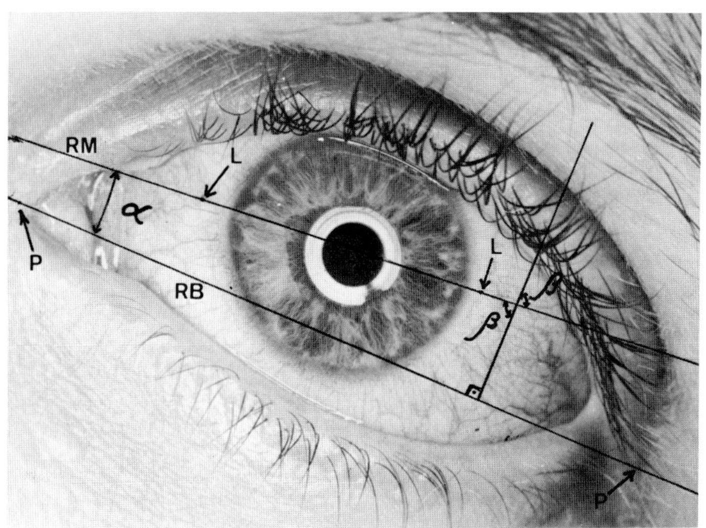

Fig. 3. Movable line (RM) and basic line (RB) for measuring the degree of eye torsion around the visual axis. A = angle made by the two lines; B = the complement of A; L = conjunctival marks near the limbus; P = natural marks on the skin.

RESULTS

Group I - The variations of the angle a for each case are shown in Tables 1 and 2 and Figures 4 and 5.

Group II - The variations of the angle a for each case are shown in Tables 3 and 4 and Figures 4 and 5.

Comparing the values of intorsion and extorsion of one eye with those of the other eye through the Student test (limit of confidence 95%), we can observe that their differences are not significant, except for the intorsion induced by 30 degrees of head tilt in the group I, which we can consider as an accident of the methodology.

Group I

Please see Tables 1 and 2.

Group II

Comparing the mean values of intorsion with those of extorsion through the Student's test (limit of confidence 95%), we can see that their differences are not significant.

1. Intorsion and extorsion of the right eye:

   Head tilt of 10 degrees: t = 0.99 (not significant)
   Head tilt of 20 degrees: t = 0.65 (not significant)
   Head tilt of 30 degrees: t = 0.18 (not significant)

2. Intorsion and extorsion of the left eye:

   Head tilt to 10 degrees: t = 0.48 (not significant)
   Head tilt of 20 degrees: t = 1.07 (not significant)
   Head tilt of 30 degrees: t = 1.42 (not significant)

COMMENTS

In order to investigate the existence and magnitude of the rotatory movements of the eye around the visual axis induced by the lateral inclination of the head, we chose the photographic method, which seemed to us sufficiently accurate. For drawing the movable line on the photos of the

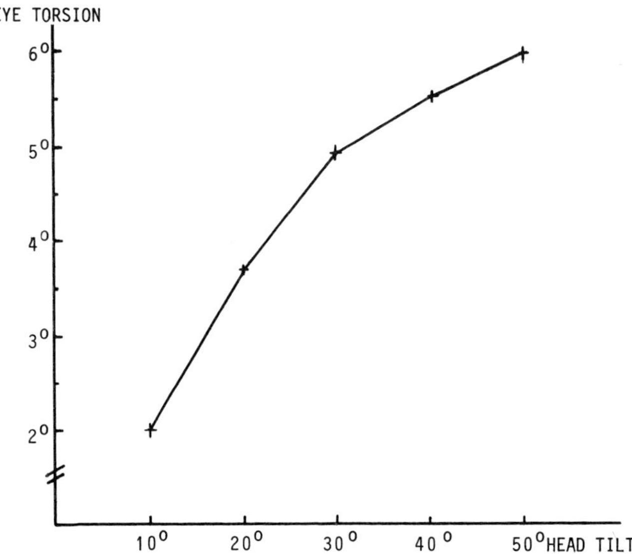

Fig. 4. Graphic representation of the amount of eye torsion (average of intorsion and extorsion of both eyes) with increasing degrees of head tilt. The value of the eye torsion with 30° of head tilt is the average of Groups I and II.

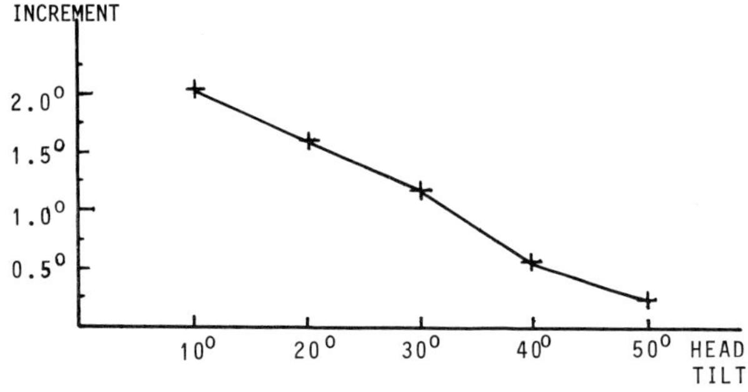

Fig. 5. Graphic representation of the increment of the eye torsion (average of intorsion and extorsion of both eyes) in the increasing steps of the head tilt. Note that the increment decreases from the zero-to-ten step of the head tilt to the forty-to-fifty step, in a linear way.

Table 1. Values of intorsion of the right (OD) and the left (OS) eyes of the 16 patients of the Group I. X = average; S = standard deviation; T = student´s test (limit of confident 95%); OU = both eyes.

Head tilt / Volunteer	10°		20°		30°	
	OD	OS	OD	OS	OD	OS
1	2.0	4.0	6.0	5.0	10.0	7.0
2	2.0	2.5	3.0	3.8	7.0	5.5
3	2.0	2,75	5.0	4.0	6.5	5.0
4	1.0	1.0	2.5	1.0	2.5	2.0
5	1.5	0,25	3.5	3.25	4.0	3.25
6	3.0	2.0	4.75	3.0	5.75	4.0
7	1.5	4.25	2.5	4.75	5.5	6.75
8	3.0	1.5	3.5	4.0	5.0	6.0
9	5.0	3.0	6.0	6.0	9.0	6.0
10	0.0	2.5	2.5	2.5	2.0	1.5
11	2.0	2.0	5.0	4.0	6.0	6.0
12	1.0	0.5	3.0	2.0	4.0	2.0
13	1.5	1.0	2.0	1.0	2.50	1.0
14	2.0	2.0	4.0	2.5	6.0	4.0
15	1.25	1.5	1.0	1.5	4.0	1.0
16	2.5	1.5	4.0	3.0	5.0	3.0
$\bar{X}$	1.95	2.02	3.67	3.20	5.29	4.00
S	1.11	1.13	1.37	1.43	2.21	2.09
t	6.96	7.21	10.79	9.14	9.62	7.69
	OU		OU		OU	
$\bar{X}$	1.98		3.44		4.65	
S	1.10		1.40		2.22	

Table 2. Values of extorsion of the right (OD) and the left (OS) eyes of the 16 patients of the Group I. X = average; S = standard deviation; T = student´s test (limit of confidence 95%); OU = both eyes.

Head tilt / Volunteer	10°		20°		30°	
	OD	OS	OD	OS	OD	OS
1	2.0	2.5	3.0	5.0	3.5	6.5
2	3.0	2.5	3.5	3.5	5.0	5.0
3	2.5	1.75	3.5	2.75	4.5	2.74
4	8.5	3.0	9.0	6.0	10.5	7.0
5	1.5	3.75	4.0	3.75	6.0	5.75
6	2.25	1.5	3.75	3.50	7.25	4.0
7	0.5	0.0	0.5	0.25	1.5	1.25
8	2.0	2.0	4.5	5.75	6.0	6.0
9	2.25	2.0	6.0	4.0	8.0	6.5
10	2.75	2.5	4.0	3.25	6.5	4.5
11	3.5	4.0	7.0	6.0	7.0	7.5
12	1.5	2.5	5.0	5.0	5.0	5.5
13	3.0	3.0	4.5	5.0	6.0	5.0
14	2.0	2.0	4.0	4.0	4.5	5.0
15	0.0	1.0	0.5	2.0	2.5	5.0
16	2.0	1.0	2.0	1.0	3.0	2.0
$\bar{X}$	2.45	2.16	4.05	3.82	5.42	4.96
S	1.84	1.02	2.15	1.84	2.25	1.75
t	5.33	8.47	7.53	8.30	9.64	11.34
	OU		OU		OU	
$\bar{X}$	2.30		3.96		5.19	
S	1.47		1.94		2.00	

Table 3. Values of intorsion of the right (OD) and the left (OS) eyes of the 16 patients of the Group II. X = average; S = standard deviation; T = student´s test (limit of confidence 95%); OU = both eyes.

Head tilt / Volunteer	30°		40°		50°	
	OD	OS	OD	OS	OD	OS
1	2.0	6.0	3.0	6.0	3.0	7.0
2	5.0	5.0	9.0	5.0	8.0	7.0
3	5.0	5.0	7.0	6.0	6.0	6.0
4	5.0	3.5	3.0	2.0	3.0	1.0
5	5.0	4.0	8.0	4.0	7.0	3.0
6	6.0	9.0	5.0	9.0	6.0	12.0
7	4.0	4.0.	2.0	5.0	2.0	5.0
8	3.0	5.0	3.0	9.0	3.0	10.0
9	5.0	6.0	8.0	10.0	9.0	8.0
10	4.0	7.0	4.0	7.0	6.0	4.0
11	4.0	5.0	5.0	6.0	6.0	7.0
12	5.0	6.0	4.0	7.0	5.0	8.0
13	6.0	9.0	7.0	8.0	9.0	13.0
14	5.0	1.0	3.0	1.0	6.0	2.0
15	5.0	6.0	5.0	4.0	5.0	4.0
16	4.0	7.0	5.0	8.0	7.0	9.0
$\overline{X}$	4.56	5.53	5.06	6.06	5.68	6.62
S	1.03	1.99	2.14	2.52	2.12	3.40
t	17.71	11.12	9.46	9.62	10.72	7.79
	OU		OU		OU	
$\overline{X}$	5.04		5.56		6.16	
S	1.64		2.35		2.83	

Table 4. Values of extorsion of the right (OD) and the left (OS) eyes of the 16 patients of the Group II. X = average; S = standard deviation; T = student´s test (limit of confidence 95%); OU = both eyes.

Head tilt / Volunteer	30°		40°		50°	
	OD	OS	OD	OS	OD	OS
1	5.0	5.0	5.0	5.0	7.0	6.0
2	5.0	7.0	7.0	8.0	2.0	5.0
3	3.0	2.0	4.0	3.0	5.0	5.0
4	7.0	6.0	9.0	5.5	9.0	7.5
5	5.0	8.0	6.5	8.0	5.0	9.0
6	6.0	6.0	5.0	7.0	5.0	8.0
7	5.0	3.0	5.0	1.0	5.0	1.0
8	6.0	3.0	3.0	5.0	4.0	5.0
9	7.0	4.0	7.0	6.0	10.0	5.0
10	5.0	7.0	5.0	9.0	9.0	11.0
11	4.0	4.0	5.0	4.0	7.0	5.0
12	5.0	1.0	3.0	4.0	3.0	5.0
13	6.0	5.0	11.0	6.0	6.0	5.0
14	5.0	11.0	4.0	5.0	5.0	7.0
15	6.0	6.0	2.0	1.0	1.0	2.0
16	4.0	7.0	7.0	8.0	8.0	9.0
$\overline{X}$	5.25	5.31	5.53	5.34	5.69	5.97
S	1.06	2.50	2.32	2.39	2.55	2.56
t	19.74	8.56	9.53	8.96	8.93	9.33
	OU		OU		OU	
$\overline{X}$	5.10		5.44		5.83	
S	2.10		2.32		2.52	

members of the group I, we made marks on the juxta limbal conjunctiva with methylene blue. When planning the photos of the group II, however, we saw tha the instillation of an irritant collyrium produces a congestion of the conjunctival vessels which supplied adequate landmarks.

In order to avoid paralactic errors, the volunteers were asked to look at the center of the camera lens with the eye to be photographed. This gave us the certitude that the visual axis was always parallel to the optic axis of the camera and thus the equatorial plane of the eye was kept in a constant angle with regard to it.

When inclining the head to one side, care was taken not to bend it forward or backward, in order to keep the eyes in the primary position.

The data obtained in group I are consistent with the existence of a torsional movement of the eye around the visual axis, in the inverse direction, when the head is inclined to one side. The statistical analysis of the results showed that the mean values that were obtained for intorsion and extorsion were highly significant, as we can see by the Student's Test. The difference between the values of the right and left eye are statistically insignificant, as well as the difference between the values of intorsion and extorsion of the same eye. These findings agree with Linwong & Herman's (5).

A second group was then submitted to the same measurements but with tilting of the head of 30 degrees, 40 degrees and 50 degrees. The aim of the inclusion of this group was to determine the increase of the eye torsion with augmenting degrees of head tilt beyond 30 degrees. An inclination of more than 50 degrees was not included because, in some people, it induces bending of the thoracic spinal column besides the bending of the cervical column, which could eventually introduce an error in the results. The results obtained with group II were the following:

Analyzing the data from groups I and II, we can see that the increment of the eye torsion from 10 degrees to 50 degrees of head tilt decreased in the linear way. (Fig 5).

The values of eye torsion that we obtained for a head tilt of 30 degrees coincide roughly with the values of Linwong &

Herman (5) and A. Scott (7).

The maximum amount of eye torsion was 13 degrees, which occurred in only one instance. There was 12 degrees of torsion in one instance, 11 degrees in 3 instances and 10 degrees in 4 instances. In all other instances, the eye torsion was smaller than 10 degrees. (Total number of instances = 448)

CONCLUSIONS

In conclusion, we can say that this study has demonstrated in a statistically significant way, that the eyes make a torsional movement around the visual axis in the inverse direction when the head is tilted to the side, probably in an attempt to keeping the vertical meridian of the retina in a vertical position. It has also demonstrated that the amplitude of this movement is widely variable among the individuals and that its increment decreases in a linear way with the increase of the head inclination, up to an inclination of 50 degrees. Furthermore, it has demonstrated that there is no difference between the values of intorsion and extorsion, or between those values for both eyes.

REFERENCES

1. Howard IP, Templeton WB: Human spatial orientation, London, John Wiley & Sons, Inc., 1966, p. 50.

2. Barany R: In: Duke-Elder WS: Textbook of Ophthalmology, Vol I, St. Louis, The C. V. Mosby Co., 1939, p. 628.

3. Cogan DG: Neurology of the ocular muscles, 2nd Ed., Springfield, Charles C. Thomas, 1956, p. 127.

4. Javal E: In Wecker L (Ed): Traite des maladies des yeux, Vol 2, Paris, Delahaye, 1866, p. 815.

5. Linwong M, Herman SJ: Cycloduction of the eyes with head tilt. Arch Ophthalmol 85:570-573, 1971.

6. Scott AB: Extraocular muscles and head tilting. Arch Ophthalmol 78:397-399, 1967.

7. Scott AB: Ocular motility, in Records ER (ed): Physiology of the Human Eye and Visual System. Hagerstown, Harper & Row, 1979, p. 610.

8. Helmholtz H von: In: Duke-Elder WS: Textbook of Ophthalmology, Vol 1, St. Louis, The C.V. Mosby Co., 1938, p. 624.

9. Hewitt RS: Torsional eye movements. Am J Ophthalmol 34:253-260, 1951.

10. Jampel RS: The action of the superior oblique muscle: an experimental study in monkey. Arch Ophthalmol 75:535-544, 1966.

11. Jampel RS: Ocular torsion and the function of the vertical extraocular muscles. Am J Ophthalmol 79:292-304, 1975.

12. Jampel RS: Ocular torsion and the law of the primary retinal meridians. In Neuro-Ophthalmology, Vol 10, Glaser JS (Ed) Symposium of the University of Miami and the Bascom Palmer Institute, 1980, p. 201-216.

13. Levine MH: Evaluation of the Bielschowsky head-tilt test. Arch Ophthalmol 82:433-439, 1969.

14. Woellner RC, Graybel A: Counter-rolling of the eye and its dependence on the magnitude of gravitational or inertial force acting laterally on the body. J Appl Physiol 14:632-634, 1959.

CONGENITAL MONOCULAR LIMITATION OF ELEVATION BY INFERIOR RECTUS ABNORMALITIES

N. Kubota and T. Maruo

ABSTRACT

We have reported ten cases caused by the abnormalities of the inferior rectus muscle, which show congenital monocular limitation of elevation, hypotropia, and a significant restriction with sursumduction. Although these cases tend to be included in double elevator palsy, we have proposed to think they are one clinical entity.

INTRODUCTION

The diseases with monocular limitation of elevation include double elevator palsy, oculomotor palsy, dysthyroid ocular myopathy, blowout fracture, and others. The causes of this condition are not only the abnormalities of the elevator muscles but also the abnormalities of the depressor muscles. The latter include dysthyroid myopathies, blowout fractures, aberrant regeneration of oculomotor nerves, and Brown's syndromes. Several cases have been reported of congenital monocular elevation palsy due to inferior rectus abnormalities. Most of these cases are thought to be included in double elevator palsy. However, we consider them one clinical entity. We observed ten cases of this abnormality and performed electromyographic studies in two cases and surgical correction of all. Electromyographic studies have shown the paradoxical innervation of the inferior rectus muscle, and histological studies have not shown any fibrosis of the inferior rectus muscle. We report the above clinical findings, differential diagnosis, and treatment of monocular elevation palsies.

CASES

We present a case example of a 17-year old girl. This patient had been aware of a congenital left hypotropia. Vision was 30/20 in the right eye with +0.5D, and 2/20 in the left eye with best correction. A left 25 degree hypotropia and 10 degree esotropia was present in the primary position. It was impossible for the left eye to elevate higher than the horizontal in attempted upgaze (Fig 1). The left lid showed pseudo-ptosis. By forced duction test, the left eye had a significant mechanical restriction toward upgaze.

STRABISMUS II
ISBN 0-8089-1424-3

Electromyographical examination revealed the superior rectus muscle and the inferior oblique muscle had a normal pattern. The peak of innervation of the inferior rectus muscle occured in attempted sursumduction. The volume of the discharge became minimal in infraduction (Fig 2). It was thought that this increase of the discharge might be caused by misinserting the electrode into the inferior oblique muscle or by a stretch reflex. We removed the inferior rectus muscle and inserted the electrode directly into the inferior rectus at the time of surgery. The result was that the same findings were obtained.

The surgery was an 8 mm recession of the left inferior rectus. The inferior rectus was fibrotic, taut, and firmly attached to the sclera. As soon as the inferior rectus was cut, the restriction to sursumduction disappeared.

After the surgery, the left hypotropia and limitation of elevation was slight, but this seemed unsatisfactory, therefore, we performed a resection of the left superior rectus. Subsequently, orthophoria in the primary position was obtained, and the limitation of elevation disappeared. The result was satisfactory (Fig 3).

Ten cases of monocular limitation of elevation by inferior rectus abnormalities are illustrated in Table 1. Electromyographic examination was also performed in case 4, and the paradoxical innervation of the inferior rectus similar to the case example was observed. Histological examination of the inferior rectus was made in case 4 and case 6, and the muscle fibers were comparatively normal.

DISCUSSION

The diseases with monocular limitation of elevation are double elevator palsy, oculomotor palsy, aberrant regeneration of oculomotor nerve, dysthyroid ocular myopathy, Brown's syndrome, inferior rectus fibrosis, aplasia of the superior rectus and inferior oblique, blowout fracture, and others. In the above diseases, such diseases as the causes of limitation of elevation are not exclusively the abnormalities of elevator but include the abnormalities of depressor, and include the following: dysthyroid ocular myopathy, blowout fracture, aberrant regeneration, Brown's syndrome, and inferior rectus fibrosis.

Now a few cases of limitation of elevation by the abnormalities of the inferior rectus are treated as a type of double elevator palsy. It is reasonable to consider that

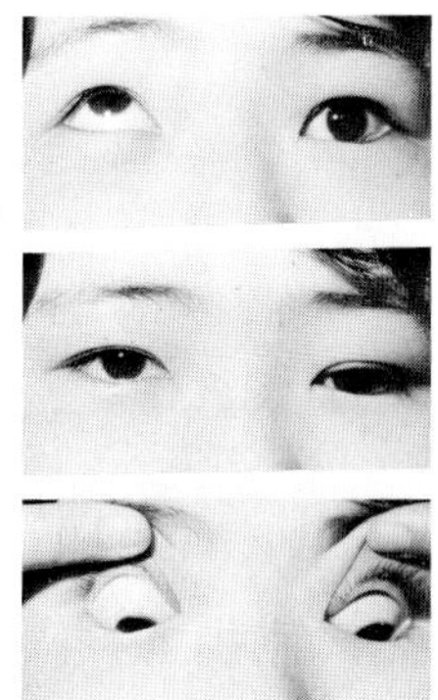

Figure 1. Case III : Preoperative findings.
Inability of voluntary elevation of the left eye.

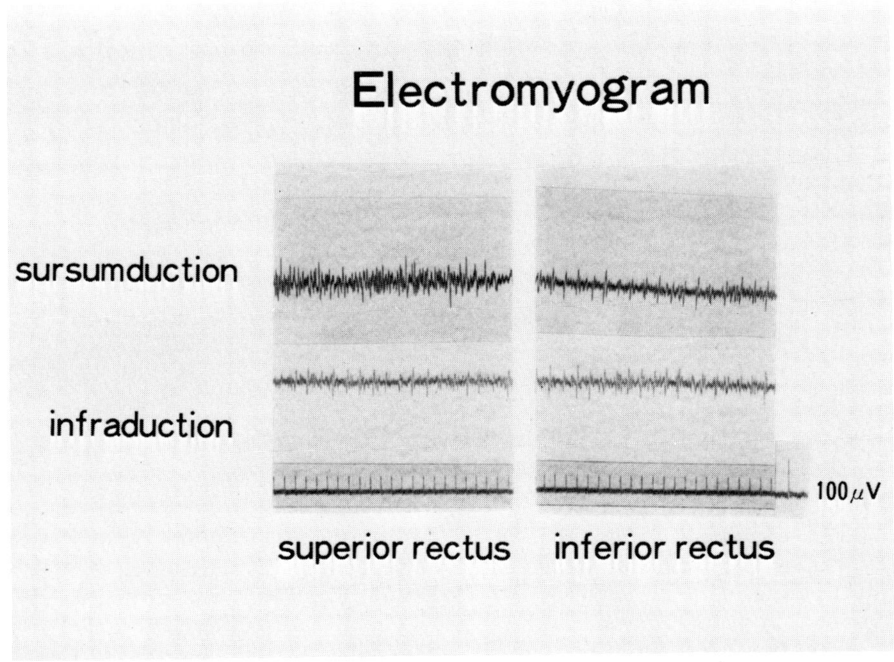

Figure 2. Electromyogram (Case VI) shows paradoxical discharge pattern in the inferior rectus muscle.

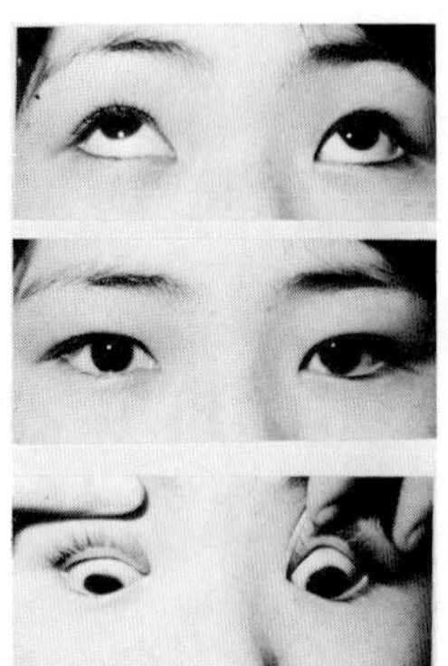

Figure 3. Case Ⅲ : Postoperative findings.
Upward gaze, though still insufficient, was attained by resection-recession of superior and inferior rectus muscles.

No.	Age	Sex	Side	Primary position		Limitation of ocular movement		Forced duction test	Vision		findings of inferior rectus		Surgery
				hypotropia	horizontal deviation	elevation	others		R	L	fibrotic change	abnormality of insertion	
1	7	F	R	+	XT	+	−	+	0.02	1.4	+	−	recession of IR
2	1	F	R	+	ET	+	−	+	abnormal fixation	normal fixation	+	−	recession of IR
3	17	F	L	+	ET	+	−	+	1.5	0.1	+	−	1)recession of IR 2)resection of SR
4	14	F	R	+	−	+	−	+	0.01	1.2	+	−	1)recession of IR 2)resection of SR
5	5	F	L	+	ET	+	−	+	1.2	0.05	+	+	recession of IR recession of MR
6	5	F	R	+	XT (previous surgery)	+	(adduction previous surgery)	+	0.5 ((latent nystagmus)	1.2	+	−	recession of IR
7	4	M	R	+	ET	+	−	+	0.5 (ametropic	0.6 smblyopia)	+	+	recession of IR resection of SR recession of MR
8	5	M	R	+	ET	+	abduction	+	0.05	1.2	+	+	recession of IR recession of MR
9	3	F	L	+	−	+	−	+	1.0	1.0	+	−	recession of IR resection of SR
10	3	M	L	+	ET	+	−	+	0.6	0.01	+	−	recession of IR resection of SR recession of MR

Table 1. Clinical findings in 10 Cases

double elevator palsy should be defined to the cases acquired by brain stem lesion because no resistance is shown in forced duction test, though doubld elevator palsy is monocular limitation of elevation. We would consider monocular limitation of elevation due to inferior rectus abnormalities, as reported at this time, to be one clinical entity.

The summary of the findings in our ten cases is as follows:

1. Eye position: The eye position in the primary position is a marked hypotropia. Many cases have more than 20 degrees hypotropia. In the horizontal eye position six cases showed hypotropia, but two cases were orthophoria and two cases were exotropia.

2. Ocular movement: Aside from the limitation of elevation, there is no trouble with ocular movements.

3. Forced duction test: There is a significant restriction with sursumduction. When the inferior rectus is cut from its insertion, the restriction is removed.

4. Pseudo-ptosis: Some cases show secondary pseudo-ptosis with the hypotropia.

5. Vision: Amblyopia is often associated.

6. Findings of the inferior rectus: The inferior rectus is taut and attached firmly to the sclear. There are findings similar to contracture or fibrosis. There are some cases associated with anomalies of insertion of the inferior rectus muscle.

7. Electromyographical findings: The superior rectus muscle and the inferior oblique muscle have a normal pattern. The following paradoxical innervation is demonstrated: the volume of the discharge of the inferior rectus muscle increases with supraduction.

8. Histological findings: The inferior rectus muscle has normal muscle fibers.

9. Treatment: The first choice is a recession of the inferior rectus muscle. According to the postoperative course, a resection of the superior rectus muscle may be added. Surgery for horizontal strabismus should be performed after that done for the vertical strabismus.

The diseases which require differential diagnosis are given in Table 2. As a history, the onset is congenital, and without the signs of oculomotor palsy, mydriasis, anomalous reflex of the pupil, ptosis, and other oculomotor disturbances. This serves as a good reference. The most important thing in diagnosis is that a significant restriction with supraduction is observed in forced duction test.

Cause	Onset	Ocular anomalies	Forced duction test	EMG findings of superior rectus
Double elevator palsy	acquired	Bell's phenomenon is often present	—	neuropathy
Superior rectus palsy (Oculomotor palsy)	congenital acquired	abnormal pupils and other third nerve involvement	—	neuropathy
Aberrant regeneration of oculomotor nerve	congenital acquired	other misdirection syndrome	+	misdirection
Dysthyroid ocular myopathy	acquired	exophthalmos	+	myopathy
Aplasia of superior rectus and inferior oblique	congenital		—	norecord
Blowout fracture	acquired	history of trauma enophthalmos	+	normal
Brown's syndrome	congenital	sign of inferior oblique muscle palsy	+	normal
Inferior rectus abnormalities	congenital		+	normal

Table 2. Differential diagnosis of monocular limitation of elevation

REFERENCES

1. Paolillo RD, Burch PG: Infantile contracture of inferior rectus muscle with resultant mechanical hypotropia. Am J Ophthalmol 68:1057-1059, 1972.

2. Rosner RS: Double elevator paralysis. Am J Ophthalmol 55:87-93, 1963.

3. McNeer KW and Jamplolsky A: Double elevator palsy caused by anomalous insertion of the inferior rectus. Am J Ophthalmol 59:317-319, 1965.

4. Scott WE, Jakson OB: Double elevator palsy: the significance of inferior rectus restriction. Am Orthopt J 27:5-10, 1977.

5. Metz HS: Double elevator palsy. Arch Ophthalmol 97:901-903, 1979.

6. Metz HS: Double elevator palsy. J Ped Ophthalmol Strabismus, 18:31-35, 1981.

7. Maruo T, Kubota N and Arimoto H: Congenital monocular elevation palsy by inferior rectus abnormality. Jpn J Clin Ophthalmol 32:581-588, 1978.

8. Jampel RS and Fells P: Monocular elevation paresis caused by a central nervous system lesion. Arch Ophthalmol 40:45-47, 1968.

9. Knapp P: The surgical treatment of double elevator paralysis. Trans Am Ophthal Soc 67:304-323, 1969.

10. Stanworth A: Unusual results of vertical muscle surgery. Br Orthop J 28:23-31, 1971.

11. Stegall FW: Differential diagnosis in ocular motility problems. Am Orthop J 19:125-135, 1969.

RESULTS OF KNAPP AND CALLAHAN PROCEDURES IN HYPOTROPIA AND PSEUDOPTOSIS

J. P. Lee, J. R. O. Collin and C. Timms

ABSTRACT

Hypotropia and ptosis, with or without pseudoptosis, has been treated surgically in 10 patients, 9 with knapp procedures, one with a Callahan procedure. Improvement obtained varied from 7 to 26 prism diopters. No overcorrections were encountered. It is concluded that these are safe and effective procedures in this situation and should be utilized prior to considering direct surgical intervention for the ptosis.

INTRODUCTION

The combination of blepharoptosis with hypotropia of the ispilateral globe is familiar to most ophthalmologists. Many authorities have emphasised the importance of first fully correcting the ocular position before embarking upon any direct attempt to relieve the ptosis. In some cases, no further surgery may be necessary, and in all cases a more accurate and cosmetically satisfactory result may be anticipated from subsequent ptosis surgery. This study chiefly concerns itself with the results of the ocular muscle surgery. It is hoped to discuss the results of the later ptosis surgery in a subsequent communication.

SUBJECTS

Ten cases are presented, these being consecutive cases treated between October 1979 and December 1981. The majority of the patients were referred to one of us (J.R.O.C) for consideration of ptosis surgery. The ages at the time of surgery ranged from five to twenty years, with a mean of 11.7 years. There were six females and four males. There were various etiologies.

Five patients had congenital ptosis of the dystrophic type with coincident hypotropia of the affected eye. Two cases had neurofibromatosis with buphthalmos and an enlarged orbit on the affected side. Two cases had third cranial nerve palsy with misdirection-regeneration: one was congenital, the other traumatic, following a motor cycle accident. One case had Marcus-Gunn jaw winking syndrome. She had undergone

STRABISMUS II
ISBN 0-8089-1424-3

CASE	INITIALS	AGE & SEX	CORRECTED V.A. O.D.	O.S.	AETIOLOGY	PREVIOUS STRABISMUS SURGERY	PREVIOUS PTOSIS SURGERY	PRE-OP ORTHOPTIC STATUS	PSEUDOPTOSIS
1	J.R.	10 F	6/9	6/9	Congenital ptosis and hypotropia	R S.R. +	Yes - ? nature	R Hypo 11° R Eso 3° Fusion on down-gaze	Yes
2	S.M.	13 F	6/9	6/9	Neuro-fibromatosis	No	No	L Hypo 60° L Eso 20°	No
3	L.H.	12 F	6/6	6/6	Congenital ptosis and hypotropia	L I.R. - 1976 L S.R. + 1979	L levator resection 1979	L Hypo 25° L Eso 2° Stereopsis on downgaze	Yes
4	F.S.	13 F	6/36	6/9	Congenital ptosis and hypotropia	No	R levator resection 1972 R Frontalis sling 1975	R Hypo 29° R Eso 5° R suppression	Yes
5	B.B.	9 M	6/24	6/5	Congenital ptosis and hypotropia	R I.R. - R S.R. + 1979	R levator resection 1979	R Hypo 9° R Eso 8° R suppression	Yes
6	M.C.	20 M	6/60	6/5	Traumatic R III palsy with misdirection. R optic nerve chiasmal damage	No	No	R Hypo 11° R Exo 25° misdirection	No
7	P.R.	11 F	P.L.	6/5	Neuro-fibromatosis	No	No	Gross R Hypo Mod R Eso	Minimal
8	J.R.	7 M	6/9	6/6	Congenital R III palsy with misdirection	1975-R LR- L MR+ 1977-R MR+ R IR- 1979-L MR+ L LR-	No	R Hypo 11° R Exo 20° R suppression	Yes
9	S.M.	14 M	6/5	6/18	Congenital ptosis and hypotropia L myopia	No	1968-L ptosis surgery 1979-L levator resection	L Hypo 30° L Exo 3° "variable L suppression"	Yes
10	J.S.	15 F	C.F.	6/5	Marcus-Gunn syndrome R myopia	No	1971-R levator resection 1979-R Frontalis sling	R Hypo 20° R Exo 18° R suppression	No

Table 1. Pre-Operative Data

previous unsuccessful ptosis surgery.

Details of pre-operative examination are presented in Table 1. Seven patients had deficient visual acuity in the affected eye. Four were amblyopic, with acuities from 6/18 to 1/36. In two cases, high myopia was an additional factor. The two cases of buphthalmos had acuities of 6/60 and light perception in the affected eyes. The case of traumatic third nerve palsy also had optic nerve and chiasmal injuries with extensive field loss in the affected eye.

Pre-operative examination showed hypotropia with various

horizontal deviations. Elevation of the affected eye was invariably poor. Six cases showed marked pseudoptosis, with elevation of the affected lid to near-normal height when the hypotropic eye fixated. One case showed minimal elevation. Four cases showed signs of binocular vision, with stereopsis in the lower field of vision and suppression on upgaze.

PREVIOUS SURGERY

Four cases (Nos. 1, 3, 5 & 8) had undergone previous extraocular muscle surgery. Three cases had undergone superior rectus resections with inferior rectus recession in two cases. Case 8, with congenital third nerve palsy, had a history of three previous procedures on the horizontal recti of both eyes.

Six cases (Nos. 1, 3, 4, 5, 9 & 10) had undergone previous ptosis surgery, usually a levator resection. Two cases also had brow suspension procedures. In three cases the amount of resection performed was known, the figures being 10, 12 and 13 mm.

SURGERY

In eight of the cases, the surgery was performed by one of us (J.P.L). Nine cases were treated by the procedure described by Knapp(1), with the horizontal recti being transplanted to the level of the superior rectus insertion. One case underwent the procedure described by Callahan(2), where the horizontal recti and superior rectus are split without being disinserted and are joined in a similar fashion to the Jensen(3) procedure for lateral rectus palsy. In five cases, a significant horizontal deviation was present. Four cases had modification of a knapp procedure with appropriate amounts of horizontal rectus recession and resection. Where a muscle was recessed the points of reattachment were measured from the superior rectus insertion.

Nine cases had pre-operative forced duction testing of the affected eye under general anesthesia prior to beginning the surgery. In six cases, this was judged to show resistance to passive elevation of the globe. Five cases were treated with inferior rectus recession (in one case at a subsequent date). The sixth case had the area of the inferior rectus explored. The muscle was found to be surrounded by a condensation of fibrous tissue. When the muscle had been dissected free, the traction test improved markedly and the muscle was therefore not recessed.

RESULTS AND COMPLICATIONS

In every case, the hypotropia was reduced as a result of surgery. The data are given in Table 2. The reduction in vertical deviation ranged from 26 to 7 prism diopters, with a mean of 15 prism diopters where additional recession-resection had been added to the basic knapp procedure, the horizontal deviation was reduced. Interestingly, the group which received additional inferior rectus recession had, on average, rather small improvement in vertical deviation, which was on average 10 prism diopters. In general, the improvement was seen in the reduction of the vertical deviation in the primary position. In all cases, elevation remained poor and the deviation increased on upgaze. In all cases, the patient or

CASE	PRE-OP STATUS	SURGERY PERFORMED	TRACTION TEST	POST-OP STATUS	CORRECTION ACHIEVED	COMPLICATION
(1) J.R.	R Hypo 11△ R Eso 3°	R Knapp 24.10.79	Not done	R Exo 8° No vertical deviation	11△	R lower lid retraction
(2) S.M.	L Hypo 60△ L Eso 20°	L Knapp. 29.11.79 LR + 6 mm MR - 5.5 mm IR - 5 mm	+	Improved		No
(3) L.H.	L Hypo 25△ L Eso 2°	L Knapp 10.3.80	-	R Eso 1°	25△	No
(4) P.S.	R Hypo 29△ R Eso 8°	R Knapp + IR Freeing 12.5.80	+	R Hypo 3△ R Eso 3°	26 △	No
(5) B.B.	R Hypo 9△ R Eso 8°	R Knapp 14.7.80	-	R Hypo 2△	7△	No
(6) M.C.	R Hypo 11△ R Exo 25°	R Knapp. 12.2.81 LR - 10 mm MR + 7 mm R I.R. - 4 mm 2.4.81	+	No deviation in Primary position	11△ Hypo 25° Exo	No
(7) P.R.	Gross R Hypo Mod R Eso	R Callahan + I.R. - 4 mm 2.4.81.	+	Less R Hypo More R Eso		No
(8) J.R.	R Hypo 11△ R Exo 20°	R Knapp IR - 3 mm LR - 4 mm MR + 5 mm	+	R Exo 10° No vertical	11△ Hypo 10° Exo	Mild peri-orbital cellulitis
(9) S.M	L Hypo 30△ L Exo 3°	L Knapp 17.9.81	-	L Hypo 4△ with vertical A.R.C. L Hypophoria 22-26△	26△	No
(10) J.S.	R Hypo 20△ R Exo 18°	R Knapp 17.12.81 LR - 3 mm MR + 3 mm IR - 3 mm	+	R Hypo Exo - ?	8△ Hypo	No

Table 2. Results

parents felt that there had been a cosmetic improvement. Later orthoptic assessment suggests that the improvement is a lasting one.

Three of the four cases in whom some fusion and binocular vision was demonstrable on downgaze had an extension of their binocular area upwards towards the primary position, while still suppression on upgaze. One patient (case 9) was found post-operatively to have vertical anomalous retinal correspondence. Pre-operative examination only suggested left suppression. This case is discussed further below.

Complications were minor. Case 1 developed lower lid retraction later treated with a scleral graft to the lower tarsus. Case 8 developed mild periorbital cellulitis which swiftly resolved on oral antibiotic therapy. No cases of post-operative uveitis or other signs of anterior segment ischaemia were encountered.

DISCUSSION

Knapp(1), in 1969, described a surgical procedure for double-elevator palsy in which the horizontal rectus muscles were detached and reattached on either side of the insertion of the superior rectus muscle of the affected eye. He reported fifteen patients in whom the correction obtained ranged from 21 to 55 prism diopters of vertical deviation. In two cases, an inferior rectus recession was also performed. He noted relatively little effect on horizontal rotations, but noted that elevation was usually limited, even where a good result was obtained in the primary position. Many surgeons with an interest in strabismus have performed the procedure, and it is highly regarded as safe and effective.

Callahan(2), in 1981, reported three cases of failed ptosis surgery in the presence of severe hypotropia of the affected eye. He elevated the affected eyes by means of a new operation, similar in principle to the Jensen(3) procedure for lateral rectus palsy, in which the superior, medial and lateral recti were split, but not detached, and united by means of non-absorbable sutures. The anterior ciliary circulation is threrby considerably less affected. The inferior rectus is also recessed. Very satisfactory results were obtained. We became aware of this procedure relatively late in this series and have therefore performed it on only one patient to date, the details of which follow:

This patient, Case 7, was a 12-year old white male with Von Recklinghausen´s neurofibromatosis. There was a right-sided ptosis, partly mechanical in nature, due to the plexiform neuroma of the upper lid. The right globe was enlarged and there were areas of scleral atrophy with staphyloma formation visible. The right acuity was light perception. Two years previously, he had had a debulking procedure on the upper lid neurofibroma. There was a gross right hypotropia with moderate right esotropia.

In view of the scleral thinning, we were rather apprehensive of scleral suturing, especially superiorly. A Callahan procedure with inferior rectus recession of 4 mm was performed on April 2, 1981, a pre-operative forced duction test having shown passive restriction of elevation. A considerable improvement in the hypotropia was obtained, but with an increase of the esotropia to greater than 45 prism diopters. He has since undergone a further upper lid debulking and a lower lid fascia lata sling with considerable cosmetic improvement.

We therefore conclude that the procedure has a worthwhile effect for hypotropia, but may enhance a pre-existing horizontal deviation. For such cases, we favor the Knapp procedure, as appropriate adjustments of the horizontal rectus muscle forces may be incorporated.

To illustrate how effective surgery can be, we would like to describe case 9, a white 14-year old girl who presented with 30 prism diopters of left hypotropia and 3 degrees of left exotropia. The refraction of the right eye was -0.25 diopters, that of the left was +0.50 -5.00 175, giving an acuity of 6/18. There was a left ptosis with 6 mm of levator function. Orthoptic testing pre-operatively showed "left suppression". A knapp procedure was performed on September 17, 1981, with considerable improvement in her ocular posture and some limitation of left elevation. Interestingly, she was then found to have a vertical form of anomalous correspondence, with anomalous fusion at left hypo 4 prism diopters, with a vertical angle on dissocation of 22-26 prism diopters. She underwent anterior levator resection on March 17, 1982, with an excellent final cosmetic result.

Various authories, writing on double elevator palsy with or without ptosis, have emphasiesed the importance of detecting inferior rectus restriction. This may be due to contracture of the muscle, or as in case 4 of this series, to a fibrous condensation around the muscle.

Scott and Jackson(4), reported a high incidence of inferior restriction, in 11 out of 15 cases of double elevator palsy, and felt that this represented secondary inferior rectus restriction. They also noted two signs which they felt were commonly associated with inferior restriction. These were an accentuated lower lid fold on upgaze of the affected eye and a deficient Bell′s phenomenon. McNeer and Jamplolsky(5), described a case in which an additional anomalous insertion of the inferior rectus was found at surgery. Division of this improved rotations and led to a good cosmetic result.

Metz(6) studied a series of 15 patients with limited vertical movement of one eye. Nine were hypotropic in the primary position. Of these, five had normal saccadic velocities in an upward direction, and a positive forced duction test. The remaining four had reduced upward saccadic velocity. Of these, only one had a positive forced duction test. In our series, six out of 10 patients had a positive forced duction test, a similar proportion to that found by Metz. Our policy was to perform muscle transpositions on all patients and an inferior rectus muscle recession if the traction test was positive. In one patient, case 6, the inferior rectus recession was performed three months later. No overcorrections were obtained, suggesting that to have performed only the Knapp procedure or the inferior rectus recession would have led to an inadequate correction. The average correction in this group was not particularly large compared with the cases with negative traction tests.

Three of our cases had previous vertical rectus muscle surgery which had been ineffective in elevating the globe. Not all of the previous records were available to us, but where they were, they showed that poor results were obtained from superior rectus strengthening procedures. The Knapp or Callahan procedures produced a far greater correction. Evidently, the superior rectus in these cases was either paretic or congenitally hypoplastic in association with levator muscle dystrophy.

Beard(7) notes that superior rectus resection is liable to increase the apparent ptosis and recommends the Knapp procedure as having less effect on the upper lid. Six of our patients had previous ptosis surgery which had been ineffective in elevating the upper lid. This was usually some form of levator resection, but in addition, case 4 had previously undergone a frontalis sling and case 10 (with Marcus-Gunn jaw-winking syndrome) had a levator excision and frontalis sling of subsequent ptosis surgery in a later communication. We agree with the authors cited that ocular alignment must always procede lid surgery.

Finally, there is the interesting finding of a vertical form of anomalous retinal correspondence in case 9. So far, no other patient in this series has shown this phenomenon. We have found three references to vertical anomalous correspondence, none of whom is similar in type to this case. Crone and LaFaut(8) described anomalous fusion in patients with congenital superior oblique paralysis. These were investigated with vertical fixation disparity plotting and were compared with patients with acquired superior oblique paresis. Patients with the congenital palsies showed an "anomalous" type of fixation disparity curve and tended to have much larger vertical fusion ranges.

Lang(9) described cases of vertical microstrabismus with a larger angle on dissociation.

Hardjowijoto(10) presented three cases where there was a small angle of hypertropia under binocular viewing conditions (2-5 prism diopters), associated with a large angle on dissociation up to 25 prism diopters, on Maddox rod testing. He speculated that in all cases of anomalous fusion there would be a small manifest deviation with anomalous correspondence associated with a larger phoria demonstrable on dissociation. Case 9 in our series does not appear to fit into any of these categories. Her deviation was a marked hypotropia and her anomalous correspondence was not demonstrated until after her Knapp procedure. The fusion state pre-operatively can only be speculated upon, as variable left suppression was the only finding.

REFERENCES

1. Knapp P: The surgical treatment of double elevator paralysis. Trans Am Ophthalmol Soc 67:304-323, 1969.

2. Callahan M: Surgically mismanaged ptosis associated with doubld elevator palsy. Arch Ophthalmol 99:108-112, 1981.

3. Jensen EDF: Rectus muscle union: a new operation for paralysis of the rectus muscles. Trans Pac Coast Oto-ophthalmol Soc 45:359-387, 1964.

4. Scott W, Jackson OB: Double elevator palsy: the significiance of inferior rectus restriction. Am Orthopt J

27:5-10, 1977.

5. McNeer K, Jamplolsky A: Doubld elevator palsy caused by anomalous insertion of the inferior rectus. Am J Ophthalmol 59:317-319, 1965.

6. Metz H: Doubld elevator palsy. Arch Ophthalmol 97:901-903, 1979.

7. Beard C: Ptosis. C V Mosby 3rd ed, p. 142, 1981.

8. Crone RA, LaFaut N: Anomalous fusion in congenital trochlear paralysis. Brit Orthopt J 28:2-10, 1971.

9. Lang J: Mikrostrabismus. Bucherei Des Augenartztes, Heft 62 Ferdinand Enke, Stuttgart, 1973.

10. Hardjowijoto S: Vertical microstrabismus with large latent deviation. In Strabismus, R Reinecke (ed). Proceedings of the third meeting of the International Strabismological Association, 1978, New York, Grune & Stratton, 1978.

SYMPTOMATIC DISSOCIATED HYPERS (DVD)--RESULTS WITH UNILATERAL SUPERIOR RECTUS RECESSIONS

T. F. Moore

ABSTRACT

Seventy-five children presenting with symptomatic Dissociated Vertical Divergence (DVD) over a nine year period were treated surgically with non-"super-maximum" (3-6mm) unilateral superior rectus recessions of the higher eye measured by prism and cover. The vast majority of the recessions were 4mm. Ten percent of the patients developed a symptomatic DVD hyper of the fellow eye at a later date requiring similar surgical treatment on that eye. Significant undercorrections occured in less than five percent of the patients.

Eleven patients presented with an isolated unilateral DVD and the surgical results with these patients were uniformly good. Another eleven patients had DVD associated with Exotropia and overcorrections of the Exotropia occurred when attempts were made to treat these disorders simultaneously. The median follow-up period for all surgically treated patients is three years.

It is our conclusion that unilateral superior rectus recessions for DVD hypers when measured to be ten prism diopters or more than the fellow eye by prism and cover is an appropriate procedure for control of symptomatic DVD Hypers.

STRABISMUS II
ISBN 0-8089-1424-3

THE USE OF SYNOPTOMETRY IN DIAGNOSIS OF EYE MOVEMENT DISORDERS

K. M. Krzystkowa and A. Kubatko-Zielinska

ABSTRACT

The results of examination with the synoptometer in 127 cases of different types of eye movement disorders are presented. The determination of the objective angle in various regions of the binocular field of gaze forms the basis of all surgical therapy, for this reason the advantages of synoptometry as compared with other methods are stressed. Synoptometry enables the objective angle to be measured in extreme areas of the binocular field of gaze. It enables quantitative measurement of muscular function, which is particularly important in pre- and postoperative evaluation. The possibility of detailed examination of cyclophoria in all directions of gaze is emphasized.

Synoptometry facilitates the differential diagnosis, establishment of the surgical indications especially in vertical ocular deviations, and follow-up examination.

The results of pre- and postoperative examination are presented in the following groups of cases: I. Post-traumatic motility disorders as a sequel to orbital trauma (47 patients), II. Neurogenic vertical eye movement disorders (50 patients), and III. Neurogenic horizontal eye movement disorders and congenital syndromes (30 patients).

INTRODUCTION

Diagnosis indications for surgical therapy, follow-up, and evaluation of results in complicated eye motility disorders are an important and often difficult problem. In paralytic squint and post-traumatic diplopia the determination of the objective angle in varioyus regions of the field of vision constitutes the basis of all surgical therapy. A number of methods may be used, but all have one or more shortcomings.

We have experienced difficulties especially in determining the indications for operations on the vertical eye muscles. The pre- and postoperative analysis often remains inadequate, and probably is an important factor in the divergency of opinion concerning the surgical procedure in

STRABISMUS II
ISBN 0-8089-1424-3

these cases.

The synoptometer, according to Cuppers, seems to be a solution to this problem (Cuppers 1972, Adelstein 1975, Cuppers a. Muhlendyck 1976). It has been constructed on haploscope principles as a synoptphore with special properties. The images are presented by means of two small mirrors of maximal pupillary size. These are situated immediately in front of the eyes and optimal observation of the corneal reflexes is possible. The main factor is that gaze in free space remains possible.

The apparatus allows precisely adjusted and reproducible excursions of the object presented with the aid of the holder arms, and because of the small size of the mirrors a wide area of the field of gaze is comprised. The deviation found is read in the usual manner, according to the horizontal and vertical directions, with measurements taken as a rule from 10 degrees to 10 degrees. Any refractive errors are corrected in the path of the rays through the apparatus.

MATERIALS AND RESULTS

Our material consists of 127 selected patients representastive of various ocular motility disorders. The age ranged from 4 to 70 years and there were 82 males and 45 females (Table I).

The causes of eye muscle disturbances are shown in Table II. The most frequent cause was trauma (59.1%), while congenital malformations accounted for 35.4%.

Table I

Material

Sex and age of 127 patients studied

Total # of Patients	Sex		Age in years					
	M	F	0-10	11-20	21-30	31-40	41-50	50+
127	82	45	23	33	34	13	15	9
100.0	64.6	35.4	18.1	26.0	26.8	10.2	11.8	7.1

Table II

Causes of eye movement disorders in 127 patients studied

Cause	# of Patients	%
Traffic accident	26	20.5
Assault	18	14.2
Fall	15	11.8
Blunt trauma	16	12.6
Congenital disturbance	45	35.4
Neurological diseases	3	2.4
Miscellaneous	4	3.1
Total	127	100.0

The time elapsing between the onset of disturbance and the first examination is shown in Table III. In our material, this period was usually from 1 to 4 weeks (41.1% of cases). The length of this period is important in the development of secondary changes in the eye muscles and in the results of surgery. For example, prolonged incarceration of the eye muscles in blowout fracture of the orbit or secondary contracture in paralytic squint give secondary changes.

The classification of our patients into three groups representing various ocular motility disorders is shown in Table IV.

Group I included 47 patients with motility disorders as sequel to orbital trauma, mainly due to incarceration of eye muscles and other soft tissues in the fracture.

Group II included 50 patients with vertical eye movement disturbances of neurogenic origin, mainly paresis of the oculomotor and/or trochlear nerve or direct muscle trauma.

Group III included 30 patients with horizontal eye motility disorders, mainly neurogenic or congenital anomalies (Duane´s retraction syndrome).

Table III

Time between first occurrence of motility disorders and examination

Time of admission after injury	Weeks		Months	Years	From Birth	Total
	1-2	3-4	2-5	0.5-5		
# of Patients	27	25	20	10	45	127
%	21.4	19.7	15.7	7.8	35.4	100.0

Complete examinations and synoptometry were performed in every case, at the beginning of treatment and before surgery to establish the indications for operation, the choice of muscle, and the method.

Table IV

Classification of 127 patients selected for study

Type of disorder	# of patients	%
Group I Injury to the orbit (mechanical cause of motility disorders)	47	37.0
Group II Neurogenic vertical eye motility disorders (paresis of trochlear or oculomotor nerves)	50	39.4
Group III Neurogenic horizontal eye motility disorders (paresis of abducent nerve and Duane's retraction syndrome)	30	23.6
Total	127	100.0

Table V

Classification of Group I
(47 patients with eye
motility disorders after orbital trauma)

Type of injury to the orbit	Blowout fracture of floor	Blowout fracture of medial wall	Fracture of upper rim and/or roof	Maxillo-malar complex fracture	Orbital haematoma	Total
# of pts	36	2	4	4	1	47
%	76.6	4.3	8.5	8.5	2.1	100.0

In patients with post-traumatic diplopia, these examinations, supplemented by X-ray, determine the need for orbital surgery to free the incarcerated muscles or eye muscle surgery only. Follow-up examinations were performed two weeks after operation, and again after six months.

Group I: Post traumatic motility disorders as a sequel to orbital trauma

In this group patients with blowout fractures predominated. Fractures of the roof and upper rim of the orbit seldom appeared (Table V). Vertical motility disorders and diplopia were the most frequent symptoms.

To show the use of synoptometry in the diagnosis of these cases, we give examples of examination before and after treatment.

In snyoptometry the characteristic picture of the vertical deviation (VD) in the upper part of the field of gaze in relation to VD in the lower part predominated (Fig 1 and 2).

To supplement synoptometry, the field of monocular foveal fixation was tested in the affected eye, using a real object (a point) and the Haidinger phenomenon (Fig 3). If the field is displaced beyond the physiological area, this suggests that there is some mechanical obstacle to motility requiring orbital surgery, that is, a need to explore the orbital floor and to free any incarcerated muscles.

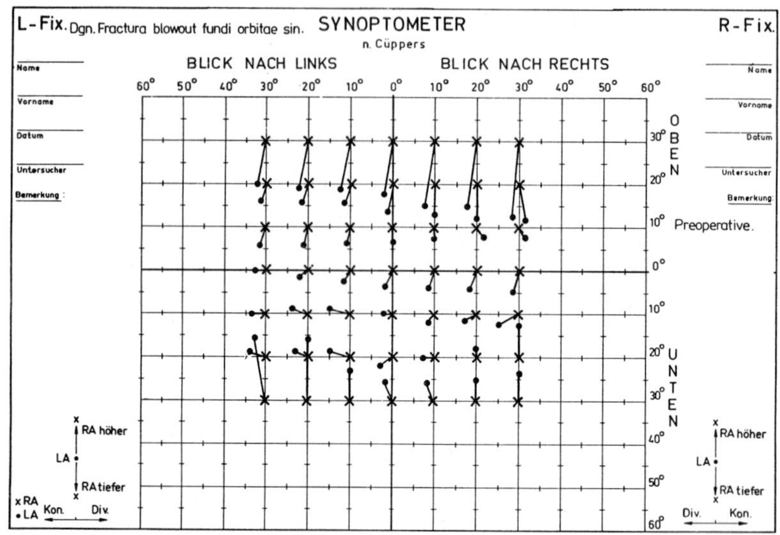

Figure 1. Synoptometer diagram of a patient with blowout fracture of the left orbit before operation.

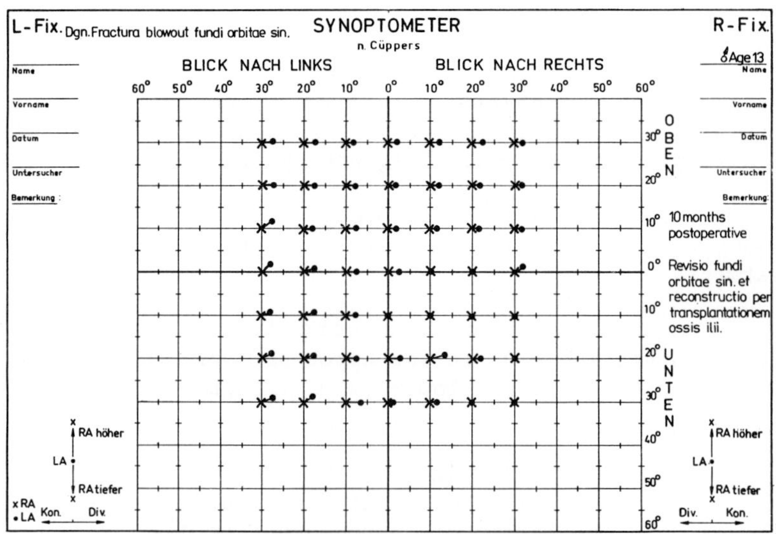

Figure 2. Synoptometer diagram of the same patient after operation.

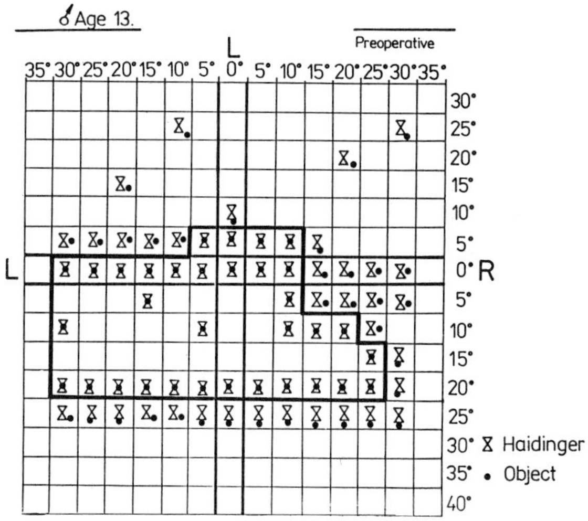

Figure 3. The field of monocular foveal fixation of the same patient displaced beyond the physiological area before operation.

Synoptometry and the demarcation of the field of monocular foveal fixation are also important in the indications for surgery on the extrinsic eye muscles in cases with persistent diplopia after orbital reconstruction: should the affected or the sound eye be operated on? If the field of monocular foveal fixation is displaced beyond the physiologically useful area, then in the first stage this field in the affected eye should be shifted to the central and lower parts of the field of gaze by operating on the muscles of this eye. If, in spite of this shift diplopia still persists, then operation on the sound eye in the second stage is indicated.

Another aspect is the value of synoptometry in examining cyclophoria, which cannot be quantitatively determined over so large a field by any other method. This is a great importance in damage to the oblique muscles.

Summarizing, the aim of surgical treatment in post-traumatic diplopia is to shift the field of monocular foveal fixation of the affected eye and the field of motor coordination of the other eye to the physiological, most useful part of the field of gaze.

In fresh injuries the freed muscles usually begin to function normally after orbital surgery, while in old fractures the prognosis is worse and often subsequent eye muscle surgery on both eyes is indicated.

Group II: Neurogenic vertical eye movement disorders (without orbital fractures)

Group II included 50 patients with vertical motility disorders which, in contradistinction to Group I, were not caused by orbital trauma. They were divided into those with paresis of the oculomotor nerve and those with paresis of the trochlear nerve (Table VI).

Total paralysis of the oculomotor nerve with typical clinical symptoms was easy to diagnose without using special

Table VI

Causes of vertical eye motility disorders in Group II (50 patients)

Type of motility disturbance / Cause	Paresis of oculomotor n.		Paresis of trochlear n.		Total	
	# of pts	%	# of pts	%	# of pts	%
Blunt trauma to the head	3	6.0	7	14.0	10	20.0
Blunt trauma to the orbit	4	8.0	5	10.0	9	18.0
Injury to the eye muscles	-	-	3	6.0	3	6.0
Congenital disorders	7	14.0	18	36.0	25	50.0
Neurological diseases	-	-	3	6.0	3	6.0
Total	14	28.0	36	72.0	50	100.0

methods. More complicated symptoms appeared in cases with partial paresis of the oculomotor nerve, i.e. paralysis of both elevator muscles, especially in cases after craniofacial trauma. The clinical picture at first seemed similar to that observed in blowout fractures of the orbit. In partial paresis of the oculomotor nerve, however, synoptometry showed the inversion of VD in the upper and lower part of the field of gaze, but this disparity changed gradually and not jerkily, which would have indicated a mechanical obstacle in the orbit (Fig 4). The positive forced duction test is here decisive. In paresis, however, passive motility is normal. In addition, the field of monocular foveal fixation in paresis is greater than in mechanical restriction of eyeball motility (Fig 5).

A detailed analysis was made of cases with paresis of the trochlear nerve. Paresis of the superior oblique muscle rapidly leads to secondary changes in the homolateral inferior oblique muscle and heterolateral vertical rectus muscles. These changes are often irreversible and inoperable. Cyclophoria and subsequent torticollis ocularis are serious consequences of paresis of the superior oblique muscle.

Synoptometry facilitates the indications for surgery as

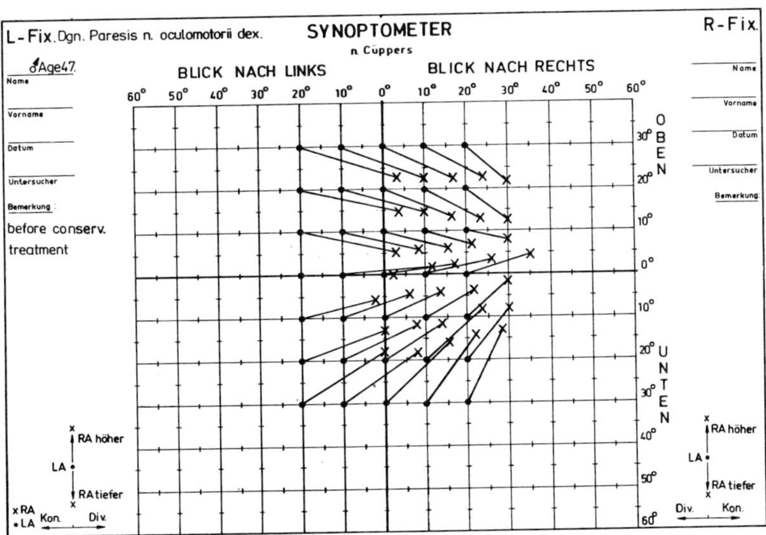

Figure 4. Synoptometer diagram of a patient with oculomotor nerve paresis after cranio-facial trauma before treatment.

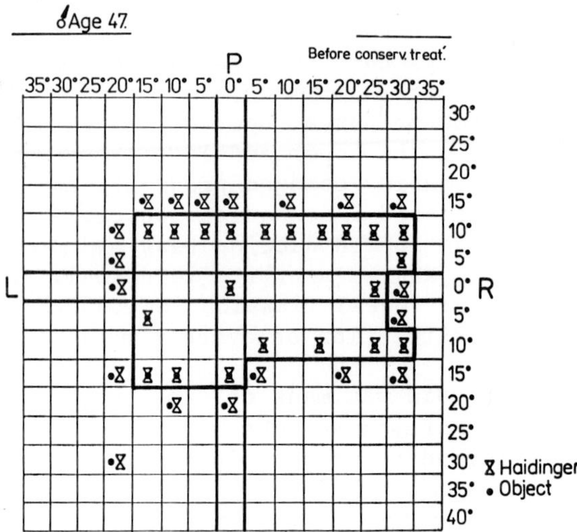

Figure 5. The field of monocular foveal fixation of the same patient before treatment.

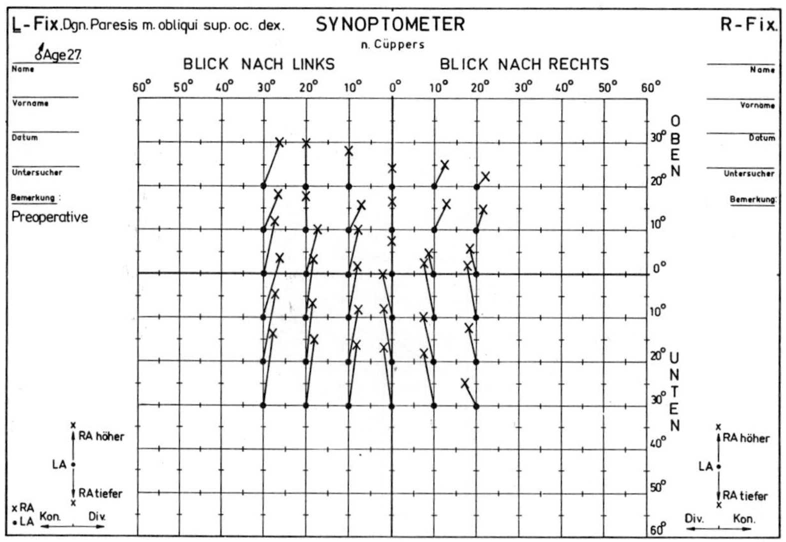

Figure 6. Synoptometer diagram of a patient with trochlear nerve paresis before operation.

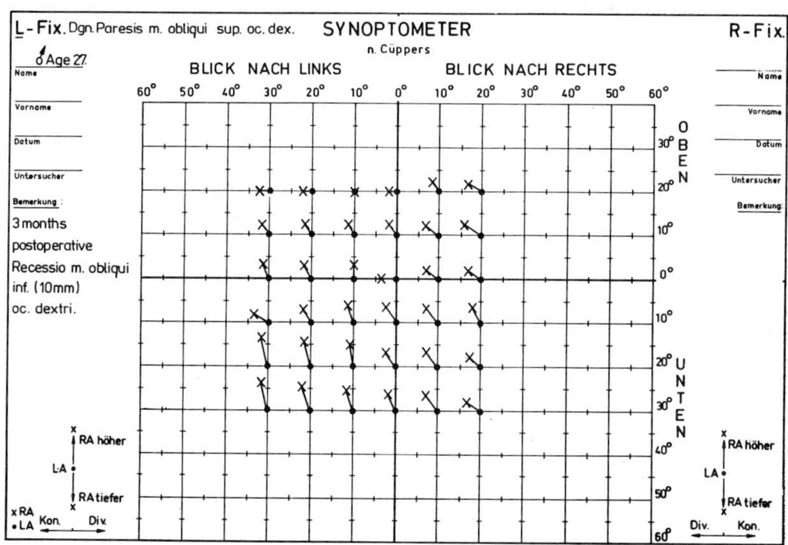

Figure 7. Synoptometer diagram of the same patient after operation.

well as the choice of the muscle to be operated on and the method. In this group also we only tried to shift the field of binocular single vision from a less to a more important functional area. In other words, the upper parts of the field of gaze may often be sacrificed in favour of the lower parts (Fig 6 and 7).

In the synoptometer diagram, the appearance and degree of secondary changes in the eye muscles should be analysed.

The VD in the upper and lower quadrants of the field of gaze on the right or left side, depending on which eye is affected, indicates secondary hyperaction of the inferior oblieque muscle, while an increase in the VD in the lower quadrant shows that there is no contracture of the inferior oblique muscle. If the VD enters far into the area of the opposite side, this suggests secondary changes in the vertical rectus muscles of the sound eye.

Sometimes, the primary paresis of the superior oblique muscle regresses, but the functioning of this muscle is inhibited by secondary contracture of the inferior oblique muscle. The forced duction test (FDT) is of decisive importance in these cases.

In our own experience, if, in a case of paresis of the superior oblique muscle, postoperative hypofunction of the weakened antagonists is observed, and the field of monocular foveal fixation is situated in the central area, the next operation should be delayed to see whether spontaneous recovery of muscle function will occur.

Group III: Patients with horizontal eye movement disorders

This group was divided into two parts: A. patients with paresis of the abducent nerve and B. those with congenital Duane´s retraction syndrome (Table VII). The clinical picture in all patients is typical and the examination findings are clear. In server paralysis of the abducent nerve, it may be difficult to perform synoptometry, especially when homolateral antagonist contracture markedly limits eye motility.

The small VD observed in the whole field of gaze is caused by the absence of abduction and hence the inability of

Table VII

Causes of horizontal eye motility disorders in Group III (30 patients)

	Paresis of abducent n.		Duane's retraction syndrome		Total	
Causes	# of pts	%	# of pts	%	# of pts	%
Blunt trauma to the head	7	23.4	-	-	7	23.4
Blunt trauma to the orbit	3	10.0	-	-	3	10.0
Neurological diseases	1	3.3	-	-	1	3.3
Congenital	-	-	19	63.3	19	63.3
Total	11	36.7	19	63.3	30	100.0

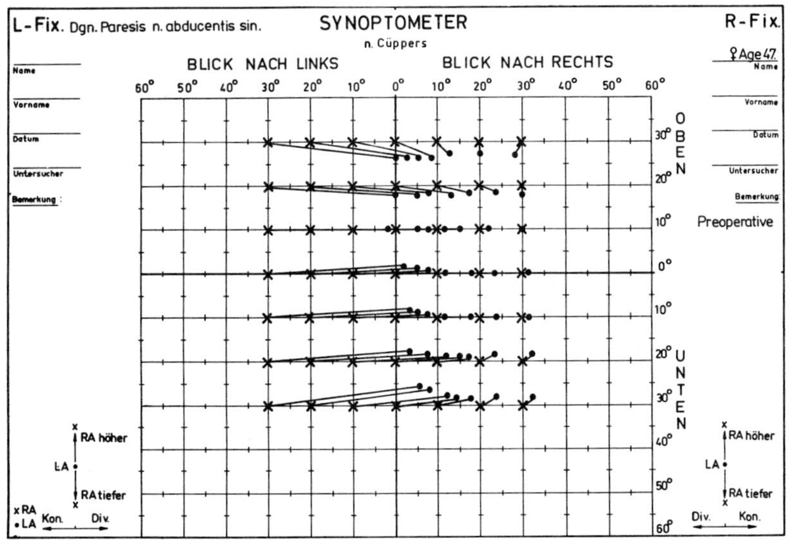

Figure 8. Synoptometer diagram of a patient with abducens nerve paresis.

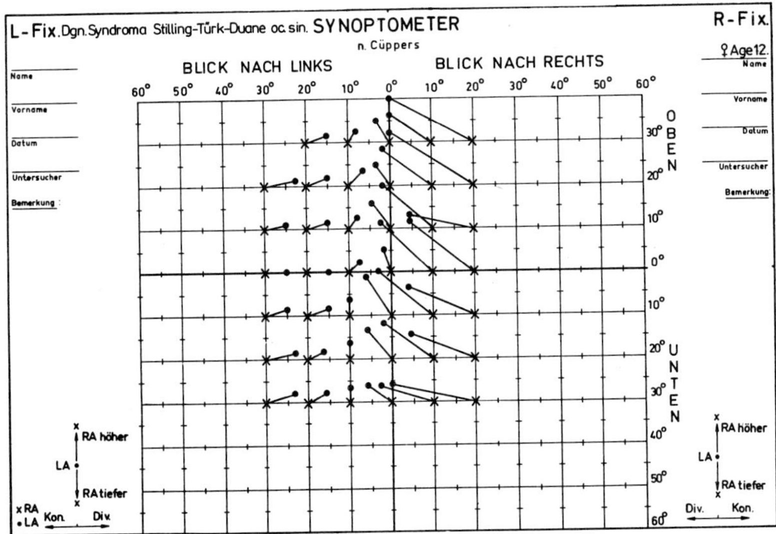

Figure 9. Synoptometer diagram of a patient with Duane's retraction syndrome.

the vertical rectus muscles to function. The manifestation of cyclophoria in peripheral areas of the field of gaze may be explained in the same way: in the adducted eye, the torsional function of both the oblique muscles which dominate in torsion of the eye is impossible. Both the discrete changes described can be detected only by synoptometry (Fig 8).

In Duane´s retraction syndrome synoptometry is not important in diagnosis, and only serves as supplementary documentation of the disturbance in horizontal and occasional vertical deviations. In the synoptometric diagram, the inversion of horizontal eye movement limitation is interesting (Fig 9). This corresponds to both abduction and adduction. The inversion area corresponds to the extent of torticollis ocularis.

As our studies have shown, synoptometry enables eye movements to be analysed precisely, and so facilitates the determination of the indications for surgery, and of the postoperative follow-up. The results of examinations are reproducible, and in the latest model registration is automatic. The main factor is, that gaze in free space remains possible when large area of the field of gaze is comprised.

REFERENCES

1. Adelstein FE: Zur qutachtlichen Beurteilung traumatisch bedingter Motilitatsstorungen. Klin Mbl Augenhk 167:258-272, 1975.

2. Cuppers C: Determination of the objective angle. Orthoptics. Proceeding of the Second International Orthoptic Congress, Amsterdam, May 1971, 65-71. Excerpta Medica, Amster dam 1972.

3. Cuppers C, Muhlendyck H: Die Verwendund des Synoptometers zur Differentialdiagnose und postoperativen Verlaufskontrolle von sog. Blowout-Frakturen. In: Das Kopftrauma aus augen arztlicher Sicht Bucherei des Augenarztes, H 68:50-70 F Enke Verlag Stuttgart 1976.

KERATITIS SICCA FOLLOWING STRABISMUS SURGERY: A NEW SYNDROME

A. M. Eisenbaum and R. A. Sargent

ABSTRACT

Two women in their mid-thirties developed keratitis sicca following multiple eye muscle operations. Both had several surgical procedures before dry eye symptoms were noted. Evidence of reduced Schirmer´s tests and clinical symptoms developed after the fourth strabismus operation in one patient and after the eighth strabismus surgery in the other patient.

In the case where bilateral keratitis sicca developed after the fourth operation, the less symptomatic eye could move freely; the more involved eye had symptoms, even after a dellen and restrictive hyperopia were corrected. The other patient´s eighth strabismus repair involved bilateral rectus muscle recessions with adjustable sutures and bare scleral closure. The eye with the greater scar dissection became more symptomatic; both eyes have slightly restricted horizontal motility.

Whether the cause of dry eye in these cases relates to loss of conjunctival goblet cells or inadequacy of corneal lubrication is not clear. To our knowledge this syndrome of postoperative keratitis sicca following multiple strabismus surgeries in middle-aged women has not been previously reported.

STRABISMUS II
ISBN 0-8089-1424-3

DISCUSSION BY W. E. GILLIES

With regard to this paper on Keratitis Sicca following strabismus surgery, one´s first question is whether the condition described is specific enough to constitute a new syndrome. Several features seem prominent in the two cases: (1) the multiple operations; (2) post-operative scarring mentioned specifically in one case or inferred from loss of movement in the other; (3) reduced Schirmers test; (4) both patients are females in their mid-thirties.

The multiple operations may be less important than scarring which may follow one badly done operation in producing a loss of lacrimal gland or conjunctival lubricating function. A similarity with the dry eye following enthusiastic removal of a dermolipoma comes to mind and an impaired Schirmers test suggests some interference with lacrimal gland secretion from scarring which has eventually involved the super-lateral fornix after repeated dissection and mobilization of the conjunctiva which may be pulled into the field of operation. Perhaps oft repeated surgery especially with repeated conjunctival recessions may cause loss of conjunctival function from scarring and shrinkage of conjunctiva but there seems no other reason why careful surgery should affect conjunctival function.

Is it significant that the two patients are young women in their thirties? Perhaps this is an early Sjogrens syndrome but no other features of that entity seem to be present.

The paper does indicate the need for great care with multiple operations for squint and the desirability of limiting surgery to one or two operations.

ANTERIOR SEGMENT ISCHEMIA CAUSED BY JENSEN'S PROCEDURE

T. Frey

ABSTRACT

The second reported case of anterior segment ischemia since introduction of this procedure in 1964 is presented. Flouroscein angiography and direct observation in the operating room showed compromised anterior ciliary arteries. The vertical rectus anterior ciliary arteries seem to be most important in maintaining adequate blood flow to the anterior segment and virtually all the transposition procedures pose a threat to the vertical ACA and have caused problems in the past. The Jensen Muscle Union Procedure remains a good method of treating lateral rectus paresis but is not without risk.

INTRODUCTION

Since Jensen, in 1964,(1) described a muscle union procedure as a means of dealing with lateral rectus paresis, this technique has gained acceptance as an effective procedure.(2-4) The rationale of apparently sparing five of seven anterior ciliary arteries has, it appears, made good safety sense; since, in the eighteen years since this procedure was introduced, only one case of anterior segment ischemia associated with this procedure has been reported.(5) Another case of anterior segment ischemia following a Jensen's muscle union is now presented with fluorescein and surgical evidence of compromised anterior ciliary arteries.

CASE REPORT

A 49-year old white male presented one year following head trauma with a history of double vision and of his eye "stuck in the corner". (Fig 1) Examination revealed a visual acuity of 20/20 in each eye. There were 50 diopters of left esotropia and inability to abduct the eye to the midline. A traction test showed minimal restriction.

The operative procedure consisted of a 6.5 mm recession of the right medial rectus and a Jensen muscle union procedure using 000000 mersiline sutures. The muscle slips were just approximated and care was taken to avoid

STRABISMUS II
ISBN 0-8089-1424-3

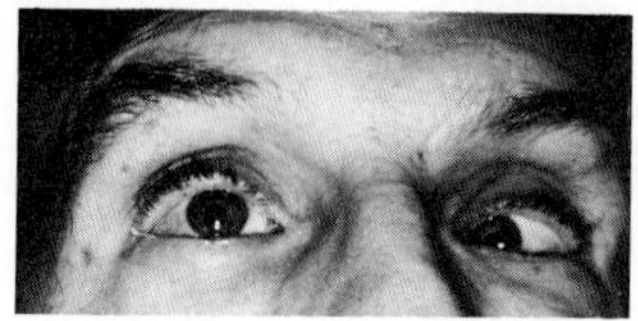

Figure 1

strangulating the vessels. On the day following surgery, the patient's visual acuity had decreased to light perception. There was dense striate keratopathy and an intraocular tension of 7 mm Hg. He was placed on oxygen and steroids. Seven hours later his low tension was barely measurable. He was taken back to the operating room and it was noted that the anterior ciliary arteries of the lateral rectus and of the inferior rectus were distended, blue and appeared thrombotic. The superior rectus arteries appeared to be functioning well. The sutures were cut and removed.

Postoperatively the patient was treated with oral and topical steroids and heparin anti-coagulation. The cornea began to clear by the following day and the tension came up to 11. Fluorescein angiography on the sixth postoperative day revealed areas of leakage superiorally from twelve o'clock to ten thirty and a larger area below extending from three o'clock to eight o'clock. (Fig 2)

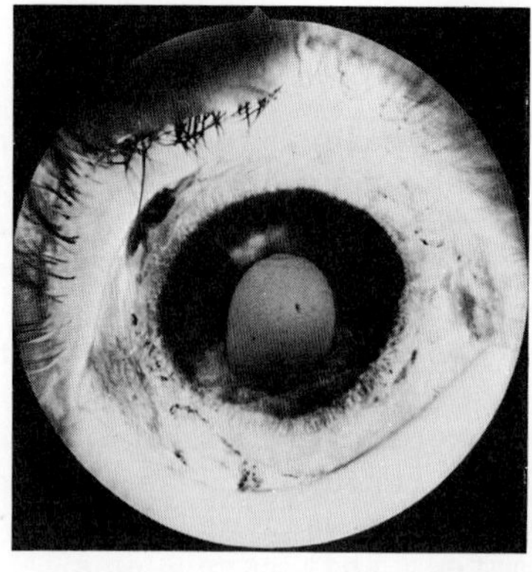

Figure 2

The patient was discharged on the sixth postoperative day on oral and topical steroids and on Persantine. One month later the patient's visual acuity was 20/20. There were still some fine circulating cells. The pupil was dilated and there were residual areas of iris atrophy corresponding to the fluorescein leakage.

DISCUSSION

The possibility of anterior segment ischemia is a threat to the patient requiring extensive and/or repeated muscle surgery. What is safe to do and when it is safe to do it are the concerns of the strabismus surgeon as he attempts to preserve the arterial supply of the anterior segment.

Hayreh and Scott(6), in 1978, used fluorescein angiography to study the blood supply to the anterior segment. The nasal iris, they felt, was supplied by the medial long posterior ciliary artery with the anterior ciliary artery (ACA) of the medial rectus playing only a subsidiary role. The temporal iris, they concluded, was supplied by the anterior ciliary arteries of the superior rectus and the inferior rectus with a less significant role being played by the lateral rectus anterior ciliary artery and the temporal long posterior ciliary artery. They felt that the major arterial circle of the iris plays only a minor role and that once blood supply was jeopardized, no appreciable collateral supply was later established.

Using the Reference Blood Flow Method in Primates, Wilcox, Keough and Connally(?) came up with similar results. Horizontal recti tenotomy initiated a compensatory blood flow to the anterior segment, resulting in no decrease in blood supply. They postulated this increased flow to be mainly via the medial long posterior ciliary, with some flow from the lateral long posterior ciliary artery and the vertical ACAs. Vertical rectus tenotomy, on the other hand, resulted in normal medial quadrant blood flow, but a reduction to 20-30% of normal flow in the vertical quadrants, and only 10% of normal flow in the lateral quadrant, suggesting the large reliance of the temporal anterior segment on the vertical ACAs. If one accepts the premise of Hayreh and Scott, and of Wilcox et al, extreme care must be taken to preserve the vertical recti ACAs and staging of this procedure should have little beneficial effect.

Anterior segment ischemia following compromised blood supply was described by Schmidt in the German literature in 1874.(7) It has been reported to complicate types of occlusive arterial disease;(?) in symmetrical arterial occlusion of the upper extremities; Pulseless disease, etc.(10) It was first reported following surgical disruption of the blood supply to the anterior segment by Wilson and Irvine(10) in a case involving retinal detachment surgery in 1955.

Girard,(11) in 1960, reported anterior segment ischemia following extensive muscle surgery. There appear to be some individuals more at risk than others to develop ischemia as a sequela of muscle surgery. Jacobs et al(12) reported a 26-year old female with leukemia who developed this problem following surgery on two rectus muscles. Ryan and Goldberg(13), in 1971, reported nine patients with sickle cell hemoglobinopathy who developed anterior segment ischemia following scleral buckling procedures. Special care has been advised in elderly patients.(5) The safest surgical procedure for lateral rectus paresis appears to be a large recess/resect operation, where four of the seven ACAs are left intact including, most importantly, the vertical ones.

In the presence of a truly paralytic lateral rectus, however, the patient is usually left with an eye that will not rotate past the midline and with a residual head turn and esotropia. Metz and Jamplolsky(14) stated that "recession-resection surgery improved ocular position but rotation beyond the midline was not possible and saccadic speed toward abduction was unchanged."

The need for some other type of operation led to the prototype Hummelsheim(15) operation and its variations. One sacrifices during this procedure four of the seven ACAs including half the vertical recti arteriols. Girard(11) reported four patients who developed anterior segment ischemia following the Hummelsheim operation.

Reinecke(16) recommends correcting the problem in two steps, doing a horizontal recess/resect and following this in six weeks with complete transposition of the vertical recti. Saunders and Sandall,(17) however, reported two patients who developed anterior segment ischemia using this approach - one nine and the other twenty years after the original surgery. They recommend leaving the lateral rectus intact and proceeding directly to a transposition procedure. Girard(11) and Hiatt(18), though, both reported patients who had medial rectus recession, vertical recti transposition and intact lateral recti who developed ischemia.

The Jensen procedure seems to offer the safest method of dealing with lateral rectus paresis, since it theoretically leaves intact five of the seven ACAs. This procedure, though, is obviously not without risk. My patient showed fluorescein and surgical evidence of compromised vertical ACAs. I have seen two other patients who developed difficulties following a Jensen procedure. The first was a 51-year old male seen in consultation several months after he had had a Jensen procedure for a sixth nerve paresis secondary to a CVA. His ophthalmologist described flare and cells and cloudy cornea with decreased visual acuity following this procedure. I performed a Jensen procedure for a traumatic sixth nerve paresis on a 51-year -ld lady who immediately postoperatively developed cells and flare and a tension 4 mm less than the other eye. She subsequently completely cleared.

It appears that there is no perfect, safe procedure to do for a sixth nerve paresis. Anterior segment ischemia has been decribed following virtually every type of operation. Being young and healthy seems to be helpful. There have been no cases reported of anterior segment ischemia in children. Girard,(11) in fact, reported eleven children who had all four recti muscles detached at one sitting and developed no problem.

Careful follow-up is necessary for a patient who has had extensive muscle surgery. Steroids may be helpful for the inflammatory response. My patient was treated with oxygen and anti-coagulation on the advice of vascular surgeons. Whether it made any difference at all in the final outcome is certainly open to conjecture; but delivering more oxygen and attempting to prevent more thromboses in a, perhaps, partially occluded vessel seems to make good sense, as does surgical intervention when the situation is deteriorating. It is consoling in reviewing the literature to find that the general rule is for the patients to get better and recover vision, though they may be left with a residual dilated irregular pupil and iris atrophy and rarely a cataract.

It is obvious that the final answer is not at hand as to the best and safest method to treat sixth nerve paresis. If preoperative evaluation shows any significant muscle force generation, a large recess/resect appears to be the safest and best procedure to be carried out. In the absence of this, a Jensen-type procedure, tying the vessels together loosely and taking great pains to avoid strangulation, still appears to be a reasonable thing to do. Careful surgery and follow-up remains the important ingredient, but no surgical procedure appears to be without risk.

REFERENCES

1. Jensen CDF: Rectus muscle union: a new operation for paralysis of the rectus muscles. Trans Pacific Coast Otolaryngol Ophthalmol Soc 45:359-387, 1964.

2. Scott WE, Werner DB, Lennarson L: Evaluation of Jensen procedures by saccades and diplopic fields. Arch Ophthalmol 97:1886-1889, 1979.

3. Selezinka W, Sandall GS, Henderson JW: Rectus muscle union in sixth nerve paralysis. Arch Ophthalmol 92:382-386, 1974.

4. Frueh BR, Henderson JW: Rectus muscle union in sixth nerve paralysis. Arch Ophthalmol 85:191-196, 1971.

5. Von Noorden GK: Anterior segment ischemia following the Jensen procedure. Arch Ophthalmol 94:845-847, 1976.

6. Hayreh SS, Scott WE: Fluorescein iris angiography. II. Disturbances in iris circulation following strabismus operation on the various recti. Arch Ophthalmol 96:1390-1400, 1978.

7. Wilcox LM Jr, Keough EM, Connally RJ: Regional ischemia and compensatory vascular dymanics following selective tenotomy in primates. Exp Eye Res 33:353-360, 1981.

8. Schmidt H: Beitrag zur kenntniss deu embolie der arteria centralis retinae. Albrecht von graefes Arch fur Ophthalmol 20:287-307, 1874.

9. Skipper E, Flint FJ: Symmetrical arterial occlusion of upper extremities, head and neck: rare syndrome. Brit Med J 2:9-14, 1952.

10. On "pulseless disease" outside of Japan. Acta Med Scand 149:161-178, 1954.

11. Wilson WA, Irvin SR: Pathologic changes following disruption of blood supply to iris and ciliary body. Trans Am Acad Ophthalmol Otolaryngol 59:501-502, 1955.

12. Girard LJ, Beltronena F: Early and late complications of extensive muscle surgery. Arch Ophthalmol 64:576-584, 1960.

13. Jacobs DS, Vastine DW, Urist MJ: Anterior segment ischemia and sector iris atrophy after strabismus surgery in a patient with chronic lymphocytic leukemia. Ophthalmol Surg 7:42-48, 1976.

14. Ryan SJ, Goldberg MF: Anterior segment ischemia following scleral buckling in sickle cell hemoglobinopathy. Am J Ophthalmol 72:35-50, 1971.

15. Metz HS, Jampolsky A: Change in saccadic velocity following rectus muscle transposition. J Ped Ophthalmol 11:129-134, 1974. 1974.

16. Hummelsheim E: Weitere Erfahrunger mit Partieller Schneubergflanzung anden Augenmuskeln. Arch Augenheilk 62:71-74, 1908.

17. Reinecke B: Personal communication.

18. Saunders RA, Sandall GS: Anterior segment ischemia syndrome following rectus muscle transposition. Am J Ophthalmol 93:34-38, 1982.

19. Hiatt RL: Production of anterior segment ischemia. J Ped Ophthalmol and Strabismus 15:197-204, 1978.

DISCUSSION BY W. E. GILLIES

Anterior Segment Ischemia following a Jensens Procedure is a recognized hazard of muscle transfer procedures especially to replace loss of function of the lateral rectus. It is perhaps remarkable that it has been so seldom reported which suggests that it only occurs in patients who differ from the normal, perhaps having some underlying pathological condition. If the results of Jensens procedure seem worthwhile, then avoidance of the complication is desirable. Fluorescein angiography of the iris may be helpful, especially if it shows a drop-out of the radial vasculature of the iris or a marked delay in filling of any segment. This would seem particularly important between the stages of a two-stage procedure. Unfortunately in a darkly pigmented iris, angiography is difficult.

COMPENSATORY MECHANISMS IN SELECTIVE TENOTOMY

L. M. Wilcox, E. M. Keough, R. J. Connolly

ABSTRACT

There is much anecdotal information and a paucity of good clinical data relating to anterior segment ischemia (ASI). To explore the vascular physiology involved in ASI, selective tenotomy was performed on primates (Macaca assamensis, Papio anubis) followed by quantitative experiments to determine blood flow (BF) to AS. The anterior ciliary arteries (ACA) were found to supply 90% of BF to AS. Cutting the ACA's would be expected to decrease BF to AS. Selective tenotomy of the horizontal recti (MR + LR) however actually caused an increase in BF to AS (Exp 2.53 ± 0.35, Control 1.41 ± 0.16) (ml/min/gm tissue). There appears to be a compensatory mechanism through the long posterior ciliary arteries especially the medial one, that protects against ASI.

The results of these experiments and their implication for the strabismus surgeon were discussed.

1. Wilcox LM, Keough EM, Connolly RJ, Hotte CE: The contution of blood flow by the anterior ciliary arteries to the anterior segment in the primate eye. Exp Eye Res 30:167-174, 1980.

2. Hodson S, Wigham C, Williams L, Mayes KR, Grahm MV: Observations on the human cornea in vitro. Exp Eye Res 32:353-360, 1981.

(No paper was submitted)

STRABISMUS II
ISBN 0-8089-1424-3

DISCUSSION BY W. E. GILLIES

There seems no doubt that some mechanism exists in children which protects against anterior segment ischemia even when all the anterior ciliary arteries are severed, presumably an anastomotic circulation from the long posterior ciliary vessels. This mechanism does not seem reliable in adults in whom the blood flow on fluorescein angiography is radial and segmental. In primates the existence of a compensatory mechanism seems confirmed. Does this mean that a compensatory mechanism may also develop in humans and that a two-stage Jensen/Hummelsheim procedure may avoid anterior segment ischemia? Some of the evidence of the previous paper is against this.

ADJUSTING ADJUSTABLE EYE MUSCLE SUTURES UNDER GENERAL ANESTHESIA

R. H. Bedrossian

ABSTRACT

Fifty-four patients had 57 operations for horizontal muscle imbalances. Sutures were adjusted under anesthesia to compensate for the difference in the ocular deviation when the patient was awake and asleep. Of fifty of these operations, the postoperative horizontal deviation was within 10 pd (or 5 degrees) of what might be expected by the manner in which the light reflex was positioned under anesthesia. Three patients were originally straight immediately after surgery and drifted to twelve diopters of esotropia six months after surgery. These patients required no additional surgery. Three patients needed a second surgery using the same technique, which resulted in the correction of the deviation. One patient remains uncorrected six months after surgery. This method of adjusting muscle sutures under anesthesia expands the use of adjustable sutures. It appears to give satisfactory results in over 90% of the operations using horizontal rectus muscle surgery.

INTRODUCTION

Many factors may enter into the development of strabismus. Resecting or recessing a muscle a specified number of millimeters for a specific degree of deviation may end with an undesirable result. The ophthalmic surgeon may modify the amount of surgery depending upon:

1. The size and position of the muscles.

2. Resistance of the eye to rotation.

3. Possible innervational factors.

Long term results of eye muscle surgery may be influenced by sensory factors which years later result in a change in deviation.

STRABISMUS II
ISBN 0-8089-1424-3

Jampolsky(1) has helped reduce the immediate postoperative surprises by using muscle sutures that are adjusted the evening of, or the day after, the surgery. This procedure is difficult to perform in younger individuals because of the discomfort which may be involved in making the adjustments and because of apprehension or lack of cooperation.

The position of the eyes in the awake patient, and in the same patient under anesthesia may be considerably different. These differences have been studied by Apt and Eisenburg.(2) Mindel(3) and France(4) have shown that depolarizing agents (especially succinyl choline) have a profound effect on the ocular muscles. These agents will considerably alter the position of the eyes due to stimulation of certain fibers of the external ocular muscles.

This study was done to determine if the outcome of eye muscle surgery can be influenced by using the corneal light reflex and the relationship between the position of the eyes in the awake and anesthetic state as a guide to adjusting muscle sutures at the time of surgery.

METHODS AND MATERIALS

This study involved fifty-seven operations. Thirty operations were done on twenty-eight patients with esotropia and twenty-seven surgeries on twenty-six patients with exotropia. Prior to surgery, the patient had muscle imbalances measured in the cardinal positions at both distance and near by the prism cover test. (If it was not possible to measure the imbalance with the prism because of the patients age, the imbalance was estimated by the Hirschberg light reflex). If any accommodative element was present, glasses were worn. The appropriate muscles were selected for surgical manipulation by the usual studies. With the light 0.75 meters away, the corneal light reflex of both the fixating and deviating eye was recorded in relation to the pupil center. This was done with each eye fixing when possible. Not included in the study are patients with evidence of a muscle paralysis.

The patients were anesthetized to plane 2 surgical anesthesia as determined by the anesthesiologist. The operating room light or a flash light was used to locate the light reflex on the cornea. This light was also positioned about 0.75 meters from the eyes. The deviation was measured by prisms. The plan was to adjust the muscle sutures so the light reflex of both eyes was in such a position that the awake deviation plus the change in position under anesthesia was corrected. An example: if the patient had 20 p.d. of esotropia while awake and 20. p.d. while asleep, the sutures were adjusted so that at the end of the surgery the eyes had no deviation (Fig 1). If there was 20 p.d. of esotropia when patient was awake and the eyes were straight under anesthesia, the position of the eyes were adjusted to 20 diopters of exotropia (Fig 2).

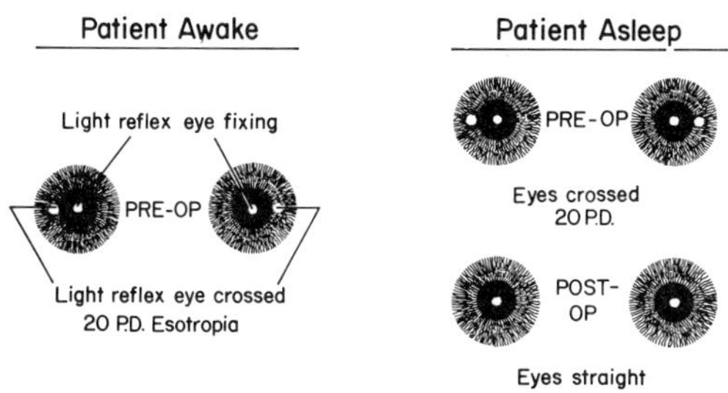

Figure 1

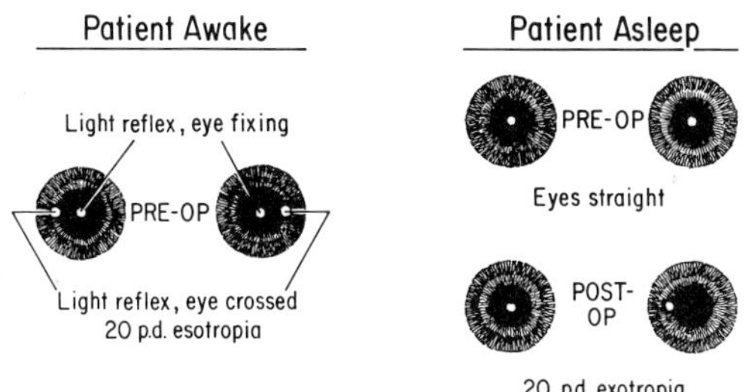

Figure 2

Anesthetic factors were considered important. Care was taken to make certain that no depolarizing agents were used during induction, or if used, their effects had worn off. Equally important was the need for a knowledgeable and cooperative anesthesiologist or anesthetist who could keep the patient at a proper and consistent depth of anesthesia.

Forced ductions were performed, and after allowing for spring back,(5) the eye position was again checked for consistent positioning. The muscles to be operated upon were isolated. If a recession-resection operation was to be done, the "recessed muscle was separated from the globe and loosely reattached with an adjustable type" of suture. The antagonist was then resected an amount that was considered appropriate for the deviation. The adjustable suture was then loosened or tightened an amount determined by the positioning of the eyes. If a marginal myectomy-resection was done, the resected muscle was the one adjusted. If bilateral recessions were done, both horizontal recti were isolated and were allowed to retract approximately similar amounts. The deviation was then measured by prism and the sutures adjusted to compensate for the difference between the awake and anesthetized position.

RESULTS

The 30 patients with esotropia were divided into three groups, those with less esotropia under anesthesia; those with the same amount of esotropia awake and asleep; those with larger amounts of esotropia when under anesthesia (Table 1). There were 20 operations for patients whose esotropia was significantly less (greater than 10 diopters) under anesthesia than when awake. Surgery resulted in 18 postoperative deviations of less than 10 p.d. of deviation six months after surgery. One patient required a second surgery because of under-correction. Seven patients were the same awake and under anesthesia. Five of these had less than 10 p.d. of deviation postoperatively, two were straight immediately after surgery and drifted to 12 diopters of esotropia at six months. These patients had no fusion and were cosmetically satisfactory and required no additional surgery. One patient required a second surgery which resulted in no residual deviation. Two patients whose deviations was less under anesthesia than awake, had residual deviations of less than 4 p.d. six months after surgery.

The 26 patients with exotropia were also divided into those whose exotropia was greater, the same, or less under anesthesia when awake. Twelve patients had a greater exotropia under anesthesia. All of these patients were within 10 p.d. of being in the orthotropic position six months after surgery. Nine patients had the same amount of deviation under anesthesia as when awake. One of the patients required a second surgery because of under correction. The last group of patients with exotropia were those who had less deviation under anesthesia. There were six patients in this category, all of whom had less than 10 diopters of deviation six months after surgery.

DISCUSSION

While the described method of adjusting sutures during muscle surgery at the time of the operation appears to provide an increased predictability of results, a number of considerations are important:

1. There is still the need for careful pre-operative evaluation and the use of good judgement in the selection of proper muscles for surgery.

2. Proper surgical techniques are necessary.

3. A competent and interested anesthesiologist is necessary to keep the patient at the proper and steady level of anesthesia.

4. If any depolarizing agents are used, it is necessary to make certain that the effects have worn off before taking any measurements.

5. The full correction of innervational factors may result in an increase in the number of consecutive exotropia's over a long period of time.

TABLE 1

POST OPERATIVE RESULTS

DEVIATION UNDER ANESTHESIA	OPERATIONS	PATIENTS	LESS THAN 10 P.D.	MORE THAN 10 P.D.
ESOTROPIA				
LESS	20	19	18	2
SAME	8	7	5	3
GREATER	2	2	2	
EXOTROPIA				
GREATER	12	12	12	
SAME	9	8	7	2
LESS	6	6	6	
TOTAL	57	54	50	7*

(*) 3 patients-12 p.d. residual esotropia
(*) 3 patients-reoperated and corrected

REFERENCES

1. Jampolsky A: Strabismus reoperation techniques. Trans Am Academy Ophthalmol Otolaryngol 79:704-717, 1975.

2. Apt L, Isenberg S: Eye position of strabismus patients under general anesthesia. Am J Ophthalmol 84:574-579, 1977.

3. Mindel J, Raab EL, Eisenkraft JB, Teusch G: Succinydicholine induced, return of the eyes to the basic deviation. Ophthalmology 87:1288-1295, 1980.

4. France NK, France TD, Woodburn JD, Burbank DP: Succinylcholine alteration of the forced duction test. Ophthalmology 87:1282-1287, 1980.

5. Jampolsky A: Spring back balance test in strabismus surgery, in Helveston, EM (ed): Symposium on Strabismus. Transactions of the New Orleans Academy of Ophthalmology. St Louis, CV Mosby Co., 1978, p. 104-111.

DISCUSSION BY W. E. GILLIES

The ideal anesthetic for the squint surgeon would be one which gave complete anesthesia in a conscious relaxed patient with no effect on muscle tone.

This paper presents a method which tries to achieve a similar effect by adjusting for the alteration in muscle tone in an unconscious patient which occurs in present techniques of general anesthesia. Unfortunately, it is difficult with modern methods of anesthesia to be sure that a patient can be held at plane 2, a convention not so often used with thiopentone based anesthesia, nor can one be sure that muscle tone will remain constant throughout an operation. Still, the results seem promising and this represents an effort to achieve more predictable results with squint surgery.

We have attempted to solve the same problem with A scan to design the operation more accurately and perhaps some fusion of the two methods may be possible.

ADJUSTABLE STRABISMUS SUTURE TECHNIQUES IN CHILDREN

J. A. Gammon and J. Forestner

ABSTRACT

Adjustable strabismus sutures are now widely used to help achieve the surgical goal. There are definite applications of adjustable strabismus methods in children who constitute the largest group with strabismus problems.

Forty children ranging in age from 6 months to 15 years underwent strabismus surgery with utilization of adjustable sutures. A simple office screening test was used to assist with patient selection and informed consent. Anesthesia techniques employing only short acting agents such as fentanyl and nitrous oxide were studied. Cooperation and interest of the anesthesiologists was important.

Postoperative ocular motility assessment was enhanced by the use of video recording of ocular alignment and motility. Adjustment of completion of the sliding suture knot was accomplished with inhalation sedation in young, uncooperative children while older children were managed with topical anesthetic drops. No complications related to the adjustable suture techniques occurred. Adjustable strabismus sutures can be utilized in children without regard to age.

INTRODUCTION

Children of all ages can be managed with the adjustable suture techniques described in this report. Various types of adjustable strabismus sutures have been used since the turn of the century.(1) We have adaptedthe two-stage technique originally described by Jampolsky(2) et al for use in children. Recent popularity of adjustable sutures follows a period of strabismus surgery directed by tables or formulas. Various recommendations relating amount of surgery to clinical measurements have been routinely employed in children. However, the surgical alingment goal often is elusive and re-operations a frequent complication. Adjustable strabismus sutures help the surgeon achieve surgical ocular alignment and may decrease reoperations.

STRABISMUS II
ISBN 0-8089-1424-3

Adjustable sutures are considered for patients when there is concern about achieving surgical alignment with conventional strabismus techniques. Successful application of adjustable sutures in adults has been reported by Jampolsky, Scott, Rosenbaum and others.(3-5) These reports have described methods applicable for cooperative adults and hae not included young children who constitute a large portion of the strabismus population. We have developed adjustable strabismus suture techniques appropriate for infants and young children. This report summarizes our experience in more than fifty children treated between August 1980 and August 1982.

PATIENT SELECTION

Successful use of adjustable sutures requires proper patient selection and preparation. Age is an important factor. In our series we discovered that most children over three years of age could be managed by the two-stage adult technique while patients younger than three years invariably required a second anesthetic postoperatively. An office screening test is employed in older children to determine their ability to cooperate and to gain their trust. After explaining the adjustable technique to the patient and parent, several drops of .5% proparacaine is used to anesthetize the eye. A force duction test is then completed by grasping the eye at the limbus with a .3 mm Castroviejo forcep. This demonstrates to the parent and child that the eye can be comfortably manipulated with only topical anesthesia. Patients unable to tolerate a forced duction test in the office are not good candidates for the two-stage adjustable suture methods. Two uncooperative children were correctly identified by this screening routine. Postop anesthesia standby is arranged for all children and has been needed in most patients under three years of age. The child's maturity and the surgeon's pursuasiveness determine the need for additional anesthesia. The use of adjustable sutures in children thus requires special planning and teamwork between surgeon, patient and anesthesiologist. With proper planning and experience, adjustable sutures can be employed in children at any age. The youngest patient in our series was six months old.

ANESTHETIC MANAGEMENT

A rapid emergence anesthetic technique is employed allowing ocular motility evaluation soon postoperatively. No preoperative medications are used. Halothane is used briefly for induction and light anesthesia is then maintained with Fentanyl and nitrous oxide. Depressants, tranquilizers and narcotics are avoided postoperatively. Using this technique most children are awake and alert one to two hours after surgery and can be examined in the recovery area.

SURGICAL TECHNIQUE

Strabismus surgery is completed using either limbal or fornix incisions. Vicryl 000000 suture on a spatula needle is used adding a millimeter of surgery to traditional formulas. The adjustable suture is preferentially employed on a recessed muscle using a sliding knot fashioned from the Vicryl material. This facilitates quick adjustment postoperatively. A small amount of dexamethasone in injected subconjunctively at the adjustable suture site. The suture ends are tucked into the fornix and the eye with the adjustable suture is patched with a sterile pad.

POSTOP OCULAR MOTILITY EXAMINATION

After the patient is fully awake and alert with brisk eye movements, an abbreviated ocular motility examination is completed. This includes a cover test and ocular rotations. The child is made comfortable by topical proparacaine and nalloxone is given intravenously if indicated to reverse residual narcotic effects evidenced indicated by drowsiness or groggy eye movements. Effective and varied fixation targets faciltiate the examination. Video recording helps to ascertain the postoperative alignment by freezing in still frame the eye movements as desired for detailed evaluation of ocular alignment and position. Magnification produced by a large 25 inch monitor is also helpful. Permanent, inexpensive records of the ocular motility are collected.

THE ADJUSTMENT

A sterile instrument kit contains two needle holders used to manipulate and tie the suture and scissors for cutting the suture. A toothed forceps may be needed to manipulate the eye or muscle. The eye is gently held open by an assistant with sterile q-tips. Loupes with an attached light source are helpful. In cooperative children, the strabismus suture is adjusted as needed to achieve the alignment goal using only topical anesthesia and pursuasion. Inhalation sedation in addition to the topical anesthesia is required in young children for suture adjustment or tying. After the knot is completed a drop of steroid-antibiotic is instilled into the palpebral fissure and the patient is discharged when recovery from the second brief anesthesia is completed.

COMPLICATIONS

Five children have required additional surgery for a reoperation rate of 10% with minimum two month followup. Other complications have not been observed. Adjustable strabismus sutures offer a second chance for ocular alignment if needed during the same hospitalization. Bold surgery is encouraged reducing undercorrections and improving the surgical outcome. These techniques require additional planning and effort by both the surgeon and the anesthesiologist. Increased patient risk and discomfort is minimal but should be considered when comparing results obtained with traditional nonadjustable methods. Pitfalls of the technique include improper patient selection, pharmacologic "posioning" of the oculomotor system which complicates postoperative examination and confusion about the desired ocular alignment goal.

CONCLUSION

Adjustable strabismus sutures can be safely used in children of all ages with appropriate planning.

REFERENCES

1. Worth C: Squint: It's Causes, Pathology and Treatment. John Bale Danielsson, London, 1903, p. 206.

2. Jampolsky A: Adjustable strabismus surgical procedures. In Syposium on Strabismus: Transactions of the New Orleans Academy of Ophthalmology. Mosby, St. Louis, 1978, p. 321-349.

3. Rosenbaum A, Metz H, Carlson M, Jampolsky A: Adjustable rectus muscle recession surgery. Arch Ophthalmol 95:817-820, 1977.

4. Scott WE, Martin-Casals A, Jackson OB: Adjustable sutures in strabismus surgery. J Pediatr Ophthalmol 14:71-75, 1977.

5. Jampolsy A: Current techniques of adjustable strabismus surgery. Am J Ophthalmol 88(3):406-418, 1979.

DISCUSSION BY W. E. GILLIES

This is an effort to achieve more predictable results with less multiple operations in the future. Unfortunately, it is still a two-stage procedure and the use of fentanyl and nitrous oxide is not free from risk. Immediate access to full resuscitation prodedures is necessary so it would need to be an operating theater procedure. A single stage procedure would be preferrable if practical.

PEDIATRIC EPIKERATOPHAKIA

K. S. Morgan, P. A. Asbell, J. G. May,
D. N. Loupe and H. E. Kaufman

INTRODUCTION

Children with cataracts have the potential for good vision, if they receive the benefits of prompt diagnosis, effective optical correction, and vigorous amblyopia therapy after surgical lens removal.(1) Epikeratophakia is a form of optical correction in which a shaped piece of donor tissue is attached to the de-epithelialized anterior cornea. The lenticule is covered with the patient's epithelium and repopulated with the patient's keratocytes, and in effect, forms a permanent, contact-len-like correction.(2)

SUBJECTS AND METHODS

The details of the preoperative examination, the surgical technique, and the postoperative care have been reported elsewhere.(3) Briefly, corneal curvatures and axial length measurements were used to compute the required power of the lenticule. The attachment of the lenticule was done in conjunction with cataract extraction or as a secondary procedure. Sutures were removed 2 to 3 weeks after surgery. By 6 weeks postoperative, a crisp retinoscopic reflex could be obtained, and overcorrection was prescribed as necessary. Patching of the contralateral eye was begun for 90% of waking hours for the preverbal children and 100% for older children. Visual acuities were assessed monthly by fixation preference, Allen cards, Snellen line charts, and visual evoked potentials.

RESULTS

Forty children, aged two months to 6.6 years, received 43 epikeratophakia grafts. Thirty-four had six months or more follow-up. Twenty-one patients had dense congenital cataracts, 12 had traumatic cataracts, four had incomplete congenital cataracts, and three had persistent hyperplastic primary vitreous.

Seventeen patients were aphakic and underwent epikeratophakia as a secondary procedure; 16 had epikeratophakia combined with cataract extraction. One

STRABISMUS II
ISBN 0-8089-1424-3

patient had cataract extraction, epikeratophakia, and a recession/resection procedure for esotropia; one had epikeratophakia and recession/resection; and five had epikeratophakia coupled with a membranectromy.

In the 34 patients with 6-31 months of follow-up, 29 of 37 grafts were successful (78%); 3 of the 8 failed lenticules were replaced, so that 29 of the 34 patients (85%) have clear grafts. The failures included three with persistent epithelial defects, three that were infected by bacteria in the immediate postoperative period, one that opacified, and one that was lost as a result of mechanical trauma within a week after suture removal.

Visual acuity was measured in 23 of the 29 patients who had successful grafts (Table 1) and at least 6 months of follow-up. Five preverbal patients were unable to cooperate in the visual evoked potential procedure and are represented (Table 1) by estimates of fixation. One patient was lost to follow-up before a final visual acuity could be obtained.

Table 1. Visual Acuity

			Visual Acuity					
				Postop Range				
Diagnosis	Number of Patients	Age Range (Months)	Preop Range	Fixation	VEP	Allen Cards	Snellen Line Chart	Followup (Months)
Congenital cataracts	16	3-56	NFF-HM	CUSUM-CSUM (5)	20/50-20/140 (3)	10/30-3/30 (4)	20/500-20/800 (4)	7-31
Incomplete congenital cataracts	4	58-78	20/120-20/400	--		--	20/60-20/200 (4)	13-26
Traumatic cataracts	8*	9-66	NFF-20/200	--	20/65-20/100 (3)	20/30 (1)	20/40-20/300 (3)	8-19

NFF - no fix and follow

CUSUM - central, unsteady, unmaintained

CSUM - central, steady, unmaintained

*One traumatic cataract patient excluded because of retinal detachment.

Unilateral congenital cataracts or PHPV

Ten patients were operated on within the first year of life. Two grafts failed; one patient was lost to follow-up; four were uncooperative in electrophysiological testing. Two patients were assessed by visual evoked potential measurements. Two had visual acuities better than 20/50 in the operated eye (20/20 in the other eye) by VEP, and one also displayed 10/30 and 18/30 in the involved eye and normal eye respectively by Allen cards. The other patient had Allen care vision of 5/30 in the operated eye. Five children were operated on within the second year of life. One graft failed. Three patients had visual acuities of 20/70 by VEP, 4/30 by Allen cards, and 20/800 by Snellen chart, respectively. One preverbal child's vision was graded as central but unsteady and unmaintained. Six children had surgery after the second year oflife. One graft failed. The average age at surgery was 41 months and postoperative visual acuties ranged from 20/140 by VEP to 20/800 by Snellen line chart.

Incomplete congenital cataracts

Four patients averaged six years of age at the time of surgery. All grafts were successful. Average preoperative vision was 20/230; postoperative visual acuity was 20/132.5

Traumatic cataracts

Nine patients were operated on at an average age of 41 months. One grat failed, one eye developed an inoperable retinal detachment, and one patient had severe preoperative corneal astigmatism and psotoperative vision not improvable to better than 20/300. The postoperative visual acuities of the other six patients averaged 20/62. Three of these patients have measurable fusion.

All the older patients with unilateral congenital cataracts or persistent hyperplastic vitreous deomonstrated some improvement in visual function as a result of removing the lens opacity (in the primary cases) or correcting a longstanding refractive error and undertaking amblyopia therapy. Our clinical impression was that these patients achieved sufficient vision to navigate, play games, color and read using only the vision from the involved eye.

No patient experienced a permanent decrease in visual acuity in the occluded eye as the result of amblyopia therapy. Transient decreases in vision in the good eye manifested by a shift in fixation preferences or poor response to visual evoked potential measurements were seen in some of the younger patients but were readily reversed when the amount of occlusion time was reduced.

Keratometry readings for early patients averaged 13.00 dioptersincrease in corneal curvature. This change was stable between the time of suture removal and 6 to 18 months after surgery. The average overrefraction needed to achieve emmetropia in these patients was +0.48 D spherical equivalent. In the most recent patients, wjho have not had 6 months of follow-up and who are, therefore, not included in the visual acuity data, the average correctin obtained was +16.36 D and the average overrefraction was -0.79 diopters. These patients received grafts in which tissue hydration was controlled by means of a cornea press.(4)

DISCUSSION

This report presents our results with a new means of visual rehabilitation for children with unilateral congenital or traumatic cataracts. Many of the original technical and surgical details of this approach have been abandoned in favor of newer ones, and many of the problems seen in the earliest patients would not have occurred with our present knowledge. Seven of the eight failed grafts occurred amont the first 19 patients; only one failure occurred in te last 21 patients. Also, we have selected patients who were ppor candidates for other types of therapy. Most of our early patients were contact lens fialures or were considered too old or too noncompliant for other forms of treatment. None of our patients with unilateral congenital cataracts were young enough at diagnosis to fit the strict selection criteria advocated by Beller, et al.(1)

Epikeratophakia corrects refractive error by changing the anterior curvature of the cornea. For aphakic children, the needed change can range from +10 to +30 diopters, depending on the size and shape of the eye. This study demonstrates that we can now add an average of 16 diopters with an epikeratophakia graft; the largest correction achieved was +25.65 diopters. We have modified the preparation of the donor tissue for shaping on the cryolathe in order to improve the predictability and increase the power of the correction.

Ideally, for the treatment of amblyopia, we need to correct the refractive error for near work. Some overcorrection was achieved in less than half of the cases. Even though our procedure required considerable correction in the spectacles in some of the early cases, we think that the quality of the image should be superior to what is obtained with all of the power in a thick spectacle or in a contact lens thatmay not be in place much of the time.

The size of the optical correction needed for an aphakic toddler is less than that needed for an aphakic neonate. With our new techniques of tissue handling it may be advisable to intentionally undercorrect the neonate so the toddler may be slightly overcorrected. The changes in the eye's refraction during this first year of life could be managed with periodic spectacle changes as is done routinely in accommodative esotropias.

There is some recent evidence that the infant eye possesses an extremely large depth of focus and that optical blur may not be as detrimental to visual acuity as it is in adults.(5) It is possible that precise corrections are not essential in very young amblyopic patients.

We have obtained good visual results in our very young patients and have also seen some improvement in older children over one year of life in whom our present amblyopia model would predict that no improvement is possible. It is probable that the critical period for visual development described by Hubel and Wiesel(6) is not an absolute threshhold,(7) but rather a sloping barrier of diminishing returns with increasing age.

It is too soon to predict the long term usefulness of epikeratophakia for these children, but the procedure does appear to be a safe and effective alternative for those who cannot wear contact lenses; it is certainly less hazardous than secondary or primary intraocular lens implants.

ACKNOWLEDGEMENTS

From the Lions Eye Research Laboratories, LSU Eye Center, LSU Medical Center School of Medicine, New Orleans, louisiana.

This study was supported in part by USPHS grants EY02580 (Dr. Kaufman), EY02377 (Dr. Kaufman), and EY05496 (Dr. Asbell) from the National Eye Institute, and an unrestricted grant from Research to Prevent Blindness, Inc., New York, NY.

REFERENCES

1. Beller R, Hoyt CS, Marg E, Odum JV: Good visual function after neonatal surgery for congenital monocular cataracts. Am J Ophthalmol 91:559-565, 1981.

2. Werblin TP, Kaufman HE, Friedlander MH, Granet N: Epikeratophakia: the surgical correction of aphakia. III.

Preliminary results of a prospective clinical trial. Arch Ophthalmol 99:1957-1960, 1981.

3. Morgan KS, Werblin TP, Asbell PA, Loupe DN, Friedlander MH, Kaufman HE: The use of epikeratophakia grafts in pediatric monocular aphakia. J Pediatr Ophthalmol Strabis 18:23-29, 1981.

4. Safir A, McDonald MB, Klyce SD, Kaufman HE: The cornea press: restoring donor corneas to normal dimensions and hydration before cryolathing. Submitted.

5. Powers MK, Dobson V: Effect of focus on visual acuity of human infants. Vision Res 22:521-528, 1982.

6. Hubel DH, Wiesel TN: The period of susceptibility to the physiological effects of unilateral eye closure in kittens. J Physiol 206:419-436, 1970.

7. von noorden GK: Stimulus deprivation amblyopia. Am J Ophthalmol 92:416-421, 1981.

DISCUSSION BY W. E. GILLIES

This is a fascinating and highly sophisticated approach to the problem posed by the child with amblyopia in an eye with unilateral cataract or aphakia. It is common knowledge that the adventurous implant surgeons are solving the problem of the badly tolerated or infrequently worn contact lens in these children by implanting lenses. This seems hazardous in view of the risks to the corneal endothelium and the lack of long-term follow-up of posterior chamber lenses where the risk to the endothelium may be less. It is well established that amblyopia can be reversed in these children if conditins are optimal and this method of epi kerato phakia seems far safer though technically complex. The results in the later cases in particular seem most impressive.

INDEX